WOMEN'S DRUG AND SUBSTANCE ABUSE

This newly revised and expanded edition of *Women's Drug and Substance Abuse: A Comprehensive Analysis and Reflective Synthesis* offers a unique analysis and synthesis of theory, empirical research, and clinical guidance for treating substance abuse among young, middle-aged, and older women of various racial and sociocultural backgrounds in the United States, 2000 to 2018. This text uses the most current research findings to examine the actions and effects of drugs, women's patterns of medical and personal use and abuse, and common mental disorders associated with drug use. The authors also present their own empirically-based assessment model as well as prevention and treatment approaches specifically designed for women. Also included in the text is a comprehensive, cross-referenced subject index. Clear, comprehensive, accessible, and fully referenced, this book will be an invaluable resource for students and for professionals in all health and social care disciplines. *Women's Drug and Substance Abuse* is the 18th clinical pharmacology text that the Pagliaros have written over the past 40 years and is the 6th that deals exclusively with drug and substance abuse.

Ann Marie Pagliaro, BSN, MSN, is currently Professor Emeritus at the University of Alberta and co-director of the Substance Abusology and Clinical Pharmacology Research Group. She was formerly a tenured, full professor in the Faculty of Nursing at the University of Alberta, where she taught and supervised undergraduate and graduate students in the area of drug and substance abuse for over 30 years.

Louis A. Pagliaro, PharmD, MS, PhD, is currently Professor Emeritus at the University of Alberta and co-director of the Substance Abusology and Clinical Pharmacology Research Group. He was formerly a tenured, full professor in both the Department of Educational Psychology and the Faculty of Pharmacy and Pharmaceutical Sciences at the University of Alberta, where he taught and supervised undergraduate and graduate students in the areas of drug and substance abuse and the biological basis of clinical psychology for over 30 years.

WOMEN'S DRUG AND SUBSTANCE ABUSE

A Comprehensive Analysis and Reflective Synthesis

SECOND EDITION

Ann Marie Pagliaro and Louis A. Pagliaro

Routledge
Taylor & Francis Group
NEW YORK AND LONDON

Second edition published 2018
by Routledge
711 Third Avenue, New York, NY 10017

and by Routledge
2 Park Square, Milton Park, Abingdon, Oxon, OX14 4RN

Routledge is an imprint of the Taylor & Francis Group, an informa business

First edition published by Taylor & Francis 2000

Library of Congress Cataloging-in-Publication Data
Names: Pagliaro, Ann M., author. | Pagliaro, Louis A., author.
Title: Women's drug and substance abuse : a comprehensive analysis and reflective synthesis / Ann Marie Pagliaro and Louis Pagliaro.
Other titles: Substance use among women
Description: Second edition. | New York : Routledge, 2017. |
Preceded by Substance use among women : a reference and resource guide / Ann Marie Pagliaro and Louis A. Pagliaro. c2000. |
Includes bibliographical references and index.
Identifiers: LCCN 2017011987 | ISBN 9781138909021 (hbk : alk. paper) |
ISBN 9781138908383 (pbk. : alk. paper) | ISBN 9781315111179 (ebk)
Subjects: | MESH: Substance-Related Disorders | Sex Factors |
Women's Health | Women | United States
Classification: LCC RC564.5.W65 | NLM WM 270 | DDC 362.29082–dc23
LC record available at https://lccn.loc.gov/2017011987

ISBN: 978-1-138-90902-1 (hbk)
ISBN: 978-1-138-90838-3 (pbk)
ISBN: 978-1-315-11117-9 (ebk)

Typeset in Bembo
by Out of House Publishing

To *all* women, particularly those whose hearts have been broken, whose hopes have been dashed, whose bodies have been wounded, whose souls have been tormented, and whose families have been injured, lost, or destroyed by their harmful use of the drugs and substances of abuse, and to the health and social care professionals, whose compassion, commitment, knowledge, and care, provide comfort, strength, support, and healing for these women and their families.

CONTENTS

ABOUT THE AUTHORS

Ann Marie Pagliaro, Professor Emeritus, University of Alberta, was formerly a tenured, full professor in the Faculty of Nursing at the University of Alberta. Teaching and supervising undergraduate and graduate students in drug and substance abuse for over 30 years, she also was director of the Pagliaro Interdisciplinary/Interagency AIDS Research Group and, later, co-director of the Substance Abusology and Clinical Pharmacology Research Group. Her primary area of undergraduate and graduate supervision was health promotion across the lifespan with a specialty clinical focus on the prevention and treatment of substance use-related disorders among children, adolescents, and women. A historical, quantitative, and qualitative researcher, her major research focus continues to be the epistemological study of drug and substance abuse.

Louis A. Pagliaro, Professor Emeritus, University of Alberta, and co-director of the Substance Abusology and Clinical Pharmacology Research Group, was formerly a tenured, full professor in the Faculty of Education, Department of Educational Psychology, and full professor in the Faculty of Pharmacy and Pharmaceutical Sciences at the University of Alberta. There, he taught and supervised undergraduate and graduate students in the areas of drug and substance abuse and the biological basis of clinical psychology, for over 30 years, while maintaining a specialty practice as a psychologist in the treatment of drug and substance use disorders. He also served a 3-year term as the elected president of the College of Alberta Psychologists. Having earned graduate degrees from the University of California (San Francisco Medical Center), Schools of Pharmacy and Medicine, and the University of Alberta, Faculty of Education, his area of clinical practice is pharmacopsychology across the lifespan, particularly the assessment and management of alcohol and substance use disorders, substance-induced disorders, and contemporaneous disorders. He also consults widely as a forensic psychologist, particularly in cases of drug and substance abuse-related crime.

The Pagliaros, full-time members of the academic staff at the University of Alberta from 1977 to 2008, taught thousands of students; published over 300 professional scientific articles; and consulted extensively for numerous governmental and professional organizations locally, nationally—including the White House Office of Drug and Substance Abuse—and internationally. Five of their previous 17 books focused explicitly on drugs and substance abuse, including *Substance Use Among Women*, which was published in 2000 by Brunner/Mazel (Taylor & Francis) and *Pagliaros' Comprehensive Guide to Drugs and Substances of Abuse* (1st and 2nd editions), which were published by the American Pharmacists Association in 2004 and 2009. Their most recent book, *Handbook of Child and Adolescent Drug and Substance Abuse: Pharmacological, Developmental, and Clinical Considerations*, was published in 2012 by John Wiley & Sons and received the "Choices Award" in 2013 as an "Outstanding Academic Title" from the Association of College and Research Libraries. *Women's Drug and Substance Abuse: A Comprehensive Analysis and Reflective Synthesis* is the 18th professional book that the Pagliaros have co-edited or co-authored since 1979. They have been married for 45 years.

ACKNOWLEDGMENTS

First, we would like to acknowledge and thank our woman colleagues, students, and patients, who, over the past 40 years, have shared their narratives with us, thereby, expanding our knowledge of women's drug and substance abuse and helping us to better understand and validate much of the information that we have provided to the readers of this text. Second, we would like to acknowledge and thank all of the women, who directly contributed to the development and production of this text, particularly five women for their special support, encouragement, and assistance: Elizabeth Graber, Editor; Nina Guttapalle, Editorial Assistant; Elizabeth Spicer, Production Editor; Penny Harper, Copy Editor; and Nicola Howcroft, Project Manager.

PREFACE AND INTRODUCTION

Popular Notion: Women generally have fewer and/or less severe forms of drug and substance abuse than men.

NOT TRUE. See the following discussion in this introduction and the related discussion in the following chapters of this text.

Women in the U.S.—regardless of age, continental or other descent, education, ethnicity, marital status, race, religion, sexual orientation, or socioeconomic status—are exposed to and actively use various drugs and substances of abuse in ways and contexts that adversely affect their health, safety, and well-being, as well as that of their families, friends, and communities. Since the publication of Pagliaro and Pagliaro (2000), *Substance Use Among Women*, the availability of drugs and substances of abuse, as well as their patterns of use among women, have undergone significant changes that are now rapidly closing the *gender gap*,[1] particularly regarding the use of alcohol, amphetamines, benzodiazepines, caffeine, cannabis (marijuana), cocaine, nicotine (tobacco smoking), methylenedioxymethamphetamine (MDMA), opiate analgesics, and z-drugs. Since the beginning of the new millennium, women also display, when compared to men, a *greater* frequency of physical dependence (i.e., *tolerance* and *withdrawal*) and psychological dependence (i.e., *craving*) with more associated harmful effects—even when their levels of use are the same, or *lower* (Hernandez-Avila, Rounsaville, & Kranzler,

[1] The "gender gap"—as related to the use of drugs and substances of abuse in the U.S.—refers to the significantly *higher* levels of drug and substance use, and associated problems, which, historically, typically were associated with men.

2004; Kinsaul & Copeland, 2013).[2] In addition, as noted by Ait-Daoud, Blevins, and Khanna (2017):

> Women are becoming the fastest-growing population of substance abusers in the United States.
>
> *(p. 285)*

These noted changes—in the observed patterns and rates of drug and substance use/abuse among women during the new millennium in the U.S.—have been associated with several factors, including: (1) increased availability of relatively inexpensive drugs and substances of abuse; (2) changes in sociocultural norms for women;[3] and (3) inadequate attention—and related lack of appropriate action/intervention—in regard to the serious nature and growing extent of drug and substance abuse among women by society, in general, and by local, state, and federal governments, in particular. Consequently, we now find ourselves in the midst of "reaping the whirlwind." In the following chapters of this text, we examine this troubling situation in depth and offer valuable insights and recommendations for its resolution.

---

[2] As explained by Greenfield, Back, and Lawson (2010), this phenomenon—often referred to as "telescoping"—is characterized by the observation that:

> When women enter substance abuse treatment, they typically present with a more severe clinical profile (e.g., more medical, behavioral, psychological, and social problems) than men, despite having used less of the substance and having used the substance for a shorter period of time compared with men.
>
> *(p. 339)*

Although "telescoping" has been widely endorsed as a useful theory that helps to explain many reported findings, researchers have provided mixed results in regard to its validity, particularly in relation to alcohol dependence (e.g., Alvanzo, Storr, & La Flair, 2011; Diehl, Croissant, & Batra, 2007; King, Bernardy, & Hauner, 2003; Sullivan, Rohlfing, & Pfefferbaum, 2010). However, for other drugs and substances of abuse (e.g., cannabis), there is a consensus that telescoping is a *significant* factor affecting women (Ehlers, Gizer, & Vieten, 2010; Khan, Secades-Villa, & Okuda, 2013). Although *not* wanting to dwell on this issue here, we feel obliged to posit, based upon our analyses of the related data, that these differences—in the belief of whether telescoping is a prominent factor for a significant number of women, who have an alcohol and or a substance use disorder—is largely a matter of semantics or perspective. For example, Lewis and Nixon (2014) observed, in their study of drinking consequences and gender differences, that regarding the "progression from drinking milestones to alcoholism," no significant telescoping effects were noted. However, regarding the "progression to treatment … marked telescoping effects were detected" among women (p. 274). Thus, we can say, with a considerable degree of certainty, that—while not occurring for all women in all contexts—"telescoping" occurs for a significant number of women in the context of the abuse of several of the drugs and substances of abuse (Pagliaro & Pagliaro, *Clinical Patient Data Files*). (Also, see related discussion in the following chapters.)

[3] Indicated by both: (1) a *decrease* in male-to-female ratios of prevalence (i.e., use) estimates for the drugs and substances of abuse; and (2) women *progressively* initiating the use of drugs and substances of abuse at *younger* ages (Keyes, Martins, & Blanco, 2010; Zilberman, Tavares, & el Guebaly, 2003).

Fortunately, a growing number of health and social care professionals—counselors, family therapists, nurses, occupational therapists, pharmacists, physicians, psychologists, social workers, sociologists, and others—are becoming increasingly concerned about drug and substance abuse among women in the U.S. and its associated harmful effects. These professionals also have voiced increasing concerns regarding the related consequences for both the families and the communities of which these women are an integral part. This text is written for these health and social care professionals, and for students, who are assimilating related knowledge and developing related clinical skills in their respective professional programs of study.

In this text, which has been carefully designed and prepared specifically for these audiences, we provide accurate, up-to-date, and, whenever possible, gender-specific research findings—obtained from both qualitative and quantitative published research sources—on the nature, extent, and associated consequences of women's drug and substance abuse across the lifespan. Attention is given to the major drugs and substances of abuse that are used by women throughout the new millennium in the U.S., their patterns of use, and related clinical considerations.

Our goal, in writing this text, is to create and present a significant and unique contribution to women's health, both individually and collectively, and to the transdisciplinary science of women's drug and substance abusology. Our express intended immediate purpose, as academic scholars and clinicians, is to help to prevent and relieve the pain and suffering experienced by women as a result of their drug and substance abuse.

It is fairly axiomatic that a comprehensive and accurate understanding of the nature and extent of women's exposure to and abuse of drugs and substances of abuse is vital for all concerned health and social care providers who have an interest in, and/or provide direct care to, women—even when drug and substance abuse may *not* be their major area of clinical practice or interest. For example, this understanding will help to inform and alert:

- *Corrections* and other *Law Enforcement Officers* to patterns of criminal and violent behavior associated with the use of various drugs and substances of abuse by women. For example, the use of alcohol, amphetamines, cocaine, or phencyclidine (PCP)—each of which, among other effects, can contribute to or exacerbate the perpetration of violent physical assaults and homicides.[4] An accurate understanding of women's drug and substance abuse is particularly important to corrections and other law enforcement officers because, in the U.S., over 25% of women are incarcerated for drug offenses and more women inmates than men self-report significant drug and substance use

[4] Variables such as age and ethnicity have been associated with *increased* rates of drug and substance abuse-related violence against women (e.g., Nowotny & Graves, 2013; Waller, Iritani, & Christ, 2012). (See related discussion in the chapters of this text.)

problems—both prior to and during incarceration (Sipes, 2012). As noted by Henderson (1998), "Drug abuse is the primary reason women enter prison and is the primary health problem of women in prison" (p. 579).

In addition, several studies (e.g., Semple, Strathdee, & Zians, 2013) have identified specific characteristics of women who become actively involved in "drug dealing"—an occupation that is often unsuspected among women by *most* law enforcement officers and, consequently, largely goes unrecognized. For example, drug use and the sale of drugs by non-criminal users is significantly greater in clubs and college bars, where those, who both use and sell illicit drugs, are most likely to be co-eds of European continental descent (Pagliaro & Pagliaro, *Clinical Patient Data Files*; Vaughn, Salas-Wright, & DeLisi, 2015; Vuolo, Kelly, & Wells, 2014).

- *Neurologists / Neuropsychologists* to the need to distinguish drug and substance use as a cause of neurocognitive dysfunction (e.g., dementia) from organic causes, or physical injuries. For example, diagnosing an *older* woman's memory loss as related to either, or both, her: (1) regular drinking of alcohol at social events several times during the week; and/or (2) use of prescription opiate analgesics several times during the day for the management of her severe osteoarthritic pain.
- *Nurses* to the use of the various drugs and substances of abuse by women and the associated occurrence of accidental injuries and other adverse health consequences that can be fatal. For example: a young woman's severe skin burns associated with "dabbing" cannabis with butane or producing methamphetamine in her kitchen; a middle-aged woman's death associated with a heroin overdosage; and an older woman's head injuries associated with alcohol intoxication and a "drunken fall" down a flight of stairs. Other consequences, including preventable infections (e.g., hepatitis C; human immunodeficiency virus [HIV]) related to the *method* used for administering various drugs and substances of abuse (e.g., sharing contaminated needles and syringes; or sharing a hookah mouthpiece during a cannabis smoking session at a local hookah bar), also may occur.

In addition, the mental effects of various drugs and substances of abuse (e.g., *psychodepression*; *psychostimulation*; or *psychodelic empathogenic effects*) may be a significant contributing risk factor in relation to a woman having "consensual," unprotected sex with multiple partners—or being a victim of drug-facilitated rape. (Also, see related discussion in Chapter 1, *Women's Opiate Analgesic Abuse*; Chapter 2, *Women's Alcohol Abuse*; Chapter 3, *Women's Prescription Sedative-Hypnotic Abuse*; Chapter 5, *Women's Amphetamine and Cocaine Abuse*; and Chapter 6, *Women's Psychodelic Abuse*.)

As noted by Wong and Mellor (2014), with an awareness of the reported, established inter-relationships among the use of the various drugs and substances of abuse, nurses should be encouraged to routinely screen for a possible history of violence (and we would add sexually transmitted diseases) among *all* women who present with substance-related disorders (i.e., *alcohol and substance use disorders* and *substance-induced disorders*). Conversely, when women present with a history involving violence and/or sexually transmitted diseases, nurses should routinely screen for drug and substance use disorders. This practice will facilitate the detection, for example, of instances of drug and substance use-related violence and, consequently, present an opportunity to make appropriate, necessary referrals to other health and social care professionals within hospital and community settings.

- *Obstetricians / Nurse Midwives* to focus more carefully on the prevention of teratogenic pathology related to women's use of drugs and substances of abuse during pregnancy,[5] particularly the fetal alcohol syndrome (FAS),[6] which may occur among the offspring of women who drink alcohol while pregnant. In this context, it is interesting to note that women, who are "OB/GYN" physicians, are reportedly more likely to value and conduct maternal screening for drug and substance abuse than are their male counterparts (Oser, Biebel, & Harris, 2011).

  In addition, the Centers for Disease Control and Prevention now recommend that testing for hepatitis C virus (HCV) infection be increased for pregnant women because of the significant rise in HCV infection in this cohort. This rise in HCV infection among women of childbearing age during the new millennium in the U.S., is specifically related to injection drug use (IDU) (Koneru, Nelson, & Hariri, 2016).
- *Pharmacists* to actual and potential pharmacotherapeutic concerns, including significant drug interactions, double doctoring, poly-pharmacy, and illicit patterns of obtaining drugs for personal abuse. For example, a mother selling her young son's mixed amphetamines (Adderall®) that were prescribed for the management of his attention-deficit/hyperactivity disorder (A-D/HD). Or, in another example, a mother using her diabetic daughter's insulin needles/syringes to self-inject methamphetamine. (See Chapter 5, *Women's Amphetamine and Cocaine Abuse*.)
- *Physicians* to "rule out" drug and substance abuse when formulating diagnoses or when clinically monitoring therapeutic responses for women, who present with conditions such as clinical depression or unexplained injuries. In this context, it can also serve as a guide for physicians to develop and use related protocols. For example, that physicians, who work in American College of Surgeons level I trauma centers, routinely conduct admission toxicology screening for drug and substance abuse for *all* older women who

[5] As identified by Wendell (2013), and thoroughly discussed in the chapters of this text, "Maternal drug use and subsequent prenatal drug exposure have reached levels of critical concern" (p. 91).

[6] The *fetal alcohol spectrum disorder* (FASD) is another term used in the published literature for the fetal alcohol syndrome. For additional related discussion, see Chapter 2, *Women's Alcohol Abuse*.

are admitted—regardless of the circumstances related to a specific admission (Ekeh, Parikh, & Walusimbi, 2014).

Physicians also can be alerted to the possibility of women "faking signs and symptoms," or "malingering," in an effort to obtain prescriptions for such desired drugs and substances of abuse as the sedative-hypnotic, alprazolam (Xanax®), the opiate analgesic, oxycodone (OxyContin®), or medicinal marijuana—for themselves, family members, friends, or to sell for needed cash. (Also, see Chapter 1, *Women's Opiate Analgesic Abuse*; Chapter 3, *Women's Prescription Sedative-Hypnotic Abuse*; Chapter 5, *Women's Amphetamine and Cocaine Abuse*; and Chapter 6, *Women's Psychodelic Abuse.*)

- *Psychologists* to consider the possibility of *substance-related disorders*, alone or in combination with other mental disorders (i.e., *contemporaneous diagnoses*), among women who require psychological or counseling services (see Chapter 7, *Identifying Women's Contemporaneous Diagnoses*). For example, the regular use or abuse of:

    - Alcohol (see Chapter 2, *Women's Alcohol Abuse*), as a possible explanation for a woman's depressive disorder
    - Caffeine (see Chapter 4, *Women's Caffeine and Nicotine Abuse*), as a possible explanation for a woman's anxiety disorder
    - Cannabis (see Chapter 6, *Women's Psychodelic Abuse*), as a possible explanation for a woman's social withdrawal or lack of interest in her family (e.g., amotivational syndrome)
    - Cocaine (see Chapter 5, *Women's Amphetamine and Cocaine Abuse*) or phencyclidine (PCP) (see Chapter 6, *Women's Psychodelic Abuse*), as a possible explanation for a woman's psychotic disorder—as has been noted by Sara, Burgess, and Malhi (2014), and many others

    In addition, psychologists will be alerted to the fact that while drugs and substances of abuse can cause or exacerbate mental disorders, they also can *mask* them. This clinical consideration becomes particularly significant when reflected upon in relation to the reported research finding that "approximately half of individuals with mental health disorders have a comorbid drug and alcohol diagnosis" (McClean, Anspikian, & Winters, 2014, p. 16). (See related discussion in Chapter 7, *Identifying Women's Contemporaneous Diagnoses.*)

- *Social Workers* to investigate potential high-risk use of drugs and substances of abuse among women and related problems in the home (e.g., child neglect; physical, mental, or sexual abuse; exposure of children to other harm, such as skin burns associated with a mother's methamphetamine production in the home or injury associated with growing large amounts of marijuana in the home [i.e., managing a home "grow-op"]) and community (e.g., participation in local neighborhood sales of drugs and substances of abuse or participating in sex-for-drug exchanges). (See Chapter 5, *Women's Amphetamine and Cocaine Abuse*, and Chapter 6, *Women's Psychodelic Abuse.*) It also alerts social workers to needed action to *decrease* potential harm to communities associated with related crime, violence, and resultant *social decay*. This intervention is crucial for breaking the intergenerational cycle of drug and substance abuse, particularly in recognition of the extremely well-documented intergenerational correlation between physical and sexual abuse among girls and resultant drug and substance abuse among women (e.g., Dunlap, Golub, & Johnson, 2009; Pagliaro & Pagliaro, 2012).

Finally, it alerts social workers to barriers, perceived or real, that prevent women—particularly visible minority women; homeless women; and bisexual, lesbian, and trans women—from obtaining needed treatment for their specific patterns of drug and substance abuse (e.g., Chen, Strain, & Crum, 2013). These formidable barriers include the paucity of woman-specific and gender identity-sensitive drug and substance abuse programming (e.g., Stewart, Gavric, & Collins, 2009). (See related discussion in Chapter 8, *Preventing and Treating Women's Drug and Substance Abuse*.)

Unfortunately, an understanding of the nature and extent of drug and substance abuse among women in the U.S. is *neither* easily, *nor* quickly, gained by those who both require and would benefit from this understanding. There are many factors that contribute to this situation. However, a particularly important factor is that the overwhelming majority of the research findings and conclusions published in professional journals, textbooks, and databases, as well as over the Internet—from *2000 to 2018*—provide little information that is *directly* applicable to women in the U.S.[7,8] For example:

1. Potentially valuable research often presents *only* equivocal or mixed results in terms of reported incidence and consequence.[9]

[7] Some of these difficulties and limitations in research design, methods, and dissemination of results are understandable because of the difficulty inherent in obtaining data from women who use various drugs and substances of abuse. Women, as a vulnerable population group, may require, in addition to informed consent, other assurances when asked to participate in research studies involving the personal use of drugs and substances of abuse. For example, the nature of the very behavior studied (i.e., use of the drugs and substances of abuse) is often illegal. Therefore, it makes it more difficult to obtain accurate reports of behavior from participants who may fear arrest, losing their jobs, or having their children taken into custody by social services.

[8] Since the publication of *Substance Use Among Women* (Pagliaro & Pagliaro, 2000), global attention to women's drug and substance abuse has increased significantly. Correspondingly, the overwhelming majority of published articles that we found during the preparation of this text—and that needed to be largely *excluded*—were studies of women from virtually every country around the world, including Canada, China, Japan, and Mexico. While we applaud the increased worldwide attention to this important area of women's health and well-being, this change has contributed to the increased difficulty in finding relevant articles that focus specifically on women living in the U.S., particularly regarding socioeconomic and sociocultural factors, as well as related prevalence of use statistics. In this context, we included *all* available data found for women living in the U.S. and deliberately omitted data regarding women living outside the U.S., including other North American countries (i.e., Canada and Mexico).

[9] These published research studies often conclude with the phrase: "more (or additional) research is necessary." Therefore, the use of potentially helpful findings is limited because of the need for study

2. Available published research findings and conclusions do *not* address women in a major way and rarely separate them from men—either in research designs or in presented conclusions and recommendations.[10]
3. Authors often demonstrate a significant bias in their conclusions and recommendations, while others appear to inaccurately minimize, or trivialize, the harm associated with using various drugs and substances of abuse.[11] For example, referring to the cult, classic movie, "Reefer Madness" (Gasnier, 1936), in an attempt to document the exaggeration of harm associated with the use of marijuana. Perhaps this bias is a way to rationalize their own use of the drugs and substances of abuse or, perhaps, to help further the social agenda for decriminalization or legalization of *all* of the drugs and substances of abuse. In any event, these biased views are often ensconced in a libertarian or secular progressive perspective that those authors are attempting to advance—without *publicly* endorsing this stance.

   Conversely, other authors may exaggerate associated harm, perhaps to dissuade use by rationalizing harsh legal penalties and consequences associated with possession and use of the various drugs and substances of abuse and, accordingly, establishing a deterrent to use. This latter biased viewpoint is often laden with moral underpinnings (i.e., that the use of a drug or substance of abuse is *not* only illegal, but immoral)—a view often ensconced in a conservative or religious perspective.[12]

---

replication or extension into more specific population groups (e.g., adolescent girls versus young women or middle-aged women versus older women). In addition, the authors rarely provide specific recommendations for replicating their studies or research questions aimed at extending their reported findings.

[10] In these studies, the population sample, while often including a significant proportion of women, is generally gender neutral when results are presented (i.e., the subjects may be identified only as, for example, "Americans of Hispanic descent," "college students," or, most commonly, "adults").

[11] Such authors may use, for example, the accurate, but misleading, argument that the harm associated with the use of marijuana in the U.S. is, in comparison, significantly less than that associated with the use of alcohol or nicotine (see related discussion in Chapter 2, *Women's Alcohol Abuse*, Chapter 4, *Women's Caffeine and Nicotine Abuse*, and Chapter 6, *Women's Psychodelic Abuse*).

[12] On this point, we tend to view drug and substance use as neither good nor bad, nor moral or immoral. As scholars, scientists, and expert clinicians rooted in several views of knowledge production (e.g., positivism, post-positivism, postmodernism, or post-postmodernism), we focus instead on evaluating the results of scientific findings based on each science's inherent assumptions, research methods, and claims to fact (i.e., their theories and inherent *truth*). Most importantly, as subscribers to the scientist-clinician model, we are particularly concerned with the contribution that a study or research program makes to the further development of knowledge and understanding leading to valuable, positive outcomes for women who personally use the drugs and substances of abuse. Thus, we are concerned with the result of the *interaction* of the use of a particular drug or substance of abuse by a particular woman in a particular context at a particular time (e.g., the use of an opiate analgesic, such as morphine, for a woman hospitalized with a broken leg to relieve her pain versus the use of morphine by a woman who is a sex trade worker to ward-off her opiate analgesic withdrawal symptoms and that results in her overdosage death). Thus, for us, it is *not* the use of a particular substance of abuse by a particular woman at a particular time that is "good" or "bad." Rather, it is

Because of this situation, health and social care providers desperately need, but do *not* currently have, a readily accessible, clearly written, and unbiased, scholarly reference on the topic of drug and substance abuse among women during the new millennium in the U.S. *Women's Drug and Substance Abuse: A Comprehensive Analysis and Reflective Synthesis* presents both a deep depth and a wide breadth of understanding, coincident with a *timely*, objective, *quantitative* analysis and subjective, *qualitative* synthesis of available research conclusions and recommendations that are completely substantiated with referenced documentation and supportive clinical examples. Thus, readers are provided with a text that enables a better understanding of women's use and abuse of the drugs and substances of abuse during the new millennium in a current and unbiased context that reflects a comprehensive, transdisciplinary interpretation and evaluation of the published research and related available data.

Since the publication of our related text in 2000, almost 2 decades ago, the needs of readers, and our own approaches to preparing professional texts for publication, have changed dramatically. For example, at that time there were no such things as "smart" and "super" cellular phones and ready—virtually instantaneous—access to full books and complete journal articles on the Internet. Consequently, at that time, the primary challenge for clinicians—our primary intended audience—was obtaining relevant published research findings that could be appropriately applied, with confidence, in the context of their respective areas of clinical practice.

Today, our major challenge, and that for our readers, has changed from too little available data to too much available data (i.e., a surfeit of data). This change has necessitated a consequent change in our approach to the preparation of our clinical pharmacology and other texts, particularly those focusing solely on the drugs and substances of abuse. We no longer have to physically go into the library "stacks" in order to retrieve relevant data because most journal abstracts and articles can be accessed through internet sites where they can be read online, saved to a file for later access, or immediately printed at minimal cost. In fact, *prepublication* copies of relevant research, reviews, and opinions are often readily available following the process of journal submission, review, and acceptance. Having turned in our electric typewriters decades ago, we have used the various editions of WordPerfect and MSWord and related software and hardware to create, revise, store, manipulate, and immediately send files of figures, tables, chapters, entire manuscripts, and completed copy-edited textbooks with the click of a "mouse."

---

the *result* of the use of the drug or substance of abuse by a woman in a certain context at a particular time that is "good" or "bad." To emphasize this point in our lectures and discussions, we have often compared a drug or substance of abuse to a writing pen, which—as an inanimate object—is *neither* inherently "good" *nor* "bad." For example, if the pen is used to write a needed text, it may be considered to be "good." However, if it is used to poke someone in the eye, it may be considered to be "bad." The pen is an inanimate object and, thus, is devoid of "goodness" or "badness." It is how it is used that makes it "good" or "bad." So, too, with the drugs and substances of abuse.

Consequently, the major challenge today is *not* the search for relevant available data of importance, but, instead, the compilation, sorting, and assimilation from a virtual mountain of readily available data—some relevant, much not; some accurate, much not; some useful, much not—into what is more valid, more reliable, more true, and most useful for clinical application *before* it is shared with the reader.

In addition to being of benefit to health and social care professionals, *Women's Drug and Substance Abuse: A Comprehensive Analysis and Reflective Synthesis* also should be of benefit to students who are assimilating knowledge in their respective fields of professional study.

Last, but not least, we trust that this text also may be of benefit to health and social care policy makers. These policy makers include, for example: the Surgeon General; politicians, such as city mayors and state governors; public health administrators, such as the members of boards of public health or healthcare authorities; and social administrators, such as directors of related women's treatment/recovery centers, both public and private. These policy makers, at all levels, must increasingly address both the direct and indirect healthcare costs and social consequences associated with women's drug and substance abuse—particularly, if they wish to appropriately deal with the related adverse impact on all segments of society in the U.S.[13]

In an effort to meet the identified knowledge needs of these health and social care professionals, students, and policy makers, this text presents the authors' distillation and interpretation of the current published clinical literature and available demographical statistical reports addressing drug and substance abuse among women in the U.S.[14] Historical and other relevant published literature (e.g., formalized theories; general review articles; significant textbooks; and helpful related websites) also have been used and cited, as appropriate.[15]

These data, obtained from a variety of computerized (e.g., CINAHL®; PubMed®; PsycINFO®) and non-computerized database sources utilizing available internet search engines (e.g., BING®; Google®; YAHOO!®), were used to

---

13 These costs and consequences are: (1) *biological* (e.g., physical injuries to body systems, such as cirrhosis of the liver related to chronic alcohol use, or lung cancer related to tobacco smoking); (2) *psychological* (e.g., emotional distress and mental disorders, such as amphetamine-related psychosis or cannabis-related memory impairment); and (3) *sociological* (e.g., child neglect and family violence related to the use of alcohol, cocaine, or methamphetamine by women and/or their intimate partners, female or male).

14 It is important to note that the *authors* have performed critical analysis and reflective interpretation of the available published data in the context of their combined 80+ years of *lived* academic experience and clinical practice in the fields of nursing, pharmacology, psychology, and public health—specifically dealing with clinical issues related to the use of the drugs and substances of abuse in the U.S. The authors used this method of analyzing and synthesizing the published data in order to help to ensure, for the reader, the appropriate evaluation of data and the best approximation of *truth* (i.e., in an earnest attempt to eliminate, or at least minimize, any potential biases).

15 The authors also performed hand searches of hardcopy databases (e.g., published journal tables of contents; reference lists of printed research articles; textbooks) in order to complement the computer searches of relevant databases and to validate and extend the conclusion(s) proffered by the original sources and their suggested leads. All cited references are fully documented and listed in alphabetical order at the end of each chapter.

more accurately reflect the diverse scientific findings, theoretical orientations, and clinically relevant views in our study of the use of drugs and substances of abuse by women in the U.S. during the new millennium. A subsequent and appropriate analysis and synthesis indicated the "best" and most parsimonious organization for these data.

Consequently, the text contains six chapters on women's use of specific drugs and substances of abuse, or groups of drugs and substances of abuse, in the U.S. The focus, formulation, and development of each of these six chapters was based on a drug or substance of abuse as being:

1. Pharmacologically classified as a member of a subclass of one of the three major classes of drugs and substances of abuse (i.e., *psychodepressant*; *psychostimulant*; or *psychodelic*)[16]
2. Identified, among members of its subclass, as *most* commonly abused by women in the U.S. during the new millennium

Based on these criteria, the following chapters were created: Chapter 1, *Women's Opiate Analgesic Abuse*; Chapter 2, *Women's Alcohol Abuse*; Chapter 3, *Women's Prescription Sedative-Hypnotic Abuse*; Chapter 4, *Women's Caffeine and Nicotine Abuse*; Chapter 5, *Women's Amphetamine and Cocaine Abuse*; and Chapter 6, *Women's Psychodelic Abuse*.

Each of the six chapters focus on the: (1) pharmacology of the selected drugs or substances of abuse discussed in the chapter; and (2) characteristics and statistics of women's medical and personal use and abuse of the drugs and substances of abuse in the U.S. during the new millennium.

Regarding *pharmacology*, for each of the drugs and substances of abuse that is presented and discussed, attention is given to its:

- Pharmacodynamics (i.e., *mechanism of action*)
- Pharmacokinetics (i.e., *absorption, distribution, metabolism, and excretion*)
- Undesired, or harmful, effects and toxicities, including: acute and chronic effects; physical and psychological dependence; and specific harmful effects and toxicities associated with maternal drug and substance use/abuse during pregnancy and lactation
- Overdosage

In addition, attention is given to high-risk groups of women—young women (NIDA, 2007); bisexual and lesbian women (Matthews, Cho, & Hughes, 2013); trans women (Hotton, Garofalo, & Kuhns, 2013); and women who are intravenous drug users (i.e., IVDUs) (Scherer, Trenz, & Harrell, 2013)—who are

---

16 This useful, accurate, and concise taxonomy was developed by the Pagliaros, over 25 years ago, and has since been used in several of their published textbooks.

identified in each chapter with attention to related research findings and strategies aimed at *reducing* their risky sexual and other behaviors associated with drug and substance abuse.

Regarding women's medical and personal drug and substance use/abuse, attention is given, whenever relevant data are available, to demographical and sociocultural comparisons by:

- Age
- Culture
- Ethnicity
- Geographic residence
- Pregnancy, lactation, and mothering/child-rearing status[17]
- Religion
- Sexual orientation
- Socioeconomic status

The Chapters

Chapter 1, *Women's Opiate Analgesic Abuse*, presents and discusses women's abuse of the *illicit* opiate analgesic, *heroin* (diacetylmorphine, "Black Tar," "H"), and the prescription opiate analgesics *oxycodone* (OxyContin®, "Hillbilly Heroin"), hydrocodone (Dicodid®, "Hyke"), buprenorphine (Buprenex®, "Tems"), and *fentanyl* (Actiq®, "China White," "Fen").

Not surprisingly,[18] during the new millennium in the U.S., women developed a myriad of patterns of opiate analgesic abuse that closely rival, and in some cases surpass, that of their male counterparts. The significantly *increasing* incidence of women's opiate analgesic abuse is often accompanied by an associated significant *increase* in the use of *higher* dosages, physical and psychological dependence, and overdosages. Also, *increasing* is the incidence of neonatal addiction associated with maternal opiate analgesic abuse during pregnancy, which is characterized by

---

[17] Regarding developmental considerations and the characteristic patterns associated with the use of the drugs and substances of abuse across a woman's lifespan and possible effects on pregnancy, lactation, and mothering, we, where necessary and appropriate, use the conventional definitions and descriptions as follows: *embryo* and *fetus*, conception to birth; *neonate*, first 30 days of life; *infant*, first year of life; *toddler*, 1 to 3 years-of-age; *preschooler*, 3 to 5 years-of-age; *child*, 5 to 12 years-of-age; *preadolescent*, 12 to 13 years-of-age; *adolescent*, 13 to 18 years-of-age (also currently widely defined as, the second decade of life, 10 to 20 years-of-age); *young women*, 18 to 35 years-of-age; *middle-aged women*, 35 to 65 years-of-age; and *older women*, 65 to 100+ years-of-age. In addition, in an attempt to avoid any confusion when presenting research findings, we provide, whenever possible, the participant age ranges as specified by the authors of the cited reference.

[18] Not surprisingly because we have previously predicted, in several publications (e.g., Pagliaro & Pagliaro, 2000) and numerous academic and professional presentations, that the *psychostimulant* epidemics of the 1980s and 1990s in the U.S., which increasingly involved women, would be followed by *psychodepressant* epidemics in the new millennium.

the neonatal withdrawal syndrome or neonatal abstinence syndrome (NAS) (e.g., McKim & Bottari, 2014; Okoroh, Gee, & Jiang, 2017).

Chapter 2, *Women's Alcohol Abuse*, discusses beverage alcohol—a legally available sedative-hypnotic that is generally purchased as beer ("brew"), wine ("vino"), and distilled spirits ("hard stuff"). Alcohol is commonly abused by women of *all* ages across the U.S. For example, alcohol and other drug and substance abuse reportedly are *highest* among women, who are college/university students in the U.S., who belong to Greek Life sororities and reside in "Greek" housing on, or near, campus (Sidani, Shensa, & Primack, 2013). Of *increasing* concern is the binge drinking noted among co-eds and their participation in "alcohol games," which are often associated with sexual assault (Clarke, Kim, & White, 2013).

Chapter 2 is dedicated to alcohol use among women because of its preferential and ubiquitous use among women across the lifespan and, consequently, the large amount of related published data that are available. As such, the information presented and discussed also is foundational for the alcohol-related discussions in the subsequent chapters of this text.

Attention also is given in this chapter to alcohol-related birth defects, which are characterized by the Fetal Alcohol Syndrome (FAS)—also commonly referred to as the Fetal Alcohol Spectrum Disorder (FASD). FAS/FASD is commonly encountered among the offspring of various specific population groups of women in the U.S. and, unfortunately, can present with life-long challenges for many of the affected offspring (May, Blankenship, & Marais, 2013). Therefore, FAS/FASD is covered in detail. This detailed coverage remains extremely relevant because, although FAS/FASD is completely preventable and its cause widely known for over 50 years, "Women continue to drink alcohol during pregnancy despite Surgeon Generals' Advisory statements and educational efforts about the dangers" (Elek, Harris, & Squire, 2013, p. 177).

Another high-risk group of women in relation to the development of alcohol use disorders (AUDs) are bisexual, lesbian, and trans women. Sociocultural and other variables, such as the "lesbian bar scene," may encourage and support drug and substance abuse among these women (Trocki & Drabble, 2008). As noted by Storm (cited by Brownworth, 2010):

> The main places for lesbians to meet off-line continue to be mostly bars and clubs … I look around my community and I see women in their 40s, 50s, and 60s still going to the bars and still getting drunk.
>
> *(p. 4)*

Chapter 3, *Women's Prescription Sedative-Hypnotic Abuse*, discusses prescription sedative-hypnotics that are commonly abused by women particularly, the *benzodiazepines* (e.g., lorazepam, Ativan®, "Zzz") and *z-drugs* (e.g., zolpidem, Ambien®, "Tic Tacs"). The use of these drugs, which are prescribed primarily to provide symptomatic relief of a variety of anxiety and sleep disorders, is not as generally noticeable because their use, unlike other drugs and substances of abuse among women (e.g., cocaine; heroin; methamphetamine), generally is hidden among older women, particularly those in residential care, who do *not* garner the attention or headlines that other women do. This form of harmful drug use is often directly related to the over-prescription of sedative-hypnotics (e.g., alprazolam [Xanax®]; zolpidem [Ambien®]) for both middle-aged and older women by physicians and, thus, is often referred to as "iatrogenic drug use"—in a similar way to what occurs, to a significant extent, in the context of prescription opiate analgesic abuse (see for example, Mercado, Jumner, & Spelke, 2017). (For additional related discussion, see Chapter 1, *Women's Opiate Analgesic Abuse.*)

Chapter 4, *Women's Caffeine and Nicotine Abuse*, presents and discusses two subclasses of psychostimulants that are legally available, non-prescription, and widely and commonly used by new millennial women in the U.S.: (1) *caffeine* ("Java," "Joe"), which is commonly available in popular beverages, including coffee, tea, and energy drinks; and (2) nicotine ("cancer sticks," "coffin nails," "Leaf"), which is commonly available in a variety of tobacco products and e-cigarettes, as well as in a number of tobacco smoking cessation products that are absorbed through the mucous membranes of the mouth (e.g., nicotine chewing gum [Nicorette Gum®] and oral sprays [NICORETTE® Quick Mist Mouth Spray]) or transdermally through skin application sites where "patches" [NicoDerm® CQ]) are placed. (Also, see related discussion in Chapter 8, *Preventing and Treating Women's Drug and Substance Abuse.*)

Chapter 5, *Women's Amphetamine and Cocaine Abuse*, presents and discusses two other psychostimulants commonly abused by women: (1) *amphetamines*, particularly methamphetamine ("Crank," "Crystal Meth"), which is illicitly available and commonly intravenously injected, or inhaled into the lungs (i.e., smoked); and (2) cocaine ("Blow," "C," "Coke"), including cocaine hydrochloride, or powder, which is usually nasally insufflated (i.e., "snorted") or intravenously injected, and cocaine base, or "crack" cocaine, which is usually vaporized and inhaled.

Violence against women that involves various drugs and substances of abuse is most often associated with the abuse of amphetamines and cocaine. (Also, see Chapter 2, *Women's Alcohol Abuse*, for a related discussion of violence against women involving alcohol abuse.) This violence commonly occurs in several major *contexts and locations*, including: (1) crack houses (Kalokhe, Paranjape, & Bell, 2012); (2) domestic residences, particularly in the embedded context of "intimate partner violence" (IPV) (Wong & Mellor, 2014); (3) homeless abodes for women "living on the street" (Meinbresse, Brinkley-Rubinstein, & Grassette, 2014); and (4) hotels/motels, automobiles, and trucks, particularly for women involved in the sex trade (Comack & Seshia, 2010; Janssen, Gibson, & Bowen, 2009).

Chapter 6, *Women's Psychodelic Abuse*, presents an overview of three subclasses of the psychodelics (i.e., amphetamine-like; LSD-like; and miscellaneous psychodelics) that are frequently abused by women, including: cannabis ("Bud," *Ganja*, marijuana); methylenedioxymethamphetamine ("Ecstasy," MDMA, "Molly"); lysergic acid diethylamide ("Acid," LSD); and phencyclidine ("Angel," HOG,

PCP). Attention is given to harmful patterns of psychodelic use by young women, particularly in the context of "clubbing" and music festivals, where use has been associated with numerous reported incidents of serious toxicities and death. In addition, in approximately 25 states, women are now able to legally buy, for medical and/or personal use, a wide variety of cannabis products for ingesting, smoking, and vaporizing—and many of these women are becoming increasingly involved in the criminal diversion of these products.[19]

Two chapters follow that focus on *identifying* and *preventing and treating* women's drug and substance abuse. Chapter 7, *Identifying Women's Contemporaneous Diagnoses*—diagnoses of an alcohol use disorder (AUD) and/or substance use disorder (SUD) and other mental disorder (OMD)—which often occur concurrently among women, such as AUD and posttraumatic stress disorder (PTSD), or cocaine use disorder and a psychotic disorder (e.g., *schizophrenia*). Attention also is given to *poly-diagnoses* identified among women (i.e., concurrent AUD, SUD, OMD, and another condition, such as HIV infection).

It is currently estimated that as many as 1 in 5 older women suffer from a contemporaneous diagnosis. In addition, in the U.S. (by percentage), significantly *more* women who are incarcerated, have contemporaneous diagnoses than men, who are incarcerated (Cusack, Herring, & Steadman, 2013). The prevalence of these diagnoses among women, and their related factors, are discussed emphasizing the importance of accurate diagnosis and treatment with attention to the inter-relationships of the presenting AUD and/or SUD and OMD (e.g., as a cause, exacerbation, or consequence, of each other).[20] For example, women with adult forms of attention-deficit/hyperactivity disorder (A-D/HD) have been reported to have significantly *higher* rates of:

1. Anorexia nervosa, bulimia nervosa, and panic disorder than do men with A-D/HD (Cumyn, French, & Hechtman, 2009)
2. Treatment for AUDs than do women without A-D/HD (Schubiner, Tzelepis, & Milberger, 2000)
3. Opiate analgesic use than do men with A-D/HD (Vingilis, Erickson, & Toplak, 2015)

---

[19] *Diversion* can be accomplished by a woman for whom the marijuana was prescribed (e.g., for relief of migraine headaches, glaucoma, or dysmenorrhea) in either the context of being: (1) *unaware*—as in the situation where one of her children takes some of her marijuana product without her permission for his own personal use; or (2) *fully aware*—as in the situation where she deliberately stock-piles her prescription marijuana in order to later share it with a friend so that they can smoke and get *high* together.

[20] Here, as well as in Chapter 8, *Preventing and Treating Women's Drug and Substance Abuse*, we have conceptualized the related data in the context of our *New Millennial Interactive Model of Women's Drug and Substance Abuse*. Essentially, this model provides a framework for examining relationships among concepts and variables that may significantly affect the nature, occurrence, and extent of drug and substance abuse among women. It also can easily incorporate related discussions in the published literature, particularly among social scientists and clinical practitioners, that are often listed under the heading of "syndemics"—diseases associated with health disparity, or synergistically interacting epidemics.

An overview of the *most* common contemporaneous diagnoses that occur among women—*anxiety disorder* (i.e., panic disorder; posttraumatic stress disorder), *eating disorder, gender dysphoria, major depressive disorder, psychotic disorder* (i.e., schizophrenia), or *sleep disorder* (Stewart, Gavric, & Collins, 2009)—are presented.

Chapter 8, *Preventing and Treating Women's Drug and Substance Abuse*, is the final chapter in the text. It presents specific prevention strategies and programs aimed at the primary, secondary, and tertiary prevention of drug and substance abuse among women. Specific strategies for women are identified and discussed, with attention to women's different reasons for *initiating* drug and substance use; *continuing* use as it becomes *increasingly* harmful to themselves, their families, and communities; and *discontinuing* use. A variety of (1) recently developed pharmacotherapeutic approaches; and (2) traditional and new forms of psychotherapy and counseling for women are described and discussed. The goal of meeting the *unique* needs of women, who may have *greater* success associated with certain types of intervention—and, by corollary, *less* success with others—is a major focus.

For example, attention is given to the role that pharmacotherapy plays in treating AUDs and SUDs among women, including: (1) substance-assisted abstinence and substitution (e.g., nicotine [Nicorette®, Nicotrol®] for tobacco cessation programs); (2) antidotes for specific acute overdosages (e.g., naloxone [Narcan®] for opiate analgesic overdosage); (3) treatment of specific withdrawal syndromes associated with the specific drugs and substances of abuse (e.g., diazepam [Valium®] to prevent or manage sedative-hypnotic withdrawal syndromes); and (4) abstinence maintenance (e.g., methadone [Dolophine®] for heroin dependence).

In regard to the pharmacotherapy of women's AUDs and SUDs, special attention is given to the significant influence of a relatively *new* direction of study by several researchers (e.g., Marteau, Aveyard, & Munafo, 2012; Ray, Bujarski, & Chin, 2012; Somogyi, Barratt, & Ali, 2014) that explores pharmacogenetic/pharmacogenomic factors as being important in regard to obtaining: (1) a better understanding of women's use of the drugs and substances of abuse; and (2) optimal therapeutic outcomes for women who harmfully use drugs and substances of abuse.

In addition to Short-Term Residential Treatment Programs and Relapse Prevention Programs (e.g., Alcoholic Anonymous and other 12-Step Programs), "family drug courts"[21] are described and discussed. These courts were originally developed to "address the poor outcomes derived from family reunification programs for substance-abusing parents" (Marlowe & Carey, 2012, p. 1). Largely established by the U.S. Department of Justice during the new millennium, they deal primarily with civil or criminal cases that involve parental rights as related to a parent's drug and substance abuse. As of December 2014, over 3,000 family drug courts were in operation across the U.S. (NIJ, National Institute of Justice, 2016).

[21] In the related published literature, these courts also are referred to as, "drug courts," "family dependency treatment courts," "family drug and alcohol courts," "family drug treatment courts," "family treatment courts," and "family treatment drug courts."

Attention also is given to theoretical and philosophical aspects of treatment for women—areas of study that are *not* usually addressed in the context of "best practices" treatment. For example, the suggestion offered by Douglas, Shilling, and Reaves (2013) that "treatment for women should be initiated within particular phases of the menstrual cycles where ovarian hormone levels are stable" (p. 125). Another example is the finding of Gibbons, Kingsbury, and Weng (2014), that racial discrimination, real or perceived, adversely affects both entry into treatment and successful completion of treatment for minority women in the U.S.—*generally*, including Latinas, lesbians, and women of African continental descent.

Our use of multiple perspectives, including various feminist viewpoints in the context of both preventing AUDs and SUDs among women and treating women who have these disorders, as well as contemporaneous diagnoses, enables us to present current, empirically-driven "best practices" and to also reflect upon changes that may *improve* prevention and treatment efforts for women in the future. As noted by Kruk and Sandberg (2013):

> A key barrier to the addiction recovery of women is the present framework of addiction treatment, as well as current drug laws, policies, and service delivery systems.
>
> *(p. 1)*

To actively address many of these related issues, we developed and present the *New Millennial Interactive Model of Women's Drug and Substance Abuse.* We specifically developed the interactive model to facilitate a better understanding among readers of the many interacting variables that influence a woman's use of the drugs and substances of abuse. Based on our comprehensive analysis and reflective synthesis of the data presented in this text, the model is comprised of *four* major variable dimensions. Specifically, attention is given to the *Woman Dimension* and its interaction with the other three dimensions—the *Drug or Substance of Abuse Dimension*, the *Societal Dimension*, and the *Time Dimension*—in order that associated, clinically significant interactions and relationships can be more fully and properly identified and understood in an actual clinical context. This approach allows for the optimal analysis of contributory factors related to the various patterns of drug and substance abuse noted among women in the U.S.—both individually (e.g., a college/university student) and in groups (e.g., homeless women; incarcerated women; older women).

Comprehensive Subject Index

The *Comprehensive Subject Index* concludes the text. This comprehensive and extensively cross-referenced subject index was carefully constructed by the authors to facilitate rapid and accurate retrieval of needed information by readers.

Concluding Remarks

By applying the wealth of knowledge presented in this text, it is our fervent hope that health and social care professionals and students will better understand the current nature and extent of drug and substance abuse among women in the U.S. during the new millennium and its effects, often painful and tragic, upon them, their families, and their communities. It also is hoped that health and social care professionals and students will be better able to: (1) provide accurate diagnoses for women who use the drugs and substances of abuse; and (2) develop appropriate and effective prevention and treatment approaches to meet the unique needs of these women. Through an understanding of the complexities of women's drug and substance abuse, as developed over the new millennium, health and social care professionals and students can better work together with women toward a shared goal of achieving optimal health and well-being for them and, by extension, for their families, friends, and communities.

> *Sedulo curavi humanas actiones—*
> *Non ridere, non lugere, neque detestare, sed intelligere.*[22]
>
> [I labor with care when faced with human actions—
> Not to ridicule, not to lament, never to detest, but to understand.]

References[23,24,25]

Ait-Daoud, N., Blevins, D., & Khanna, S. (2017). Women and addiction. *Psychiatric Clinics of North America*, 40(2), 285–297. doi: 10.1016/j.psc.2017.01.005

Alvanzo, A. A., Storr, C. L., & La Flair, L. (2011). Race/ethnicity and sex differences in progression from drinking initiation to the development of alcohol dependence. *Drug and Alcohol Dependence*, 118(2–3), 375–382. doi:10.1016/j.drugalcdep.2011.04.024

Brownworth, V. (2010, June 16). *Lesbians and substance abuse.* Retrieved from Curve Magazine—Web Articles 2010—USA, pp. 1–18: www.curvemag.com/Curve-Magazine/Web-Articles-2010/Lesbians-and-Substance-Abuse

[22] Benedictus de Spinoza (1632–1677), *Tractatus Politicus*, published anonymously in Latin, 1670.

[23] As per publisher style, only the first three authors are listed for each reference.

[24] Several times the number of references listed were found, obtained, and analyzed by the authors during the preparation of this chapter. However, only the references that were cited at least once in the body of the text are included in the list. Major reasons for *not* citing other references, include that they: (1) did *not* provide any additional unique data; (2) were *not* well researched or written (i.e., were evaluated as *not* being valid or reliable); (3) were based predominantly, or exclusively, on animal studies; (4) provided usage statistics from outside the U.S.; and/or (5) were redundant with, or *not* as recent as, the already cited references.

[25] The reference citation, "Pagliaro & Pagliaro, *Clinical Patient Data Files*," refers to unpublished data collected, with permission, over the last 50 years by the authors, in the formal course of their professional academic roles as clinician scientists and professors—by permission from their patients, research subjects, and students, from the 1970s to date.

Chen, L. Y., Strain, E. C., & Crum, R. M. (2013). Gender differences in substance abuse treatment and barriers to care among persons with substance use disorders with and without comorbid major depression. *Journal of Addiction Medicine*, 7(5), 325–334. doi:10.1097/ADM.0b013e31829b7afe

Clarke, N., Kim, S.-Y., & White, H. R. (2013). Associations between alcohol use and alcohol-related negative consequences among black and white college men and women. *Journal of Studies on Alcohol and Drugs*, 74, 521–531.

Comack, E., & Seshia, M. (2010). Bad dates and street hassles: Violence in the Winnipeg Street sex trade. *Canadian Journal of Criminology and Criminal Justice*, 52(2), 219–230.

Cumyn, L., French, L., & Hechtman, L. (2009). Comorbidity in adults with attention-deficit hyperactivity disorder. *The Canadian Journal of Psychiatry*, 54(10), 673–683.

Cusack, K. J., Herring, A. H., & Steadman, H. J. (2013). PTSD as a mediator between lifetime sexual abuse and substance use among jail diversion participants. *Psychiatric Services*, 64(8), 776–781. doi:10.1176/appi.ps.000052012

de Spinoza, B. (1677/1862). *Tractatus theologico-politicus, tractatus politicus.* (R. U. Elwes, Trans.) London and New York, NY: George Routledge and Sons.

Diehl, A., Croissant, B., & Batra, A. (2007). Alcoholism in women: Is it different in onset and outcome compared to men? *European Archives of Psychiatry and Clinical Neuroscience*, 257(6), 344–351. doi:10.1007/s00406-007-0737-z

Douglas, H. A., Shilling, E. A., & Reaves, D. L. (2013). Women and addiction: Exploring the role of psychology and hormones. In J. Marich (Ed.), *The psychology of women: Diverse perspectives from the modern world. Psychology of emotions, motivations and actions* (pp. 125–143). Hauppauge, NY: Nova Science.

Drug Courts. (2016, May 13). Retrieved October 2, 2016, from National Institute of Justice: nij.gov/topics/courts/drug-courts/pages/welcome.aspx

Dunlap, E., Golub, A., & Johnson, B. D. (2009). Normalization of violence: Experiences of childhood abuse by inner-city crack users. *Journal of Ethnicity in Substance Abuse*, 8(1), 15–34. doi:10.1080/15332640802683359

Ehlers, C. L., Gizer, I. R., & Vieten, C. (2010). Linkage analyses of cannabis dependence, craving, and withdrawal in the San Francisco family study. *American Journal of Medical Genetics Part B: Neuropsychiatric Genetics*, 153B(3), 802–811 doi:10.1002/ajmg.b.31050

Ekeh, A. P., Parikh, P. P., & Walusimbi, M. (2014). The prevalence of positive drug and alcohol screens in elderly trauma patients. *Substance Abuse*. 35(1), 51–55. doi:10.1080/08897077.2013.797539

Elek, E., Harris, S. L., & Squire, C. M. (2013). Women's knowledge, views, and experiences regarding alcohol use and pregnancy: Opportunities to improve health messages. *American Journal of Health Education*, 44(4), 177–190. doi:10.1080/19325037.2013.768906

Gasnier, L. J. (Director). (1936). *Reefer madness* [motion picture].

Gibbons, F. X., Kingsbury, J. H., & Weng, C. (2014). Effects of perceived racial discrimination on health status and health behavior: A differential mediation hypothesis. *Health Psychology*, 33(1), 11–19. doi:10.1037/a0033857

Greenfield, S. F., Back, S. E., & Lawson, K. (2010). Substance abuse in women. *Psychiatric Clinics of North America*, 33(2), 339–355. doi:10.1016/j.psc.2010.01.004

Henderson, D. J. (1998). Drug abuse and incarcerated women. *Journal of Substance Abuse Treatment*, 15(6), 579–587. doi:10.1016/S0740-5472(97)00319-X

Hernandez-Avila, C. A., Rounsaville, B. J., & Kranzler, H. R. (2004). Opioid-, cannabis- and alcohol-dependent women show more rapid progression to substance abuse treatment. *Drug and Alcohol Dependence*, 74(3), 265–272.

Hotton, A. L., Garofalo, R., & Kuhns, L. M. (2013). Substance use as a mediator of the relationship between life stress and sexual risk among young transgender women. *AIDS Education and Prevention: An Interdisciplinary Journal*, 25(1), 62–71. doi:10.1521/aeap.2013.25.1.62

Janssen, P. A., Gibson, K., & Bowen, R. (2009). Peer support using a mobile access van promotes safety and harm reduction strategies among sex trade workers in Vancouver's Downtown Eastside. *Journal of Urban Health*, 86(5), 804–809. doi:10.1007/s11524-009-9376-1

Kalokhe, A. S., Paranjape, A., & Bell, C. E. (2012). Intimate partner violence among HIV-infected crack cocaine users. *AIDS Patient Care and STDs*, 26(4), 234–240. doi:10.1080/apc.2011.0275

Keyes, K. M., Martins, S. S., & Blanco, C. (2010). Telescoping and gender differences in alcohol dependence: New evidence from two national surveys. *The American Journal of Psychiatry*, 167(8), 969–976. doi:10.1176/appi.ajp.2009.09081161

Khan, S. S., Secades-Villa, R., & Okuda, M. (2013). Gender differences in cannabis use disorders: Results from the National Epidemiologic Survey of Alcohol and Related Conditions. *Drug and Alcohol Dependence*, 130(1–3), 101–108. doi:10.1016/j.drugalcdep.2012.10.015

King, A. C., Bernardy, N. C., & Hauner, K. (2003). Stressful events, personality, and mood disturbance: Gender differences in alcoholics and problem drinkers. *Addictive Behaviors*, 28(1), 171–187.

Kinsaul, J. A., & Copeland, A. L. (2013). The role of telescoping in the development of smoking in women. In J. Marich (Ed.), *The psychology of women: Diverse perspectives from the modern world. Psychology of emotions, motivations and actions* (pp. 109–123). Hauppauge, NY: Nova Science.

Koneru, A., Nelson, N., & Hariri, S. (2016, July 22). Increased hepatitis C virus (HCV) detection in women of childbearing age and potential risk for vertical transmission—United States and Kentucky, 2011–2014. *MMWR, Morbidity and Mortality Weekly Report*, 65(28), 705–710.

Kruk, E., & Sandberg, K. (2013, December 20). Home for body and soul: Substance using women in recovery. *Harm Reduction Journal*, published on-line. doi:10.1186/1477-7517-10-39

Lewis, B., & Nixon, S. J. (2014). Characterizing gender differences in treatment services. *Alcoholism: Clinical and Experimental Research*, 38(1), 275–284. doi:10.1111/acer.12228

Marlowe, D. B., & Carey, S. M. (2012, May). Need to know: Research update on family courts. *NADCP, National Association of Drug Court Professionals*, 1–10, 12.

Marteau, T. M., Aveyard, P., & Munafo, M. R. (2012). Effect on adherence to nicotine replacement therapy of informing smokers their dose is determined by their genotype: A randomised controlled trial. *PLoS One*, 7(4). doi:10.1371/journal.pone.0035249

Matthews, A. K., Cho, Y. I., & Hughes, T. (2013). The relationships of sexual identity, hazardous drinking, and drinking expectancies with risky sexual behaviors in a community sample of lesbian and bisexual women. *Journal of the American Psychiatric Nurses Association*, 19(5), 259–270. doi:10.1177/1078390313505644

May, P. A., Blankenship, J., & Marais, A. S. (2013). Maternal alcohol consumption producing fetal alcohol spectrum disorders (FASD): Quantity, frequency, and timing of drinking. *Drug and Alcohol Dependence*, 133(2), 502–512. doi:10.1016/j.drugalcdep.2013.07.013

McClean, J. M., Anspikian, A., & Winters, B. N. (2014). Factors that affect treatment initiation among individuals with serious mental illness and substance abuse disorder. *Addictive Disorders & Their Treatment*, 13(1), 16–24.

McKim, J., & Bottari, M. (2014, March 30). *Cases of newborns with addictions soaring*. Boston, MA: The New England Center for Investigative Reporting.

Meinbresse, M., Brinkley-Rubinstein, L., & Grassette, A. (2014). Exploring the experiences of violence among individuals who are homeless using a consumer-led approach. *Violence and Victims*, 29(1), 122–136.

Mercado, M. C., Sumner, S. A., & Spelke, M. B. (2017, March 6). Increase in drug overdose deaths involving fentanyl—Rhode Island, January 2012–March 2014. *Pain Medicine*, [Epub ahead of print]. doi: 10.1093/pm/pnx015

NIDA, National Institute on Drug Abuse. (2007, October 1). *Meeting reviews roles of drug abuse and risky behavior in HIV.* Retrieved December 10, 2014, from National Institute on Drug Abuse (NIDA): www.drugabuse.gov/news-events/nida-notes/2007/10/meeting-reviews-roles-drug-abuse-risky-behavior-in-hiv

NIJ, National Institute of Justice. (2016, May 13). *Drug courts*. Retrieved August 30, 2016, from National Institute of Justice (NIJ): www.nij.gov/topics/courts/drug-courts/pages/welcome.aspx

Nowotny, K. M., & Graves, J. L. (2013). Substance use and intimate partner violence victimization among White, African American, and Latina women. *Journal of Interpersonal Violence*, 28(17), 3301–3318. doi:10.1177/0886260513496903

Okoroh, E. M., Gee, R. E., & Jiang, B. (2017, February 6). Neonatal abstinence syndrome: Trend and expenditure in Louisiana Medicaid, 2003–2013. *Maternal* and *Child Health Journal* [Epub ahead of print] doi: 10.1007/s10995-017-2268-1

Oser, C., Biebel, E., & Harris, M. (2011). Gender differences in provider's use of a standardized screening tool for prenatal substance use. *Journal of Addiction Medicine*, 5(1), 36–42. doi:10.1097/ADM.0b013e3181ccec2e

Pagliaro, A. M., & Pagliaro, L. A. (2000). *Substance use among women: A reference and research guide*. Philadelphia, PA: Brunner/Mazel.

Pagliaro, L. A., & Pagliaro, A. M. (2012). *Handbook of Child and Adolescent Drug and Substance Abuse*. Hoboken, NJ: Wiley & Sons.

Ray, L. A., Bujarski, S., & Chin, P. F. (2012). Pharmacogenetics of naltrexone in Asian Americans: A randomized placebo-controlled laboratory study. *Neuropsychopharmacology*, 37(2), 445–455. doi:10.1038/npp.2011.192

Sara, G. E., Burgess, P. M., & Malhi, G. S. (2014). Stimulant and other substance use disorders in schizophrenia: Prevalence, correlates and impacts in a population sample. *Australian and New Zealand Journal of Psychiatry*, 48(11), 1036–1047. doi:10.1177/0004867414533838

Scherer, M., Trenz, R., & Harrell, P. (2013). The role of drinking severity on sex risk behavior and HIV exposure among illicit drug users. *The American Journal on Addictions*, 22(3), 239–245. doi:10.1111/j.1521-0391.2012.12006.x

Schubiner, H., Tzelepis, A., & Milberger, S. (2000). Prevalence of attention-deficit/hyperactivity disorder and conduct disorder among substance abusers. *Journal of Clinical Psychiatry*, 61(4), 244–251.

Semple, S. J., Strathdee, S. A., & Zians, J. (2013). Correlates of drug dealing in female methamphetamine users. *Journal of Urban Health*, 90(3), 529–541. doi:10.1007/s11524-012-9748-9

Sidani, J. E., Shensa, A., & Primack, B. A. (2013). Substance and hookah use and living arrangement among fraternity and sorority members at US colleges and universities. *Journal of Community Health*, 38(2), 238–245. doi:10.1007/s10900-012-9605-5

Sipes, L. A. (2012, February 6). *Statistics on women offenders.* Retrieved December 10, 2014, from corrections.com, pp. 1–3: www.corrections.com/news/article/30166-statistics-on-women-offenders

Somogyi, A. A., Barratt, D. T., & Ali, R. L. (2014). Pharmacogenomics of methadone maintenance treatment. *Pharmacogenomics*, 15(7), 1007–1027. doi:10.2217/pgs.14.56

Stewart, S. H., Gavric, D., & Collins, P. (2009). Women, girls, and alcohol. In K. T. Brady, S. E. Back, & S. F. Greenfield (Eds.), *Women and addiction: A comprehensive handbook* (pp. 341–359). New York, NY: Guilford.

Sullivan, E. V., Rohlfing, T., & Pfefferbaum, A. (2010). Pontocerebellar volume deficits and ataxia in alcoholic men and women: No evidence for "telescoping." *Psychopharmacology (Berlin)*, 208(2), 279–290. doi:10.1007/s00213-009-1729-7

Trocki, K., & Drabble, L. (2008, November). Bar patronage and motivational predictors of drinking in the San Francisco Bay Area: Gender and sexual identity differences. *Journal of Psychoactive Drugs*, (Supplement 5), 345–356.

Vaughn, M. G., Salas-Wright, C. P., & DeLisi, M. (2015). A typology of drug selling among young adults in the United States. *Substance Use & Misuse*, 50(3), 403–413. doi:10.3109/10826084.2014.984850

Vingilis, E., Erickson, P. G., & Toplak, M. E. (2015). Attention deficit hyperactivity disorder symptoms, comorbidities, substance use, and social outcomes among men and women in a Canadian sample. *BioMed Research International*. doi:10.1155/2015/982072

Vuolo, M., Kelly, B. C., & Wells, B. E. (2014). Correlates of prescription drug market involvement among young adults. *Drug and Alcohol Dependence*, 143, 257–262. doi:10.1016/j.drugalcdep.2014.08.002

Waller, M. W., Iritani, B. J., & Christ, S. L. (2012). Relationships among alcohol outlet density, alcohol use, and intimate partner violence victimization among young women in the United States. *Journal of Interpersonal Violence*, 27(10), 2062–2086. doi:10.1177/0886260511431435

Wendell, A. D. (2013). Overview and epidemiology of substance abuse in pregnancy. *Clinical Obstetrics and Gynecology*, 56(1), 91–96.

Wong, J., & Mellor, D. (2014). Intimate partner violence and women's health and wellbeing: Impacts, risk factors and responses. *Contemporary Nurse*, 46(2), 170–179. doi:10.5172/conu.2014.46.2.170

Zilberman, M., Travares, H., & el-Guebaly, N. (2003). Gender similarities and differences: The prevalence and course of alcohol- and other substance-related disorders. *Journal of Addictive Diseases*, 22(4), 61–74. doi:10.1300/J069v22n04_06

1

WOMEN'S OPIATE ANALGESIC ABUSE

The abuse of opiate analgesics has significantly *increased* among young, middle-aged, and older women, across the U.S., since the beginning of the new millennium. Although there are seven major *licit* prescription opiate analgesics that are mainly abused—*buprenorphine, fentanyl,*[1] *hydrocodone*, *hydromorphone*, *methadone, morphine*, and *oxycodone*[2]—there is only one major *illicit* non-prescription opiate analgesic that is mainly abused—*heroin*. Medically prescribed primarily for the relief of *moderate to severe* pain, women generally abuse these opiate analgesics to achieve: (1) an intense feeling of euphoria; (2) an overall warm and pleasant feeling, or *rush*; or (3) a sleepy, dream-like state, commonly known as "*being on-the-nod*." In addition, women, who are regular, long-term opiate analgesic users, also commonly use the opiate analgesics to: (4) prevent or self-manage the opiate analgesic withdrawal syndrome.

We begin with an overview and discussion of the basic pharmacology of the opiate analgesics with attention to their similarities and differences regarding:

1. *Pharmacodynamics*, or mechanisms of action
2. Dosage formulations and methods of use

---

[1] N.B. *Fentanyl* is a prescription opiate analgesic that is *less* often prescribed for non-hospitalized, or outpatients, because of its *high* potency and risk for overdosage. However, *illicitly* manufactured fentanyl is readily available and easily obtained "on the street"—the current primary source in the U.S. for this prescription opiate analgesic. In this context of use, illicitly produced fentanyl is almost always clandestinely mixed with street heroin (Gladden, Martinez, & Seth, 2016; Pagliaro & Pagliaro, *Clinical Patient Data Files*). (Also, see related discussion in the "Fentanyl" section at the end of this chapter.)

[2] Over the new millennium, several other prescription opiate analgesics (e.g., codeine, loperamide, and tramadol) also have been abused by women in the U.S. However, these opiate analgesics are *not* discussed in detail in this text because they are either: (1) *less* frequently abused by women; and/or (2) *less* likely to be associated with significant harmful effects and toxicities. We refer readers, who require additional information that may be specific to each of these drugs, to Pagliaro and Pagliaro (2009).

3. *Pharmacokinetics,* or absorption, distribution, metabolism, and excretion
4. Undesired, or harmful, effects and toxicities[3]

We then present and discuss women's medical and personal use and abuse of the opiate analgesics.

Pharmacology

The opiate analgesics comprise three subgroups, or *families*: (1) *natural pure agonists*; (2) *synthetic pure agonists*; and (3) *synthetic mixed agonists/antagonists* (see Table 1.1). The first, and original family, includes opium and its pure natural derivatives—codeine (Codeine Contin®)[4] and morphine (MS Contin®). The second family includes several *synthetic* modifications of morphine, such as fentanyl (Actiq®), heroin (diacetylmorphine), methadone (Dolophine®), and oxycodone (OxyContin®). These synthetic modifications have chemical structures and pharmacologic actions that resemble their natural parent drug, morphine. The third family comprises the *synthetic mixed agonists/antagonists*—buprenorphine (Buprenex®), nalbuphine (Nubain®), and pentazocine (Talwin®).

Opium is prepared from the dried resin of the unripe seed pod of the poppy plant (*Papaver somniferum*)—the poppy that causes sleep. The crude resin, often called "poppy tears" (*lachryma papaveris*), is scrapped off the poppy pod, which was lanced soon after the flower petals began to fall to release the raw opium. The opium alkaloids[5] are then extracted from the resin by various methods. Raw opium contains approximately 10% morphine by weight. Morphine is considered the *standard* against which *all* other opiate analgesics are compared regarding strength (i.e., *potency*) and therapeutic effectiveness (i.e., *efficacy*). The relative potencies of the various opiate analgesics—the average dosages that are required to generally provide equivalent pain relief, or *equal efficacy*—are listed in Table 1.2.

Pharmacologically, opiate analgesics have been traditionally referred to as *narcotic analgesics* reflecting their major therapeutic indication—to relieve pain. They also have been simply called, *narcotics*. Derived from the Greek word, *narke*, narcotic means a lack of feeling or sensation—a feeling of numbness. However, the

[3] These effects also are denoted in the published literature as, *adverse drug reactions, adverse drug events, or adverse drug experiences.*

[4] Brand/trade names are denoted by the symbol, "®." They are included to facilitate clinical practice application for readers who comprise a wide range of health and social care professionals. The inclusion of a brand/trade name is *not* meant to endorse an opiate analgesic, nor is it meant to suggest that the pharmacology and other data presented are preferentially associated with that brand/trade name—unless explicitly stated.

[5] In addition to morphine (10% to 15%) and codeine (1% to 3%), opium alkaloids also contain *noscapine* (i.e., *narcotine*; 4% to 8%), *papaverine* (1% to 3%), and *thebaine* (1% to 2%). The concentrations vary depending on the country of origin, the amount and type of nitrogen-based fertilizers used to cultivate the opium plants, the number of times that a pod is lanced, and the techniques used to lance the opium seed pod so that the opium resin, or "latex," can run out (Annett, 1920).

TABLE 1.1 Opiate Analgesics

OPIATE ANALGESICS		
Reasons for Women's Personal Use/Abuse: To achieve dreams (*pipe dreams*); euphoria; pain relief; a *warm rush*; and a sleepy, dreamlike state (being *on-the-nod*). Also, used to prevent/self-manage the opiate analgesic withdrawal syndrome.		
Generic Name	*Trade or Brand Name(s)®*	*Common Street Name(s)*
Pure agonists, natural		
Opium	—	Doda; Poppy
Opium derivatives:		
Codeine[a]	Codeine Contin®; Ratio-Codeine®	Codies; Cough Syrup; School Boy; T3
Morphine	M.O.S.®; MS Contin®	Drug Store; Good Ole M; Hospital Heroin; Morph; MS
Pure agonists, semi-synthetic and synthetic		
Fentanyl	Actiq®; Duragesic®	Fen; Murder 8; Perc-O-Pop
Heroin	—	Black Tar; Brown; Capital H; Charley; Horse; Junk; Shit
Hydrocodone[b]	OxyContin®	Hyke; Tuss; Vikes
Hydromorphone	Dilaudid®	Delaud; Dillies; Hillbilly
Levorphanol	Levo-Dromoran®	—
Meperidine	Demerol®	Dems; Mep
Methadone	Dolophine®	Adolph; Dollies; Done; Wafer
Oxycodone[c]	OxyContin®	Cotton; Oxycotton; Poor Man's Heroin; Percs
Oxymorphone	Numorphan®	—
Propoxyphene	Darvon®	Footballs; Yellows
Mixed agonists/antagonists, synthetic		
Buprenorphine	Buprenex®	Tems
Butorphanol	Stadol®	—
Nalbuphine	Nubain®	Nubian
Pentazocine	Talwin®	Big T; Ts
Tramadol	Ultram®	—

N.B. Some brand/trade names for specific opiate analgesics are included in this table even though they may no longer be *licitly* manufactured or marketed in North America. These specific opiate analgesics may have been discontinued by the manufacturer because they were: (1) replaced with a generic version; or (2) officially withdrawn from the market by FDA regulation. These specific opiate analgesics remain available from other countries or illicit producers within North America and are easy to obtain by purchase over the Internet.

[a] Codeine is usually available as one of the ingredients of a multiple-ingredient product (e.g., *Empirin #4* [codeine and aspirin]; *Tylenol #3* [codeine and acetaminophen]).

[b] Usually available as one of the ingredients of a multiple ingredient product (e.g., Vicodin® [hydrocodone and acetaminophen]).

[c] Also available in multi-ingredient combination products, such as Percocet® (oxycodone and acetaminophen).

TABLE 1.2 Average Dosages (i.e., *Potency*) of Opiate Analgesics Required to Achieve Equivalent Pain Relief (i.e., *Efficacy*)

Opiate analgesic	*Average dosage*	
Generic Name *(Trade or Brand Name®)*	*IM (mg)*	*PO (mg)*
Butorphanol *(Stadol®)*	2	—
Codeine	120	200
Fentanyl *(Actiq®)*	0.2	—
Hydrocodone	—	60
Hydromorphone *(Dilaudid®)*	1.5	7.5
Levorphanol *(Levo-Dromoran®)*	2	4
Meperidine *(Demerol®)*	75	300
Methadone *(Dolophine®)*	10	20
Morphine	10	30
Nalbuphine *(Nubain®)*	10	—
Oxycodone *(OxyContin®)*	15	20
Oxymorphone *(Numorphan®)*	1	15
Pentazocine *(Talwin®)*	60	180

N.B. These are single, average dosage laboratory equivalents. Consequently, for women who use/abuse opiate analgesics, there may be significant inter-individual variability.

general use of the term, *narcotic*, has caused much confusion because of its *legal* meaning.

Legally, the term, narcotic, is used to denote *all* the various drugs and substances of abuse that are listed under the U.S. and international Narcotic Acts and Laws. For example, cannabis, cocaine, heroin, and lysergic acid diethylamide (*LSD*), are all *legally* classified as narcotics. However, of the four drugs and substances of abuse listed in this example, only heroin is *pharmacologically* classified as a narcotic based upon its chemical structure and pharmacological action.

Adding to the confusion, the opiate analgesics are often referred to as *opioids*—a term that is also used to denote the: (1) opiate analgesic *antagonist*, naloxone (Narcan®); and (2) opiate analgesic-like substances that are naturally found in the body (i.e., *endogenous* opioid peptides). Thus, to minimize the confusion associated with the use of these various terms, we selected to use the term, *opiate analgesic*, throughout this book, for *any* "natural or synthetic drug or substance that exerts morphine-like actions upon the human brain and spinal cord."

Pharmacodynamics: Mechanism of Action

The opiate analgesics have an interesting mechanism of action. Rather than *raising* the pain threshold to achieve analgesia and pain relief, they *modify* the brain's *interpretation* of painful stimuli by depressing central nervous system (CNS) activity. Thus, the sensation of pain is still experienced, but it does *not* seem to "hurt so much."

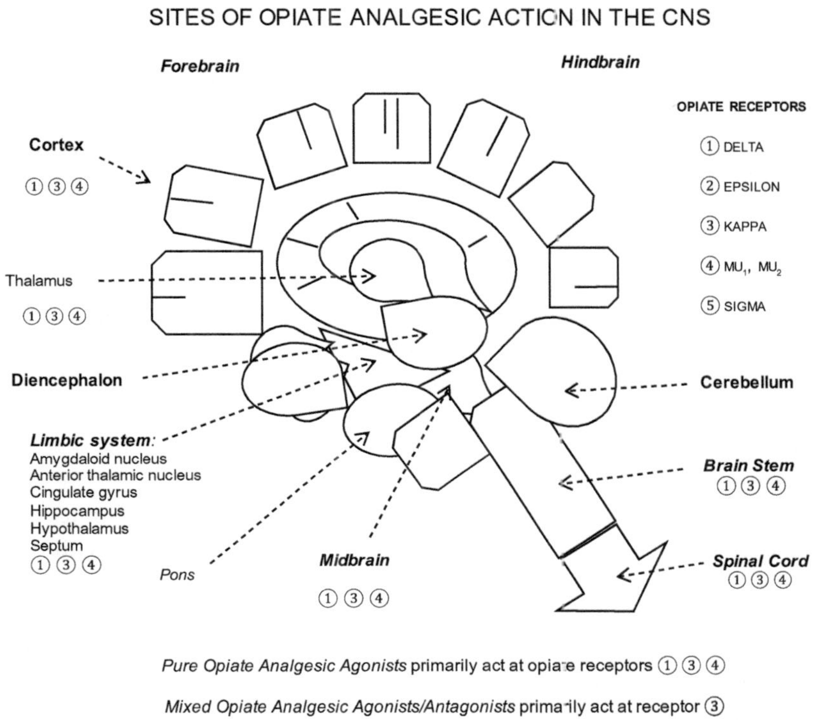

FIGURE 1.1 Opiate Analgesic Receptor Sites in the Brain and Spinal Cord

The endogenous opioid peptides were identified in the brain during the 1970s and were named *dynorphins, endorphins, and enkephalins.* Various opiate analgesic receptors also were discovered within the body and were extensively studied. Although the receptor classification system that evolved from this research remains incomplete, *three* major groups of opiate analgesic receptors were pharmacologically characterized and named *delta*, *kappa*, and *mu*.[6] The *highest* concentrations of these receptors are found in the hypothalamus; limbic system;[7] midbrain, which also includes the *ventral tegmental area* (VTA); spinal cord and thalamus (see Figure 1.1). These *G-protein-coupled* receptors (i.e., *delta, kappa,* and *mu*) are essential to the analgesic actions of the opiate analgesics.

The similarities and differences in the pharmacology and toxicology (i.e., undesired, or harmful, effects and toxicities) of the opiate analgesics are due

[6] Three other receptors (i.e., *sigma* [σ], *epsilon* [ε], and *nociceptin* receptors) have been identified and studied. However, their *full* role regarding the mechanisms of opiate *analgesic* action in humans remains controversial. Nociceptin receptors are found in the brain and spinal cord. They appear to be associated with anxiety, mental depression, and the development of *tolerance*.

[7] The limbic system includes the amygdala, cingulate gyrus, dentate gyrus, and hippocampus.

primarily to their similarities and differences in selectivity for, and binding to, the *delta*, *kappa*, and *mu* opiate analgesic receptors (Gharagozlou, Demirci, & Clark, 2002; Inturrisi, 2002; Okada, Tsuda, & Bryant, 2002; Zuurmond, Meert, & Noorduin, 2002).

Pure opiate analgesics (e.g., morphine) appear to exert their analgesic action primarily at the *mu* receptors found in the brain, spinal cord, and intestinal tract. These receptors are associated with analgesia and euphoria. *Mu* receptors also are associated with: constipation; pupil contraction (i.e., *miosis*); respiratory depression; and the development of physical dependence. Mixed opiate analgesics (e.g., butorphanol [Stadol®]) act primarily at the *kappa* receptors, which are associated with sedation and spinal analgesia, as well as miosis. *Synthetic* opiate analgesics, including meperidine (Demerol®), appear to act at the *delta* receptors, which are located primarily in the limbic system of the brain.[8] Delta receptors are associated with an exaggerated feeling of mental depression or unhappiness (i.e., *dysphoria*), hallucinations, and other *psychotomimetic* effects.

Pharmacologically, drugs that *stimulate* any of the opiate analgesic receptors (i.e., *delta*, *kappa*, or *mu* receptors) have been designated as *agonists*. Those that *block* the opiate analgesic receptors have been designated as *antagonists* (i.e., naloxone [Narcan®]; naltrexone [Trexan®]). Opiate analgesics that *stimulate* one receptor and *block* another have been designated as *mixed agonists/antagonists* (i.e., buprenorphine [Buprenex®]) (see Table 1.1).

The mechanism of action of the opiate analgesic antagonist, *naloxone* (Narcan®), is particularly important regarding opiate analgesic overdosage. Naloxone can bind to and block *all* opiate analgesic receptors and, thus, prevent opiate analgesics from attaching to these receptors and eliciting their analgesic and other effects. Its attraction to and ability to bind to *mu* receptors, readily reverses the respiratory depression associated with opiate analgesic overdosage. Naloxone's affinity for *mu* receptors is at least tenfold higher than its affinity for *kappa* receptors. This greater affinity may also explain why it readily reverses the respiratory depression that occurs with opiate analgesic overdosage involving the mixed agonists/antagonists (e.g., butorphanol [Stadol®]), but only minimally reverses the analgesia that occurs with the stimulation of the *kappa* receptors in the spinal cord.

Naloxone (Narcan®) is the *only* essentially pure opiate analgesic antagonist currently available for the treatment of opiate analgesic overdosage.[9] In response to

[8] The limbic system of the brain influences both the: (1) autonomic nervous system (ANS) (i.e., the part of the CNS that controls involuntary body activity such as heart rate, dilation of the pupils [i.e., *mydriasis*], and the occurrence of goose-flesh); and (2) endocrine system (i.e., the body system that controls hormone production and secretion in the body). The limbic system is generally activated by states of physiological arousal and motivated behavior.

[9] Although *naltrexone* (Trexan®) also is available, it is used more specifically for the treatment of opiate analgesic dependence. For example, naltrexone has been used in *rapid and ultra-rapid opioid detoxification* treatment centers that promise quick, painless, *same-day detoxification* for people who are

the significant increase in opiate analgesic overdosage deaths in the U.S. during the new millennium, the FDA approved the use of a single dose naloxone auto-injector (Evzio®). Formulated for *intramuscular* (IM) or *subcutaneous* (SC) use, it is indicated for the management of opiate analgesic overdosage for children, adolescents, and adults (A naloxone, 2014). It has a usual duration of action of 1 to 2 hours.[10] Naloxone has *no* other pharmacologic action other than its antagonism of the opiate analgesic agonists and has *not*, itself, been associated with any overdosage toxicity. Thus, there are virtually *no* contraindications for its use. However, cautious use is indicated because, along with its rapid reversal of the respiratory depression associated with opiate analgesic overdosage, it also can precipitate an *acute* opiate analgesic withdrawal syndrome when administered to women who are physically dependent on opiate analgesics. (Also, see the later sections, *Undesired, or Harmful, Effects and Toxicities*, "Physical and Psychological Dependence," and *Overdosage*.)

Pharmacokinetics: Absorption, Distribution, Metabolism, and Excretion

Opiate analgesics can be orally ingested as capsules (e.g., propoxyphene, Darvon®), liquids (e.g., methadone, Dolophine®), or tablets (e.g., codeine). In addition, opiate analgesics can be: vaporized and inhaled into the pulmonary system by *Chasing the Dragon* (e.g., heroin; opium); nasally insufflated or *snorted*, as a powder (e.g., heroin; hydrocodone); *transmucosally* absorbed by sucking a lozenge (e.g., fentanyl, Actiq®);[11] or *sublingually* absorbed by placing a sublingual tablet under the tongue (e.g., buprenorphine, Buprenex®). They can be intravenously injected

---

physically dependent on opiate analgesics. However, the procedures involving its use (e.g., administration of a general anesthetic followed by high-dose opiate analgesic antagonists that induce severe withdrawal without the *patient* having to *experience* it) generally pose significant risks for the patient, including several documented fatalities (Hamilton, Olmedo, & Shah, 2002). We do *not* generally recommend this form of opiate analgesic detoxification treatment. See Chapter 8, *Preventing and Treating Women's Drug and Substance Abuse*, for additional explanation and discussion.

10 Naloxone is *not* well-absorbed by oral ingestion and, therefore, has traditionally been intravenously, intramuscularly, or subcutaneously injected. However, because of the identified risks (i.e., possible needle-stick injuries involving medical staff members) associated with injecting naloxone for opiate analgesic users who have overdosed—a high-risk population for HIV, hepatitis, and other serious infections—researchers explored other methods of administration that would be both expedient and safe. The result of this research was the development of a *needleless* intranasal method of use that appears to be effective in approximately 75% of pre-hospital treatment cases (Robinson & Wermeling, 2014; Weber, Tataris, & Hoffman, 2012). In November 2015, the FDA approved this route of administration and made it available to care givers, family members, and first responders under the formulation and product name of *Narcan Nasal Spray®* (National Institute on Drug Abuse, 2015a; U.S. Food and Drug Administration, 2015). Narcan Nasal Spray® is dispensed in a box containing two individual doses of naloxone (4 mg each in 0.1 ml of nasal spray solution) in self-contained, single use disposable nasal spray units (Nordrum, 2015).

11 Actiq®, the *fentanyl lollipop*, is a solid drug matrix of fentanyl on a plastic stick. It was designed to facilitate easy removal from the mouth, where it is buccally, transmucosally absorbed, in the event of early signs of fentanyl overdosage (i.e., respiratory depression) during medical use.

(i.e., *mainlined*) as an *aqueous*, or water-soluble solution (e.g., heroin; pentazocine, Talwin®) or they can be subcutaneously injected or *popped* under the skin (e.g., heroin). They also can be absorbed through the various skin layers (e.g., epidermis, dermis) by the application of a transdermal delivery system or *skin patch* (e.g., fentanyl, Duragesic®).

These different formulations and methods of use, or administration, can affect the pharmacokinetics—absorption, distribution, metabolism, and excretion—of the various opiate analgesics in several ways.

Absorption

The absorption of the various opiate analgesics depends on their:

1. Dosage formulation (e.g., oral tablet or transdermal delivery system)
2. Method of use/route of administration (e.g., intravenous injection; pulmonary inhalation)
3. Purity, presence of adulterants, and method of production (e.g., a tablet that is too tightly compressed, or otherwise incorrectly formulated, may not break up or dissolve in the stomach or intestines when orally ingested and, thus, reduce or prevent the absorption of its active ingredients into the systemic circulation)

Following oral ingestion, opiate analgesics are mainly absorbed from the intestines, where absorption can be more erratic and unpredictable when compared to other methods of use. Absorption also is slowed and less complete from the GI tract because of *first-pass hepatic metabolism*. Consequently, opiate analgesic blood concentrations that are achieved after oral ingestion are often half, or less than half, of those achieved when the same dose of the opiate analgesic is intravenously injected—a method that insures *immediate* and *complete* absorption and effects. It is important to note that, when compared to intravenous injection, absorption following SC injection into the fatty tissues under the skin layers or IM injection into muscle tissues also is more variable and produces less rapid blood concentrations than does IV injection. These and other basic pharmacological differences often affect women's selection of an opiate analgesic and its dose and method of use.

In addition to intravenous injection, other methods of opiate analgesic use that may largely avoid *first-pass hepatic metabolism*, include:

- Buccal transmucosal absorption from the inner cheek (e.g., buprenorphine, Belbuca®)
- Intranasal instillation (e.g., heroin nose drops) and intranasal insufflation (e.g., crushing hydrocodone tablets and snorting the powder)[12]

---

[12] Transmucosal absorption also is the mechanism used for intranasal drug delivery (e.g., nasal drops; nasal sprays). Increasingly, intranasal administration of opiate analgesics (e.g., butorphanol [Stadol

- Pulmonary inhalation (e.g., *Chasing the Dragon*)
- Subcutaneous injection (e.g., *Chipping*)
- Sublingual absorption from under the tongue (e.g., buprenorphine, Subutex®)
- Transdermal absorption (e.g., applying a fentanyl, Duragesic®, transdermal delivery system, or "skin patch"); or the use of an iontophoretic transdermal system, such as Ionsys®, for the delivery of fentanyl
- Transmucosal buccal absorption (e.g., fentanyl [Actiq®] *lollipop* or "lozenge on a stick")

The various methods used for delivering *morphine* can be used to help illustrate some factors that may affect the choice and use of opiate analgesics. Following intravenous injection, morphine is readily and completely absorbed within seconds and, avoiding first-pass hepatic metabolism, quickly achieves maximal blood concentrations. However, although morphine is well-absorbed after oral ingestion, it takes *longer* to be absorbed when compared to intravenous injection and achieves maximal blood concentrations more slowly. In addition, only approximately 40% of an oral dosage of morphine is delivered to the systemic circulation and *mu* receptor sites because of significant first-pass hepatic metabolism. Thus, to achieve morphine blood concentrations and desired effects that are comparable to those achieved with intravenous injection, an oral dosage of morphine that is approximately *twice* as high as the intravenous dosage is generally required.

Distribution

The various opiate analgesics, once absorbed into the systemic circulation, have different distribution characteristics. These differences may help to explain why some women prefer one opiate analgesic over another. For example, morphine, which is not as fat soluble (i.e., lipophilic) as heroin, does *not* cross the blood-brain barrier as readily and, thus, does *not* achieve its onset of opiate analgesic action as rapidly. This distribution characteristic may explain why women, who abuse opiate analgesics, generally prefer heroin over morphine (Pagliaro & Pagliaro, *Clinical Patient Data Files*). (Also, see following section *Metabolism and Excretion* for further discussion.)

Metabolism and Excretion

Morphine and other opiate analgesics are largely metabolized into several inactive products by the liver before being excreted by the kidneys. Some opiate analgesics, such as small amounts of codeine and most of a dose of heroin (diacetylmorphine), are first metabolized into morphine before they are further metabolized into inactive

NS®]; fentanyl [Lazanda®]) have been advocated and used to manage breakthrough cancer pain (Dietrich & Gums, 2012; Grassin-Delyle, Buenestado, & Naline, 2012).

metabolites and excreted by the kidneys. The metabolism of most opiate analgesics is relatively rapid. Thus, their duration of action, on average, is 4 to 5 hours.

Consequently, women who require an opiate analgesic for the management of moderate to severe pain following an injury or a surgical procedure, generally require its administration every 4 to 5 hours to maintain adequate pain relief. This time frame for metabolism and excretion also helps to explain why women who are physically dependent on opiate analgesics must use them daily, at intervals as short as every 3 to 5 hours,[13] to prevent the onset of the *opiate analgesic withdrawal syndrome* (for further discussion, see later section, *Undesired, or Harmful, Effects and Toxicities*, "Physical and Psychological Dependence").

Urine screening for opiate analgesic use detects codeine and morphine (either as *free drug* or as *conjugated metabolite*), as well as the active metabolites dihydrocodeine, dihydromorphone, and hydromorphone.

Popular Notion: Finding morphine and codeine in the results of a woman's urine drug test indicates that she recently used both opiate analgesics.
NOT TRUE.

Heroin use may be *suspected* when both morphine and codeine are found in the results of a urine screen because heroin is metabolized to morphine. However, a small amount of codeine also is metabolized to morphine. Therefore, rapid screening assays *cannot* be used to differentially determine whether codeine, heroin, or morphine has been used.[14,15]

Heroin has a rapid onset of action after intravenous injection (i.e., within 10 seconds) and is a potent inducer of histamine release that dilates the blood vessels

---

13 For example, when heroin is available, women who "mainline," generally, "shoot up"—on average—4 times per day (Pagliaro & Pagliaro, *Clinical Patient Data Files*).

14 To precisely determine that a certain opiate analgesic has been used, a more specific chemical assay using gas chromatography with mass spectroscopy (GC-MS) or high pressure liquid chromatography (HPLC) must be used. These assays are significantly more complex, time consuming, and costly to perform than are the rapid screening assays. However, they are more accurate.

15 Urine screening for *illicit* or problematic patterns of opiate analgesic use can produce both *false positive* and *false negative* results. For example, codeine is widely available in cough and cold products and combination analgesic products. If any of these products, or if sufficient poppy seeds are consumed (poppy seeds also contain very small amounts of morphine), morphine can be detected in the urine for 2 to 4 days and yield positive urine screens for morphine and codeine—*false positive* results regarding *illicit* opiate analgesic use. False negative tests also can occur. For example, increasingly, specific adulterants (e.g., Absolute Detox®; Stealth®) are being used by *illicit* opiate analgesic users, including those in treatment programs, to produce false *negative* urine test results to avoid detection of their opiate analgesic use (Cody, Valtier, & Kuhlman, 2001; Dasgupta, 2015; Stolberg & Gerth, 2000). These products are widely advertised and are easily obtained by means of purchase from vendors over the Internet (Hoyle, 2002; Pagliaro & Pagliaro, *Clinical Patient Data Files*).

of the skin and, through this mechanism, increases feelings of body warmth (i.e., a *rush*). Heroin crosses the blood-brain barrier more rapidly than morphine and produces greater *euphoric* effects when used in equivalent amounts. However, once in the brain, heroin is chemically changed (i.e., hydrolyzed) back into morphine. Heroin functions essentially as a pro-drug with a short half-life of elimination (i.e., 2 to 6 minutes) because it is rapidly metabolized from diacetylmorphine to 6-acetylmorphine and morphine—both of which are pharmacologically active (Clarification, 2016).

Undesired, or Harmful, Effects and Toxicities

The opiate analgesics are associated with many undesired, or harmful, effects and toxicities that are generally related to their patterns of use—irregular, *short-term* use or regular, *long-term* use.[16] The toxicities associated with the opiate analgesics can be immediate (i.e., *acute*) or can develop over time (i.e., *chronic*). Acute toxicity occurs more commonly and can be quite severe, while chronic toxicity occurs *less* commonly and is usually relatively mild.[17] The risk of morbidity and mortality for women who use the opiate analgesics is primarily associated with *acute* toxicity. Generally, there is little direct residual physiological damage associated with the regular, long-term use of the opiate analgesics.[18] Persistent constipation commonly occurs with regular, long-term opiate analgesic use, particularly when orally ingested. As the opiate analgesic management of non-cancer pain significantly increased during the new millennium, the incidence of constipation related to opiate analgesic use (i.e., *opioid-induced constipation*, or OIC) correspondingly increased, particularly among older women (Weber, 2016).[19]

---

[16] The difference between a *desired* pharmacological effect associated with the use of an opiate analgesic and an *undesired*, or *harmful*, effect or *toxicity* often is related to the context of use. For example, the development of an undesired effect, such as constipation, for a woman being successfully treated for a severe, non-productive cough, with a cough syrup containing an opiate analgesic versus a woman with severe diarrhea who takes an opiate analgesic, or a derivative anti-diarrhea product, for its desired constipating effects.

[17] In fact, *chronic* toxicity associated with the opiate analgesics is generally considered to be *lower* than that observed for any other group of psychodepressants, as well as for most of the other drugs and substances of abuse.

[18] For example, although deficits in executive cognitive functioning may occur with periods of opiate analgesic abuse, residual impairment among former opiate analgesic users has *not* been noted. This observation is in stark contrast to former amphetamine users who, although abstinent, continue to display deficits in executive cognitive functioning related to their former periods of amphetamine abuse (Ersche, Clark, & London, 2006; Pagliaro & Pagliaro, *Clinical Patient Data Files*). (Also, see related discussion in Chapter 5, *Women's Amphetamine and Cocaine Abuse.*)

[19] When additional opiate analgesic-related gastrointestinal (GI) symptoms (e.g., abdominal pain; bloating; dry mouth; gastric stasis; nausea; and vomiting) are combined with OIC, the resultant spectrum/syndrome of GI complaints is commonly referred to as, "opioid-induced bowel dysfunction" (OIBD) (Leppert, 2015).

Significant recent and developing pharmacotherapeutic advances in the treatment of OIC/OIBD have primarily focused on *peripheral-acting mu-opiate analgesic receptor antagonists* (PAMORAs) (Holder & Rhee, 2016; Leppert, 2015).[20] Their clinical use in patients with advanced/severe OIC/OIBD symptoms, who do *not* respond well to traditional oral laxatives, has resulted in significant relief of adverse GI symptoms without compromising related opiate analgesia. The use of PAMORAs is associated with several undesired, or harmful, effects, which are *not* dose-related, including: fecal impaction; bowel obstruction; and bowel perforation. In addition, with regular, long-term opiate analgesic use, tolerance does *not* develop to these undesired, or harmful, effects (Jones, Prommer, & Backstedt, 2015).

Other major harmful effects related to the use of opiate analgesics also include those associated with: physical and psychological dependence; the opiate analgesic withdrawal syndrome; and overdosage. In addition, serious harmful effects also are associated with women's opiate analgesic use during pregnancy and lactation. These effects are discussed in the following sections.

Physical and Psychological Dependence

Several of the opiate analgesics, including heroin, methadone (Dolophine®), and propoxyphene (Darvon®), were specifically developed to provide analgesia *without* causing physical or psychological dependence. However, it is now generally known that the regular, long-term use of *any* opiate analgesic, including the synthetic derivatives, that are capable of producing pain relief, is associated with the development of both physical and psychological dependence, characterized by: (1) tolerance;[21] (2) craving; and (3) the opiate analgesic withdrawal syndrome when opiate analgesic use is abruptly discontinued.[22]

As noted by the National Institute on Drug Abuse:

---

[20] Naloxegol (Movantik®) prevents opiate analgesics from binding to *mu* opiate analgesic receptors in the GI tract (Garnock-Jones, 2015). It was approved for adult use by the FDA in September 2014 (U.S. Food and Drug Administration, 2014a). As such, it became the *first* orally ingested drug in this new pharmacological classification of drugs developed for the treatment of OIC (Anantharamu, Sharma, & Gupta, 2015; Corsetti & Tack, 2015). These PAMORAs (Jones, Prommer, & Backstedt, 2015) are PEGylated derivatives of naloxone that are specifically developed to have negligible penetration of the CNS, when orally ingested. Consequently, they block the constipating effects associated with the use of the opiate analgesics, but *not* the analgesic effects. As such, their use is particularly indicated for adults with chronic, non-cancer pain who require opiate analgesic pharmacotherapy. Common undesired, or harmful, effects associated with naloxegol, include: abdominal pain, diarrhea, and excessive gas and flatulence (U.S. Food and Drug Administration, 2014a).

[21] Tolerance is identified when the desired actions or effectiveness of an opiate analgesic diminishes over time requiring more and more of the opiate analgesic to be used in an attempt to achieve the desired actions.

[22] In an effort to prevent associated signs and symptoms of the opiate analgesic withdrawal syndrome, continued use, or a gradual reduction in the amount used, is necessary.

> An estimated 2.1 million people in the United States suffer from substance use disorders related to prescription opioid pain relievers in 2012 and an estimated 467,000 are addicted to heroin.
>
> *(Volkow, 2014, p. 1)*

Tolerance, Withdrawal, and Craving. Tolerance is the need to use *increasingly* higher dosages, or amounts, of an opiate analgesic more often, or at more frequent intervals, in order to achieve desired actions that were experienced with *initial use.* Tolerance develops within a few months of regular, long-term opiate analgesic use. Replacing the usual opiate analgesic with a different opiate analgesic generally does *not* help to achieve desired effects (e.g., analgesia; euphoria) due to the common occurrence of *cross-tolerance* (i.e., when tolerance occurs to one of the opiate analgesics, such as heroin, tolerance to the other opiate analgesics, such as morphine, also occurs). In addition, for many of the opiate analgesics, including heroin and methadone, the *higher* the dosage of the opiate analgesic used, the *more* severe the physical dependence and the associated opiate analgesic withdrawal syndrome upon abrupt discontinuation of use.

Popular Notion: If women take their opiate analgesics exactly as prescribed, they can avoid the development of tolerance.
NOT TRUE.

As noted by Volkow and McLellan (2016) from the NIDA:

> There is lingering *misunderstanding* among some physicians about the important differences between physical dependence and addiction. The repeated administration of any opioid almost inevitably results in the development of tolerance and physical dependence.
>
> *(p. 1)*

The *euphorigenic* action that opiate analgesics produce among non-tolerant people is generally reduced, or eliminated, as tolerance develops. It is important to note that tolerance is only one component of *physical dependence.*[23] *Craving* is a characteristic of *psychological dependence. Craving*—the memory of, and the desire for, the feeling of euphoria—appears to be one of the major factors underlying the

[23] Physical dependence is associated with both: (1) the development of *tolerance*; and (2) a characteristic *opiate analgesic withdrawal syndrome*, which occurs when regular, long-term use of an opiate analgesic is abruptly discontinued and which resolves "immediately" when its use is resumed.

high potential for abuse of the opiate analgesics—the physical and psychological dependence associated with regular, long-term opiate analgesic use.

To once again achieve the desired euphorigenic actions, women who are opiate analgesic abusers, and who are tolerant, may greatly *increase* the amount of the opiate analgesic they use—and, consequently, place themselves at *increased* risk for overdosage and death associated with *severe* respiratory depression. In addition, among women who are regular, long-term users, the *higher* the dosage of the opiate analgesic used, the *more* severe is the physical dependence, and, thus, the more *severe* the associated opiate analgesic withdrawal syndrome. Consequently, an increased desire to avoid the opiate analgesic withdrawal syndrome develops and this desire becomes a powerful, and very often persuasive, motive for continued opiate analgesic use. (See the following section for additional discussion of the opiate analgesic withdrawal syndrome.)

Opiate Analgesic Withdrawal Syndrome. The *opiate analgesic withdrawal syndrome* occurs when regular, long-term opiate analgesic use is abruptly discontinued and is *immediately* relieved when opiate analgesic use is resumed. Signs and symptoms of the opiate analgesic withdrawal syndrome generally include: abdominal pain, chills with goose flesh (i.e., "going cold turkey"), diarrhea, fever, irritability, muscle aches and jerks (i.e., "kicking the habit"), running nose, sleeplessness, sweating, vomiting, watery eyes, worrying, and yawning.[24] In severe cases, *terrifying* hallucinations, convulsions, and coma may occur.

The signs and symptoms of opiate analgesic withdrawal usually *begin* within 8 to 16 hours following the last time that an opiate analgesic was used and *resolve* after 2 to 12 days. The occurrence and severity largely depend on the: (1) specific opiate analgesic used;[25] (2) the length of time that the opiate analgesic was regularly used; (3) dosage used (higher versus lower); and (4) the method of use (intravenous injection versus oral ingestion). Although many women, who have undergone opiate analgesic withdrawal, generally report the experience as being *extremely* painful and difficult, most cases are relatively *mild* in terms of the physical stress that is experienced.[26]

---

[24] These signs and symptoms are *not* generally life-threatening and have often been likened to those experienced during a severe case of the *flu* (Pagliaro & Pagliaro, *Clinical Patient Data Files*).

[25] Reportedly, methadone (Dolophine®) has the *most* severe withdrawal syndrome when compared to other opiate analgesics at equivalent dosages (Hiltunen & Eklund, 2002; Pagliaro & Pagliaro, 2009).

[26] Despite the objective documentation of the relatively *mild*, undesired effects associated with the opiate analgesic withdrawal syndrome, the conscious attempt to avoid or diminish these effects is, reportedly, one of the major reasons, after "to achieve feelings of euphoria," for their continued regular, long-term use (Pagliaro & Pagliaro, *Clinical Patient Data Files*). As such, when their favorite opiate analgesic is not available, women will use whatever opiate analgesic is available to them to avoid or diminish the undesired effects even if they would not generally otherwise use that opiate analgesic (e.g., codeine) because they "don't like it" or think it is "junk" or "shit." Loperamide is one-such opiate analgesic. It was developed and approved by the FDA as an antidiarrheal. Because it acts primarily at the intestinal opiate analgesic mu-receptor in the myenteric plexus of the GIT, its potential for abuse is officially labeled as "low." Consequently,

In addition, the opiate analgesic withdrawal syndrome is *not* usually fatal, even if managed without medical assistance (i.e., quitting "cold turkey"). Fatalities that may occur among women who are undergoing opiate analgesic withdrawal are usually the result of such complicating factors as poly-drug or substance abuse, heart disease, or depression leading to suicide. (For specific details regarding the treatment of opiate analgesic withdrawal, see Chapter 8, *Preventing and Treating Women's Drug and Substance Abuse*.)

Toxicities Associated with Method of Use

In addition to direct toxicities associated with the use of opiate analgesics, there are several significant undesired, or harmful, effects that are specifically associated with its method of use, particularly the *intravenous* injection of the opiate analgesics (Bangsberg, Rosen, & Aragon, 2002; Ciccarone, 2009; Ciccarone & Bourgois, 2003; Pieper & Templin, 2001; Schoener, Hopper, & Pierre, 2002; Williamson, Archibald, & Van Vliet, 2001).[27] These effects include: abscesses at injection sites (e.g., cellulitis); damage to veins (e.g., thrombophlebitis) and resultant scarring of the skin (i.e., needle tracks; "railroad tracks");[28] and other undesired effects (see following list).

- Aneurysm
- Blood infection (e.g., bacteremia; sepsis; septicemia)
- Blood vessel damage, inflammation, or infection (e.g., thrombophlebitis; thrombosis; venous insufficiency [chronic]; venous sclerosis)
- Brain and spinal cord infection
- Endocarditis[29]
- Gangrene[30]

---

it is widely available "over-the-counter," without a prescription. However, at higher dosages, it can readily cross the blood-brain barrier resulting in central systemic effects, including euphoria, respiratory depression, and relief of the opiate analgesic withdrawal syndrome. Consequently, in response to the opiate analgesic epidemic during the second decade of the new millennium, it has become commonly known as "poor man's methadone" (Daniulaityte, Carlson, & Falck, 2013; Dierksen, Gonsoulin, & Walterscheid, 2015). The abuse of loperamide has been associated with physical and psychological dependence, respiratory depression, and life-threating ventricular dysrhythmias (MacDonald, Heiner, & Villarreal, 2015; Marraffa, Holland, & Sullivan, 2014; Spinner, Lonardo, & Mulamalla, 2015).

27 Except in cases of opiate analgesic withdrawal involving *high* dosages or methadone use.

28 Commonly used anatomic sites for intravenous injection of the various drugs and substances of abuse, in decreasing order of use, include the: antecubital fossa, or forearm at the bend of the elbow, and, foot, leg, breast, groin, and neck (Pagliaro & Pagliaro, *Clinical Patient Data Files*).

29 Infective endocarditis related to intravenous injection has increased significantly during the new millennium, with the highest rates reported for young women of European continental descent.

30 Often requires removal of the infected body tissue, or, depending on the extent of the infection, when involving an extremity, amputation of the affected finger(s) or hand, and toe(s) or foot.

- Infections (e.g., hepatitis B virus [HBV]; hepatitis C virus [HCV];[31,32] HIV)
- Muscular infection (e.g., myonecrosis; myositis; pyomyositis)
- Soft-tissue infection or inflammation (e.g., cellulitis; cutaneous venous ulcer;[33] necrotizing fasciitis)
- Tetanus
- Wound botulism

Not directly caused by the opiate analgesics, themselves, these infections and other undesired effects are caused by: (1) the adulterants used by dealers to *cut* the opiate analgesic in order to increase its weight and street value; (2) crushing and injecting drugs intended for oral use together with related excipients; (3) infection caused by using unsterile, shared needles and syringes; and (4) improper injection techniques and resultant local tissue and vessel damage.

Obviously, these serious complications do *not* occur when opiate analgesics are *swallowed*, *smoked*, or *snorted*. However, these other methods of use may be associated with their own undesired, or harmful, effects. For example, during the past decade, the intranasal use (i.e., *snorting*) of the opiate analgesics, particularly hydrocodone-acetaminophen tablets, has been associated with: (1) erosion of the lateral nasal walls, nasopharynx, and soft palate; (2) fungal invasion of the nasal surfaces; (3) inflammation of the nasal passages and sinuses; (4) bacterial infection of the nasal surfaces with a resultant runny nose containing a mixture of mucus and pus (i.e., *mucopurulent exudate*); and (5) perforation of the nasal septum (Alexander, Alexander, & Valentino, 2012; Sloan & Klimkina, 2009; Yewell, Haydon, & Archer, 2002). In addition, severe, life-threatening asthmatic attacks have been associated with the intranasal insufflation, or *snorting*, of heroin by women who have pre-existing asthma (Krantz, Hershow, & Prachand, 2003; Pagliaro & Pagliaro, *Clinical Patient Data Files*).

Pregnancy, Neonatal Abstinence Syndrome, Breast-Feeding, and Mothering

In their study of women of reproductive age, who were enrolled in Medicaid in selected states in the U.S. from 2008 to 2012, Ailes, Dawson, and Lind (2015)

---

31 Often a precursor to cirrhosis of the liver or cancer of the liver (i.e., hepatocellular carcinoma) either of which may be fatal or require liver transplantation. The most common cause of hepatitis C in North America is the sharing of contaminated needles among women who use drugs and substances of abuse.

32 In 2016, the CDC announced that hepatitis C virus (HCV) infection had its most significant increase among women of childbearing age *and* cautioned about an increased risk in the U.S. for mother-to-child transmission. The increased rates of HCV were identified as being *directly* related to increased intravenous drug use (IVDU) among women of childbearing age in the U.S. (Koneru, Nelson, & Hariri, 2016). Although under development, there is no hepatitis C vaccine currently available (Ahlen & Frelin, 2016; Ogholikhan & Schwarz, 2016). However, there are several available and effective treatment options (see Zeuzem, 2017).

33 Often is a chronic condition affecting the lower extremities that can be extremely debilitating.

found that approximately 40% of the women received a prescription for an opiate analgesic from their prescribers. In a similar study of women of reproductive age (i.e., 15 to 45 years-of-age), who were enrolled in Medicaid from 2008 to 2013 in New York state, approximately 20% filled a prescription for an opiate analgesic at their neighborhood pharmacy (Gallagher, Shin, & Roohan, 2016).

Pregnancy. Opiate analgesics have been medically used to provide women with pain relief just prior to, or during, labor and delivery. Bateman, Hernandez-Diaz, and Rathmell (2014, p. 1216), in a review of data from 534,500 women in the U.S., who completed their pregnancies while enrolled in a commercial insurance plan, found that "76,742 (14.4%) were dispensed an opiate analgesic (primarily codeine, hydrocodone, and oxycodone) at some point during their pregnancies."

The short-term medical use of opiate analgesics for a specific indication for women, who are pregnant, is relatively safe for themselves and their fetuses, as well as their neonates and infants. The *short-term* medical use of opiate analgesics by mothers who are breast-feeding also is relatively safe for both mothers and their breast-fed neonates or infants. However, *caution* is required because expected psychodepressant actions (e.g., drowsiness; slowed respirations) may occur among mothers and their breast-fed neonates and infants, as well as physical dependence if mothers use *higher dosages,* dose themselves at more frequent intervals than prescribed, or continue their use, long-term/chronically. Other related concerns are discussed in the following sections.

It is important to recognize that opiate analgesics are medically and personally used and abused by *many* women in the U.S., who are pregnant. For example, Heil, Jones, and Arria (2011) found, in their study of a *large* sample of women who abused opiate analgesics, that 90% had a history of admission for drug or substance abuse treatment and 86% reported having had an "unintended" pregnancy. As emphasized by Jumah (2016), "opioids are now the most common reason for seeking treatment for illicit substances during pregnancy" (p. 35).

Clearly, health and social care professionals require accurate knowledge about: (1) women's use of opiate analgesics during pregnancy; (2) propensity for abuse; and (3) potential effects on pregnant women, themselves, and their developing embryos/fetuses, neonates, and infants.[34] However, in this context, health

[34] However, as with alcohol use/abuse during pregnancy and its association with possible FAS/FASD (see Chapter 2, *Women's Alcohol Abuse*, for related discussion), mothers are *not* always accurate historians regarding reporting their personal use of drugs and substances of abuse during pregnancy. Thus, frequently, in order to confirm or evaluate cases of possible maternal opiate analgesic use/abuse, biological testing of neonates for Neonatal Abstinence Syndrome (NAS), including the testing of biological specimens collected from neonatal cord blood, hair, meconium, and urine, is required (Cotten, 2012; Eichel & Johannemann, 2014; Lozano, Garcia-Algar, & Vall, 2007; Murphy-Oikonen, Montelpare, & Southon, 2010) and *highly* recommended in order to achieve optimal treatment outcomes (Pagliaro & Pagliaro, *Clinical Patient Data Files*).

and social care professionals would be well-advised to heed the cautionary advice of Krans and Patrick (2016):

> Efforts to penalize women and negative consequences for disclosing substance use to health care providers are harmful and may prevent women from seeking prenatal care and other beneficial health care services during pregnancy.
>
> *(p. 4)*

Neonatal Abstinence Syndrome. Opiate analgesics cross the placental barrier. Thus, their use just prior to, or during, labor and delivery may result in drowsiness, lethargy, or other expected pharmacologic actions (e.g., respiratory depression; constipation) among neonates. Although women's opiate analgesic abuse during pregnancy has *not* been directly associated with congenital malformations, or birth defects, it does place neonates at a significant risk for NAS that is directly associated with *decreasing* neonatal opiate analgesic blood concentrations following birth.[35]

> In his first three weeks of life, Brayden suffered through a form of newborn drug dependency called Neonatal Abstinence Syndrome. He trembled and wailed inconsolably, clenching his muscles and sometimes gasping for breath as he went through withdrawal.
>
> *(Wilson & Shiffman, 2015, p. 2)*

Although first formally identified over 40 years ago, by Finnegan, Connaughton, and Kron (1975), the incidence of NAS and its related clinical sequelae have continued to increase virtually unabated into the new millennium.

INCIDENCE OF NAS. Of concern is the consistent observation that the incidence of NAS in the U.S. has *increased* significantly during the new millennium. For example: Ko, Patrick, and Tong (2016) noted that:

> The overall NAS incidence increased 300% from 1.5 per 1,000 hospital births in 1999, to 6.0 per 1,000 hospital births in 2013.
>
> *(p. 799)*

---

[35] Interestingly, Oei, Xu, and Abdel-Latif (2012, p. F193), in their study of the characteristics of dopamine D2 receptor gene (DRD2) polymorphisms in heroin- or methadone-exposed and drug-free control neonates and the relationship to NAS, found that the:

(1) A2A2 allele is more common in *drug-exposed* neonates
(2) 141ins allele is significantly more common in *drug-exposed* neonates *and* in *drug-free control* neonates with *less* severe postnatal withdrawal

These findings help to further our understanding of NAS and its characteristic signs and symptoms as well as its potential mechanisms of action.

Similarly, as identified by McQueen and Murphy-Oikonen (2016):

> The incidence of the neonatal abstinence syndrome has increased substantially in the past decade. In 2012, the syndrome was diagnosed in 21,732 infants in the United States, which represents an increase by a factor of 5 during the previous 12 years.
>
> *(p. 2468)*

The associated reported rates of NAS per 1,000 hospital live births were *highest* in the states of Kentucky (i.e., 15.0), Vermont (i.e., 33.3), and West Virginia (i.e., 33.4).[36] As found by Lind, Petersen, and Lederer (2015), in their two-year study (2010–2011) of 242 neonates confirmed as having NAS, over 235 of the neonates (i.e., over 97%) required admission to a Neonatal Intensive Care Unit (NICU) for an average of 26 days. Fortunately, all neonates in this study survived.[37]

The occurrence of NAS is significantly *increased* among neonates whose mothers: (1) regularly abused opiate analgesics during pregnancy; or (2) abused opiate analgesics during the last trimester (Desai, Huybrechts, & Hernandez-Diaz, 2015).[38] As reported by Lind, Petersen, and Lederer (2015), the mothers, who participated in their study of maternal opiate analgesic use during pregnancy, provided the following reasons, listed in *descending* order:[39]

1. Illicit personal use (133 mothers, or 55%)
2. Drug abuse treatment (100 mothers, or 41%)
3. Chronic pain (52 mothers, or 22%)
4. Unknown or unspecified (25 mothers, or 10%)

---

[36] These reported *increases* in the rates of NAS in the U.S. are consistent with an earlier report by Patrick, Schumacher, and Benneyworth (2012). In their retrospective analysis of a nationally representative sample of newborns with NAS, they found that the rate of incidence increased from 1.20 per 1,000 hospital births in 2000 to 3.39 per 1,000 hospital births in 2009 (p. 1934).

[37] However, as in Brayden's case, survival is *not* equivalent to "safely and happily ever after." As noted in the related NBC/Reuters report:

> Reuters identified 110 cases since 2010 that are similar to Brayden's: Babies and toddlers whose mothers used opioids during pregnancy and who later died preventable deaths.
>
> Being born drug-dependent didn't kill these children. Each recovered enough to be discharged from the hospital. What sealed their fates was being sent home to families ill-equipped to care for them.
>
> Like Brayden, more than 40 of the children suffocated. Thirteen died after swallowing toxic doses of methadone, heroin, oxycodone or other opioids.
>
> *(Wilson & Shiffman, 2015, p. 3)*

[38] Other major health risks for women, who are physically dependent on opiate analgesics and are pregnant or breast-feeding, are the use of *illicit* opiate analgesics that contain adulterants or that are self-injected (see earlier discussion of "Undesired, or Harmful, Effects and Toxicities Associated with Method of Use").

[39] The total percentage exceeds 100% because some of the mothers provided *more* than one reason for their opiate analgesic use during pregnancy.

SIGNS AND SYMPTOMS OF NAS. Signs and symptoms associated with NAS include: abruptio placentae; body temperature instability; disruption of maternal-infant attachment or bonding;[40] body temperature instability; body weight loss; *excessive*, high pitched crying; *excessive* sucking; feeding difficulties; fever; hyperactive reflexes; growth restriction; *increased* muscle tone; *increased* number of stools; *increased* respiratory rate; irritability; myoclonic jerks; nasal stuffiness; preterm delivery; respiratory distress; seizures; sleep/wake abnormalities; small head circumference; sneezing; tremors; vomiting; and yawning (Jansson & Velez, 2012; Ko, Patrick, & Tong, 2016; Osborn, Jeffery, & Cole; 2010a, 2010b; Pagliaro & Pagliaro, 2002; Pagliaro & Pagliaro, *Clinical Patient Data Files*; Uebel, Wright, & Burns, 2015).

The incidence and signs and symptoms of NAS vary widely depending upon the type of opiate analgesic used and the context of use (e.g., concomitant use of other drugs and substances of abuse). Thus, the intensity of the signs and symptoms does *not* always reflect the *amount* or *duration* of maternal opiate analgesic use during pregnancy. Although the opiate analgesics, methadone and morphine, are widely used for the medical management of neonates at risk for the opiate analgesic withdrawal syndrome, there is *no* consensus as to the *best* approach for their pharmacological medical management (Pagliaro & Pagliaro, 2002). (See following discussion.)

TREATMENT OF NAS. In association with the *increasing* rate of opiate analgesic abuse among women in the U.S. during the new millennium, the rates of NAS also have significantly *increased*—as foreseen or expected (Davies, Gilbert, & Johnson, 2016). In response, several treatment approaches, both pharmacological and non-pharmacological (e.g., breast-feeding and mothering; counseling; education; psychotherapy; supportive care, including creating a gentle, soothing environment with minimal stimulation to calm and soothe infants with NAS). For example, as identified by McQueen and Murphy-Oikonen (2016, p. 366):

> The strongest evidence from systematic reviews for improving outcomes [e.g., severity of NAS; length of hospital stay] is in support of breast-feeding, with emerging evidence that favors "rooming-in."

However, in general, response to non-pharmacological treatment strategies has been severely limited—most researchers (e.g., Kocherlakota, 2014; Pagliaro & Pagliaro, *Clinical Patient Data Files*) report that positive response rates, in the context of NAS, are significantly *less* than 50%. Thus, the primary focus of therapy for NAS is on pharmacotherapy.

Various opiate analgesics (e.g., methadone [Dolophine®]) have been used to maintain maternal opiate analgesic dependence during pregnancy and to decrease the risk for neonatal opiate analgesic physical dependence and associated

---

[40] Also, see related discussion in later section, "Mothering."

NAS (e.g., Brown, Hayes, & Thornton, 2015; Osborn, Jeffery, & Cole, 2010a).[41] Currently, it appears that the use of sublingual *buprenorphine* (Buprenex®), a mixed opiate agonist/antagonist (see earlier discussion), is preferred because it is associated with a significantly:

1. *Milder* form of NAS, such as lower incidents of preterm labor and of neonatal respiratory distress (Jansson & Velez, 2012; Jones, Kaltenbach, & Heil, 2010; Pagliaro & Pagliaro, 2009, 2012; Thomas, Fullerton, & Kim, 2014; Unger, Jagsch, & Jones, 2011; Wilder & Winhusen, 2015)
2. *Less* severe maternal opiate analgesic physical dependence that is relatively easier to manage than that associated with methadone use (Gaalema, Heil, & Badger, 2013)
3. *Longer* mean gestational age, *larger* head circumference, *longer* body length, and *heavier* body weight at birth for neonates whose mothers received buprenorphine maintenance pharmacotherapy when compared to neonates whose mothers received methadone maintenance pharmacotherapy during pregnancy (Brogly, Saia, & Walley, 2014)
4. *Shorter* hospital stay (i.e., fewer days in the hospital) for neonates born to mothers who received buprenorphine maintenance pharmacotherapy when compared to mothers who received methadone maintenance pharmacotherapy (Pritham, Paul, & Hayes, 2012)

If a neonate requires additional pharmacotherapy for the medical management of NAS (i.e., in addition to an opiate analgesic, such as buprenorphine or methadone), a sedative-hypnotic can be added to reduce the severity of opiate analgesic withdrawal. In related systematic reviews performed for the Cochrane Database, Osborn, Jeffery, and Cole (2005, 2010b) found that the use of a barbiturate (i.e., *phenobarbital*) provided superior results when compared to a benzodiazepine (i.e., diazepam) in terms of the "reduction in treatment failure." We, too, have endorsed this approach in the context of managing seizures associated with NAS (see, for example, Lemke, 2002).

Pharmacological intervention typically involves the following sequential process:

1. Selection of specific pharmacologic intervention
2. Dosage adjustment—generally starting at a lower dosage and increasing as clinically indicated by scores on selected NAS evaluation instruments (e.g., *Finnegan Neonatal Abstinence Scoring Tool*; *Finnegan Neonatal Abstinence Syndrome Scale—Short Form*; *MOTHER NAS Scale*; *Neonatal Narcotic Withdrawal Index*; and *Neonatal Withdrawal Inventory* [Finnegan, Connaughton, & Kron, 1975;

[41] Methadone is currently the most frequently prescribed medication for the maintenance of opiate analgesic physical and psychological dependence during pregnancy (Hudak & Tan, 2012) (see related discussion in Chapter 8, *Preventing and Treating Women's Drug and Substance Abuse*).

Green & Suffet, 1981; Jones, Seashore, & Johnson, 2016; Lipsitz, 1975; Maguire, Cline, & Parnell, 2013; Zahorodny, Rom & Whitney, 1998]).

3. Stabilization of dosage (i.e., maintenance of optimal dose for a minimum of 48 hours)
4. Discharge, generally after 48 to 72 hours, depending upon *improved* clinical response (e.g., adequate improvement in signs and symptoms of NAS and normalization of feeding behavior; reflex response; sleep patterns; stool production; and other expected neonatal/infant behaviors) (Pagliaro & Pagliaro, *Clinical Patient Data Files*)

BREAST-FEEDING. The safety of opiate analgesic use among mothers who are breast-feeding has *not* been established. Opiate analgesics have been detected in breast milk in amounts that can cause expected pharmacologic actions among neonates and infants, such as constipation and both CNS and respiratory depression. Neonates and infants also may develop opiate analgesic physical dependence and are at risk for experiencing opiate analgesic withdrawal if maternal use of opiate analgesics or breast-feeding is abruptly discontinued.

Generally, women who are breast-feeding should *not* use opiate analgesics (Pagliaro & Pagliaro, 2012). However, there are other views on this topic. For example, Welle-Strand, Skurtveit, and Jansson (2013, p. 1060), in a national cohort study of 124 Norwegian women treated with either methadone or buprenorphine maintenance pharmacotherapy during pregnancy, found that "breast fed neonates exposed to methadone prenatally had significantly lower incidence of NAS requiring pharmacotherapy (53% vs. 80%)."[42]

MOTHERING. The abuse of opiate analgesics by mothers has been associated with extremely distressing consequences, including poor maternal-infant and child bonding and severe neglect and abuse of infants and children. As found by Nair, Black, and Schuler (1997), in their randomized, longitudinal cohort study of 152 mother/infant dyads for evidence of disruption of primary caregiving or neglect during the first 28 months of life, maternal heroin use during pregnancy was the *most* significant factor associated with disruption of maternal care giving. This trend has continued in the U.S. through the new millennium. However, as noted by McQueen and Murphy-Oikonen (2016), for neonates suffering from NAS (also, see related discussion in the previous and following sections):

> Breast-feeding and rooming-in are promising nonpharmacologic strategies that may also improve outcomes for infants and mothers, including maternal satisfaction with and involvement in the care of the newborn.
>
> *(p. 2477)*

[42] The confounding variable in this study and analysis is, of course, the potential residual effects of prenatal methadone exposure on NAS—in the absence of subsequent breast-feeding.

Other extremely deleterious effects upon "mothering"—from neglect to active physical abuse of infants, children, and adolescents—have been associated with the use of opiate analgesics by mothers as well as other women (Pagliaro & Pagliaro, *Clinical Patient Data Files*). For example:

> A woman from Ohio was sentenced to 51 years in prison for the "horrific" crime of allowing her drug dealer to have sex with her 11-year-old daughter to obtain heroin to feed her addiction … Prosecutors said the girl was raped, sodomized, and forced to perform oral sex with the encounters sometimes videotaped … The girl's grandmother told the courtroom she doesn't know if the young girl will ever recover from the ordeal.
>
> *(Russell, 2016, p. 1)*

Also, consider, for example, the following related case report:

> On Nov. 15, 2015, Child Protective Services investigators removed a 6-year-old boy, a 4-year-old girl and a 2-year-old girl from Hutt and McIver's home because there was heroin in the house, as well as needles and rat droppings. CPS employees noticed marks, bruising and cuts on the younger girl's body, indicative of heroin injection. The oldest child was interviewed a month later and described being choked by McIver and then injected with "feel good medicine." … The 2-year-old girl tested positive for heroin through a hair follicle test two months later.
>
> *(Ocker, 2016, pp. 1–2)*

In a related manner, we have noted, and previously reported (e.g., Pagliaro & Pagliaro, 2004, 2012), that mothers and grandmothers have used opium derivatives administered to infants and young children to manage perceived problem behaviors, including: crying; inability to fall asleep; and irritable behavior related to teething; or to sedate them for a long drive or flight. One particularly interesting example involved the rather common cultural practice in one Ukrainian-American community for "babas" (i.e., grandmothers) to use the opium poppies that they raised in their gardens—grown primarily to harvest the seeds to use in baking (e.g., poppy seed bread and cakes)—packaged in a sachet and utilized as a pacifier to settle neonates and to help them to sleep and, primarily among infants, to manage their teething pain (Pagliaro & Pagliaro, *Clinical Patient Data Files*).

Unfortunately, in the context of our forensic consulting, we also have encountered the administration of heroin, and other psychodepressants, to infants and young children by mothers, and others responsible for their care (e.g., a mother's boyfriend; girlfriend; or "fiancé"), to facilitate sexual assault (Pagliaro & Pagliaro, *Clinical Patient Data Files*).

Overdosage

Over the first decade of the new millennium, 1997 to 2009, the rate of hospitalizations in the U.S. related to opiate analgesic overdosage *increased* sharply and significantly from 2 per 100,000 U.S. population to 15 per 100,000 population (Unick, Rosenblum, & Mars, 2013). As identified by Williams and Bisaga (2016, p. 813),

> The United States is facing a vast epidemic of opioid-related deaths. More than 2.4 million Americans have a severe opioid-use disorder (OUD)[43] involving dependence on pain medications, heroin, or both, and rates of drug-overdose deaths in this country have outpaced mortality from motor vehicle accidents since 2013.

Approximately, 16,000 people in the U.S. die annually because of a prescription opiate-analgesic overdosage and an additional number of approximately 8,000 die annually because of heroin-related overdosages (i.e., approximately 65 people daily) (National Institute on Drug Abuse, 2015a). We expect that these numbers will continue to increase significantly over the next 20 years, together with related prescription opiate analgesic deaths and emergency department visits, as increasing numbers of baby boomers reach age 65+ (Colliver, Compton, & Gfroerer, 2006; Gossup & Moos, 2008; Han, Gfroerer, & Colliver, 2009a, 2009b; Nordrum, 2016; Pagliaro & Pagliaro, *Clinical Patient Data Files*; Wu & Blazer, 2011).

Deaths associated with opiate analgesic overdosage, in the U.S., *increased over* 200% from 2000 to 2014 (Rudd, Aleshire, & Zibbell, 2016). These deaths have been reported among all groups of women, with the highest increased risk reported for: (1) women of European descent; (2) women veterans with AUDs and/or SUDs; and (3) homeless woman veterans suffering from physical or sexual abuse (Carroll Chapman & Wu, 2014; Ilgen, Bohnert, & Ignacio, 2010; Pagliaro & Pagliaro, *Clinical Patient Data Files*).[44] It also has been reported that "overdosage deaths in the U.S. are rising fastest among middle-aged women, and their drug of choice is usually prescription painkillers" (Stobbe, 2013, p. 1).

"Mothers, wives, sisters, and daughters are dying at rates we have never seen before," said Dr. Thomas Frieden, director of the Centers for Disease Control and Prevention. The CDC (2013, p. 1), goes on to warn that approximately 20 women die *every* day from an opiate analgesic overdosage in the U.S. and, for every woman who dies of an opiate analgesic overdose, another 30 are treated at emergency departments for related misuse or abuse. The concomitant use of alcohol and/or benzodiazepines (e.g., alprazolam, Xanax®; diazepam, Valium®) are frequently associated with cases of opiate analgesic overdosage and death (Jones, Paulozzi, &

---

[43] This term is used in the 5th edition of the DSM taxonomy (i.e., *DSM5*).

[44] Geographically, the *highest* reported increases in these opiate analgesic overdosage deaths occurred in the Appalachian and Southwestern states (Park & Bloch, 2016).

Mack, 2014). As illustrated in the sad, but rather prototypical, overdosage suicide death of actor Jim Carrey's girlfriend:

> White took her own life at age 28 by overdosing on Carrey's and her own prescription medication (a combination of sleeping pills, painkillers, and beta blockers).
>
> *(Jancelewicz, 2016, p. 1)*

The opiate analgesic antagonist, naloxone (Narcan®),[45] can literally bring a woman, who has overdosed on an opiate analgesic, back from death's doorstep.[46] However, death due to acute *heroin* overdosage is a relatively common event and has been increasing since the early1990s—from fewer than 1,000 per year to more than 10,000 per year (National Institute on Drug Abuse, 2015b; Ochoa, Hahn, & Seal, 2001; Rudd, 2014). As noted by Jones, Logan, and Gladden (2015, p.1), "Heroin use and overdose deaths have increased significantly in the United States"—quadrupling from 2002 to 2013 (Nordrum, 2015) and more than tripling from 2010 to 2014 (Rudd, Aleshire, & Zibbell, 2016). As part of the response to this situation, the FDA approved the use of a hand-held naloxone auto-injector (Evzio®) in 2014 (U.S. Food and Drug Administration, 2014b).

In some of these cases, death is often a rapid event in which the needle and syringe may be found still attached to the user's injection site (e.g., inner arm or top of hand) (Pagliaro & Pagliaro, *Clinical Patient Data Files*). However, the *largest* number of annual overdosage deaths, as well as the *highest* rate of increase in overdosage death in the U.S. during the first decade of the new millennium (i.e., 2000 to 2011) involved the *prescription* opiate analgesics, particularly oxycodone (OxyContin®) (Brown, 2011; Centers for Disease Control and Prevention, 2013; Girion, Glover, & Smith, 2011; Rudd, 2014).

> Between 1999 and 2010, OPR [*opioid pain reliever*, or opiate analgesic] overdose deaths increased more than fivefold among women (a total of 47,935 OPR overdose deaths during that period).
>
> *(Mack, Jones, & Paulozzi, 2013, p. 2)*

---

[45] Naloxone (Narcan®) is a relatively inert drug that has *no* other action than to competitively bind to endogenous opiate analgesic receptor sites, and, subsequently, prevent the opiate analgesics from binding to the sites and eliciting their expected therapeutic and toxic effects. (Also, see previous related discussion in the earlier *Pharmacology* section, "Pharmacodynamics: Mechanism of Action.")

[46] N.B. It is *extremely* important to note that naloxone reverses, *solely*, the actions of the opiate analgesics. Naloxone does *not* reverse the actions of any other drugs and substances of abuse (or any other drugs) that may have been consumed as part of an overdosage. Other drugs and substances of abuse that may be involved in an overdosage *must* be appropriately individually identified and dealt with (e.g., by specific antidote; gastric lavage) as per established clinical protocols.

As noted by Nora Volkow, Director of the National Institute on Drug Abuse:

> We are seeing an increase in the number of people who are dying from overdoses, predominantly after abuse of prescribed opioid analgesics. This disturbing trend appears to be associated with a growing number of prescriptions in and diversion from the legal market.
>
> *(Volkow & McLellan, 2016, p. 8)*

Several others have reported similar findings. For example, as reported by Frieden and Houry (2016): "Death from prescription-opioid overdose has dramatically increased in the United States, quadrupling in the past 15 years" (p. 10). Of particular relevance to this text, and to the context of this discussion, is the reported finding that, "Women ages 45 to 54 have the highest risk of dying from a prescription painkiller overdose" (Centers for Disease Control and Prevention, 2013, p. 2).

Most heroin users are poly-drug and substance users. Thus, overdosages, as previously noted, also may be caused by the *synergistic* effects[47] of heroin and another psychodepressant (e.g., alcohol; benzodiazepine) or heroin and a psychostimulant (e.g., cocaine),[48] which may have been used concurrently by the same, or by a different, method of use (Jones, Paulozzi, & Mack, 2014; Pagliaro & Pagliaro, 2009; Sharp & Melnik, 2015; Sporer, 1999). This is *not* a new phenomenon. For example, consider the following obituary notice:

> Last week, on a day that superficially seemed to be less lonely than most, Janis Joplin [popular 1960s singer of such well-known classics as, "Piece of my Heart" and "Me & Bobby McGee"] died on the lowest and saddest of notes. Returning to her Hollywood motel room after a late-night recording session and some hard drinking with friends at a nearby bar, she apparently filled a hypodermic needle with heroin and shot it into her left arm. The injection killed her.
>
> *(Obituaries, 1970, p. 54)*

Over the last 30 years, increasingly pure supplies of heroin (i.e., higher relative concentrations of heroin in actual street samples) became generally available in North America. These supplies of heroin were associated with literally

---

47 Synergistic drug effects occur when two or more drugs, including the drugs and substances of abuse, work together to produce, either: (1) an *effect* that neither drug can produce on its own; or (2) an *effect size* that is significantly greater than the sum of the individual drug effects when added together. For example, fatal overdosages involving either alcohol, alone, or a benzodiazepine, alone, are relatively rare. However, when both alcohol and benzodiazepines are orally ingested together, overdosages are much more common—including fatal overdosages.

48 When injected intravenously, the combination of heroin and cocaine is commonly referred to on-the-street as a "speedball." (Also, see Chapter 5, *Women's Amphetamine and Cocaine Abuse*.)

TABLE 1.3 Common Body System Signs of Acute Opiate Analgesic Overdosage

Body system	*Common signs*
Cardiovascular System	Hypotension; shock
Central Nervous System	Stupor or coma. Seizures may occur with meperidine (Demerol®) or propoxyphene (Talwin®)[a]
Ophthalmic System	Generally, pupils are constricted (i.e., *miosis*), or may be dilated (i.e., *mydriasis*) with meperidine (Demerol®) and with an extreme lack of oxygen related to extreme hypoxia
GI System	Constipation
Reflex System	Diminished or absent reflexes (e.g., abdominal reflex; ankle jerk; quadriceps knee jerk; and radial brachialis)
Respiratory System	Decreased or absent respirations with cyanosis caused by *increased* concentrations of *reduced* hemoglobin in the blood resulting in a deficiency of oxygen and an excess of carbon dioxide
Thermoregulation System	Subnormal body temperature

[a] Convulsions also may occur when breathing is slowed, or ceases, because of hypoxemia.

thousands of deaths as noted earlier.[49] In many of these cases, the deaths were the result of users not making allowances for the increasingly pure supplies of heroin that they were obtaining (i.e., they failed to reduce their *usual dosages*). The signs and symptoms of acute opiate analgesic overdosage are listed in Table 1.3.

In addition, during the second decade of the new millennium, a significant *increase* in overdosage deaths was identified among intravenous heroin users in the U.S. However, chemical analyses conducted by both the CDC and DEA, determined that fentanyl, *and its analogs*, which were added to the street heroin, were the *most* frequent cause of the significant increase in overdosage deaths (Gladden, Martinez, & Seth, 2016; Peterson, Gladden, & Delcher, 2016).[50]

The *highest* increase in these fentanyl-related overdosage deaths occurred in eight "high burden" states—Florida, Kentucky, Maine, Maryland, Massachusetts, New Hampshire, North Carolina, and Ohio. For example, for women in the "high-burden" states, the percentage increase in fentanyl-related overdosage deaths from 2013 to 2014 was 104% versus 11% for women in "low-burden" states (Gladden, Martinez, & Seth, 2016). Overall, the number of fentanyl-related overdosage deaths in the U.S. *increased* significantly from approximately 3,000 deaths,

[49] N.B. Not only has the *number* of heroin-related overdosage deaths increased significantly among women in the U.S., but also the *rate* of heroin-related deaths. For an example, from 2010 to 2013, the rate of heroin overdosage deaths among women in the U.S. *tripled* (from 0.4 to 1.2 per 100,000) (ASAM, American Society of Addiction Medicine, 2016, p. 3).

[50] Generally, overdosage deaths are not identified separately (i.e., as distinct from heroin or opiate analgesic overdosages) in national statistical reports.

in 2010, to approximately 6,000 deaths, in 2014 (NIDA, 2015c, 2016b). (Also, see related discussion in the later section, "Fentanyl.")

Women's Medical and Personal Opiate Analgesic Use and Abuse

During the new millennium, in the U.S., women's opiate analgesic abuse involved the medical and personal abuse of:

1. *Illicitly* obtained prescription opiate analgesics (e.g., oxycodone [OxyContin®]; hydrocodone [Dicodid®]; buprenorphine [Buprenex®]; fentanyl [e.g., Fentora®])
2. *Illicitly produced and purchased* opiate analgesics (e.g., "street" heroin or other illicit, clandestinely produced, opiate analgesics)

Women's Medical Opiate Analgesic Use/Abuse

The opiate analgesics continue to be medically prescribed for basically the same indications that they were prescribed for during the 19th and 20th centuries: (1) treatment of severe, unproductive cough; (2) management of diarrhea; and (3) relief of moderate to severe pain.[51] Although capable of inducing sleep, the opiate analgesics are *not* generally used for this indication because of their high potential for physical and psychological dependence and the availability of safer and more effective sedative-hypnotics (see Chapter 3, *Women's Prescription Sedative-Hypnotic Abuse*).

> Americans, constituting only 4.6% of the world's population, have been consuming 80% of the global opioid supply, and 99% of the global hydrocodone supply.
>
> *(Manchikanti & Singh, 2008, p. 563)*

---

[51] The use of prescription opiate analgesics grew exponentially over the first 2 decades of the new millennium. As reported by Manchikanti (2007, p. 399):

> Opioid pill prescribing grew 533% from 1997 to 2005 with hydrocodone becoming the leading prescribed medication and oxycodone the top retailed opioid by weight in the United States.

While much of this growth was due to the medical management of *moderate to severe* cancer pain, much also was due to the largely inappropriate management of *chronic, nonmalignant* pain. "Baby Boomers," now in their 60s and 70s, have become "Zoomers" and are willing to press the therapeutic envelope, as are many of their healthcare providers, to manage pain without regard for long-term efficacy or the development of physical and psychological dependence (Backer & Fiellin, 2017; Pagliaro & Pagliaro, *Clinical Patient Data Files*; Pergolizzi, Boger, & Budd, 2008; Trescot, Helm, & Hansen, 2008).

Perhaps *not* surprisingly, the use and abuse of opiate analgesics by women in the U.S. has *never* been as common as it has been since the beginning of the new millennium (Jones, Logan, & Gladden, 2015). Volumes of published data, statistical reports, and authoritative claims are readily available to document this ever-growing and serious problem.

Generally, most women briefly use opiate analgesics as medically prescribed by their physicians for the management of a specific indication (e.g., pain) and do *not usually* develop harmful patterns of use. However, many women *abuse* their prescribed opiate analgesics by using them *more* frequently than prescribed, and in *larger* amounts than prescribed. These women usually go on to develop a pattern of *compulsive use*—a particularly harmful pattern of use. To maintain the compulsive use of their prescription opiate analgesics, they often resort to "double doctoring" and other *illicit* means to ensure a constant supply. For example, as identified by Maremmani (2010):

> Women are at higher risk of abusing opioids through a pathway of initial prescription painkiller use, and later to resort to street methadone to cope with prescription pain killer addiction.[52]
>
> *(p. 89)*

For example, in a large international study, Winstock (2016) found that prescription opiate analgesic abuse was *highest* in the U.S. He also reported a somewhat unexpected finding and related recommendation:

> Our study showed that less than 50% of patients in receipt of prescription opioids had ever been warned about the risks of addiction, so [as a request to his medical colleagues], please have that conversation upfront when you start prescribing. Informed patients are safer patients.
>
> *(p. 19)*

In 2016, in partial response to the continuing, and escalating, epidemic of prescription opiate analgesic abuse, the CDC released new guidelines for the prescription of opiate analgesics (Dowell, Haegerich, & Chou, 2016).

> Popular Notion: The *typical* opiate analgesic addict in the U.S. is a young man of European descent, with a criminal history, and often on welfare, or "living on the street."
>
> NOT TRUE.

---

[52] Among a large sample of incarcerated women, Proctor (2012) found that opiate analgesic dependence was especially common among U.S. women of either African continental descent or American Indian descent.

Women's Personal Opiate Analgesic Use/Abuse

Generally, during the new millennium, women across the lifespan illicitly abused opiate analgesics to achieve such desired psychodepressant actions as a: (1) feeling of extreme euphoria; (2) warm and pleasant feeling, or *rush*; or (3) sleepy, dream-like state (*being on-the-nod*). Many women also abused illicit opiate analgesics to, (4) prevent, or self-manage, the unpleasant effects associated with the opiate analgesic withdrawal syndrome (see the previous Pharmacology section in this chapter, *Undesired, or Harmful, Effects and Toxicities*: "Physical and Psychological Dependence," opiate analgesic withdrawal syndrome).

In addition, as identified by McHugh, Devito, and Dodd (2013), women, when compared to men, report *higher* licit and illicit use of the opiate analgesics "to cope with negative affect and pain" (p. 38). In this regard, drug and substance abuse, particularly prescription opiate analgesic abuse, has been widely documented as a *major* public health concern in the U.S., especially for *older* women (Blazer & Wu, 2009a, 2009b; Culberson & Ziska, 2008; Lofwall, Brooner, & Bigelow, 2005; Lofwall, Schuster, & Strain, 2008; Tsui, Herman, & Kettavong, 2010).

Other specific, significant differences between women and men, who abuse opiate analgesics, have been identified, including differences that may affect treatment selection and response. For example, Back, Payne, and Wahlquist (2011), in their sample of 892 adults screened for the *National Institute on Drug Abuse Clinical Trial Network*, found that women:

1. Tested significantly *more* positive for amphetamines, methamphetamine, and phencyclidine
2. Had significantly more current and past medical problems
3. Displayed significantly greater *craving* for opiate analgesics

As with several other drugs and substances of abuse (e.g., alcohol, see Chapter 2, *Women's Alcohol Abuse*), women demonstrate a "telescoping" effect regarding their use of the opiate analgesics. Although women begin to use opiate analgesics at about the same age as men, they experience an *accelerated* progression—from initial use to compulsive use—with associated *increasingly* harmful effects for self and family members. It is during this time that many women, usually after several *unsuccessful* attempts to achieve resumed nonuse of the opiate analgesics, seek professional assistance and treatment (Greenfield, Back, & Lawson, 2010; Hernandez-Avila, Rounsaville, & Kranzler, 2004; Pagliaro & Pagliaro, *Clinical Patient Data Files*). We now consider patterns of women's abuse of *heroin* and other *illicit* prescription drugs during the new millennium.

Heroin Abuse

A relatively *new* and unique phenomenon regarding women's heroin use, which has developed over the new millennium in the U.S., is the increasing *acceptance* of its use and abuse. In this context, women find themselves in a situation in which heroin: (1) is readily available; and (2) its use is *not* generally frowned upon (i.e., an increasing percentage of women during the new millennium, as indicated by U.S. usage statistics, consider the use of heroin—particularly *non-intravenous* methods of use—just as socially acceptable as the use of many other commonly available drugs and substances of abuse, such as alcoholic beverages, tobacco cigarettes, and marijuana). The *rapid* rise in heroin use and abuse among women has been largely due to the "unanticipated consequences" of government interventions[53] set in the context of a "perfect storm" (i.e., the convergence of several individual factors that, together, strongly encouraged and supported women's heroin use). As reported by the National Institute on Drug Abuse (2014, p. 1):

> For a few years, NIDA and other Federal partners have been sounding the alarm over the rise in heroin use, particularly among people with addictions to prescription opioids who switch to heroin because it is cheaper and easier to obtain. Half a million Americans are now addicted to heroin, and four out of five recent heroin initiates had previously used prescription opioids non-medically.

Similarly, and following the same line of reasoning, Case and Deaton (2015) noted:

> Tighter controls on opioid prescription brought some substitution into heroin and, in this period, the U.S. saw falling prices and rising quality of heroin, as well as availability in areas where heroin had been previously largely unknown.
>
> *(p. 15081)*

As shared by Mars, Bourgois, and Karandinos (2014), in their ethnographic study of transitions from "opioid pills to heroin injecting" in Philadelphia and San Francisco:

> From accounts of younger/recent heroin injectors in this study, it is evident that since the rise of the opioid pill epidemic, the barriers to heroin use and to injection have been reduced by the normalized pervasiveness of these pharmaceuticals. The widespread availability of opioid analgesics outside sanctioned channels and, paradoxically, medical and regulatory attempts to curb this through monitoring and limiting prescribing, appear to be

---

[53] Specifically, responding to an epidemic of opiate analgesic abuse, the FDA issued several rules, and Congress passed several laws, intended to limit the illicit production, and often inappropriate overprescription, of opiate analgesics, particularly oxycodone (OxyContin®). (See related discussion within this chapter.)

> drawing a new generation into higher risk heroin injecting. Unlike those substances previously labeled "gateway drugs," opioid pills seem to have a direct relationship with progression to heroin initiation.
>
> *(p. 264)*

Several characteristic behaviors have been identified that favor injectable heroin use among women. In this regard, women are *more* likely than men to:

- Have a current sexual partner who also injects heroin intravenously
- Have their heroin intravenously injected by their sexual partner(s)
- Have their first intravenous injection of heroin made by their sexual partner
- Be influenced to intravenously inject heroin by pressure exerted by their sexual partner(s)
- Inject their heroin, or other opiate analgesics, first thing in the morning

(Back, Lawson, & Singleton, 2011; Greenfield, Back, & Lawson, 2010; Pagliaro & Pagliaro, Clinical Patient Data Files; *Pagliaro, Pagliaro, & Thauberger, 1993)*

A decade into the new millennium, Holscher, Reissner, and Di Furia (2010) identified that there was *no* difference between women and men in the U.S. regarding the age of onset of regular, long-term heroin use. Attracted to the opiate analgesics when offered by a sexual partner, friends, or acquaintances, many women become *hooked* and continue to seek and use opiate analgesics in an effort to obtain their desired effects.

In addition, *pooling* data from the annual *National Survey on Drug Use and Health* (NSDUH) for 2002 through 2011, Muhuri, Gfroerer, and Davies (2013, p. 1) found that the:

> Heroin incidence rate was 19 times higher among those who reported prior nonmedical pain reliever use [i.e., prescription opiate analgesic use] than those who did not.

Heroin is often used in place of prescription opiate analgesics, particularly by women of European[54] descent residing in suburban and rural areas because it is "more readily accessible and much less expensive" (Cicero, Ellis, & Surratt, 2014a, p. 821).

[54] A noted exception are young women of Hispanic descent (Pagliaro & Pagliaro, *Clinical Patient Data Files*; Park & Bloch, 2016). As noted by Park and Bloch (2016):

> Heroin addiction has been "passed down from generation to generation in small cities around New Mexico" by "grandparents who have been heroin users for years, and it is passed down to younger generations; it's almost like a way of life."
>
> *(p. 7)*

It also is abused by mothers, often with associated undesired, or harmful, effects, and toxicities:

> Mom whose 5-month-old baby died from drinking formula laced with heroin gets up to eight-year prison term[55]
>
> *(Associated Press, 2016, p. 1)*

It has been commonly recognized by both government agencies and drug and substance abuse professionals, that during the *second* decade of the new millennium, "a growing heroin epidemic is impacting states across the U.S." (Whitman, 2015, p. 2). Rates of heroin addiction and overdosage have *increased* at particularly alarming rates in Indiana, Kentucky, and New Jersey.

Opium and heroin production is *higher* than ever (Table 1.4). Transshipped from Asia to Colombian sources to North America for distribution at specified geographical locations, heroin is readily available in both *higher* concentrations and purity in the U.S. than at any other previous time in history (Ciccarone, 2009).[56] Its distribution and commerce in the U.S. is largely controlled by ethnically defined criminal gangs.[57] The ready availability of this high-grade heroin, at relatively *low* prices, contributed to a significant *increase* in intranasal use (i.e., *snorting*), particularly among young adults living in suburban areas.

A *re-emerging* trend from the 1970s is the more casual, non-intravenous, non-daily, social use of heroin. During the 1970s, this pattern of use was often referred to as *chipping.* Rather than intravenously injecting, or "mainlining," the heroin, it is *subcutaneously* injected, in much the same way as insulin is injected by women with diabetes. However, women who are more *casual* heroin users are still *more* likely

---

55 Also, see related discussion in earlier section, *Undesired, or Harmful, Effects and Toxicities*, "Pregnancy, Breast-Feeding, and Mothering."

56 Currently, in the U.S., the average concentration of injectable forms of heroin at street level is approximately 10% to 27%—in comparison to approximately 7% during the 1980s. The purity of street-level Colombian heroin typically ranges from 25% to 80% pure, while Mexican black tar heroin typically ranges from 14% to 60% pure with the highest purity found in cities along the U.S.-Mexico border (e.g., El Paso, Texas) (Pagliaro & Pagliaro, 2012). Heroin purity, at street level, varies significantly in the U.S. from city to city and from time to time—depending upon availability and demand (Pagliaro & Pagliaro, *Clinical Patient Data Files*). For example, in 2008 heroin street-level purity in San Francisco was reported as 8.5% while in Philadelphia it was reported as 60% (Mars, Bourgois, & Karandinos, 2014).

57 For example: the importation and distribution of heroin in Seattle Washington is mostly controlled by Chinese gangs; a significant amount of the retail-level heroin distribution and sales along the northeastern coast is controlled by Dominican gangs, based primarily in New York City; most of the importation and distribution of heroin from Mexico into the Southwestern U.S. is controlled by Mexican gangs (e.g., *Sinaloan Cowboys*); much of the smuggling of heroin into the U.S. from southeastern Asia is by Nigerian gangs, based primarily in Chicago; and much of the distribution of Asian heroin that is transshipped through the Port of Los Angeles is controlled by Thai gangs (*Drug trafficking in the United States* (ND); National Drug Intelligence Center, 2001; Pagliaro & Pagliaro, 2009, 2012; Pagliaro & Pagliaro, *Clinical Patient Data Files*).

TABLE 1.4 Average Annual Opium Poppy Cultivation and Related Opium/Heroin Production Estimates by Country

Country	*Opium poppy cultivation (hectares)*[a]	*Opium/heroin production estimates (metric tons)*[b]	*Comments*
Afghanistan	157,000	7,700 opium 907 heroin	*Largest* producer of opium in the world. Major source of funding for the *Taliban*—and major source of income for Afghani farmers.[c,d]
Burma (Union of Myanmar)	28,500	410 opium	Most of the opium (i.e., 90%) is cultivated in the *Shan* state. Mainly trafficked to China.
Colombia	394	10 opium	Almost *all* of the opium is processed into heroin for the U.S. market. Major supplier of heroin to states that are *east* of the Mississippi River.
India	—	2,000 opium	World's *largest* producer of *licit* opium for use by pharmaceutical companies.
Laos	1,900	17 opium	—
Mexico	19,200	325 opium 18 (heroin) 50 (*black tar heroin*)	Major supplier of heroin to the U.S., particularly to states *west* of the Mississippi River.
Pakistan	2,300	48 opium	—
U.S.	0	0	World's *largest* consumer of both Colombian heroin and Mexican heroin.

Data sources: Afghanistan opium, 2008; Central Intelligence Agency, 2010; Office of National Drug Control Policy, 2010; Pagliaro & Pagliaro, 2009; UNODC, 2011.

[a] One hectare is equal to 10,000 square meters or 2.471 acres.

[b] One metric ton is equal to 1,000 kilograms or 2,205 pounds.

[c] The major source of both opium and heroin and the development of tens of thousands of new addicts during the first decade of this century has been largely related to the long-standing U.S. military involvement in Afghanistan. In 2000, the Taliban issued a religious edict making opium production contrary to their fundamentalist view of Islam. With strict penalties, including beheading for growing poppies or producing, selling, or using opium, the opium market was decimated (Afghanistan, Opium … 2001), falling to under 200 metric tons. However, following the October 2001 invasion of Afghanistan by U.S. and British troops, it rapidly recovered and rebounded to an all-time high (Glaze, 2007; Rebuilding Afghanistan, 2005; UNODC, 2002). By 2009, Afghanistan was, by far, the *largest* producer of opium in the world. As noted at a press conference by Mylven Levitsky, a member of the International Narcotics Control Board (INCB), "Afghanistan is the source of over 90% of the illicit opium in the world" (Rizvi, 2009, p. 1).

[d] It should be noted that we have long (i.e., for over 2 decades) advocated that the hundreds of hectares of opium that is cultivated in areas in which it is easily visible (even from a plane with the naked eye when in blossom) should be completely eradicated on an annual basis by appropriate chemicals such as defoliants (i.e., "weed killers"), which can readily, and effectively destroy them. This effort would result in a significant *increase* in the "street" cost of heroin and, consequently, significantly decrease "street" availability and use. Unfortunately, although relatively easy to accomplish and at a very modest financial cost, the Government of Afghanistan, as well as their western allies (including the U.S.), have been totally unwilling to take this action because of resultant antagonism of the tribes that cultivate and make most of their money through opium sales.

to *Chase the Dragon* (i.e., smoke their heroin). They also intranasally insufflate, or *snort*, their heroin (Katz, Dart, & Bailey, 2011; Pagliaro & Pagliaro, 2009, 2012; Stern, 2011). Women, during the new millennium, may also use transmucosal opiate analgesic nasal sprays, or what is known on the street as, "heroin nose drops." Consequently, only approximately 40% of new millennium women intravenously inject their heroin. As noted by Stanos, Bruckenthal, and Barkin (2012, p. 683):

> A study of prescription opioid abusers in a drug rehabilitation program found that 80% tampered with opioid tablets to accelerate drug release by chewing or administering the drug intranasally or intravenously.

During the new millennium, particularly troubling is the noted change in the attitudes of women toward the use of opiate analgesics—including heroin and its *non-oral* routes of administration—for which there is apparent increasingly tacit acceptance that now ranks with "snorting a line of coke" or "smoking a joint" (Pagliaro & Pagliaro, *Clinical Patient Data Files*).

As noted by the Substance Abuse and Mental Health Services Administration (SAMHSA, 2009), based on national data:

> Nearly 2 million individuals in the U.S. have opioid abuse or dependence, with the majority reporting abuse of prescription opioids.
>
> *(p. 1)*

Illicit Prescription Opiate Analgesic Abuse

For women, illicit prescription opiate analgesic use and abuse has *soared* during the new millennium (Brady, McCauley, & Back, 2016; Pagliaro & Pagliaro, 2009; Pagliaro & Pagliaro, *Clinical Patient Data Files*). For example, Green, Grimes Serrano, and Licari (2009, p. 65), in a study of almost 30,000 assessments of participants entering 202 drug abuse treatment centers in the U.S. between 2005 and 2008, found that:

1. Women were *more* likely than men to report the *use* of any prescription opiate analgesic (i.e., 32.1% versus 29.8%)
2. Women were *more* likely than men to report *abuse* of any prescription opiate analgesic (i.e., 15.4% versus 11.1%).

As further supported by Greenfield, Back, and Lawson (2010), "Two large epidemiological surveys found that women engage in the nonmedical use of prescription opioids more often than men" (p. 339).

This significant increase has been noted among *every* demographic of women in the U.S. Factors that have been related to the prescription, and subsequent abuse, of opiate analgesics by women include:

- Chronic, noncancer pain, including arthritis and back pain
- Concurrent affective disorders (e.g., depression) (See related discussion in Chapter 7, *Identifying Women's Contemporaneous Diagnoses*)
- Current, acute moderate to severe pain
- History of alcohol abuse
- Inability to fall and/or stay asleep
- Increased severity of pain

(Barth, Moran-Santa Maria, & Lawson, 2013; Brady, McCauley, & Back, 2016; Jamison, Ross, & Michna, 2010; Tsui, Herman, & Kettavong, 2010)

The U.S. Department of Health and Human Services (SAMHSA, 2014) reported that, for every age cohort of adults examined at admission for treatment of prescription opiate analgesic abuse, the percentage of women was significantly *higher* than the percentage of men. As noted by the SAMHSA (2014):

> Within the 65 or older age group, the proportion of female admissions reporting primary abuse of prescription pain relievers was nearly 3 times that of their male counterparts (7.2 verses 2.8 percent).
>
> *(p. 5)*

Double-Doctoring, or Physician Shopping

In the U.S., women, particularly those who have several identified characteristics (see *specific variables or correlates* on the following page), are significantly *more* likely to engage in the practice of "double-doctoring," or "physician shopping." This practice is commonly used by women to obtain multiple opiate analgesic prescriptions from several prescribers for the same medical condition (e.g., back pain, *real* or *feigned*). In a comprehensive study of data obtained from over 146 million opioid prescriptions dispensed by 76% of U.S. retail pharmacies, during 2008, McDonald and Carlson (2013) found that "doctor shoppers":

- Comprised approximately 1% of all prescription purchases
- On average, obtained 32 prescriptions for opiate analgesics
- On average, filled their prescriptions for opiate analgesics at 10 different pharmacies
- Bought approximately 2% of all opiate analgesic prescriptions (4% of "weighed amounts")
- Often paid for their prescriptions in cash to avoid detection

In addition to "double doctoring" or "doctor shopping," women, who obtain medical prescriptions for chronic pain relief, are significantly *more* likely than men to *hoard* their unused opiate analgesics (i.e., from previous prescriptions for themselves or family members) (Back, Payne, & Waldrop, 2009).

Specific variables or correlates, reportedly associated with women's abuse of the prescription opiate analgesics include the following correlates, identified by Green, Grimes Serrano, and Licari (2009):

- *Younger* than 54 years-of-age
- *Active* alcohol use disorder
- History of drug overdosage
- Residence in a non-western state

Interestingly, in a later study, Cicero, Surratt, and Kurtz (2012) identified a few other correlates:

- *Older* than 45 years-of-age
- Chronic, severe (debilitating) pain[58]
- Contemporaneous diagnoses[59]

Specific Prescription Opiate Analgesics Most Abused by Women

The *four* prescription opiate analgesics that are *most* abused by new millennial women in the U.S. are: (1) oxycodone; (2) hydrocodone; (3) buprenorphine; and (4) fentanyl. Oxycodone (OxyContin®) and hydrocodone (Dicodid®; Hycodan®) are the *most* widely abused prescription opiate analgesics in the U.S. (Cicero, Inciardi, & Munoz, 2005). Illicitly used primarily to achieve euphoric effects, or a "rush," and to prevent or manage the opiate analgesic withdrawal syndrome, their use, abuse, and associated toxicities *skyrocketed* during the 1990s and has remained high ever since. It has been estimated that 99% of the world's production of oxycodone and hydrocodone during the new millennium has been consumed in the U.S. (Winstock, 2016).

Oxycodone. OxyContin®, the extended-release formulation of oxycodone, was approved by the FDA in 1995. Generally considered to have a *lower* abuse potential because of its slow-release properties, its widespread abuse began in 2000 and continued throughout the first decade of the new millennium as users learned

58 Several studies and reports have noted that: (1) the most common sources of chronic, recurrent pain among people in the U.S. are lower back pain, approximately 38 million Americans; and osteoarthritis, approximately 17 million Americans; (2) the prevalence of chronic, recurrent pain is significantly higher among women (34.3%) than men (26.7%); and (3) the prevalence of chronic, recurrent pain *increases* with increasing age (Johannes, Le, & Zhou, 2010, p. 1230; Volkow, 2014, p. 2).

59 In addition, as noted by Shei, Rice, and Kirson (2015), in their study of 9,291 adults with a diagnosis of opiate analgesic abuse in the U.S, those with the *highest* healthcare costs (i.e., on average, 8 times higher) were women with contemporaneous diagnoses. As we have previously noted, this group of women also is much harder to effectively treat. (See Chapter 7, *Identifying Women's Contemporaneous Diagnoses*, for additional details and related discussion.)

that crushing and "snorting" the extended-release tablets enabled them to achieve a *rapid* release of the OxyContin® and *high* blood OxyContin® levels (Aquina, Marques-Baptista, & Bridgeman, 2009; Cicero, Inciardi, & Munoz, 2005; Pagliaro & Pagliaro, 2009). In 2010, the *most* potent strength tablet of OxyContin® (i.e., 160 mg) was discontinued and a new formulation was introduced that made crushing and dissolving the extended-release tablets more difficult (MacLaren, 2015). These changes resulted in only *moderate* success in terms of decreasing or eliminating OxyContin® abuse and in little to no success in terms of decreasing opiate analgesic abuse, overall. As noted by Cicero and Surratt (2012):

> Although 24% found a way to defeat the tamper-resistant properties of the abuse-deterrent formulation, 66% indicated a switch to another opioid, with "heroin" the most common response. These changes appear to be causally linked, as typified by one response: "Most people that I know don't use OxyContin to get high anymore. They have moved on to heroin [because] it is easier to use, much cheaper, and easily available."
>
> *(p. 189)*

Oxycodone abuse is *highest* in rural and suburban regions of the Western U.S. (Cicero, Surratt, & Inciardi, 2007) with most abusers being middle-aged men of European descent (Jones, Vosburg, & Manubay, 2011). However, a significant number of oxycodone abusers are women (Pagliaro & Pagliaro, *Clinical Patient Data Files*). Carise, Dugosh, and McLellan (2007), in their analysis of approximately 28,000 participants admitted to 157 addiction treatment programs in the U.S. from 2001 to 2004, found that approximately 5% used OxyContin® which was predominantly obtained from nonmedical sources. In comparing past-year Oxy-Contin® users to past-year other opiate analgesic users, Martins, Storr, and Zhu (2009) found that OxyContin® users were more likely to be 18 to 25 years-of-age and to have a concurrent mental health problem.

Hydrocodone. In the U.S., women of European descent, 20 years-of-age to 40 years-of-age, are the *most* common abusers of hydrocodone (Pagliaro & Pagliaro, 2009). As reported by Cicero, Ellis, and Surratt (2013, p. 2639), "hydrocodone users were generally risk-aversive women, elderly people, noninjectors, and those who prefer safer modes of acquisition than dealers (i.e., doctors, friends, or family members)."

Between 2014 and 2015, the FDA approved two extended-release formulations of hydrocodone, Hysingla ER® and Zohydro ER®, for the medical management of chronic, severe pain (Extended-Release, 2014, 2015). To address the potential risk for the abuse of these products, they were formulated with several abuse-deterrent properties. For example, whether the tablets were coarsely or finely ground, the resultant powder was formulated to fall out of the nostrils when intranasally administered, or snorted. In addition, when attempts are made to dissolve the tablets for intravenous injection, a viscous gel is formed that is difficult to inject. In addition, as part of a *Risk Evaluation and Mitigation Strategy* (REMS) program, the FDA mandated that pharmaceutical manufacturers make training programs for the optimal use of these formulations available to prescribers.

Buprenorphine. Buprenorphine (Buprenex®) is a synthetic opiate analgesic that was synthesized in the late 1970s for the medical management of *moderate to severe* pain. It binds primarily as an agonist with *high* affinity to *mu* receptors and dissociates slowly from the *mu* receptors. Consequently, buprenorphine produces expected opiate analgesic agonist effects, particularly at *low* to *moderate* dosages. However, at *higher* dosages it can reach a ceiling effect and, subsequently, work as an opiate analgesic antagonist (Buprenorphine, 2016).

Buprenorphine also binds as an antagonist at *kappa* receptors. Because of its *mixed* agonist/antagonist actions, it is medically used for the management of *acute* opiate analgesic detoxification, stabilization, and long-term maintenance of resumed *non-use* of opiate analgesics (Connery, 2015; Greenwald, Comer, & Fiellin, 2014; Hard, 2014; Soyka, 2015) (see *earlier* related discussion). (Also see related discussion in Chapter 8, *Preventing and Treating Women's Drug and Substance Abuse.*) Naloxone (also, see related discussion in the earlier section, *Undesired or Harmful Effects and Toxicities*, "Overdosage") is generally combined with a sublingual dosage form of buprenorphine (i.e., Suboxone®, sublingual film; Zubsolv®, sublingual tablet) to *minimize* the risk for diversion and abuse of buprenorphine (Smith, Bailey, & Woody, 2007).

Combination buprenorphine and naloxone continues to be diverted and illicitly used in the U.S. primarily to self-manage the signs and symptoms of the opiate analgesic withdrawal syndrome (Lofwall & Walsh, 2014; Schuman-Olivier, Albanese, & Nelson, 2010; Yokell, Zaller, & Green, 2011). Reportedly, buprenorphine abusers are more likely to be intravenous drug users while those who use the buprenorphine/naloxone combination product to get "high" are *non-injection* drug users (Bazazi, Yokell, & Fu, 2011).

Among buprenorphine abusers who seek drug and substance abuse treatment in the U.S., 6% reported injecting buprenorphine "to get high" (Cicero, Surratt, & Inciardi, 2007). Going further, Dart (2011) found that 45.5% of intravenous buprenorphine users and 16.3% of combination buprenorphine/naloxone users reported use within the previous month. The abuse of buprenorphine, particularly, combination buprenorphine/naloxone, is significantly limited in the U.S., by the ready availability of *high*-quality heroin "on the streets." Women, who do abuse buprenorphine, tend to be younger and of European descent (Pagliaro & Pagliaro, *Clinical Patient Data Files*). In addition, Cicero, Ellis, and Surratt (2014b) found that:

> Buprenorphine is rarely preferred for its inherent euphorigenic properties, but rather serves as a substitute for other drugs, particularly heroin, or as a drug used, preferable to methadone, to self-medicate withdrawal sickness or wean off opioids.
>
> *(p. 98)*

Fentanyl. Fentanyl is an *extremely* potent prescription opiate analgesic that is 50 to 100 times *more* potent than morphine (see Table 1.2). It is currently approved by the FDA for the management of surgical/postoperative pain, severe pain, and breakthrough cancer pain. Fentanyl is manufactured by several pharmaceutical companies and is available in many dosage formulations for medical use in the U.S., including:[60]

- Effervescent buccal tablet (Fentora®)
- Injectable formulation for IM or IV use (Sublimaze®)
- Nasal spray (Lazanda®)
- Transdermal delivery system (Duragesic®), as well as a newer *iontophoretic* transdermal system (Ionsys®)
- Transmucosal "lozenge on a stick" (Actiq® "lollipop")

Fentanyl, because of its potency and variety of available formulations, has been widely abused in the U.S. It also is often added to heroin to increase the potency and "kick" of heroin—and is misrepresented and sold as alprazolam, hydrocodone, oxycodone, and other drugs and substances of abuse. As noted by the NIDA, "The fake pills are much cheaper than the real versions" (NIDA, 2016a, p. 1). More importantly, because buyers are generally unaware of what they are purchasing, "hundreds of people have overdosed on fentanyl across the nation since 2013, often because of using heroin that has been laced with the much stronger substance" (National Institute on Drug Abuse, 2016b, p. 1).

References[61,62,63]

A naloxone. (2014, June 9). A naloxone auto-injector (Evzio). *The Medical Letter*, 56(1444), 45–46.

[60] The major source of illicit fentanyl, which is used by street addicts in the U.S.—usually unknowingly as an "additive" to street heroin (see earlier related discussion)—is produced in chemical laboratories in Mexico (Gladden, Martinez, & Seth, 2016; Peterson, Gladden, & Delcher, 2016). In addition, China has increasingly become a major fentanyl producer and exporter nation. A large amount of the fentanyl, which is illicitly produced in China, is smuggled into the U.S. from both Canada and Mexico (Pagliaro & Pagliaro, *Clinical Patient Data Files*).

[61] As per publisher style, only the first three authors are listed for each reference.

[62] Several times the number of references listed were found, obtained, and analyzed by the authors during the preparation of this chapter. However, only the references that were cited at least once in the body of the text are included in the list. Major reasons for *not* citing other references, include that they: (1) did *not* provide any additional unique data; (2) were *not* well researched or written (i.e., were evaluated as *not* being valid or reliable); (3) were based predominantly, or exclusively, on animal studies; (4) provided usage statistics from outside the U.S.; and/or (5) were redundant with, or *not* as recent as, the already cited references.

[63] The reference citation, "Pagliaro & Pagliaro, *Clinical Patient Data Files*," refers to unpublished data collected, with permission, over the last 50 years by the authors, in the formal course of their professional academic roles as clinician scientists and professors, from their patients, research subjects, and students, from the 1970s to date.

Afghanistan opium survey 2008: Executive summary. (2008, August). 1–32. United Nations, Office on Drugs and Crime.

Afghanistan, opium and the Taliban. (2001, February 15). Retrieved from Opioids.com, pp. 1–5: http://opioids.com/afghanistan/index.html

Ahlen, G., & Frelin, L. (2016). Methods to evaluate novel hepatitis C virus vaccines. *Methods in Molecular Biology*, 1403, 221–244. doi: 10.1007/978-1-4939-3387-7_11

Ailes, E. C., Dawson, A. L., & Lind, J. N. (2015). Opioid prescription claims among women of reproductive age—United States, 2008–2012. *MMWR, Morbidity & Mortality Weekly Report*, 64, 37–41. Retrieved from www.ncbi.nlm.nih.gov/pubmed/25611168

Alexander, D., Alexander, K., & Valentino, J. (2012). Intranasal hydrocodone-acetaminophen abuse induced necrosis of the nasal cavity and pharynx. *Laryngoscope*, 122(11), 2378–2381. doi:10.1002/lary.23542

Anantharamu, T., Sharma, S., & Gupta, A. K. (2015). Naloxegol: First oral peripherally acting mu opioid receptor antagonists for opioid-induced constipation. *Journal of Pharmacology and Pharmacotherapeutics*, 6(3), 188–192. doi:10.4103/0976-500X.162015

Annett, H. E. (1920). Factors influencing alkaloidal content and yield of latex in the opium poppy (Papaver somniferum). *Biochemical Journal*, 14(5), 618–636.

Aquina, C. T., Marques-Baptista, A., & Bridgeman, P. (2009). OxyContin abuse and overdose. *Postgraduate Medicine*, 121(2), 163–167. doi:10.3810/pgm.2009.03.1988

ASAM, American Society of Addiction Medicine. (2016). *New release: Opioid addiction 2016 facts and figures*. American Society of Addiction Medicine.

Associated Press. (2016, September 8). Mom whose baby drank formula laced with heroin gets prison. *Fox News*. Plymouth, MA: Fox News.

Back, S. E., Lawson, K. M., & Singleton, L. M. (2011). Characteristics and correlates of men and women with prescription opioid dependence. *Addictive Behaviors*, 36(8), 829–834. doi:10.1016/j.addbeh.2011.03.013

Back, S. E., Payne, R. L., & Wahlquist, A. H. (2011). Comparative profiles of men and women with opioid dependence: Results from a national multisite effectiveness trial. *The American Journal of Drug and Alcohol Abuse*, 37(5), 313–323. doi:10.3109/00952990.2011.596982

Back, S. E., Payne, R., & Waldrop, A. E. (2009). Prescription opioid aberrant behaviors: A pilot study of gender differences. *The Clinical Journal of Pain*, 25, 477–484.

Bangsberg, D. R., Rosen, J. I., & Aragon, T. (2002). Clostridial myonecrosis cluster among injection drug users: A molecular epidemiology investigation. *Archives of Internal Medicine*, 162(5), 517–522.

Barth, K. S., Moran-Santa Maria, M., & Lawson, K. (2013). Pain and motives for use among non-treatment seeking individuals with prescription opioid dependence. *The American Journal on Addictions*, 22(5), 486–491. doi:10.1111/j.1521-0391.2013.12038.x

Bateman, B. T., Hernandez-Diaz, S., & Rathmell, J. P. (2014). Patterns of opioid utilization in pregnancy in a large cohort of commercial insurance beneficiaries in the United States. *Anesthesiology*, 120(5), 1216–1224. doi:10.1097/ALN.0000000000000172

Bazazi, A. R., Yokell, M., & Fu, J. (2011). Illicit use of buprenorphine/naloxone among injecting and non-injecting opioid users. *Journal of Addiction Medicine*, 5, 175–180.

Blazer, D. G., & Wu, L. T. (2009a). Nonprescription use of pain relievers by middle-aged and elderly community-living adults: National Survey on Drug Use and Health. *Journal of the American Geriatrics Society*, 57, 1252–1257.

Blazer, D. G., & Wu, L. T. (2009b). The epidemiology of substance use and disorders among middle-aged and elderly community adults: National survey on drug use and health. *American Journal of Geriatric Psychiatry*, 17, 237–245.

Brady, K. T., McCauley, J. L., & Back, S. E. (2016). Prescription opioid misuse, abuse, and treatment in the United States: An update. *The American Journal of Psychiatry*, 173(1), 18–26. doi:10.1176/appi.ajp.2015.15020262

Brogly, S. B., Saia, K. A., & Walley, A. Y. (2014). Prenatal buprenorphine versus methadone exposure and neonatal outcomes: Systemic review and meta-analysis. *American Journal of Epidemiology*, 180(7), 673–686. doi:10.1093/aje/kwu190

Brown, E. (2011, November 1). *Prescription painkillers outpace heroin, cocaine in OD deaths.* Retrieved from Los Angeles Times, pp. 1–2: http://articles.latimes.com/2011/nov01/news/la-heb-prescription-drug-overdose-deaths-20111101

Brown, M. S., Hayes, M. J., & Thornton, L. M. (2015). Methadone versus morphine for treatment of neonatal abstinence syndrome: A prospective randomized clinical trial. *Journal of Perinatology*, 35(4), 278–283. doi:10.1038/jp.2014.194

Buprenorphine buccal film (Belbuca) for chronic pain. (2016). *The Medical Letter*, 58(1492), 47–48.

Carise, D., Dugosh, K. L., & McLellan, A. T. (2007). Prescription OxyContin abuse among patients entering addiction treatment. *American Journal of Psychiatry*, 164(11), 1750–1756.

Carroll Chapman, S. L., & Wu, L.-T. (2014, March 1). Suicide and substance use among female veterans: A need for research. *Drug and Alcohol Dependence*, 136, 1–10. doi:10.1016/j.drugalcdep.2013.11.009

Case, A., & Deaton, A. (2015, December 8). Rising morbidity and mortality in midlife among White non-Hispanic Americans in the 21st century. *Proceedings of the National Academy of Science*, 112(49), 15078–15083. Retrieved from www.pnas.org/cgi/doi/10.1073/pnas.1518393112

Centers for Disease Control and Prevention. (2013, July 2). Prescription painkiller overdoses. *CDC Vitalsigns*, 1–4.

Central Intelligence Agency. (2010, January 3). *The world factbook*. Retrieved from Central Intelligence Agency, pp. 1–17: www.cia.gov/library/publications/the-world-factbook/

Ciccarone, D. (2009). Heroin in brown, black and white: Structural factors and medical consequences in the US heroin market. *International Journal of Drug Policy*, 20(3), 277–282.

Ciccarone, D., & Bourgois, P. (2003). Explaining the geographical variation of HIV among injection drug users in the United States. *Drug and Substance Misuse*, 38(14), 2049–2063.

Cicero, T. J., Ellis, M. S., & Surratt, H. L. (2012). Effect of abuse-deterrent formulation of OxyContin®. *The New England Journal of Medicine*, 367(2), 187–189.

Cicero, T. J., Ellis, M. S., & Surratt, H. L. (2013). Factors influencing the selection of hydrocodone and oxycodone as primary opioids in substance abusers seeking treatment in the United States. *Pain*, 154(12), 2639–2648. doi:10.1016/j.pain.2013.07.025

Cicero, T. J., Ellis, M. S., & Surratt, H. L. (2014a). The changing face of heroin use in the United States: A retrospective analysis of the past 50 years. *JAMA Psychiatry*, 71(7), 821–826. doi:10.1001/jamapsychiatry.2014.366

Cicero, T. J., Ellis, M. S., & Surratt, H. L. (2014b, September 1). Factors contributing to the rise of buprenorphine misuse: 2008–2013. *Drug and Alcohol Dependence*, 142, 98–104. doi:10.1016/j.drugalcdep.2014.06.005

Cicero, T. J., Inciardi, J. A., & Munoz, A. (2005). Trends in abuse of oxycontin and other opioid analgesics in the United States: 2002–2004. *The Journal of Pain*, 662–672.

Cicero, T. J., Surratt, H. L., & Inciardi, J. (2007). Use and misuse of buprenorphine in the management of opioid addiction. *Journal of Opioid Management*, 3, 302–308.

Cicero, T. J., Surratt, H. L., & Kurtz, S. (2012). Patterns of prescription opioid abuse and comorbidity in an aging treatment population. *Journal of Substance Abuse Treatment*, 42(1), 87–94. doi:10.1016/j.jsat.2011.07.003

Clarification: Half-life of heroin. (2016). *The Medical Letter*, 58(1489), 32.

Cody, J. T., Valtier, S., & Kuhlman, J. (2001). Analysis of morphine and codeine in samples adulterated with Stealth. *Journal of Analytical Toxicology*, 25(7), 572–575.

Colliver, J. D., Compton, W. M., & Gfroerer, J. C. (2006). Projecting drug use among aging baby boomers in 2020. *Annals of Epidemiology*, 16, 257–265.

Connery, H. S. (2015). Medication-assisted treatment of opioid use disorder: Review of the evidence and future directions. *Harvard Review of Psychiatry*, 23(2), 63–75. doi:10.1097/HRP.0000000000000075

Corsetti, M., & Tack, J. (2015). Naloxegol: The first orally administered, peripherally acting, mu opioid receptor antagonist, approved for the treatment of opioid-induced constipation. *Drugs of Today (Barcelona)*, 51(8), 474–489. doi:10.1358/dot.2015.51.8.2364896

Cotten, S. W. (2012). Drug testing in the neonate. *Clinics in Laboratory Medicine*, 32, 449–466.

Culberson, J. W., & Ziska, M. (2008). Prescription drug misuse/abuse in the elderly. *Geriatrics*, 63(9), 22–31.

Daniulaityte, R., Carlson, R., & Falck, R. (2013). "I just wanted to tell you that loperamide WILL WORK": A web-based study of extra-medical use of loperamide. *Drug and Alcohol Dependence*, 130(1–3), 241–244. doi:10.1016/j.drugalcdep.2012.11.003

Dart, R. C. (2011). 5th Annual Scientific Meeting Presentation. Evaluation of ADFs using RADARS system data. Retrieved from www.radars.org/Home2/Annual Meeting/RADARSSystem2011AnnualMeeting.aspx

Dasgupta, A. (2015, February 1). *How people try to beat drug testing—Issues with urinary adulterants and their detection.* Retrieved from Clinical Laboratory News, pp. 1–4: www.aacc.org/publications/cln/articles/2015/february/drug-testing.aspx

Davies, H., Gilbert, R., & Johnson, K. (2016). Neonatal drug withdrawal syndrome: Cross-country comparison using hospital administrative data in England, the USA, Western Australia and Ontario, Canada. *Archives of Disease in Childhood. Fetal and Neonatal Edition*, 101(1), F26–F30. doi:10.1136/archdischild-2015–308948

Desai, R. J., Huybrechts, K. F., & Hernandez-Diaz, S. (2015). Exposure to prescription opioid analgesics in utero and risk of neonatal abstinence syndrome: Population based cohort study. *BMJ, British Medical Journal*, h2102. doi:10.1136/bmj.h2102

Dierksen, J., Gonsoulin, M., & Walterscheid, J. P. (2015). Poor man's methadone: A case report of loperamide toxicity. *The American Journal of Forensic Medicine and Pathology*, 36(4), 268–270. doi:10.1097/PAF.0000000000000201

Dietrich, E., & Gums, J. G. (2012). Intranasal fentanyl spray: A novel dosage form for the treatment of breakthrough cancer pain. *Annals of Pharmacotherapy*, 46(10), 1382–1391. doi:10.1345/aph.1R069

Dowell, D., Haegerich, T. M., & Chou, R. (2016, March 18). CDC guideline for prescribing opioids for chronic pain—United States, 2016. *MMWR, Morbidity and Mortality Recommendations and Reports*, 65(1), 1–49. doi:10.15585/mmwr.rr6501e1

Drug Trafficking in the United States. (ND). Retrieved from usdoj.gov: www.usdoj.gov/dea/pubs/intel/01020/index.html

Eichel, M. M., & Johannemann, T. R. (2014). Implementation of universal maternal drug screening to identify neonatal abstinence syndrome candidates. *Newborn and Infant Nursing Reviews*, 14, 17–22.

Ersche, K. D., Clark, L., & London, M. (2006). Profile of executive and memory function associated with amphetamine and opiate dependence. *Neuropsychopharmacology*, 31(5), 1036–1047. doi:10.1038/sj.npp.1300889

Extended-Release hydrocodone (Hysingla ER) for pain. (2015). *The Medical Letter*, 57(1468), 71–72.

Extended-Release hydrocodone (Zohydro ER) for pain. (2014). *The Medical Letter*, 56(1444), 45–46.

Finnegan, L. P., Connaughton, J. F., & Kron, R. E. (1975). Neonatal abstinence syndrome: Assessment and management. *Addictive Diseases*, 2, 141–158.

Frieden, T. R., & Houry, D. (2016, March 15). Reducing the risks of relief—The CDC Opioid-Prescribing Guideline. *The New England Journal of Medicine*, 374(16), 1501–1504. doi: 10.1056/NEJMp1515917

Gaalema, D. E., Heil, S. H., & Badger, G. J. (2013, November 1). Time to initiation of treatment for neonatal abstinence syndrome in neonates exposed in utero to buprenorphine or methadone. *Drug and Alcohol Dependence*, 133(1), 266–269. doi:10.1016/jdrugalcdep.2013.06.004

Gallagher, B. K., Shin, Y., & Roohan, P. (2016, April 29). Opioid prescriptions among women of reproductive age enrolled in Medicaid—New York, 2008–2013. *MMWR, Morbidity and Mortality Weekly Report*, 65(16), 415–417. doi:10.15585/mmwr.mm6516a2

Garnock-Jones, K. P. (2015). Naloxegol: A review of its use in patients with opioid-induced constipation. *Drugs*, 75(4), 419–425. doi:10.1007/s40265-015-0357-2

Gharagozlou, P., Demirci, H., & Clark, J. D. (2002). Activation profiles of opioid ligands in HEK cells expressing delta opioid receptors. *BMC Neuroscience*, 3(1), 19.

Girion, L., Glover, S., & Smith, D. (2011, September 17). *Drug deaths now outnumber traffic fatalities in U.S., data show.* Retrieved from Los Angeles Times, pp. 1–3: http://articles.latimes.com/2011/sep/17/local/la-me-drugs-epidemic-20110918

Gladden, R. M., Martinez, P., & Seth, P. (2016, August 26). Fentanyl law enforcement submissions and increases in synthetic opioid-involved overdose deaths—27 states, 2013–2014. *MMWR, Morbidity and Mortality Weekly Report*, 65(33), 837–843.

Glaze, J. A. (2007, October). *Opium and Afghanistan: Reassessing U.S. counternarcotics strategy.* Retrieved from Strategic Studies Institute, U.S. Army War College: www.strategicstudiesinstitute.army.mil/pdffiles/pub804.pdf.

Gossop, M., & Moos, R. (2008). Substance misuse among older adults: A neglected but treatable problem. *Addiction*, 103, 347–348.

Grassin-Delyle, S., Buenestado, A., & Naline, E. (2012). Intranasal drug delivery: An efficient and non-invasive route for systemic administration: Focus on opioids. *Pharmacology & Therapeutics*, 134(3), 366–379. doi:10.1016/j.pharmthera.2012.03.003

Green, M., & Suffet, F. (1981). The Neonatal Narcotic Withdrawal Index: A device for the improvement of care in the abstinence syndrome. *The American Journal of Drug and Alcohol Abuse*, 8, 203–213.

Green, T. C., Grimes Serrano, J. M., & Licari, A. (2009). Women who abuse prescription opioids: Findings from the Addiction Severity Index-Multimedia Version Connect Prescription Opioid database. *Drug and Alcohol Dependence*, 103(1–2), 65–73. doi:10.1016/j.drugalcdep.2009.03.014

Greenfield, S. F., Back, S. E., & Lawson, K. (2010). Substance abuse in women. *Psychiatric Clinics of North America*, 33(2), 339–355. doi:10.1016/j.psc.2010.01.004

Greenwald, M. K., Comer, S. D., & Fiellin, D. A. (2014, November 1). Buprenorphine maintenance and mu-opioid receptor availability in the treatment of opioid use disorder: Implications for clinical use and policy. *Drug and Alcohol Dependence*, 144, 1–11. doi:10.1016/j.drugalcdep.2014.07.035

Hamilton, R. J., Olmedo, R. E., & Shah, S. (2002). Complications of ultrarapid opioid detoxification with subcutaneous naltrexone pellets. *Academic Emergency Medicine*, 9(1), 63–68.

Han, B., Gfroerer, J. C., & Colliver, J. D. (2009a). *An examination of trends in illicit drug use among adults aged 50 to 59 in the United States.* Rockville, MD: Substance Abuse and Mental Health Services Administration, Office of Applied Studies.

Han, B., Gfroerer, J. C., & Colliver, J. D. (2009b). Substance use disorder among older adults in the United States in 2020. *Addiction*, 104(1), 88–96.

Hard, B. (2014, November 28). Management of opioid painkiller dependence in primary care: Ongoing recovery with buprenorphine/naloxone. *BMJ Case Reports,* 207308. doi:10.1136/bcr-2014–207308

Heil, S. H., Jones, H. E., & Arria, A. (2011). Unintended pregnancy in opioid-abusing women. *Journal of Substance Abuse Treatment*, 40(2), 199–202.

Hernandez-Avila, C. A., Rounsaville, B. J., & Kranzler, H. R. (2004). Opioid-, cannabis- and alcohol-dependent women show more rapid progression to substance abuse treatment. *Drug and Alcohol Dependence*, 74(3), 265–272.

Hiltunen, A. J., & Eklund, C. (2002). Withdrawal from methadone maintenance treatment. Reasons for not trying to quit methadone. *European Addiction Research*, 8(1), 38–44.

Holder, R. M., & Rhee, D. (2016, March 6). Novel oral therapies for opioid-induced bowel dysfuntion in patients with chronic noncancer pain. *Pharmacotherapy,* 36(3), 287–299. doi:10.1002/phar.1711

Holscher, F., Reissner, V., & Di Furia, L. (2010). Differences between men and women in the course of opiate dependence: Is there a telescoping effect? *European Archives of Psychiatry and Clinical Neuroscience*, 260(3), 235–241. doi:10.1007/s00406-009-0053-x

Hoyle, J. (2002). Stealth advertising on the Internet: Scumware. *Journal of the American Dental Association*, 133(4), 427.

Hudak, M. L., & Tan, R. C. (2012). Neonatal drug withdrawal. *Pediatrics*, 129(2), e540–e560.

Ilgen, M. A., Bohnert, A. S., & Ignacio, R. V. (2010). Psychiatric diagnoses and risk of suicide in veterans. *Archives of General Psychiatry*, 67, 1152–1158.

Inturrisi, C. E. (2002). Clinical pharmacology of opioids for pain. *The Clinical Journal of Pain*, 18(4 Suppl), S3–S13.

Jamison, R. N., Ross, E. L., & Michna, E. (2010). Substance misuse treatment for high risk chronic pain patients on opioid therapy: A randomized trial. *Pain*, 150(3), 390–400. doi:10.1016/j.pain.2010.02.033

Jancelewicz, C. (2016, July 6). *Jim Carrey girlfriend autopsy report: Suicide note reveals tragic details.* Retrieved July 11, 2016, from National | Globalnews.ca, pp. 1–3: http://globalnews.ca/news/2806388/jim-carrey-girlfriend-autopsy-report-suicide-note-reveals-tragic-details/

Jansson, L. M., & Velez, M. (2012). Neonatal abstinence syndrome. *Current Opinion in Pediatrics*, 24(2), 252–258. doi:10.1097/MOP.0b013e32834fdc.3a

Johannes, C. B., Le, T. K., & Zhou, X. (2010). The prevalence of chronic pain in United States adults: Results of an internet-based survey. *The Journal of Pain*, 11(11), 1230–1239. doi:10.1016/j.jpain.2010.07.002

Jones, C. M., Logan, J., & Gladden, R. M. (2015, July 10). Vital signs: Demographic and substance use trends among heroin users—United States, 2002–2003. *MMWR, Morbidity and Mortality Weekly Report*, 64(26), 719–725.

Jones, C. M., Paulozzi, L. J., & Mack, K. A. (2014). Alcohol involvement in opioid pain reliever and benzodiazepine drug abuse—Related emergency department visits and drug-related deaths—United States, 2010. *MMWR, Morbidity and Mortality Weekly Report*, 63(40), 881–885.

Jones, H. E., Kaltenbach, K., & Heil, S. H. (2010). Neonatal abstinence syndrome after methadone or buprenorphine exposure. *The New England Journal of Medicine*, 363(24), 2320–2331.

Jones, H. E., Seashore, C., & Johnson, E. (2016). Psychometric assessment of the Neonatal Abstinence Scoring System and the MOTHER NAS Scale. *The American Journal on Addictions*, 25, 370–373.

Jones, J. D., Vosburg, S. K., & Manubay, J. M. (2011). Oxycodone abuse in New York City: Characteristics of intravenous and intranasal users. *American Journal on Addictions*, 20(3), 190–195. doi:10.1111/j.1521-0391.2011.00120.x

Jones, R., Prommer, E., & Backstedt, D. (2015, July 6). Naloxegol: A novel therapy in the management of opioid-induced constipation. *American Journal of Hospice and Palliative Care*, 33(9), 875–880. doi: 10.1177/1049909115593937

Jumah, N. A. (2016). Rural, pregnant, and opioid dependent: A systematic review. *Substance Abuse Research and Treatment*, 10(S1), 35–41. doi:10.4137/SART.s34547

Katz, N., Dart, R. C., & Bailey, E. (2011). Tampering with prescription opioids: Nature and extent of the problem, health consequences, and solutions. *The American Journal of Drug and Alcohol Abuse*, 37(4), 205–217. doi:10.3109/00952990.2011.569623

Ko, J. Y., Patrick, S. W., & Tong, V. T. (2016, August 12). Incidence of neonatal abstinence syndrome—28 states, 1999–2013. *MMWR, Morbidity and Mortality Weekly Report*, 65(31), 799–802.

Kocherlakota, P. (2014). Neonatal abstinence syndrome. *Pediatrics*, 134(2), e547–e561.

Koneru, A., Nelson, N., & Hariri, S. (2016, July 22). Increased hepatitis C virus (HCV) detection in women of childbearing age and potential risk for vertical transmission—United States and Kentucky, 2011–2014. *MMWR, Morbidity and Mortality Weekly Report*, 65(28), 705–710. doi:10.15585/mmwr.mm6528a2(http://dx//doi.org/10.15585/mmwr.mm6528a2

Krans, E. E., & Patrick, S. W. (2016). Opioid use disorder in pregnancy: Health policy and practice in the midst of an epidemic. *Obstetrics & Gynecology*, 128(1), 4–10. doi:10.1097/AOG.0000000000001446

Krantz, A. J., Hershow, R. C., & Prachand, N. (2003). Heroin insufflation as a trigger for patients with life-threatening asthma. *Chest*, 123(2), 510–517.

Lemke, R. P. (2002). Drug dosing for neonates. In L. A. Pagliaro, & A. M. Pagliaro (Eds.), *Problems in pediatric drug therapy* (4th ed., pp. 531–554). Washington, DC: American Pharmaceutical Association.

Leppert, W. (2015, April 16). Emerging therapies for patients with symptoms of opioid-induced bowel dysfunction. *Drug Design, Development and Therapy*, 9, 2215–2231. doi:10.2147/DDDT.S32684

Lind, J. N., Petersen, E. E., & Lederer, P. A. (2015). Infant and maternal characteristics in neonatal abstinence syndrome—Selected hospitals in Florida, 2010–2011. *MMWR, Morbidity and Mortality Weekly Report*, 64(8), 213–216.

Lipsitz, P. J. (1975). A proposed narcotic withdrawal score for use with newborn infants: A pragmatic evaluation of its efficacy. *Clinical Pediatrics*, 14, 592–594.

Lofwall, M. R., Brooner, R. K., & Bigelow, G. E. (2005). Characteristics of older opioid maintenance patients. *Journal of Substance Abuse Treatment*, 28, 265–272.

Lofwall, M. R., Schuster, A., & Strain, E. C. (2008). Changing profile of abused substances by older persons entering treatment. *Journal of Nervous and Mental Disease*, 196, 898–905.

Lofwall, M. R., & Walsh, S. L. (2014). A review of buprenorphine diversion and misuse: The current evidence base and experiences from around the world. *Journal of Addiction Medicine*, 8(5), 315–326. doi:10.1097/ADM.0000000000000045

Lozano, J., Garcia-Algar, O., & Vall, O. (2007). Biological matrices for the evaluation of in utero exposure to drugs of abuse. *Therapeutic Drug Monitoring*, 29, 711–734.

MacDonald, R., Heiner, J., & Villarreal, J. (2015). Loperamide dependence and abuse. *BMJ Case Reports, pii*, brc2015209705. doi:10.1136/bcr-2015–209705

Mack, K. A., Jones, C. M., & Paulozzi, L. J. (2013). Vital signs: Overdoses of prescription opioid pain relievers and other drugs among women—United States, 1999–2010. *MMWR, Morbidity and Mortality Weekly Report*, 62(26), 537–542.

MacLaren, E. (2015). *Oxycodone history and statistics*. Retrieved March 12, 2016, from Drugabuse.com, pp. 1–23: http://drugabuse.com/library/oxycodone-history-and-statistics/

Maguire, D., Cline, G. J., & Parnell, L. (2013). Validation of the Finnegan Neonatal Abstinence Syndrome Tool—short form. *Advances in Neonatal Care*, 13, 430–437.

Manchikanti, L. (2007). National drug control policy and prescription drug abuse. *Pain Physician*, 10, 399–424.

Manchikanti, L., & Singh, A. (2008). Therapeutic opioids: A ten-year perspective on the complexities and complications of the escalating use, abuse, and nonmedical use of opioids. *Pain Physician*, 11(2 Supplement), S63–S88.

Maremmani, M. (2010). Differential substance abuse patterns distribute according to gender in heroin addicts. *Journal of Psychoactive Drugs*, 42(1), 89–95.

Marraffa, J. M., Holland, M. G., & Sullivan, R. W. (2014). Cardiac conduction disturbance after loperamide abuse. *Clinical Toxicology (Philadelphia)*, 52(9), 952–957. doi:10.3109/15563650.2014.969371

Mars, S. G., Bourgois, P., & Karandinos, G. (2014, March). "Every 'never' I ever said came true": Transitions from opioid pills to heroin injecting. *International Journal on Drug Policy*, 25(2), 257–266. doi:10.1016/j.drugpo.2013.10.004

Martins, S. S., Storr, C. L., & Zhu, H. (2009). Correlates of extramedical use of OxyContin versus other analgesic opioids among the US general population. *Drug and Alcohol Dependence*, 99(1–3), 58–67. doi:10.1016/j.drugalcdep.2008.06.013

McDonald, D. C., & Carlson, K. E. (2013, July 17). Estimating the prevalence of opioid diversion by "Doctor Shoppers" in the United States. *PLoS ONE*, 8(7), 1–25, e69241. doi:10.1371/journal.pone.0069241

McHugh, R. K., Devito, E. E., & Dodd, D. (2013). Gender differences in a clinical trial for prescription opioid dependence. *Journal of Substance Abuse Treatment*, 45(1), 38–43. doi:10.1016/j.jsat.2012.12.007

McQueen, K., & Murphy-Oikonen, J. (2016, Deember 22). Neonatal abstinence syndrome. *The New England Journal of Medicine*, 375(25), 2468–2479. doi:10.1056/NEJMra1600879

Muhuri, P. K., Gfroerer, J. C., & Davies, M. C. (2013, August). *Associations of nonmedical pain reliever use and initiation of heroin use in the United States*. Retrieved March 3, 2016, from CBHSQ (Center for Behavioral Health Statistics and Quality) Data Review: http://archive.samhsa.gov/data/2k13/DataReview/DR006/nonmedical-pain-reliever-use-2013.htm

Murphy-Oikonen, J., Montelpare, W. J., & Southon, S. (2010). Identifying infants at risk for neonatal abstinence syndrome: A retrospective cohort comparison study of 3 screening approaches. *The Journal of Perinatal and Neonatal Nursing*, 24, 366–372.

Nair, P., Black, M. M., & Schuler, M. (1997). Risk factors for disruption in primary caregiving among infants of substance abusing women. *Child Abuse & Neglect*, 21(11), 1039–1051.

National Drug Intelligence Center. (2001, May). *Heroin. California Central District Drug Threat Assessment*, pp. 1–8. Retrieved from National Drug Intelligence Center: www.justice.gov/ndic/pubs0/668/heroin.htm

NIDA, National Institute on Drug Abuse. (2014, June 24). *What can we do about the heroin overdose epidemic?*, pp. 1–6. Retrieved June 26, 2014, from www.drugabuse.gov/about-nida/noras-blog/2014/06/what-can-we-do-about-heroin-overdose-epidemic

NIDA, National Institute on Drug Abuse. (2015a, November 18). *FDA approves naloxone nasal spray to reverse opioid overdose*, pp. 1–4. Retrieved January 12, 2016, from www.drugabuse.gov/news-events/news-releases/2015/11/fda-approves-naloxone-nasal-spray-to-reverse-opioid-overdose

NIDA, National Institute on Drug Abuse. (2015b, December). *Overdose death rates*. Retrieved February 21, 2016, from www.drugabuse.gov/related-topics/trends-statistics/overdose-death-rates

NIDA, National Institute on Drug Abuse. (2015c, March 18). *U.S. and British Columbia issue alerts on fentanyl*. Retrieved May 5, 2016, from National Institute on Drug Abuse (NIDA): www.drugabuse.gov/emerging-trends/us-british-columbia-issue-alerts-fentanyl

NIDA, National Institute on Drug Abuse. (2016a, May 5). *Fake prescription drugs laced with fentanyl*. Retrieved May 5, 2016, from National Institute on Drug Abuse (NIDA), pp. 1–2: www.drugabuse.gov/emerging-trends/fake-prescription-drugs-lacedfentanyl

NIDA, National Institute on Drug Abuse. (2016b, July 9). *Surge in fentanyl overdose deaths*. Retrieved May 5, 2016, from National Institute on Drug Abuse (NIDA): www.drugabuse.gov/emerging-trends-surge-in-fentanyl-overdose-deaths

Nordrum, A. (2015, July 7). *Deaths from heroin overdoses have quadrupled over past decade in US, CDC says*. Retrieved March 19, 2016, from IBTimes: www.ibtimes.com/deaths-heroin-overdoses-have-quadrupled-over-past-decade-us-cdc-says-1998702?rel=rel2

Nordrum, A. (2016, January 21). *Addiction 2016: As heroin use escalates, a new drug to reverse overdoses hits US drugstores*. Retrieved from IBTimes.com: www.ibtimes.com/addiction-2016-heroin-use-escalates-new-drug-reverse-overdoses-hits-us-drugstores-2271924

Obituaries. (1970, October 19). *Time Magazine*, p. 54.

Ochoa, K. C., Hahn, J. A., & Seal, K. H. (2001). Overdosing among young injection drug users in San Francisco. *Addictive Behaviors*, 26(3), 453–460.

Ocker, K. (2016, October 31). Mom gave kids heroin as "feel-good medicine," charges say. *The News Tribune*, 1–2. Parkland, WA. Retrieved November 1, 2016

Oei, J. L., Xu, H. X., & Abdel-Latif, M. E. (2012). Dopamine D2 receptor gene polymorphisms in newborn infants of drug-using women. *Archives of Disease in Childhood. Fetal and Neonatal Edition*, 97, F193–F198. doi:10.1136/archdischild-2011–300235

Office of National Drug Control Policy. (2010, January 6). *Heroin facts & figures*, pp. 1–8. Retrieved from www.whitehousedrug policy.gov/DrugFact/heroin/heroin_ff.html

Ogholikhan, S., & Schwarz, K. B. (2016). Hepatitis vaccines. *Vaccines (Basel)*, 4(1), pii: E6. doi: 10.3390/vaccines4010006

Okada, Y., Tsuda, Y., & Bryant, S. D. (2002). Endomorphins and related opioid peptides. *Vitamins and Hormones*, 65, 257–279.

Osborn, D. A., Jeffery, H. E., & Cole, M. J. (2005, July 20). Sedatives for opiate withdrawal in newborn infants. *Cochrane Database of Systematic Reviews* (3: CD002053). doi:10.1002/14651858.CD002053.pub2

Osborn, D. A., Jeffery, H. E., & Cole, M. J. (2010a, October 6). Opiate treatment for opiate withdrawal in newborn infants. *Cochrane Database of Systematic Reviews* (10:CD002059). doi:10.1002/14651858.CD002059.pub3

Osborn, D. A., Jeffery, H. E., & Cole, M. J. (2010b, October 6). Sedatives for opiate withdrawal in newborn infants. *Cochrane Database of Systematic Reviews* (10: CD002053). doi:10.1002/14651858.CD002053.pub3

Pagliaro, A. M., Pagliaro, L. A., & Thauberger, P. C. (1993). Knowledge, behaviours, and risk perception of intravenous drug users in relation to HIV infection and AIDS: The PIARG Projects. *Advances in Medical Psychotherapy*, 6, 1–28.

Pagliaro, L. A., & Pagliaro, A. M. (Eds.). (2002). *Problems in pediatric drug therapy* (4th ed.). Washington, DC: American Pharmaceutical Association.

Pagliaro, L. A., & Pagliaro, A. M. (2004). *Pagliaros' comprehensive guide to drugs and substances of abuse* (1st ed.). Washington, DC: American Pharmacists Association.

Pagliaro, L. A., & Pagliaro, A. M. (2009). *Pagliaros' comprehensive guide to drugs and substances of abuse* (2nd ed.). Washington, DC: American Pharmacists Association.

Pagliaro, L. A., & Pagliaro, A. M. (2012). *Handbook of child and adolescent drug and substance abuse.* Hoboken, NJ: Wiley & Sons.

Park, H., & Bloch, M. (2016, January 19). *How the epidemic of drug overdose deaths ripples across America.* Retrieved July 16, 2016, from The New York Times: www.nytimes.com/interactive/2016/01/07/us/drug-overdose-deaths-in-the-us.html

Patrick, S. W., Schumacher, R. E., & Benneyworth, B. D. (2012). Neonatal abstinence syndrome and associated health care expenditures: United States, 2000–2009. *JAMA: Journal of the American Medical Association*, 307(18), 1934–1940. doi:10.1001/jama.2012.3951

Pergolizzi, J., Boger, R. H., & Budd, K. (2008). Opioids and the management of chronic severe pain in the elderly: Consensus statement of an International Expert Panel with focus on the six clinically most often used World Health Organization Step III opioids (buprenorphine, fentanyl, hydromorphone, methadone, morphine, oxycodone). *The Pain Practitioner*, 8(4), 287–313. doi:10.1111/j.1533-2500.2008.00204.x

Peterson, A. B., Gladden, R. M., & Delcher, C. (2016, August 26). Increases in fentanyl-related overdose deaths—Florida and Ohio, 2013–2015. *MMWR, Morbidity and Mortality Weekly Report*, 65(33), 844–849. doi:10.15585/mmwr.mm6533a3

Pieper, B., & Templin, T. (2001). Chronic venous insufficiency in persons with a history of injection drug use. *Research in Nursing & Health*, 24(5), 423–432.

Pritham, U. A., Paul, J. A., & Hayes, M. J. (2012). Opioid dependency in pregnancy and length of stay for neonatal abstinence syndrome. *Journal of Obstetric, Gynecologic, & Neonatal Nursing*, 41(2), 180–190. doi:10.1111/j.1552-6909.2011.01330.x

Proctor, S. L. (2012). Substance use disorder prevalence among female state prison inmates. *American Journal of Drug & Alcohol Abuse*, 38(4), 278–285. doi:10.3109/00952990.2012.668596

Rebuilding Afghanistan: Weekly Activity Update. (2005, February 24). Retrieved from http://web.archive.org/web/20070509070349/www.usaid.gov/locations/asia_near_east/Afghanistan/weeklyreports/022405_report.html

Rizvi, H. (2009, February 19). *Afghanistan still world's opium capital.* Retrieved from RAWA News, pp. 1–2: www.rawa.org/temp/runews/rawanews.php?id=936

Robinson, A., & Wermeling, D. P. (2014). Intranasal naloxone administration for treatment of opioid overdose. *American Journal of Health-System Pharmacy*, 71(24), 2129–2135. doi:10.2146/ajhp130798

Rudd, R. A. (2014, October 3). Increases in heroin overdose deaths—28 States, 2010 to 2012. *MMWR, Morbidity and Mortality Weekly Report*, 63(39), 849–854.

Rudd, R. A., Aleshire, N., & Zibbell, J. E. (2016). Increases in drug and opioid overdose deaths—United States, 2000–2014. *MMWR, Morbidity and Mortality Weekly Report*, 64(50), 1378–1382.

Russell, A. (2016, July 20). *Ohio woman sentenced to 51 years for letting drug dealer rape her 11-year-old daughter for heroin*. Retrieved July 16, 2016, from National | Globalnews.ca: http://globalnews.ca/news/2836699/ohio-woman-sentenced-to-51-years-for-letting-drug-dealer-rape-her-11-year-old-daughter-for-heroin/

SAMHSA, Substance Abuse and Mental Health Services Administration, Center for Behavioral Health Statistics and Quality. (2014, April 3). *The TEDS Report: Gender differences in primary substance of abuse across age groups.* Rockville, MA.

SAMHSA, Substance Abuse and Mental Health Services Administration, Office of Applied Studies. (2009). *Results from the 2008 National Survey on Drug Use and Health: National Findings (HHNSDUH Series H-36, HHS Publication No. SMA 09-4434).* Rockville, MA.

Schoener, E. P., Hopper, J. A., & Pierre, J. D. (2002). Injection drug use in North America. *Infectious Disease Clinics of North America*, 16(3), 535–551.

Schuman-Olivier, Z., Albanese, M., & Nelson, S. E. (2010). Self treatment: Illicit buprenorphine use by opioid-dependent treatment seekers. *Journal of Substance Abuse Treatment*, 39(1), 41–50.

Sharp, M. J., & Melnik, T. A. (2015). Poisoning deaths involving opioid analgesics—New York State, 2003–2012. *MMWR Morbidity and Mortality Weekly Report*, 64(14), 377–380.

Shei, A., Rice, J. B., & Kirson, N. Y. (2015). Characteristics of high-cost patients diagnosed with opioid abuse. *Journal of Managed Care & Specialty Pharmacy*, 12(10), 902–912. doi:10.18553/jmcp.2015.21.10.902

Sloan, P. A., & Klimkina, O. (2009). Intranasal abuse of prescription hydrocodone/acetaminophen results in oronasal fistula: A case report. *Journal of Opioid Management*, 5(6), 383–385.

Smith, M. Y., Bailey, J. E., & Woody, G. E. (2007). Abuse of buprenorphine in the United States: 2003–2005. *Journal of Addictive Diseases*, 26(3), 107–111.

Soyka, M. (2015). Buprenorphine-naloxone buccal soluble film for the treatment of opioid dependence: Current update. *Expert Opinion on Drug Delivery*, 12(2), 339–347. doi:10.1517/17425247.2014.953479

Spinner, H. L., Lonardo, N. W., & Mulamalla, R. (2015). Ventricular tachycardia associated with high-dose chronic loperamide use. *Pharmacotherapy*, 35(2), 234–238. doi:10.1002/phar.1540

Sporer, K. A. (1999). Acute heroin overdose. *Annals of Internal Medicine*, 130(7), 584–590.

Stanos, S. P., Bruckenthal, P., & Barkin, R. L. (2012). Strategies to reduce the tampering and subsequent abuse of long-acting opioids: Potential risks and benefits of formulations with physical or pharmacologic deterrents to tampering. *Mayo Clinic Proceedings*, 87(7), 683–694.

Stern, A. (2011, November 17). *Afghan heroin traffic thrives in war: Russia*. Retrieved from Reuters.com, p. 1: www.reuters.com/assets/print?aid=USTRE7AG2LM20111117

Stobbe, M. (2013, July 2). *The big story: Drug overdose deaths spike among middle-aged women*. Retrieved from Atlanta Press (AP), pp. 1–5: http://bigstory.ap.org/article/drug-overdose-deaths-spike-among-middle-aged-women

Stolberg, S. G., & Gerth, J. (2000, November 16). High-tech stealth being used to sway doctor prescriptions. *New York Times*, pp. A1, A22.

Thomas, C. P., Fullerton, C. A., & Kim, M. (2014). Medication-assisted treatment with buprenorphine: Assessing the evidence. *Psychiatric Services*, 65(2), 158–170. doi:10.1176/appi.ps.201300256

Trescot, A. M., Helm, S., & Hansen, H. (2008). Opioids in the management of chronic non-cancer pain: An update of American Society of the Interventional Pain Physicians' (ASIPP) Guidelines. *Pain Physician*, 11(2 Supplement), S5–S62.

Tsui, J. I., Herman, D. S., & Kettavong, M. (2010). Physician introduction to opioids for pain among patients with opioid dependence and depressive symptoms. *Journal of Substance Abuse Treatment*, 39(4), 378–383. doi:10.1016/j.jsat.2010.06.012

U.S. Food and Drug Administration. (2014a, September 16). *Press Announcements > FDA approves Movantik for opioid-induced constipation.* Retrieved October 3, 2016, from FDA.gov: www.fda.gov/NewEvents/Newsroom/PressAnnouncements/ucm414620.htm

U.S. Food and Drug Administration. (2014b, April 3). *Press Announcements > FDA aproves new hand-held auto-injector to reverse opioid overdose.* Retrieved December 23, 2016, from FDA News Release: www.fda.gov/NewsEvents/Newsroom/PressAnnouncements/ucm391465.htm

U.S. Food and Drug Administration. (2015, November 18). *Press Announcements > FDA moves quickly to approve easy-to-use nasal spray to treat opioid overdose.* Retrieved October 3, 2016, from FDA.gov: www.fda.gov/NewsEvents/Newsroom/PressAnnouncements/ucm473505.htm

Uebel, H., Wright, I. M., & Burns, I. (2015). Reasons for rehospitalization in children who had neonatal abstinence syndrome. *Pediatrics*, 136(4), e811–e820.

Unger, A., Jagsch, R., & Jones, H. (2011). Randomized controlled trials in pregnancy: Scientific and ethical aspects. Exposure to different opioid medications during pregnancy in an intra-individual comparison. *Addiction*, 106(7), 1355–1362.

Unick, G. J., Rosenblum, D., & Mars, S. G. (2013). Intertwined epidemics: National demographic trends in hospitalizations for heroin- and opioid-related overdoses, 1993–2009. *PLoS One*, 8, e54496.

UNODC, United Nations Office on Drugs and Crime. (2002). *Afghanistan, opium poppy survey, 2002.* Retrieved from www.unodc.org/pdf/afg/afg_opium_survey_2002.pdf

UNODC, United Nations Office on Drugs and Crime. (2011). *World drug report 2011.* Retrieved from www.unodc.org/unodc/en/data-and-analysis/WDR-2011.html

Volkow, N. D. (2014, May 14). *America's addiction to opioids: Heroin and prescription drug abuse.* Retrieved March 12, 2016, from National Institute on Drug Abuse (NIDA): www.drugabuse.gov/about-nida/legislative-activities/testimony-to-congress/2016/americas-addiction-to-opioids-heroin-prescription-drug-abuse

Volkow, N. D., & McLellan, A. T. (2016, March 31). *Opioid abuse in chronic pain.* Retrieved March 30, 2016, from NEJM Resident E-Bulletin: resebulletin@nejm.org

Weber, H. C. (2016). Opioid-induced constipation in chronic noncancer pain. *Current Opinion in Endocrinology, Diabetes and Obesity*, 23(1), 11–17. doi:10.1097/MED.0000000000000220

Weber, J. M., Tataris, K. L., & Hoffman, J. D. (2012). Can nebulized naloxone be used safely and effectively by emergency medical services for suspected opioid overdose? *Prehospital Emergency Care*, 16(2), 289–292. doi:10.3109/10903127.2011.640763

Welle-Strand, G. K., Skurtveit, S., & Jansson, L. M. (2013). Breastfeeding reduces the need for withdrawal treatment in opioid-exposed infants. *Acta Paediatrica*, 102(11), 1060–1066. doi:10.1111/apa.12378

Whitman, E. (2015, April 10). *US heroin epidemic growing rates of addiction and overdose reported in New Jersey, Kentucky, Indiana.* Retrieved April 19, 2016, from IBTimes.com: www.ibtimes.com/us-heroin-epidemic-growing-rates-addiction-overdose-reported-new-jersey-kentucky-1877064?rel=rel2

Wilder, C. M., & Winhusen, T. (2015). Pharmacological management of opioid use disorder in pregnant women. *CNS Drugs*, 29(8), 625–636. doi:10.1007/s40263-015-0273-8

Williams, A. R., & Bisaga, A. (2016). From AIDS to opioids—how to combat an epidemic. *The New England Journal of Medicine*, 375(9), 813–815.

Williamson, N., Archibald, C., & Van Vliet, J. S. (2001). Unexplained deaths among injection drug users: A case of probable Clostridium myonecrosis. *CMAJ: Canadian Medical Association Journal*, 165(5), 609–611.

Wilson, D., & Shiffman, J. (2015, December 7). U.S. News. *Newborns die after going home with moms fighting drug addiction*. Lehighton, PA: NBC News. Retrieved from www.nbcnews.com/news/us-news/newborns-die-after-going-home-moms-fighting-drug-addiction-n475531

Winstock, A. R. (2016, January 12). *The Global Drug Survey 2015 Findings—What did we learn from GDS2015?* Retrieved from Global Drug Survey, pp. 1–27: www.globaldrugsurvey.com/the-global-drug-survey-2015-findings/

Wu, L.-T., & Blazer, D. G. (2011). Illicit and nonmedical drug use among older adults: A review. *Journal of Aging and Health*, 23(3), 481–504. doi:10.1177/0898264310386224

Yewell, J., Haydon, R., & Archer, S. (2002). Complications of intranasal prescription narcotic abuse. *The Annals of Otology, Rhinology, and Laryngology*, 111(2), 174–177.

Yokell, M. A., Zaller, N. D., & Green, T. C. (2011). Buprenorphine and buprenorphine/naloxone diversion, misuse, and illicit use: An international review. *Current Drug Abuse Reviews*, 4(1), 28–41.

Zahorodny, W., Rom, C., & Whitney, W. (1998). The Neonatal Withdrawal Inventory: A simplified score of newborn withdrawal. *Journal of Developmental and Behavioral Pediatrics*, 19, 89–93.

Zeuzem, S. (2017). Treatment options in hepatitis C. *Deutsches Arzteblatt International*, 114(1-02), 11–21. doi: 10.3238/arztebl.2017.0011

Zuurmond, W. W., Meert, T. F., & Noorduin, H. (2002). Partial versus full agonists for opioid-mediated analgesia—focus on fentanyl and buprenorphine. *Acta Anaesthesiologica Belgica*, 53(3), 193–201.

2

WOMEN'S ALCOHOL ABUSE

This chapter presents and discusses *alcohol*. Both legal and widely available in various forms (e.g., beers, wines, and distilled spirits), this *non-prescription* sedative-hypnotic, has been *increasingly* used and abused by women in the U.S. over the first 2 decades of the new millennium. This chapter presents an overview and discussion of the pharmacology of alcohol and its medical and personal use and abuse among women across the lifespan. (For a discussion of *prescription* sedative-hypnotics, see Chapter 3, *Women's Prescription Sedative-Hypnotic Abuse*.)

Alcohol

Alcohol—whether purchased at corner liquor stores, popular restaurants and upscale clubs, or made in carefully hidden *stills*[1] or bath tubs using *old family recipes*—is one of the most widely used drugs and substances of abuse in the U.S. Often used and abused by women for its dose-dependent *disinhibition euphoria* and to decrease social and sexual inhibitions, alcohol also is used and abused to achieve a sense of well-being; to relax; or to relieve anxiety, tension, and stress—to "cope" with "life's pains, disappointments, and impossible tasks."[2] Unfortunately,

[1] Traditional handmade copper *moonshine stills* and distillation supplies, once only a cultural icon for Appalachia and remote country sites, are now advertised over the Internet for ready delivery from, for example, the Ozark Mountains of Arkansas.

[2] The full quote from Sigmund Freud (1939/1989) is:

> Life, as we find it, is too hard for us; it brings too many pains, disappointments and impossible tasks. In order to bear it we cannot dispense with palliative measures ... There are perhaps three such measures: powerful deflections, which cause us to make light of our misery; substitutive satisfaction, which diminish it; and intoxicating substances, which make us insensitive to it.

women's alcohol abuse is associated with more harm than their abuse of *all* the other drugs and substances of abuse *combined*. This chapter presents and discusses women's alcohol abuse with attention to the pharmacology of alcohol—its *pharmacodynamics* (i.e., mechanism of action); *pharmacokinetics* (i.e., absorption, distribution, metabolism, and excretion); and *adverse drug reactions, or events/experiences* (i.e., related undesired, or harmful, effects and toxicities). It also presents and discusses women's medical and personal abuse of alcohol.

There are several reasons for our decision to separate alcohol from the other sedative-hypnotics, particularly the *benzodiazepines* and *z-drugs*, and discuss it in its own chapter. These reasons include alcohol's:

- Long history of medical and personal abuse by women
- Identification as a neurotoxin in humans
- Discontinued medical use as a sedative-hypnotic during the last century
- Cultural inculcation into U.S. social gatherings, parties, and celebrations
- Potential for significant physical, mental, and social harm, including severe, and irreversible teratogenic effects when used by women during pregnancy—Fetal Alcohol Syndrome/Fetal Alcohol Spectrum Disorder (FAS/FASD)
- Current use by more than 80% of women in the U.S.

We begin with the basic pharmacology of alcohol emphasizing recent research findings in women's pharmacology.

Pharmacology

The word, *alcohol*, generally refers to beverage alcohol—*ethyl alcohol* or *ethanol* (Figure 2.1).[3]

Beverage alcohol is a colorless, flammable, and volatile liquid that is produced by the process of fermenting various carbohydrate foodstuffs, including fruits, grains, and vegetables with the use of yeasts.[4,5] Like other sedative-hypnotics, alcohol

[3] A distinction must be made between beverage alcohol and other types of alcohol—*methanol* and *isopropyl* alcohol, or common rubbing alcohol. The confusion has resulted from the use of the term *alcohol* in chemistry to describe any organic compound made from hydrocarbons (i.e., chemical structures consisting only of carbon [C] and hydrogen [H] atoms in which hydroxyl groups [OH] are substituted for an equal number of hydrogen atoms). *Methanol*, also known as methyl alcohol, or wood alcohol, is traditionally produced from fermenting wood and further distilling the product, but is now primarily chemically synthesized for commercial use. It is particularly toxic to the optic nerve and, if ingested, can cause permanent blindness—as well as death.

[4] Yeasts are single cell fungi (genus, *Saccharomyces*) that are capable of fermenting (i.e., digesting or decomposing) carbohydrates (e.g., cellulose; starches; sugars) to ultimately produce alcohol, carbon dioxide, and water.

[5] The concentration of the alcohol that is produced is limited to approximately 16% because higher concentrations kill the yeast and, consequently, halt the fermentation process. To *increase* the alcohol concentration, for example, to 18%, as is done to produce sherry and other fortified wines, more alcohol is simply added to the already fermented product. Even higher concentrations of alcohol

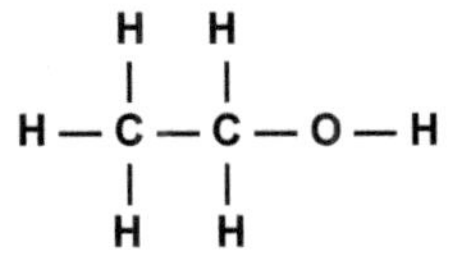

CH_3CH_2OH

FIGURE 2.1 Alcohol Molecule

produces a *progressive*, dose-related depression of the central nervous system (CNS) that ranges from *mild* sedation to *deep* sleep. Rarely, a loss of consciousness, or coma, may occur that can be fatal. These effects are generally predictable and depend on: (1) the type of alcoholic beverage ingested (e.g., beer versus whiskey); (2) its "proof," or percent of alcohol (e.g., a can of beer [approximately 5%] versus a gin and tonic or a double bourbon [approximately 40%]); and (3) the amount ingested (e.g., 1 can of beer or a 6-pack of beer) per unit of time (e.g., hour, day, or week). (See Table 2.1.)

Pharmacodynamics: Mechanisms of Action

The exact mechanism of action by which alcohol depresses the entire CNS remains a mystery. However, research over the last several decades has resulted in *two* major plausible theories:

1. Alcohol readily crosses the blood-brain barrier and disrupts the function of membrane lipids, or fats, in the brain, as well as glucose metabolism
2. Alcohol acts at specific receptor sites in the brain (i.e., gamma aminobutyric acid [$GABA_A$] receptor sites; and N-Methyl-D-aspartate [NMDA] receptor sites) (Pagliaro & Pagliaro, 2009; Peoples, Li, & Weight, 1996)

While either theory may contribute to alcohol's actual mechanism of action, research in glucose metabolism supports the first theory, which also explains alcohol's effects on learning and memory.[6] Research in support of the second theory suggests that alcohol acts to *enhance* GABAergic inhibition primarily by modifying the

(concentrations of 20%, or higher) can be obtained by distilling the fermented product to obtain distilled spirits such as brandy and whiskey.

6 Glucose, also known as dextrose, is the most important sugar involved in body function. The metabolism of glucose provides energy for cells, particularly neurons, which use glucose as their primary source of energy. Thus, the brain requires glucose to function. *Low* blood glucose concentrations (i.e., hypoglycemia) are associated with such signs and symptoms as acute fatigue, malaise, and feeling "rundown" or "weak." Severe hypoglycemia, because of its direct effects on the function of the CNS, can result in: blurred or double vision, headache, marked irritability, mental disturbances, and seizures. Unless immediately corrected, these signs and symptoms can progress to delirium (i.e., confusion and disorientation, including illusions and hallucinations), coma, and death.

TABLE 2.1 Common Types of Alcoholic Beverages Drunk by Women in the U.S.

Type of Beverage	*Alcohol Content (Average)*	*Characteristics and General Comments*
Ale, beer, and malt liquor		
Ale, Brown or Pale	4% to 7%	Brown- or amber-colored beer. Often sweet, with a fruity taste. Contains *more* malt, hops, and flavor than other beers and is fermented at *high* temperatures, using yeast (*Saccharomyces cerevisiae*) that floats in the mash (i.e., "top fermentation").
Beer (common)	4% to 7%	Beer is the *oldest* and most widely drunk alcoholic beverage in the world. Prepared by brewing and fermenting cereal grains, it is usually flavored with hops (i.e., the female flower clusters of *Humulus lupulus*) to give beer its characteristic bitter taste.
• Draft Beer	4% to 7%	Usually pasteurized, it is filtered to remove any active yeast to prevent containers from exploding during shipping.
• Lager Beer	4% to 6%	A type of German beer made with relatively small amounts of hops and *lower* temperatures during the fermentation process. The yeast (*Saccharomyces uvarum*) used sinks to the bottom of the mash (i.e., "bottom fermentation"). From the German, *lagern*, "to store," lager beers are typically aged for 2 to 6 months to allow time for natural sedimentation.
• Porter Beer	4% to 5%	Dark-brown beer brewed from charred or browned malt. It was originally brewed for porters, hence the name, and has a decidedly bitter taste.
• Stout	5% to 10%	Strong dark beer brewed with roasted barley, or malt, and hops.
Malt Liquor	5% to 10%	Aged like lager, but is carbonated and has *higher* alcohol content and more calories.
Wine, sparkling wine, and champagne		
Common Wines	9% to 16%	Wines are generally prepared by fermenting grapes (also see *fruit wines*). The fermenting and aging process is considerably longer than that for beers. Consequently, wines have a *higher* alcohol concentration than beers.
Fortified Wines		
• Dessert Wines	20%	Dessert wines (e.g., Madeira; Port; Sherry) are *fortified* wines to which a distilled spirit (e.g., brandy) has been added to raise the alcohol concentration.
• Vermouth	18%	A dry, sweet fortified wine flavored with aromatic bark, flowers, herbs, and roots (also see *Dessert Wines*). Two principal varieties are the Italian *sweet red* and the French *dry white* vermouths.

TABLE 2.1 *(cont.)*

Type of Beverage	*Alcohol Content (Average)*	*Characteristics and General Comments*
Fruit Wines	7% to 15%	Wines fermented from fruits such as apples, cherries, or plums—instead of grapes.
Red Wines	12%	Red wines (e.g., Merlot; Pinot Noir) range in color from purple red (young or immature wine) to deep shades of red. The reddish color depends on the pigment contained in the skins of the grapes that are used to make them.
Regional Wines	12%	Wines are often named after the region from where the grapes are grown and the wine is produced (e.g., Red *Burgundy* wine comes from Burgundy, a region in eastern France; White *Piesporter* wine comes from the *Piesport* region of Germany).
Sparkling Wines and Champagne	12%	*Sparkling wines* are naturally carbonated by corking before the yeast dies. Champagnes are usually associated with the sparkling white wines produced only in the Champagne provincial wine region of northeast France. The term, however, is commonly used to denote *all* white wines that are carbonated (i.e., "sparkling wines").
Varietal Wines	12%	Most wines are produced form one variety, or single species of grape.
White Wines	12%	White wines (e.g., *Pinot Grigio*; *Sauvignon Blanc; Soave*) vary in color from clear pale yellows to golden yellows and can be dry, sweet, or semi-sweet. The color of white wine is affected by the color of the pigments in the skins of the grapes that were used to produce it. However, white wines are also made with "skinless" red grapes.
Distilled Spirits[a]		
Brandy	40% (80 proof)	Distilled from wine or fruit juice (e.g., *eau-de-vie*; schnapps).
Cognac	40% (80 proof)	Cognac derives its name from the French town of *Cognac*. To be officially labeled as "cognac," the spirits must be: distilled from grapes, particularly the Saint-Emilion variety; produced around the town of Cognac; be distilled twice in copper pots; and be aged in French oak barrels for a minimum of 2 years. Usually, cognacs from different years or different vineyards or distillers are blended to obtain a characteristic "brand" of bouquet or taste.

TABLE 2.1 *(cont.)*

Type of Beverage	*Alcohol Content (Average)*	*Characteristics and General Comments*
Gin	40% to 50%	Distilled from corn or rye and water, gin is filtered through anise, caraway seeds, or juniper berries to soften the flavor and provide its distinctive taste. Colorless.
Liqueurs	15% to 55%	Distilled spirits infused with cream, flowers, fruits, herbs, or spices. They are often *not* included as distilled spirits because of their added sugar and consequent sweetness.
Rum	40% (80 Proof)	Distilled from fermented sugar cane juice or syrup and, sometimes, molasses. *Light* rum is aged in stainless steel tanks and is generally filtered during the blending process to preserve its colorless appearance. *Dark* rum is aged in oak barrels to obtain its characteristic color. Coloring rums using burnt sugar, caramel, or molasses also is sometimes done to further enhance the color of dark rum. Rums are generally aged for a minimum of 1 year.
Tequila	40% (80 proof)	Made from the blue agave plant, primarily found around Santiago de Tequila, a town in Jalisco, Mexico.
Vodka	35% to 50% (70 to 100 proof)	"A little water," from the Russian, *voda*, "water." Originally distilled from fermented wheat mash. *Pure* alcohol, almost 190 proof, it is diluted with various amounts of water to achieve the desired concentration, or proof. It is *not* aged. There is *no* difference between marketed vodkas except the proofs, the prices, or added coloring or flavoring agents.
Whiskeys	40% to 68% (80 to 136 proof)	Distilled from grain (e.g., corn or rye) or potatoes. Also, made from malted barley.
• Bourbon	40% (80 proof)	Distilled from over 50% corn. An American "spirit," it is based on traditional recipes and developed in large part by Irish and Scottish immigrants. Typically diluted to 60% (i.e., 120 proof) and aged in new, charred oak barrels for 2 years or longer. The name "bourbon" is taken from Bourbon County, Kentucky, where it was originally developed. Also, called *Bourbon Whiskey*. Bourbon can be straight (i.e., unblended) or blended. *Blended* bourbon must contain at least 51% straight bourbon, but may also contain added coloring, flavoring, or other distilled spirits. *Straight* bourbon whiskey produced in the State of Tennessee is generally referred to as *Tennessee Whiskey*.

TABLE 2.1 *(cont.)*

Type of Beverage	*Alcohol Content (Average)*	*Characteristics and General Comments*
• Corn Whiskey	40% (80 proof)	Distilled from over 80% corn. Typically produced in the U.S. as "moonshine." Colorless.
• Rye • American Rye • Canadian Rye	40% (80 proof)	Also, referred to as rye whiskey. In the U.S., it is fermented and distilled using over 50% rye grain in the mash. However, in Canada, the rye grain content of the mash can range from 10% to 100%. Like bourbon, it is diluted to 60% (i.e., 120 proof) and aged in *new* charred oak barrels for 2 years or longer. In addition, Canadian rye must be aged for a minimum of 3 years in wooden barrels, but *not* necessarily new charred oak barrels. Use of rye imparts a spicy or fruity taste to the whiskey. Rye also is drier and less sweet than bourbon.
• Scotch	40% (80 proof)	*Single* malt scotch is *only* distilled from fermented barley malt at a single distillery in Scotland. Traditionally, it is cooked over a peat fire and stored for at least 3 years in barrels that were *not* charred, but were originally filled with sherry (see *Fortified/Dessert Wines*). Also referred to as "Scotch Whiskey." *Blended* malt scotch whiskey is prepared by mixing (blending) single malt scotch from 2 or more different distilleries in Scotland. Caramel coloring is typically added to scotch prior to bottling to provide a rich and well-aged appearance. No other additives are legally allowed.

[a] Known simply as *spirits*, and in North America as *hard liquor*, distilled spirits contain at least 20% alcohol and *no* added sugar (see *Liqueurs*). Alcohol concentration can range from 20% to 95% with 40% (i.e., 80 proof) being the standard in North America.

membrane environment of the $GABA_A$ receptor complex. This action significantly *increases* the affinity of the $GABA_A$ receptor complex for both *endogenous* GABA and *exogenous* sedative-hypnotics (e.g., alcohol, barbiturates, and benzodiazepines), thus, enhancing GABAergic inhibition. (For further related discussion of the $GABA_A$ receptor complex, see Chapter 3, *Women's Prescription Sedative-Hypnotic Abuse.*)

Regardless of the actual mechanism of action, the blood alcohol concentrations (BACs) that are associated with the amount of alcohol ingested during a drinking episode *highly* correlate with the *direct* and *progressive* depression of the CNS (Pagliaro & Pagliaro, 2009).[7] (See Table 2.2.)

[7] The ingestion of a typical serving of alcohol (i.e., beer, wine, distilled spirits) increases the BAC by approximately 0.02 gram % (i.e., 20 mg/100 ml of blood) in the average adult (traditionally calculated based on a 21-year-old male of European descent who weighs 70 kg).

TABLE 2.2 Women's Blood Alcohol Concentration (BAC) and Physical and Mental Effects[a]

Increasing BAC Level (gram % or grams per 100 ml)	*Physical Effects*	*Mental Effects*
0.01 to 0.03	Generally, normal appearance.	Generally, normal behavior.
0.03 to 0.06	Feel warm and relaxed *with mild* impairment of coordination and diminished ability to perform fine motor tasks.	*Mild* euphoria (e.g., feelings of intense excitement and happiness) with *decreased* inhibitions and *increased* sociability and talkativeness. *Mild decrease* in alertness and concentration.
0.06 to 0.08	*Increasing* loss of coordination with both a *slight* loss of balance and speaking ability.	*Mild* impairment of reasoning and memory with *intensification* of emotions. *Increased* disinhibition euphoria with apparent "stimulant effect" on behavior and extroversion. *Lowered* interest in sex.
0.08 to 0.10	*Mild* impairment of hearing, speech, and vision with *slight* drowsiness.	*Mild* impairment of both judgment and self-control with *increased* accident probability or incidence.
0.10 to 0.15	*Continued* loss of coordination with marked impairment of balance, slowed reaction time, and *slightly* slurred speech.	*Increased* emotional instability with euphoria being increasingly replaced with the opposite feeling of *dysphoria* (e.g., anxiety, depression, disquiet, restlessness, or unease). *Significant* impairment in judgment and ability to make good decisions with up to tenfold *increase* in probability/incidence of accidents.
0.15 to 0.20	*Significant* drowsiness, slurred speech, and prolonged reaction times. *Significant* visual impairment with blurred vision, *reduced* glare recovery, and *decreased* peripheral vision.	*Significant* impairment of perception. *Gross* intoxication with further deterioration of judgment and up to thirtyfold *increase* in probability, or incidence, of accidents.
0.20 to 0.30	*Severe* motor and speech impairment with an appearance of a "sloppy drunk"—appears *smashed*.	*Significant* mental confusion—may be dazed or disoriented.

TABLE 2.2 (*cont.*)

Increasing BAC Level (gram % or grams per 100 ml)	*Physical Effects*	*Mental Effects*
	May require assistance to stand upright or to walk. *Impaired* gag reflex with risk of choking on food or own vomit. Risk of serious injury related to falls, walking into traffic, being attacked, robbed (i.e., being "rolled"), or raped.	*Loss* of normal understanding. *Significant* pain tolerance ("feeling no pain"). Memory loss and *alcoholic blackouts.* May become stuporous, or achieve a state of near-unconsciousness ("a drunken stupor").
0.30 to 0.35	*Total* loss of motor control. *Significantly* depressed, or absent, reflexes. Incontinence, or loss of voluntary bladder control, "totally pissed." *Significantly* slowed heart and respiratory rates.	Level of consciousness diminishes to a state of stupor, a complete lack of mental alertness, or a condition of significantly impaired ability to respond to external environmental stimuli. Level of consciousness diminishes to coma, or an extremely deep stupor—a condition in which the person cannot be aroused by external environmental stimuli (e.g., talking to the person, calling the person by name, or gently shaking the woman to arouse her). *Total* lack of response to painful stimuli, such as pinching the skin or pricking the skin with a pin or needle (i.e., level of surgical anesthesia).
0.35 to 0.40+	*Impaired* circulation of the blood throughout the body. *Death*, usually due to respiratory arrest. LD_{50} = 0.4 grams %	*Severe* CNS depression and unconsciousness.

Modified from: Pagliaro & Pagliaro (2012, pp. 19–20).

[a] The BACs listed and their associated effects are meant to provide a general guideline. Variability from one woman to another does occur and can be significant, particularly in the context of genetics, *acquired tolerance*, and the concomitant use of other drugs.

Lower BACs associated with the start of a drinking episode are generally accompanied with excitement, happiness, and increased mental and physical activity. In fact, historically, these observed behaviors led researchers to commonly *misclassify* alcohol as a CNS stimulant, or psychostimulant. However, the stimulant-like behaviors were later found to be due to alcohol's *general depression* of the CNS and it is now, accurately, pharmacologically designated as a psychodepressant.[8]

The relatively *low* BACs achieved at the beginning of a drinking episode, first diminish the medulla's control over the *higher* cortical (i.e., executive functioning) centers of the brain impairing thinking and psychomotor performance. Social norms and related inhibitions, such as being polite or wearing clothes in public, also are impaired. There also is an incremental loss in discrimination (i.e., the ability to make fine distinctions), fine motor movement, concentration, memory performance, and conscious control over behavior.[9] Wide fluctuations in mood, with frequent emotional outbursts, also may occur.

As the BAC *increases*, the state of disinhibition euphoria is progressively impaired as the actions/control of the cerebral cortex are increasingly diminished.[10] As a consequence, aggressive and other violent or pugilistic behavior may occur (e.g., bar fights). In this regard, women, when compared to men, are *equally* at risk for physically assaulting someone when they are drinking (Rothman, McNaughton Reyes, & Johnson, 2012; Timko, Moos, & Moos, 2009).

Instances of domestic violence, or intimate partner violence (IPV), often involve alcohol use—both acute intoxication and regular, long-term abuse, which is often associated with chronic alcohol use disorders (AUDs) (Pagliaro & Pagliaro, *Clinical Patient Data Files*; Stuart, Meehan, & Moore, 2006; Stuart, Moore, & Ramsey, 2004; Stuart, Temple, & Follansbee, 2008). This violence, including acts of sexual aggression perpetrated by women's intimate partners, depends upon both the: (1) pharmacologic actions of alcohol; and (2) the perpetrator's innate personality predisposition to engage in violent behavior (Abbey, 2011). For example, in their study of substance use before and during pregnancy and associated links to IPV, Martin, Beaumont, and Kupper (2003) found that:

> Before pregnancy, women who were physically assaulted by their partners were somewhat more likely to drink alcohol and use illicit drugs compared

---

[8] Alcohol also has been commonly (and correctly) classified as a neurotoxin.

[9] The behavioral reaction to *disinhibition*, occurring at *lower* doses, is unpredictable and is determined by individual factors, including a woman's mental set and the setting in which the drinking occurs. Mental set and environmental setting become less important when *increasing* amounts of alcohol are consumed because sedation dominates and behavioral activity *decreases*. As alcohol ingestion increases, *all* drinkers experience progressive psychomotor incapacitation. Thus, for example, at *low* alcohol dosages/BACs, some women may appear as "happy drunks," get on a table in a bar, take off their clothes, and dance naked without a care in the world. However, as alcohol dosages/BACs increase, all drinkers become sleepy drunks and soon fall asleep or "pass out."

[10] These psychodepressant actions are dependent upon such factors as gender, genetics, lean body weight, liver function, and alcohol tolerance.

> to women who did not experience such violence … After the women became pregnant, the links between women's experiences of intimate partner violence and their use of substances became stronger, with the women who experienced each type of partner violence being more likely to use both alcohol and illicit drugs.
>
> (p. 599)

Alcohol use—at any level—generally does *not* increase, or improve, cognitive or psychomotor performance.[11] However, with *moderate* to *heavy* alcohol ingestion: (1) visuospatial performance bias, which generally favors men, *disappears*; and (2) episodic memory performance bias, which generally favors women, is *maintained*. These observed actions may be mediated by the effects of alcohol on *sex hormones*, which, for example, facilitate the conversion of testosterone to estrogen (e.g., Yonker, Nilsson, & Herlitz, 2005).

When the BAC exceeds 0.1 gram %, usually within the first 1 to 2 hours after initiating a drinking episode (or approximately *4* drinks for women and *5* drinks for men),[12] further psychodepression occurs: judgment is impaired; coordination decreases; reaction time slows; and vision blurs. For this reason, the legal limit of *intoxication* in the U.S. is a BAC of 0.08 gram % (i.e., 0.08 gram of alcohol per 100 ml of blood) (DUI/DWI laws, 2010). (For further related discussion, see later section, "Motor Vehicle Crashes.")

It is interesting to note that the psychodepressant actions associated with the ingestion of alcohol appear to be *more* marked when the BAC is *increasing* rather than when it is *decreasing*.[13] As the ingestion of alcohol *increases*, the function of the CNS becomes increasingly impaired as a *general anesthesia* ultimately prevails. Several other body systems also are affected by acute alcohol ingestion, including: respiratory function; temperature regulation; sexual performance; and urinary output. (See later section, *Undesired, or Harmful, Effects and Toxicities*.)

---

11 A noted exception is the case of a woman with alcoholism who is experiencing the *alcohol withdrawal syndrome*. In this case, "a bit of the hair of the dog that bit her" (i.e., an alcoholic drink) would *increase* her BACs, relieve the signs and symptoms of the alcohol withdrawal syndrome, and, consequently, improve her performance—at least temporarily. Thus, an experienced surgeon or pianist might perform better in this context "with a drink" rather than "without a drink," but *not* better than if she were sober (Pagliaro & Pagliaro, *Clinical Patient Data Files*).

12 In the U.S., a standard drink is typically considered to be 0.5 ounces, or 15 grams, of alcohol. In relation to commonly consumed alcoholic beverages, this amount of alcohol is roughly equivalent to: 12 ounces (360 ml) of beer; 6 ounces (180 ml) of wine; or 1 ounce (30 ml) of 80-proof distilled spirits. Given these equivalencies, it is easy to see the truth in the adage, "a drink is a drink is a drink" (i.e., ultimately, it matters less what alcoholic beverage one drinks and more on how many drinks one has during a drinking episode).

13 This is probably due to the body's attempts to preserve homeostasis, or equilibrium, within the body (i.e., a state of dynamic equilibrium in response to both internal and external environmental changes). As such, it is more difficult to accommodate, or adapt to new changes (e.g., *increasing* BACs in the body) than those which occur after the body has adapted, or already made necessary changes (e.g., when BACs are *decreasing*).

Pharmacokinetics: Absorption, Distribution, Metabolism, and Excretion

Alcohol displays interesting and unique pharmacokinetics, from absorption to excretion. These processes are discussed in the following sections.

Absorption

Although only small amounts of alcohol (i.e., 10% to 20%) are directly absorbed from the stomach, absorption is rapid, and virtually complete (i.e., 80% to 90%) from the small intestine. Any remaining amounts of alcohol are absorbed in the colon (i.e., in total, virtually 100% of orally ingested alcohol is absorbed from the GI tract). The time from the last drink of alcohol to the *maximal* BAC usually ranges from 30 to 90 minutes, depending on gastric emptying time.

Gastric emptying time can be *prolonged* by the type and amount of food present in the stomach and, thus, *slow* both the rate by which alcohol is released into the small intestine and, in turn, the rate by which the BAC increases. The presence of food in the stomach also can *slow* the absorption of alcohol by diluting the alcohol and blocking absorption by covering some of the gastric mucosa through which alcohol is normally absorbed. In contrast, gastric emptying time can be *increased* (i.e., speeded-up) by ingesting an alcoholic beverage with a carbonated beverage (e.g., a "shot of whiskey" followed by a "beer chaser"; a "gin and tonic"; a "rum and coke"). This process involves: (1) distending the stomach; (2) relaxing the pyloric sphincter between the distal end of the stomach and the small intestine; and, consequently, (3) promoting the *rapid* release of stomach contents into the small intestines—where alcohol is primarily absorbed. The result, generally consciously intended by the drinker, is to achieve *higher* BACs and associated *desired* effects more rapidly.

However, regardless of the rate of absorption, *any* amount of alcohol that is orally ingested, under normal conditions, is eventually *completely* absorbed. This rule may be a deadly one regarding college/university students who participate in "drinking games," such as: "funneling" (i.e., pouring large amounts of alcohol through a funnel attached to a tube held in the mouth by a student or a sorority "pledge," who gulps it down as quickly as possible). These *games* are most often associated with university fraternity, or "frat," parties and "Spring Break" celebrations where college/university women also commonly participate. Another example is the heavy drinking that is frequently associated with sport championship celebrations (e.g., a favorite team winning the "Orange Bowl" or the "Super Bowl"). Unfortunately, these drinking games and sport celebrations can end in fatal alcohol overdosages.[14]

---

[14] In many of these cases, the victim simply "passes out" (as a natural consequence of increasing alcohol concentrations), alone on the beach or in her hotel room (while her friends continue to party). However, the alcohol continues to be absorbed and, if a sufficient BAC is subsequently achieved, associated respiratory depression—and death—can occur (Pagliaro & Pagliaro, *Clinical Patient Data Files*).

Distribution

Alcohol is a small molecule (see Figure 2.1) that readily dissolves in water (i.e., it is hydrophilic). It is *not* protein-bound. Thus, it easily crosses biological membranes. For example, alcohol crosses from the GI tract into the blood stream and from the blood stream across the blood-brain barrier into the CNS. Crossing the "placental barrier" and "fetal-blood-brain barrier," alcohol also is freely distributed to the fetus when consumed by women who are pregnant, easily achieving *fetal* BACs equivalent to those of the mother.

Figure 2.2 illustrates the basic principles of the transfer of free drugs across the human placenta and the fetal blood-brain barrier and the effects of other factors, including protein binding—the binding of free drug to protein—that *prevents* its cross-membrane transfer. These are important principles for health and social care professionals to understand because they explain the possible effects of women's

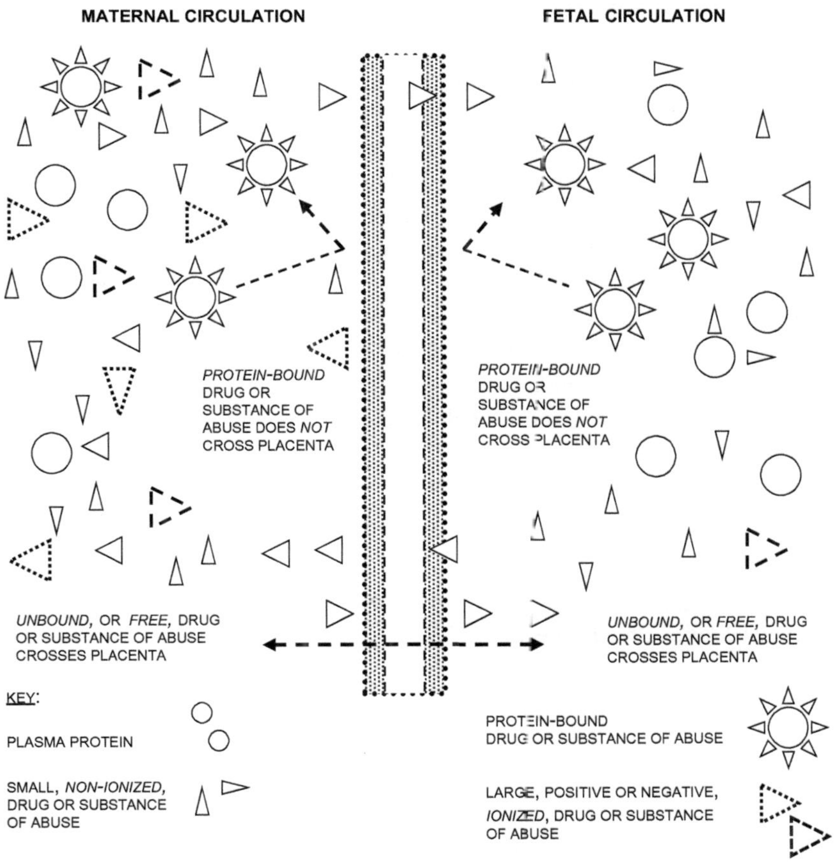

FIGURE 2.2 Transfer of Drugs and Substances of Abuse Across the Human Placenta

alcohol, or other drug or substance of abuse, on developing embryos and fetuses (also see later discussion in the section, *Fetal Alcohol Syndrome/Fetal Alcohol Spectrum Disorder* [FAS/FASD]).

Although *highly* soluble in water, alcohol is *not* well-distributed into fatty (i.e., adipose) tissues. Thus, the distribution of alcohol is generally different for women when compared to men. On average, women achieve *higher* BACs per drink consumed than do men of the same age, weight, and physical condition. This difference accounts for the observations that:

1. Men, on average, can drink *more* than women before showing signs and symptoms of drunkenness
2. Binge drinking, on average for men, consists of consuming *5* drinks at one sitting, while for women, it consists of consuming *4* drinks at one sitting (also see *later* section, *Binge Drinking*)

Metabolism and Excretion

Approximately 95% of ingested alcohol undergoes hepatic metabolism at a constant rate (Pagliaro & Benet, 1975) (see Figure 2.3). The remaining 5% of ingested alcohol that is *not* metabolized in the liver is excreted in unchanged form in the urine and breath. Alcohol has no nutritional value (e.g., vitamins and minerals) and, thus, only provides empty calories when metabolized. The energy released per gram of alcohol is approximately 7 kilocalories (kcal).

The rate of metabolism is linear with time and is minimally affected by variation in blood concentration. For the average 21-year-old, 70 kg, male of European descent, the rate of metabolism is approximately 10 to 20 ml of 100% alcohol per hour. Thus, it takes approximately 1 hour to metabolize a "typical drink" (i.e., approximately 30 ml of whiskey or another distilled spirit; 180 ml of wine; or 360 ml of beer).[15] If a larger amount of alcohol is ingested per hour than is metabolized, the BAC increases along with its corresponding psychodepressant actions, including desired and undesired, or harmful, effects and toxicities.

> <u>Popular Notion</u>: A woman who is drunk can quickly "sober up" by drinking several cups of *strong* coffee.
>
> NOT TRUE.

[15] N.B. It is particularly relevant to recognize that the early human studies on alcohol pharmacokinetics, including metabolism, predominantly (and often exclusively) used men as subjects. However, among women, the pharmacokinetics, including metabolism, can vary significantly. For example, women have been found, on average, to have a smaller volume of distribution and less first-pass metabolism than men (Baraona, Abittan, & Dohmen, 2001).

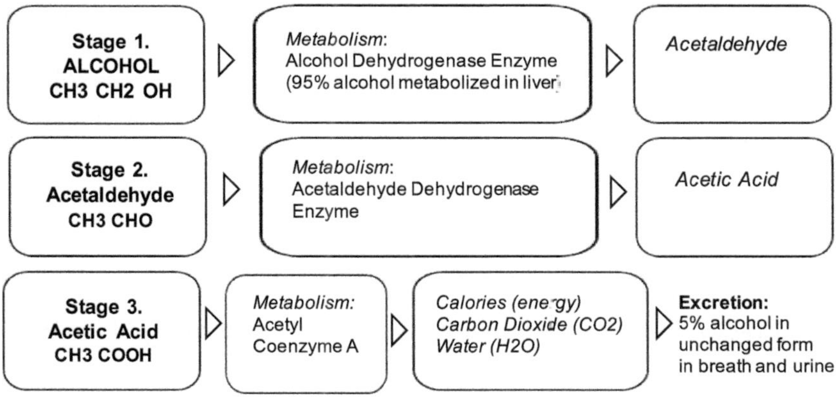

FIGURE 2.3 Alcohol Metabolism and Excretion: Three Stages

There are several factors (e.g., ingestion of fructose, or fruit sugar, and some vitamins) that may, *theoretically*, alter the rate of alcohol metabolism and, thus, hasten its elimination. However, *none* of these factors has proved clinically significant. Thus, even though it is commonly thought that drinking coffee or walking around can increase the elimination of alcohol and, thus, increase the process of sobering-up after a heavy drinking episode, it does *not*.

It also has been thought that caffeine in coffee (or energy drinks) can *counteract* drunkenness or *prolong* the *desired* effects of alcohol.[16] The only thing that these actions accomplish is to change a drowsy woman, who is drunk, into a wide-awake woman, who is drunk. Of course, the more time that is devoted to these activities, the more time passes in which alcohol can be slowly, but steadily, eliminated and, thus, make these *ineffective* activities appear to be effective.

Presently, there is *no* practical way to *increase* the rate of alcohol metabolism. Once alcohol is ingested, absorbed, and distributed throughout the body, its ultimate elimination from the body primarily depends on its *slow and steady* rate of metabolism by the liver. This process may be impaired among women who have liver disease (e.g., cirrhosis of the liver) or genetic polymorphism of both *alcohol*

---

[16] Interestingly, McKetin, Coen, and Kaye (2015), in their comprehensive review of 62 related studies reported that those who drank alcohol mixed with caffeinated energy drinks (AEDs) found that AEDs "*increased* stimulation and alertness, offset fatigue from drinking, and facilitated drinking" (p. 15). We would hasten to add that while these findings may help to account for a noted *increase* in the related consumption of alcohol/caffeine beverages, it does *not* necessarily confirm the reported effects (i.e., believing these reports of behavior to be true while potentially reinforcing the related behavior among AED consumers does not make them true to the external objective observer). Several studies (e.g., Ferreira, de Mello, & Pompeia, 2006; Marczinski, 2014; Marczinski & Fillmore, 2006) support our observations and interpretations.

dehydrogenase and *aldehyde dehydrogenase* (i.e., the enzymes involved in the hepatic metabolism of alcohol and in the occurrence of the *Asian Flush*).

Genetic polymorphism also may account, in part, for the variations in alcohol metabolism and elimination rates observed among women of certain continental descents (e.g., Jewish women versus American Indian and Alaska Native women) (Pagliaro & Pagliaro, 1992).

Undesired, or Harmful, Effects and Toxicities

Delker, Brown, and Hasin (2016, p. 13), based on their epidemiologic overview of alcohol consumption in the U.S., concluded that:

> In the United States, AUD accounts for a high and potentially preventable proportion of overall disability and mortality.

In this context, many researchers, including ourselves, have noted that during the new millennium, women in the U.S. are at particular risk for experiencing this "disability and mortality." For example:

> Females had an increased risk for all-cause mortality conferred by drinking compared with males, especially in heavy drinkers.
>
> *(Wang, Xue, & Wang, 2014, p. 373)*

> Women with moderate to heavy alcohol intake had a significantly increased risk of total mortality compared with men in multiple subpopulations.
>
> *(Zheng, Lian, & Shi, 2015, p. 773)*

> Additionally, lesbian and bisexual women were more likely than exclusively heterosexual women to report alcohol-related problems (e.g., arguments, angry relationship partners, occupational or legal problems).
>
> *(Green & Feinstein, 2012, p. 265)*

With its *desired* psychotropic actions (as previously noted), and certain other *positive* qualities (e.g., pleasant color, taste, *bouquet*; satisfies one's thirst), it is surprising to some—and often overlooked by many others—that women's alcohol abuse is associated with *more* harm than all of the other drugs or substances of abuse combined (Pagliaro & Pagliaro, 2009).[17] "All the available gender studies on alcohol show greater severity of alcohol-related damage, including brain damage,

[17] Consistently, during the new millennium, alcohol consumption has been cited as the third leading cause of death in the U.S. (Centers for Disease Control and Prevention, 2004, 2012b).

in females compared with males" (Mancinelli, Vitali, & Ceccanti, 2009, p. 77). In addition, many physiological functions—body temperature; CNS, respiratory, and urinary function; as well as sex and sleep—are *directly* affected by BAC.

Popular Notion: When a woman comes in shivering from the cold, a "little sip" of brandy or whiskey can warm her right up!

NOT TRUE. All she will get is a warm feeling in her stomach.

In fact, regarding body temperature, *acute* alcohol ingestion generally causes peripheral vasodilation (and the characteristic warm *flush* that occurs), which results in a *decrease* in body temperature. The resultant vasodilation, particularly of the blood vessels located near the skin surface, cool the body down in a way like the cooling coils in an automotive radiator, that cool the engine down. Thus, the fallacy of a woman taking a drink to warm herself up.

Regarding CNS function, for example, Bickel, Moody, and Mueller (2013, p. 1), in a non-gender study, noted "significant executive dysfunctioning" among alcohol-dependent women. Regarding respiratory function, *moderate* amounts of alcohol may *stimulate* or *depress* respirations.[18] In addition, the ingestion of *large* amounts of alcohol (e.g., BAC = 0.4 gram % or *higher*) can generally be *fatal* because of severe depression of respirations and associated cardiac functions. In an example regarding sleep, the ingestion of alcohol *slows* the electroencephalogram (EEG) activity toward slow-wave sleep, depressing rapid eye movement (REM) sleep and, thus, inhibiting dreaming. Finally, regarding the urinary system, alcohol *directly* and *indirectly* exerts a diuretic effect (i.e., increases urine production and, consequently, urination), by two principal mechanisms:

1. *Directly*, by its suppressant action on the production and secretion of antidiuretic hormone by the hypothalamus and pituitary gland, respectively, which *increases* the reabsorption of water in the distal convoluted tubules of the kidneys
2. *Indirectly*, by the large quantity of liquid ordinarily ingested as alcoholic beverages, particularly beer

[18] However, health and social care providers should understand that the: (1) "protective" effect of carbon dioxide on breathing—the increase in ventilation induced by the decreased availability of oxygen supply to the body tissues (i.e., *hypoxic ventilatory response/drive*); and (2) increasing ventilation induced by increased levels of carbon dioxide in the blood (i.e., *hypercapnic ventilator response/drive*) are *always* depressed by alcohol intoxication (Roeggla, Roeggla, & Roeggla, 1995; Sahn, Lakshminarayan, & Pierson, 1975; White, Lindsey, & Vincente, 1981).

Although, these actions and effects may result in the loss of a woman's ability to hold her urine (i.e., *urinary incontinence*), alcohol does *not* appear to directly harm the structure or function of the kidneys.[19]

As identified in Table 2.3, there are *many* undesired, or harmful, effects and toxicities—both acute and chronic—*directly* and *indirectly* associated with women's alcohol abuse. We begin with an overview and discussion of physical and psychological dependence, including: (1) alcoholism; and (2) the alcohol withdrawal syndrome and associated sequelae—*hangovers* and *delirium tremens* (*DTs*). We then present and discuss *eight* particularly *serious* alcohol-related health conditions that are commonly associated with women's alcohol abuse: (1) FAS/FASD;[20] (2) breast cancer; (3) depression and suicide; (4) heart disease (e.g., coronary artery disease); (5) liver disease (e.g., alcoholic hepatitis; cirrhosis of the liver); (6) motor vehicle crashes; (7) Wernicke-Korsakoff's Syndrome; and (8) physical and sexual abuse.

Alcohol has a *high* abuse potential, characterized by the development of *alcoholism*, a medical disease that is associated with the physical development of: (1) *tolerance*, or the need to drink more and more alcohol to achieve desired psychodepressant actions; and (2) the occurrence of an *alcohol withdrawal syndrome* when regular, long-term alcohol abuse is abruptly discontinued, which can be immediately relieved when alcohol drinking is resumed.

Regular, long-term alcohol use also is associated with psychological dependence—*craving* and *loss of control*.

Popular Notion: The ability to hold her liquor more than others indicates a woman's *immunity* to alcoholism.

NOT TRUE. The ability to "hold her liquor" is, actually, a demonstration of *acquired tolerance*—a characteristic sign of alcoholism.

---

[19] The urinary incontinence that is often associated with heavy drinking episodes occurs primarily as a direct result of the psychodepressant actions of alcohol—the drinker falls into a deep sleep, or "passes out," and, losing urinary bladder control, wets herself while asleep. This alcohol-related effect is most often noted among older women drinkers who are homeless (Pagliaro & Pagliaro, *Clinical Patient Data Files*).

[20] The term, *Fetal Alcohol Spectrum Disorder* (FASD), is now commonly used in lieu of the term, *Fetal Alcohol Effects*, a term that was used to identify neonates, infants, and children who exhibit fewer of the characteristics deemed necessary, by definition or convention, to establish a diagnosis of FAS (Caruso & ten Bensel, 1993; Ginsberg, Blacker, & Abel, 1991; Smitherman, 1994). Other diagnostic labels and definitions also have been used in this regard in the published clinical literature, including alcohol-related birth defects (ARBD) and alcohol-related neurodevelopment disorder (ARND) (Harris, Osborn, & Weinberg, 1993; Pagliaro & Levin, 1979; Sampson, Streissguth, & Bookstein, 1997; Sokol & Clarren, 1989). All such related terms are now generally subsumed by, or included within, the FASD.

TABLE 2.3 Acute and Chronic Toxicities Related to Women's Alcohol Use/Abuse

Acute Toxicities	*Chronic Toxicities*	*Acute/Chronic Toxicities*
Academic and work performance, *decreased*	Alcoholism	Absenteeism from school, social engagements, and work, *increased*
Date rape, *increased* risk (facilitation of perpetration)	Alcohol withdrawal syndrome with cessation of alcohol abuse	Abusive and aggressive behavior, physical and/or mental (e.g., child abuse or neglect; abuse of boyfriend, girlfriend, significant other, or spouse)
Eye movements, *diminished*	Anemia	Accidents, general (e.g., drownings; falls)
Hallucinations	Cardiac dysrhythmias	Alcoholic blackouts
Hangover	Cardiovascular disease	Alcoholic ketoacidosis
Homicide involvement—both as perpetrator or victim, *increased*	Diabetes mellitus	Amnesia
Hypokalemia	Dysmenorrhea, *increased*	Cognitive dysfunction
Hypothermia	Hypertension	Coma
Hypoventilation	Immune response, *decreased*	Criminal behavior, *increased*
Incontinence	Hypertriglyceridemia	Domestic violence (e.g., intimate partner violence, IPV), *increased*
Motor vehicle crashes, *increased*	Korsakoff's psychosis	Dysfunctional mothering, *increased*
Peripheral vasodilation, including flushed, or reddened face, neck, and chest	Malnutrition	FAS/FASD among offspring of women of reproductive age who drink during pregnancy
Psychomotor impairment	Peripheral neuropathy	Feelings of guilt regarding drinking
Psychosis	Physical dependence	Gastritis
Respiratory depression	Psychological dependence	Hypoglycemia
Risk taking behavior, *increased*	Sick days, increased	Memory dysfunction
Sexual activity, increased—due to *decreased* social inhibitions	Wernicke's encephalopathy	Mental depression
Sexual assault, *increased*—due to *decreased* social inhibitions—perpetrator or victim	Women's contemporaneous diagnoses (e.g., alcohol use disorder and major depressive disorder)	Neurotoxicity

TABLE 2.3 (*cont.*)

Acute Toxicities	*Chronic Toxicities*	*Acute/Chronic Toxicities*
Sexually transmitted diseases, *increased*		Self-neglect
Short-term memory, *impaired*		Social problems (e.g., arguments with colleagues, family members, and neighbors; criminal charges; financial difficulties)
Slurred speech		Suicide, *increased* (attempted or completed suicide)
Social inhibitions, *decreased*		Victimization (e.g., physical assault, sexual assault), *increased*
Violent behavior (e.g., homicide, physical assault, and rape), *increased*		Women's contemporaneous diagnoses, *increased*
Vomiting		Work performance and productivity, *decreased*

Modified from Pagliaro & Pagliaro (2012, pp. 21–22).

The extent to which physical and psychological dependence develop—as well as their associated physical, psychological, and social consequences—are directly related to the specific pattern and context in which alcohol is consumed. Infrequent use, or *low to moderate* social use of alcohol in small amounts (i.e., one or two drinks on holidays and special occasions or fewer than *5* drinks a week for women [7 drinks a week for men]) is generally associated with *few* or *no* harmful effects for most women.[21]

However, both physical and psychological dependence, in the form of increasingly serious forms of *alcoholism*, have been identified with regular, long-term moderate to heavy drinking over months and years. Tolerance develops to many of the physiological and psychological effects of alcohol. Thus, many women begin to drink increasingly more frequently and in larger amounts in an effort to obtain the desired effects that were initially achieved with infrequent, low to moderate

[21] Exceptions, for example, include women who are: (1) alcoholics that are now abstinent (i.e., have achieved a pattern of resumed nonuse); (2) receiving disulfiram (Antabuse®) pharmacotherapy to manage their alcohol use pattern of abuse or compulsive use (see Chapter 8, *Preventing and Treating Women's Drug and Substance Abuse*); and (3) pregnant (see related discussion in the later section, "Fetal Alcohol Syndrome/Fetal Alcohol Spectrum Disorder").

amounts of drinking. Alcohol also is used in an effort to prevent, or *ward off*, the signs and symptoms associated with low or abstinent BACs—the alcohol withdrawal syndrome.

For most women who drink alcohol, alcoholism, generally, is *not* easily defined nor is it often accurately recognized at an early stage. A simple, yet accurate, definition of alcoholism that we developed and find useful is:

> *Alcoholism* is a condition associated with patterns of alcohol use that result in *increasing* harm to a woman—as measured by related negative changes in her: physical and mental health; work performance and productivity; family relationships and responsibilities; and social life.

The incidence of alcoholism is approximately 15% of the entire adult population in the U.S. (i.e., approximately, 1 in 7 adults). The development of alcoholism is characterized as being: (1) progressive, in that it becomes more serious with time; (2) chronic, in that it is continuous; and (3) insidious, in that most women are unable to recognize, without assistance from others, that their use of alcohol is resulting in significant personal and social harm as presented in the definition.

Complex in nature, we have, for some time, considered *alcoholism* as actually consisting of several forms of "alcoholism," or as perhaps, more accurately, a syndrome with various "degrees of alcoholism." Alcoholism also can be characterized by many specific, related signs and symptoms, including: alcoholic "blackouts" (i.e., inability to account for specific periods of time when drinking); drinking alone; drinking increasingly more alcohol, more frequently to achieve initial desired effects (i.e., tolerance to alcohol); gulping down drinks; sneaking drinks; drinking in the morning, or "starting the day with a drink"; and personality and behavioral changes.

Approximately one-third of adults in the U.S. will develop alcoholism or another alcohol use disorder (AUD) sometime during their lifetime (Hasin, Stinson, & Ogburn, 2007). Women who have alcoholism usually can be characterized as belonging to one of two major groups: (1) *bender* or *binge* drinkers—women who drink *heavily* for short periods of time (e.g., weekends); and (2) *daily* drinkers—women who drink *heavily* every day or whenever alcohol is available to them.

Women in the U.S., who develop alcoholism, reportedly begin to display certain alcohol-related behavioral problems that continue to progress and become more serious over time. These problem behaviors are significantly different than those observed for men who develop alcoholism. For example, McCutcheon, Agrawal, and Heath (2011), in their study using diagnostic interviews of 8,605 participants from the *Collaborative Study on the Genetics of Alcoholism*, found that:

> Women were more likely than men to report drinking larger amounts or for longer periods of time than intended, spending so much time drinking or

> recovering that there was little time for anything else, and continued drinking despite physical and psychological problems, and less likely than men to report social or interpersonal problems due to drinking.
>
> *(p. 1985)*

Approximately one-sixth of women, who identify that they have alcoholism, manage to "cure themselves." However, *most* women with alcoholism have alternating periods of complete abstinence and heavy drinking. If these women do *not* receive some form of external intervention (see Chapter 8, *Preventing and Treating Women's Drug and Substance Abuse*), their alcoholism is likely to follow a typical pattern that becomes increasingly harmful over time. This pattern of use has been described as beginning when the first major problems associated with alcohol abuse are recognized by those other than the woman, herself (e.g., adult children; employer; friend; parent; physician, or other health and social care provider; sibling; spouse or significant partner).

In the U.S., these problems usually are *first* recognized among women who have developed alcoholism by the time they are 28 to 33 years-of-age. However, the great majority of these women do *not* generally seek treatment until they are approximately 40 years-of-age. Unfortunately, many of these women die between 55 years-of-age to 65 years-of-age because of such alcohol-related conditions as:

- Accidents
- Heart disease
- Cancer of the breast
- Cirrhosis of the liver with liver failure and related effects, including esophageal varices, and associated bleeding, or hemorrhage
- Depression and suicide

(See, for example, Table 2.3.)

Alcohol Withdrawal Syndrome. The alcohol withdrawal syndrome is characterized by a period of *rebound hyperexcitability* that may be quite *severe* for some women who are regular, long-term heavy drinkers and may lead to convulsions and even death. Alcohol, like many other sedative-hypnotics, can *suppress* epileptic convulsions, or seizures. However, when ingestion is discontinued, this anticonvulsant action may be followed by *hyperexcitability* that lasts for several days.[22]

Hangovers. Fortunately, for most women who drink alcohol, a milder form of the alcohol withdrawal syndrome, commonly known as a "hangover," occurs.

---

22 Whether women who have alcoholism have epilepsy or not, they may have seizures when their regular, long-term use of alcohol is discontinued for a period. During alcohol withdrawal, the associated seizures peak approximately 8 to 12 hours after their last drink.

Hangovers are typically identified by the following characteristics that generally follow heavy drinking episodes: anxiety; cognitive deficits, particularly deficits in attention and memory; depressed mood; dry mouth; fatigue; general malaise; headache (often severe); hypersensitivity to light and sound; nausea; and thirst.

In addition, as identified by several researchers (e.g., Ling, Stephens, & Heffernan, 2010; McKinney, 2010; Prat, Adan, & Perez-Pamies, 2008), hangovers also are associated with:

- Impaired job performance
- Poor academic achievement
- Potentially dangerous situations involving daily activities (e.g., child care, rearing, and supervision; driving a car; or operating heavy machinery)
- Reduced productivity
- Workplace absenteeism

Hangovers often are self-managed by woman drinkers, themselves. For example, a commonly used remedy is to take *a little hair from the dog that bit me*[23]—have a "Bloody Mary" cocktail (tomato juice and vodka) for breakfast or a "Screwdriver" cocktail (orange juice and vodka)—to which vitamins, protein powder, and a raw egg may be added. These and other approaches that are used to self-manage hangovers are not recommended because they tend to promote, or reinforce, harmful drinking patterns that are likely to result in, or sustain, alcoholism (Pagliaro & Pagliaro, 2012; Piasecki, Robertson, & Epler, 2010).

Readers should recognize that up to 25% of adult drinkers, regardless of beverage type or personal characteristics, may be relatively resistant to the common signs and symptoms of a hangover (Howland, Rohsenow, & Allensworth-Davies, 2008, p. 758; Howland, Rohsenow, & Edwards, 2008). This observation, reportedly, is most likely due to genetic factors. The observed resistance to the signs and symptoms of a hangover (i.e., alcohol-related aversive reactions) may—contrary to first thought—actually *increase* the risk for developing alcoholism or other alcohol use disorders because their absence may likely *encourage*, rather than *deter*, further alcohol use (Pagliaro & Pagliaro, *Clinical Patient Data Files*; Smith & Barnes, 1983).

Syndrome of Delirium Tremens (DTs). In a small percentage of abstinent drinkers, CNS *hyperexcitability* is accompanied by a period of agitation (*severe*), confusion, delirium, disorientation, fever, grand mal seizures, hallucinations (often bizarre and extremely frightening), insomnia, irritability, nausea, psychomotor agitation, restlessness, sleep disorders, tachycardia, tremulousness, and a variety of other associated physiological effects (e.g., fever; mydriasis; or diaphoresis). This group of signs and symptoms has been generally identified as the *Syndrome of Delirium Tremens*

---

23 The common expression for treating a hangover originated from that associated with the ancient practice of treating a rabid or other dog bite by placing some "hair from the dog that bit you" in the wound.

(*DTs*).[24] This particularly *severe* form of the alcohol withdrawal syndrome is characterized by signs and symptoms that appear to be moderated, at least in part, by a *decrease* in GABA inhibitory function and an *increase* in glutamatergic excitatory function (Malcolm, 2003).[25]

Women, who are at risk for DTs, include those who have a history of regular, long-term heavy drinking and other severe pre-existing medical conditions, including cardiovascular disease and seizure disorders. Cardiovascular collapse may occur if DTs is left untreated, and may be fatal. Women, who demonstrate characteristic signs and symptoms of this syndrome, require immediate, medical emergency treatment services. Medical management of DTs generally involves hospitalization to provide cautious administration of long-acting benzodiazepines (e.g., diazepam, Valium®), careful monitoring of body systems, and appropriate supportive care (Pagliaro & Pagliaro, 2009; Yost, 1996).

Recovery from DTs generally occurs within 3 to 5 days following the onset of signs and symptoms. However, up to 10% of people, who have alcoholism, *die* during an untreated episode of DTs.

Fetal Alcohol Syndrome/Fetal Alcohol Spectrum Disorder. Alcohol, a known human teratogen, readily crosses the maternal placental barrier from the maternal systemic circulation to the developing fetal systemic circulation and, consequently, results in exposure of the developing fetus to alcohol and its potential undesired, or harmful, effects and toxicities. The most *severe* teratogenic effects associated with alcohol use during pregnancy are displayed in the FAS/FASD (Pagliaro & Pagliaro, 1987) (see Figure 2.4). In the U.S., the FAS/FASD:

- Is the leading cause of developmental disabilities (CDC, 2012a; Floyd, Weber, & Denny, 2009; Marchetta, Denny, & Floyd, 2012)
- Is the third *most* commonly known cause of mental retardation
- Is the *most* common preventable cause of mental deficiency (Pagliaro & Pagliaro, 1995, 1997, 2000, 2012)
- May be identified in up to 3% of live births (May, Baete, & Russo, 2014; May, Keaster, & Bozeman, 2015; Mengel, Searight, & Cook, 2006)
- Is *only* caused by women's alcohol use during pregnancy

The detection of maternal alcohol use during pregnancy is an integral part of the diagnosis of FAS/FASD. However, retrospective self-report of alcohol use during pregnancy is *not* always reliable. As noted by Joya, Friguls, and Ortigosa (2012), "pregnant women tend to underreport alcohol drinking by

---

[24] Historically, this syndrome also was known by other names, including: *Alcoholic Delirium* and *Rum Fits*.

[25] This explanation is consistent with the observed clinical efficacy of the benzodiazepines (e.g., chlordiazepoxide [Librium®], diazepam [Valium®]) in managing the signs and symptoms of the alcohol withdrawal syndrome.

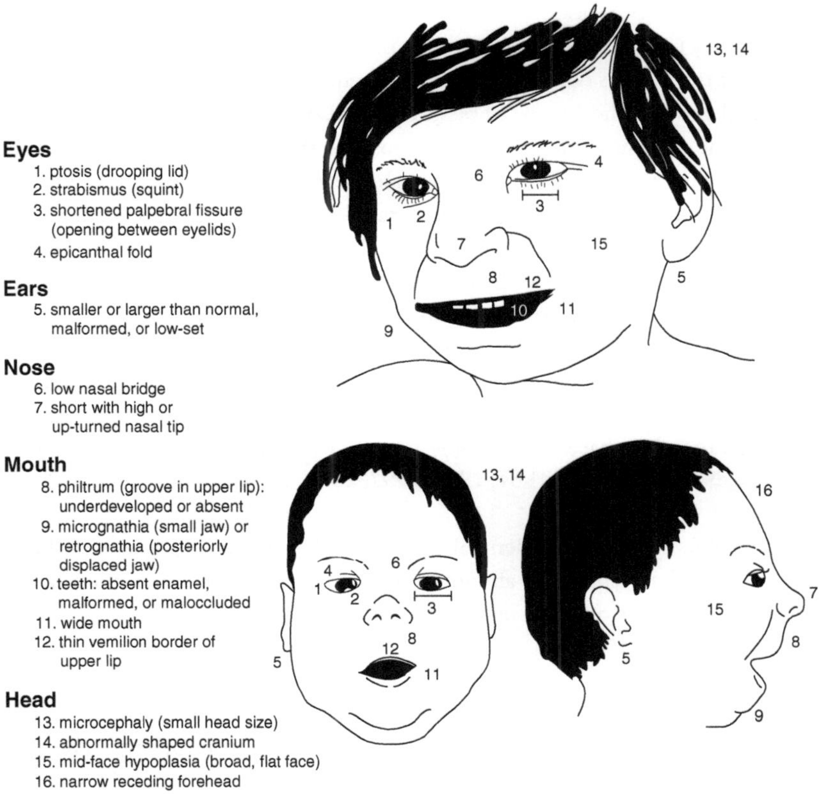

FIGURE 2.4 FAS/FASD: Infant and Child Cranial and Facial Characteristics

questionnaires" (p. 209). Thus, several researchers (e.g., Crunelle, Yegles, & van Nuijs, 2014; Pragst & Yegles, 2008) have recommended the analytical laboratory analysis of maternal hair samples for the presence and level of fatty acid ethyl esters and/or ethyl glucuronide to determine whether alcohol was consumed during pregnancy and the associated level of alcohol use (e.g., low, moderate, or heavy drinking).[26]

[26] N.B. A wide variety of "biomarkers" have been identified and used to obtain better biological assessments of women's alcohol use during the gestational period. These *indirect* measures of maternal BACs have been used in place of *direct* measures because alcohol has a relatively short and variable half-life of elimination (i.e., is subject to significant genetic and dose-dependent effects) and, consequently, is only of value in terms of determining acute intoxication or relatively recent alcohol use. The biomarkers that have been used generally measure either maternal alcohol-induced pathology or derivatives of non-oxidative alcohol metabolism. They include: alanine aminotransferase; acetaldehyde-derived conjugates; aspartate aminotransferase; fatty acid ethyl esters; ethyl glucuronide; ethyl sulfate; gamma glutamyl transferase; mean corpuscular volume; and phosphatidylethanol (Joya, Friguls, & Ortigosa, 2012).

Serum microRNAs also have served as biomarkers of women's alcohol use during pregnancy (e.g., Gardiner, Gutierrez, & Luo, 2016). In addition, some researchers also suggest the analysis of neonatal biological samples (e.g., hair; meconium), as well as placental and umbilical cord samples. Kvigne, Randall, and Simanton (2012) have suggested the analysis of neonatal BACs, positing that *increased* fetal alcohol dehydrogenase activity (as determined by increased alcohol elimination rates) would be indicative of their mother's regular, long-term alcohol use during pregnancy.

The safety of women's alcohol ingestion during pregnancy (i.e., from conception to birth) has *not* been well-documented and appears to be *highly* variable. The ingestion of up to *2* drinks per day by pregnant women has been generally considered to be *safe* for the fetus. However, because of the serious and irreversible, long-term physical and psychological defects (e.g., behavioral problems; developmental deficits, including learning deficits) associated with FAS/FASD, we have long recommended that women *completely avoid* the use of alcohol during pregnancy (Pagliaro & Pagliaro, 1987, 1996, 1997, 2000, 2002, 2003, 2009, 2012).

> In 2005, the Surgeon General issued an advisory urging women who are or might be pregnant to abstain from alcohol consumption to eliminate the risk for FASDs or other negative birth outcomes.
>
> *(Tan, Denny, & Cheal, 2015, p. 1042)*

Despite these recommendations, a significant number of pregnant women in the U.S. consume alcohol and many of these women knowingly engage in patterns of binge drinking while pregnant (Marchetta, Denny, & Floyd, 2012; Tan, Denny, & Cheal, 2015). In a large sample of "women with pregnancies that resulted in a live birth," 14% (i.e., approximately, 1 in 7) engaged in preconception binge drinking. These women tended to be single and of European descent. They also were found to be more likely to continue to *both* drink alcohol and smoke tobacco cigarettes during their pregnancies (Naimi, Lipscomb, & Brewer, 2003).

In addition, May, Keaster, and Bozeman (2015, p. 118), in their study of the mothers of 1,278 children, found that the mothers of children with FAS were significantly *more* likely to have:

- Increased depression
- Later recognition that they were pregnant
- Lower educational achievement
- Reported marijuana and methamphetamine use during their pregnancy

Montag (2016), in a review of published FASD studies, additionally noted significant correlations with other factors:

- Lower socioeconomic status
- Older age

- Single/unmarried
- Unemployed

> Among pregnant women aged 15 to 44 in 2012–2013, an annual average of 9.4 percent reported current alcohol use, 2.3 percent reported binge drinking, and 0.4 percent reported heavy drinking.
>
> *(SAMHSA, 2014, p. 37)*

Drinking patterns and rates among pregnant women also may, however, be *significantly* affected by age cohort. For example, Ethen, Ramadhani, and Scheurle (2009) reported alcohol drinking during pregnancy for over 30% of women who were 30 years-of-age or older. In addition, Denny, Tsai, and Floyd (2009) reported alcohol drinking during pregnancy for 17.7% of women who were 35 to 44 years-of-age as did the CDC in their analyses of data from the 2006 to 2010 *Behavioral Risk Factor Surveillance System* (BRFSS):

> Among pregnant women, the highest prevalence estimates of reported alcohol use were among those aged 35–44 years.
>
> *(p. 529)*

As more recently identified by Wilsnack, Wilsnack, and Wolfgang Kantor (2013), pregnant women in their thirties and forties are *more* likely to drink than are pregnant teens and women in their twenties.

While published data since 1977 have implicated FAS with *high* maternal BACs during a critical time of embryonic or fetal development, the average daily alcohol consumption during pregnancy may *not* be as important as maximal concentrations obtained during binge drinking at critical periods. For example, alcohol consumption during pregnancy, particularly during the first trimester, has been associated with an *increased* risk for miscarriage (Avalos, Roberts, & Kaskutas, 2014).

Available data suggest that *neuronal apoptosis*,[27] induced by maternal alcohol consumption during pregnancy, may be the underlying pathophysiologic basis for the development of the FAS/FASD and its associated neurobehavioral deficits and impairments (Olney, Wozniak, & Jevtovic-Todorovic, 2002). In this case, the third trimester of pregnancy, which correlates with the beginning of the brain growth spurt period, would appear to be the time of *maximal* vulnerability for the development of FAS/FASD (Ikonomidou, Bittigau, & Koch, 2001).

Producers and marketers of alcohol have included warnings to women in their advertising that drinking alcohol during pregnancy should be avoided because

[27] Neuronal apoptosis is the process by which brain cells *disintegrate* into particles that are consumed by other cells (e.g., leukocytes, macrophages). Thus, the process of brain growth and development is prevented, inhibited, or slowed.

of the possible risk for FAS/FASD. In addition, concerned groups have worked to encourage the display of signs—in bars and liquor stores—warning pregnant women *not* to drink during pregnancy because of the noted association between alcohol use and birth defects. During the new millennium, the use of alcohol has been identified as a form of child abuse and neglect and has resulted in legal action, in some jurisdictions, against women who excessively drink during pregnancy and, subsequently, give birth to infants with FAS/FASD.

As noted by the *National Institutes on Alcohol Abuse and Alcoholism* (NIAAA), "State and Federal governments have established various policies in response to the risks associated with drinking during pregnancy" (Pregnancy and alcohol, 2015, p. 1). As further explained by Thomas, Cannon, and French (2015, p. 68):

> U.S. states have enacted a wide range of laws to address health challenges associated with alcohol use during pregnancy. Some have taken punitive approaches that restrain women's behavior, and some have taken supportive approaches aimed at improving women's health and supporting healthy pregnancies.[28]

Although these and other prevention efforts have been made, the incidence of FAS/FASD in the U.S. remains at a significantly *high* level and, unfortunately, is *increasing* among women of American Indian descent (see Table 2.4) (Eustace, Kang, & Coombs, 2003; Hanson, Winberg, & Elliott, 2012; Pagliaro & Pagliaro, 2009, 2012).[29] As identified in several studies and reports (e.g., Hanson, Winberg, & Elliott, 2012; Khan, Robinson, & Smith, 2013), including data from the Indian Health Services (IHS), in some Alaska Native and American Indian communities/

---

[28] For further related discussion, see the *Alcohol Policy Information System* (Hilton, 2014; Thomas, Cannon, & French, 2015).

[29] The significant variance noted in the reported incidence of FAS/FASD in Table 2.4 is primarily the result of *five* major factors: (1) genetics; (2) culture (societal drinking patterns); (3) year that the assessment was performed (i.e., societal drinking patterns change over time); (4) the criteria used to define FAS/FASD (e.g., all cases versus only clinically severe cases); and (5) experience and competence of researchers or research assistants (e.g., nurses; occupational speech therapists; physicians; psychologists) to note *mild* cases and be able to rule out potentially overlapping conditions and syndromes that may affect appropriate diagnoses of FAS/FASD (e.g., Aarskog-Scott syndrome; Dubowitz syndrome; fetal anticonvulsant syndrome; toluene embryopathy; and Williams syndrome). These factors are supported by several findings reported in the related published literature. For example, as identified by Chasnoff, Wells, and King (2015), "high rates of missed diagnoses and misdiagnosis" are commonly observed regarding FAS/FASD (p. 264). Rojmahamongkol, Cheema-Hasan, and Weitzman (2015) found that "pediatricians underrecognize FASDs, lack confidence in making this diagnosis, and are unfamiliar with the diagnostic criteria" (p. 197). Finally, several researchers have provided additional insights into the reasons for these related observations in reported incidence of FAS/FASD. For example, Douzgou, Breen, and Crow (2012, p. 812) found that "classification of FASD was difficult in children under a year old when data on growth and development were limited." Others (e.g., Cook, Courtney, & Lilley, 2016) provided revised guidelines to facilitate the diagnosis of FAS/FASD.

TABLE 2.4 Reported Incidence of FAS/FASD in the U.S. and Other Countries, Continents, and Geographic Areas

Country, Continent, or Other Geographic Area (Ethnic or Racial Group)	*Incidence per 1,000 Live Births*[a]	*References*
Australia		
(Aboriginal Australians)[b]	120	Fitzpatrick, Latimer, & Carter, 2015
(Mixed Population Groups)[c]	0.7 to 5[d]	Harris & Bucens, 2003
Canada		
(Aboriginal Peoples)	25 to 46	Asante & Nelms-Matzke, 1985
	100	Square, 1997
	190	Robinson, Conry, & Conry, 1987
(Mixed Population Groups)	0.6	Habbick, Nanson, & Snyder, 1996
	7 to 14	Williams, Odaibo, & McGee, 1999
	14 to 44	Thanh, Jonsson, & Salmon, 2014
Croatia		
(Mixed Population Groups)	67	Petkovic & Barisic, 2013
Europe		
(Mixed Population Groups)	2 to 3	Hill, Hegemier, & Tennyson, 1989
Italy		
(Mixed Population Groups)	4 to 12	May, Fiorentino, & Coriale, 2011
South Africa		
(Mixed Population Groups)	44	CDC, 2003
	68 to 92	May, Gossage, & Marais, 2007
	75 to 170	May, Blankenship, & Marais, 2013
	182 to 259[e]	May, de Vries, & Marais, 2016
United States		
(Alaska Natives)	3 to 5[f]	Egeland, Perham-Hester, & Gessner, 1998
(American Indians)	3	Chavez, Cordero, & Becerra, 1988
	4 to 8	Duimstra, Johnson, & Kutsch, 1993
	10	May, Hymbaugh, & Aase, 1983
	5 to 30	May, 1991
(Mixed Population Groups)	0.3[g]	Fox, Pettygrove, & Cunniff, 2015
	0.3 to 1.5[h]	CDC, 2002
	0.5 to 2	May & Gossage, 2001
	1	Rosett, Weiner, & Lee, 1983
	1.3	Bertucci & Krafchik, 1994
	2[i]	Abel, 1995
	2 to 3	Hill, Hegemier, & Tennyson, 1989
	2 to 7	May, Gossage, & Kalberg, 2009
	9	Sampson, Streissguth, & Bookstein, 1997
	11 to 25	May, Keaster, & Bozeman, 2015
	14 to 36	May, Baete, & Russo, 2014

TABLE 2.4 *(cont.)*

Country, Continent, or Other Geographic Area (Ethnic or Racial Group)	*Incidence per 1,000 Live Births*[a]	*References*
Western World		
(Mixed Population Groups)	0.3[j]	Abel & Sokol, 1991
	1 to 2	Clarren & Smith, 1978
Worldwide		
(Mixed Population Groups	2	Abel & Sokol, 1987

[a] Although most often reported as "incidence per 1,000 births," a variety of measurement criteria were used by the various authors (e.g., incidence per 1,000: live births; pregnancies; or children sampled).

[b] Western Australia.

[c] Northern Australia.

[d] Highest among Aboriginal Australians.

[e] Data obtained from a *highly* rural, agricultural, and *low* socioeconomic region.

[f] Significant variance by year of birth.

[g] *Highest* among women of Alaska Native descent and American Indian descent.

[h] *Highest* among women of African continental descent, Alaska Native descent, and American Indian descent.

[i] *Highest* among women of African continental descent, Alaska Native descent, and American Indian descent.

[j] Incidence of 0.3 among women of European continental descent and 0.5 among women of African continental descent.

reservations, women's use of alcohol during pregnancy has *exceeded* 50%, particularly during the first trimester.

> Popular Notion: Children with FAS/FASD will "outgrow" most of their associated mental and physical deficits during adolescence and young adulthood.
>
> NOT TRUE. FAS/FASD is a *permanent* life-long syndrome/disorder.

The developmental deficits that are generally associated with FAS/FASD—both mental and physical—do *not* end in infancy, but persist into childhood, adolescence, and throughout adulthood (Pagliaro & Pagliaro, 2012; Smitherman, 1994; Spohr, Willms, & Steinhausen, 1993, 2007; Streissguth, Randels, & Smith, 1991). Unfortunately, even with early identification and intervention, "the growth and neurological disabilities associated with alcohol consumption during pregnancy persist—even when the child grows up in a good home" (Karp, Qazi, & Hittleman, 1993, p. 101).

For example, common problems include: behavioral problems, such as a higher incidence of attention-deficit/hyperactivity disorder (A-D/HD), conduct disorder (CD), and externalizing behavior (e.g., acting out, aggressiveness, delinquency, and hostility) (Bada, Das, & Bauer, 2007; Pagliaro & Pagliaro, 2002, 2012; Sood, Delaney-Black, & Covington, 2001). These behavioral problems are *not* easily managed, even with appropriate pharmacotherapy or psychotherapy.

While the life-long effects of FAS/FASD require *increased* attention, greater focus on prevention of the disorder and, when it is identified, appropriate and effective treatment is required. In this regard, we have long concurred with Streissguth, Randels, and Smith (1991) that, for infants and children affected with FAS/FASD—and their parents and caregivers—less frustration and optimal behavioral outcomes during later adolescence and adulthood are most likely to be achieved with:

- Realistic expectations for performance during childhood and adolescence
- Availability of more appropriate educational and healthcare services

As noted over 25 years ago by Karp, Qazi, and Hittleman (1993), and many others (e.g., Spohr, Willms, & Steinhausen, 2007), FAS/FASD is a *permanent disease* in the literal sense (i.e., it *cannot* be reversed or cured).[30] Thus, it is essential that prevention and treatment programs be developed to assist women of reproductive age, including adolescent girls, to understand the: (1) risks associated with alcohol use during pregnancy; and (2) need to discontinue use, particularly, if they are sexually active (and do *not* appropriately use available methods of birth control), or are pregnant. Attention also is needed regarding relapse prevention for women who have histories of abusive or compulsive use of alcohol, including binge drinking, and for whom abstinence during pregnancy may be difficult to achieve or maintain.

Mothering. A woman's affectionate care of her neonate, infant, toddler, preschooler, child, or adolescent comprises natural[31] and uniquely learned *physical*, *mental*, and *sociocultural* behaviors, as well as concurrent behavioral responses from her offspring, that lead to the healthy and optimal development of her offspring. Unfortunately, for women, who abuse alcohol and other drugs and substances of

[30] However, although FAS/FASD, as a teratogenic effect, is life-long and incurable, it *is* treatable, and important advances have been made in this regard (Bertrand, 2009). As noted by Chudley, Conry, and Cook (2005), infants, children, and adolescents who have been diagnosed with FAS/FASD have an opportunity to achieve optimal outcomes with the help of specialized core teams of experts in the disorder, including: (1) nurses and social workers with expertise in case management and coordination of core team member activities; (2) physicians specially trained in diagnosis and medical management of FAS/FASD; (3) clinical infant, child, and adolescent psychologists; (4) occupational therapists; and (5) speech language pathologists. These core team members, along with parents and caregivers, child care workers, family therapists, and teachers can help infants, children and adolescents who are diagnosed with FAS/FASD achieve optimal personal outcomes.

[31] Natural, or "innate" responses are generally associated with maternal instinct, as well as various ovarian and pituitary hormones (e.g., estradiol, oxytocin).

abuse, mothering abilities can be lost—or destroyed, often with decidedly deleterious, and often inter-generational, effects among offspring, particularly daughters (Pagliaro & Pagliaro, *Clinical Patient Data Files*).

A "special bulletin" for health and social care professionals, published by the U.S. Department of Health and Human Services, identified several deleterious outcomes associated with ineffective or inconsistent parenting due to a parent's alcohol and other drug or substance abuse:

- Physical or mental impairment
- Reduced capacity to respond to a child's cues and needs
- Difficulties regulating emotions and controlling anger and impulsivity
- Disruptions in healthy parent-child attachment
- Spending limited funds on alcohol and drugs rather than food or other household needs
- Spending time seeking out, manufacturing, or using alcohol or other drugs
- Incarceration, which can result in inadequate or inappropriate supervision of children
- Estrangement from family and other social supports

(Child Welfare Information Gateway, 2014, p. 3)

As aptly noted by Connors, Bradley, and Whiteside Mansell (2003) in their longitudinal national study of women and their children from 50 publicly-funded residential substance abuse treatment programs:

> Findings from this study suggest that children whose mothers abuse alcohol or other drugs confront a high level of risk and are at increased vulnerability for physical, academic, and socioemotional problems. Children affected by maternal addiction are in need of long-term supportive services.
>
> *(p. 744)*

A related "fact sheet" published by the WHO, "Child Maltreatment and Alcohol," identified that:

1. Numerous studies have established that alcohol is a significant contributory factor to child maltreatment
2. In the USA, 35% of offenders of parental child abuse had consumed either alcohol or drugs at the time of the incident

(Butchart, Poznyak, & Bellis, 2006, pp. 1, 3)

As illustrated in the following two vignettes:

> A one-year-old baby covered in vomit and feces was discovered in the backseat of a car when officers in West Virginia pulled over a driver for a

> suspected DUI … the driver of the vehicle—the child's mother—was too intoxicated to answer when she was asked for the child's name.
>
> *(Sung, 2016, p. 1)*

> Lehnardt told her Alcoholics Anonymous sponsor of a wild night in April that led to the mother losing custody of her children … she allowed the teens to smoke pot and drink booze in her home. The mother also joined the groups in a game of naked Twister. According to the police report, the mother left the game to have sex with an 18-year-old in the bathroom. The report said Lehnardt awoke around 3:30 am to find her daughter's 16-year-old boyfriend having sex with her [16 year-old-daughter].
>
> *(Frisk, 2016, p. 1)*

Breast Cancer. Several studies have identified a relationship between regular, long-term alcohol abuse and some forms of cancer, particularly rectal cancer among men (e.g., Mizoue, Tanaka, & Tsuji, 2006; Slattery, Wolff, & Herrick, 2010),[32] and breast cancer among women (Aronson, 2003; Cao, Willett, & Rimm, 2015; Feigelson, Jonas, & Robertson, 2003).[33] The association between *light* to *moderate* alcohol consumption and breast cancer has been consistently supported (Brooks & Zakhari, 2013; Cao, Willett, & Rimm, 2015; Liu, Nguyen, & Colditz, 2015). Noting that breast tissue is particularly susceptible to carcinogens between menarche and first full-term pregnancy, Liu, Colditz, and Rosner (2013) evaluated data from over 91,000 parous women in the *Nurses' Health Study II.* They found that, "Alcohol consumption between menarche and first pregnancy was consistently associated with a significant *increased* risk of proliferative benign breast disease and breast cancer" (p. 1571).

However, as noted by Zakhari and Hoek (2015, p. 7), breast cancer is "a heterogeneous and polygenic disease which is further influenced by epigenic mechanisms." Consequently, even if alcohol is a *directly* related causative factor in the development of breast cancer, it is only *one* of several significant contributory factors (e.g., genetic risk/predisposition [polymorphisms]; hormonal status; nutritional factors; and other co-carcinogens, such as tobacco smoking) (Pagliaro & Pagliaro, 2009; Scoccianti, Lauby-Secretan, & Bello, 2014).

---

[32] It is believed that the congeners of alcohol (i.e., chemicals that impart a pleasant aroma and flavor to the fermented beverage), which are formed during the brewing process, may be the major contributory factor for the increased risk for rectal cancer associated with the drinking of beer. This hypothesis is substantiated by the observation of significantly less risk (i.e., lower associated incidence of rectal cancer) when alcohol is consumed in the form of wine or distilled spirits (Pedersen, Johansen, & Gronbaek, 2003).

[33] Heavy alcohol consumption (i.e., 4 or more drinks per day) also is associated with a significant *increased* risk for esophageal, oral, and pancreatic cancers (Pelucchi, Tramacere, & Boffetta, 2011). Wu, Li, and Qureshi (2015) found that *increased* alcohol intake also was associated with an *increased* risk for developing cutaneous basal cell carcinoma.

Depression and Suicide. Using criteria specified in the *Diagnostic and Statistical Manual of Mental Disorders* (DSM), diagnoses of alcohol use disorder and major depressive disorder occur commonly among both women and men who are regular, long-term drinkers. (See related discussion in Chapter 7, *Identifying Women's Contemporaneous Diagnoses.*) This combination of disorders is *highly* correlated with the risk for suicide attempts and completions. As noted by Bailey, Patel, and Avenido (2011, p. 614), "Individuals with severe clinical depression and alcohol use disorders are at high risk [for suicide] if untreated." Whether depression precedes, or follows, alcohol abuse has *not* yet been fully determined. Very likely, it differs among different women—preceding for some, following for others, and co-occurring for still others (Pagliaro & Pagliaro, 2012). Suicide attempts are typically 5 to 10 times *higher* for women who have alcoholism when compared to women who do *not.*

Heart Disease. Regular, long-term use of alcohol is associated with the development of arteriosclerosis and dilated cardiomyopathies,[34] including damage to the heart muscle, or myocardium. Many women are surprised that the long-term, regular use of alcohol is associated with cardiovascular disease, including heart attacks. However, in fact, women, who have alcoholism, die from cardiovascular disease *more* often than from any other alcohol-related pathology. Regular, long-term alcohol use also is associated with inflammation of the stomach and pancreas (i.e., *gastritis* and *pancreatitis*).

Although some published research studies support claims that the daily consumption of relatively small amounts of alcohol (i.e., 1 or 2 glasses of red wine) may *reduce* the risk for coronary artery disease, there is significant evidence that the regular, long-term ingestion of *large* quantities of alcohol predisposes women, who drink, to coronary artery disease and such related conditions as angina pectoris, congestive heart failure, and hypertension (Lee & Regan, 2002). Cardiac dysrhythmias also are common among women who are heavy drinkers.

Liver Disease. The regular, long-term abuse of alcohol produces both *reversible* and *irreversible* changes in liver structure and function resulting in hepatitis and cirrhosis of the liver—the seventh *most* common cause of death in the U.S. (Rehm, Taylor, & Mohopatra, 2010).

> Among females in 2009, American Indians or Alaska Natives were the most likely to die of chronic liver disease and cirrhosis—at the rate of 22 per

[34] Cardiomyopathy is a disease of the heart muscle that involves electrical dysfunction of the heart. Associated signs and symptoms include: chest pain; dizziness; fainting; fatigue; and shortness of breath. Dilated cardiomyopathy is characterized by: dilation of the lower chambers of the heart (i.e., right and left ventricles); increase in myocardial mass; and thinning of the walls of the chambers of the heart. Regular long-term *heavy* alcohol use causes a non-ischemic, dilated cardiomyopathy among men and women of all continental descents in the U.S. In its early stages, there are usually *no* signs and symptoms. However, in its latter stages, heart failure, ventricular dysrhythmias, and sudden death can occur (Jefferies & Towbin, 2010; Piano, 2002).

> 100,000. Rates for females who are Hispanic (9 per 100,000), while non-white-Hispanic (6 per 100,000), black non-Hispanic (5 per 100,000), and Asian or Pacific Islander (3 per 100,000) were considerably lower.
>
> *(Clayton, Brooks, & Kornstein, 2014, p. 90)*

Motor Vehicle Crashes. Motor vehicle crashes are a leading cause of death in the U.S. Drunk driving, once clearly and predominantly associated with young men, has increasingly become commonly associated with women. As noted by Glaser (2013):

> In the nine years between 1998 and 2007, the number of women arrested for drunken driving rose 30%, while male arrests dropped more than 7%.[35]
>
> *(p. 1)*

Thus, although more men than women in the U.S. drive while impaired and are arrested for driving under the influence (DUI), the observed trend and trajectory during the new millennium support the increases noted among women and the decreases noted among men (e.g., Robertson, Liew, & Gardner, 2011; Schwartz, 2008; Schwartz & Davaran, 2013). In addition, this observation is consistent with the *increased* rates of binge drinking identified among women (see later section, "Binge Drinking") and the association noted between binge drinking and driving (Naimi, Nelson, & Brewer, 2009). These changes have been bolstered by associated changes in related enforcement efforts: (1) change in state drunk driving laws that *reduce* the requisite BAC for intoxication from 0.10 gram % to 0.08 gram %;[36] and (2) *increased* use of specialized DUI-enforcement efforts, such as "Check Stops" (Schwartz, 2008; Schwartz & Davaran, 2013).

Wernicke-Korsakoff Syndrome. Wernicke-Korsakoff Syndrome is a major syndrome associated with the regular, long-term heavy abuse of alcohol (i.e., *severe* alcoholism). However, this syndrome, comprised of Wernicke's encephalopathy and Korsakoff's psychosis, is *not* directly caused by alcohol, itself, but by a vitamin B_1 (i.e., thiamine) deficiency. This vitamin deficiency occurs because of inadequate nutrition[37]—a condition that is commonly observed among women who have

---

35 The Federal Bureau of Investigation, cited by McCutcheon, Agrawal, and Heath (2011, p. 1895), similarly reported that, "Women accounted for an increasing proportion of individuals arrested for DUI. Arrests of women for DUI rose 31% but decreased 11% for men between 2000 and 2009."

36 Interestingly, Jones and Harding (2013), in a study involving data from a forensic laboratory in Wisconsin, found that 35% of women arrested, and, subsequently, tested for DUI, had a BAC *higher* than 0.40 gram %.

37 It has long been asserted that the diuretic effect associated with alcohol (and the large related amounts of fluid generally consumed—for example, in the context of drinking beer) contribute to this syndrome by promoting the additional loss, by urinary excretion, of the water-soluble, vitamin B1 (thiamine) (Pagliaro & Pagliaro, *Clinical Patient Data Files*).

severe chronic alcoholism. *Severe* chronic alcoholism can occur among women of *all* continental descents and socioeconomic backgrounds. However, it is particularly prevalent among "homeless" women, who "live on the street," or in hostels that are provided by the Salvation Army or other charities and social agencies.

Korsakoff's psychosis is characterized by *increasing* memory impairment as *severe* brain damage occurs. Because the syndrome is characterized by ataxia, confusion, diplopia, disorientation, hallucinations, hypotension, memory failure, and muscular spasticity (i.e., common signs and symptoms associated with acute alcohol intoxication), it is often confused with the acute state of alcohol intoxication—particularly, by law enforcement officers. The treatment for this condition involves thiamine (i.e., vitamin B_1) replacement, the establishment of proper nutrition, and supportive care. However, even with appropriate treatment, the prognosis for this condition is poor—primarily, because of continued alcohol abuse. Only 20% of people diagnosed as having Korsakoff's psychosis are cured, 30% have little to moderate improvement, and 50% demonstrate *no* improvement (Pagliaro & Pagliaro, *Clinical Patient Data Files*).

Physical and Sexual Abuse. Sexual performance generally *decreases* as a direct response to *increases* in alcohol ingestion. However, of all of the commonly used drugs and substances of abuse, *alcohol* is by far the one that is *most* often used for the perpetration of sexual assault, including date rape (Madea & MuBhoff, 2009; Pagliaro & Pagliaro, 2009, 2012).[38] Alcohol intoxication places women at *increased* risk for victimization (e.g., date rape; sexual assault) (McCauley, Calhoun, & Gidycz, 2010; Parkhill, Norris, & Davi, 2014; Testa, Hoffman, & Livingston, 2010).[39] As noted by Shorey, Moore, and McNulty (2016):

> Research has demonstrated substance use, most notably alcohol use, to be associated with female dating violence victimization.
>
> *(p. 509)*

This is quite common, particularly among young women, including college/university students who binge drink (Gilmore, Stappenbeck, & Lewis, 2015; Mouilso, Fischer, & Calhoun, 2012; Pagliaro & Pagliaro, 2009, 2012). As noted in a related "Fact Sheet," from the Centers for Disease Control and Prevention:

---

[38] Other sedative-hypnotics are often associated with alcohol use in the perpetration of date rape, including, for example, methaqualone (Quaalude®), which allegedly was used by the actor and comedian, Bill Cosby (Carpentier, 2015; Michaelson, 2015).

[39] In addition, a medical/social history of IPV and/or childhood sexual abuse has been identified by several researchers (e.g., Hannan, Orcutt, & Miron, 2015; Hughes, Johnson, & Wilsnack, 2001; Ullman & Sigurvinsdottir, 2015) as a significant risk factor for the development of women's harmful patterns of alcohol use. Unfortunately, this pattern reflects a tragic cycle of alcohol use and harm (i.e., alcohol abuse leads to sexual abuse that leads to alcohol abuse, that leads to further sexual abuse, and so on).

> Binge drinking is a risk factor for sexual assault, especially among young women in college settings. Each year, about 1 in 20 college women are sexually assaulted. Research suggests that there is an increase in the risk of rape or sexual assault when both the attacker and victim have used alcohol prior to the attack.
>
> *(CDC, 2016, p. 1)*

As further noted by Shorey, Moore, and McNulty (2016):

> Findings from the current study demonstrated that the odds of dating violence victimization on college women (psychological, physical, and sexual) were increased on drinking days, heavy drinking days, and as the number of drinks increased by the victim.
>
> *(p. 516)*

Alcohol intoxication also *promotes* risky sexual behavior among women of *all* continental descents in the U.S., including bisexual women and lesbians (George, Davis, & Masters, 2014; Hughes, Szalacha & Johnson, 2010). For example, Sales, Brown, and Vissman (2012), in a review of 32 studies examining the association between alcohol use and sexual risk behaviors among women of African descent found that: "increased use of alcohol is associated with increased sexual risk practices among African-American females" (p. 117) with associated increased risk of STDs, including HIV infection.

Intimate partner violence (IPV) has been *positively* correlated with drug and substance abuse among women and their intimate partners (Afifi, Henriksen, & Asmundson, 2012). (Also, see related discussion in Chapter 5, *Women's Amphetamine and Cocaine Abuse.*) Alcohol intoxication and AUDs are the drug and substance abuse disorders that are *most* strongly associated with IPV (Smith, Homish, & Leonard, 2012). Several studies (e.g., Devries, Child, & Bacchus, 2014) suggest the possibility of the *bi-directional* nature of these observed relationships. For example, in some cases, women who suffer IPV are victims or, less often, perpetrators, because of their own, or their partner's abuse of alcohol. In other cases, women may abuse alcohol as a "self-medication" to cope, or deal with, their experience of IPV.

Overdosage

Alcohol overdosages are generally self-limiting among women, who are regular, long-term heavy drinkers, because they usually end their heavy drinking episodes by simply falling asleep. (Also, see earlier section, *Pharmacokinetics*, "Absorption," for related discussion of "drinking games.")[40] However, a troubling trend, over

[40] Also, commonly associated with acute, non-fatal overdosages of alcohol are hangovers that occur during the post-drinking recovery phase. (See additional related discussion in the earlier section, "Hangovers.")

the last 2 decades, is the *increasing* number of fatalities associated with women's concurrent abuse of alcohol and other psychodepressants. As reported by Jones, Paulozzi, and Mack (2014), working on behalf of the FDA and CDC, "alcohol was involved in 22.1% of opiate pain reliever and 21.4% of benzodiazepine drug-related deaths" (p. 881). The synergistic *CNS* and *respiratory* depressant actions of alcohol, when concurrently used with opiate analgesics and/or benzodiazepines, accounts for these *increased* mortality rates.

Women's Medical and Personal Alcohol Use and Abuse

Women's alcohol abuse has generally demonstrated many historical patterns during the last century and the first 2 decades of the new millennium in the U.S. Although for men, drinking any form of "hard liquor" was culturally accepted and fostered as a *desired* behavior associated with masculinity, or "manliness," and *proved* by the ability to drink everyone else under the table—for women it was an "un-lady-like" behavior that was *frowned* upon by society. "Proper" women often sipped fancy alcoholic drinks at social functions or carefully hid their bottles of alcohol and secretly drank alone in their homes.

Some of these sociocultural differences in men's and women's alcohol use and other traditional role expectations have continued into the 21st century, particularly among men and women of Hispanic descent. However, for most women in the U.S., the new millennium has coincided with new freedoms—including the freedom to "drink like men."

Women's Medical Alcohol Use/Abuse

Since its introduction to North America by European explorers and traders, alcohol was used to treat such varied conditions as the common cold and "rheumatism." Until approximately 70 years ago, alcohol was medically classified as a *CNS stimulant* and was administered by nurses by the "syringeful" when "rapid stimulation" was required" (Pagliaro, 1986, p. 10). It also was thought to possess nutritive and other benefits.

For the last 50 years, the *only* medical use for alcohol, other than its use as a topical antiseptic at injection sites, has been its use as a vehicle for the preparation of various pharmaceutical formulations (i.e., alcohol-containing solutions and elixirs). In response to both public and healthcare provider demands for *alcohol-free* liquid pharmaceutical products, particularly those formulated for children and older adults, who may have difficulty swallowing, the use of alcohol for the preparation of various pharmaceutical products has *decreased* significantly.[41] However,

[41] A commensurate reduction in the alcohol content of personal care products (e.g., aftershave; mouth wash) also has occurred during the new millennium. However, the reason for this reduction is to *deter* the use of these products by chronic, "skid-row" women, who are alcoholics and who often

several prescription and non-prescription (i.e., over-the-counter) pharmaceutical formulations currently contain alcohol, including many:

- Liquid cough and cold formulations, such as Ambenyl®, Benylin®, Dilaudid Cough Syrup®, Novahistine®, Robitussin®, and Vicks®
- Liquid vitamin drops, such as Ce-Vi-Sol®, Geritol®, and Nu-Iron®
- Mouth washes, such as Cepacol®, Colgate®, and Listerine®

Health and social care professionals should be aware of the alcohol content of these and other pharmaceutical drug products, particularly when working in settings[42] where women, who are regular, long-term abusers of alcohol, may substitute these products when beverage alcohol is unavailable to them. For example, when they are unable to purchase alcohol, obtain some from a friend, or are restricted from using it (e.g., when jailed or enrolled in drug treatment programs). In addition, it is particularly important for health and social care professionals to be aware of these data if women with drinking histories are initiating or being treated with *disulfiram* (Antabuse®) therapy, which requires a total restriction of the use of alcohol, because of the associated possibility of triggering an alcohol-induced *disulfiram reaction* (see Chapter 8, *Preventing and Treating Women's Drug and Substance Abuse*).

Women's Personal Alcohol Use/Abuse

Over the last 15 years, approximately 80% of adults in the U.S. regularly consumed alcoholic beverages. Over 25% of these men and women reported having consumed alcohol on more than 100 days during the past year (Alcohol Use USA, 2010). The incidence of alcoholism (see later discussion) is approximately 15% of the *entire* U.S. adult population.

Drinking among women in the U.S. during the new millennium, and its related harmful effects and toxicities, is rapidly closing the gender gap and increasingly reflects, as noted by Schmidt (2014) and many others (e.g., Pagliaro & Pagliaro, *Clinical Patient Data Files*), women's "equal right to drink" (see earlier discussion).[43]

desperately resort to drinking them to get "totally plastered" or avoid "getting sick" (i.e., to get drunk or to prevent, or self-manage, the alcohol withdrawal syndrome) at times when they are otherwise unable to obtain their usual wine, whiskey, or other alcoholic beverages (Pagliaro & Pagliaro, *Clinical Patient Data Files*). Because of the limited availability of personal care products that contain alcohol, a related concern is women resorting to drinking household cleaning products that contain alcohol (e.g., ("decanting" Lysol® Disinfectant Spray) for the same reasons.

42 These settings include, for example: convenience stores; grocery stores; and pharmacies—particularly those located in, or near, alcohol-free Indian reservations and inner city neighborhoods (Pagliaro & Pagliaro, *Clinical Patient Data Files*).

43 This view is not universally endorsed. For example, Roberts (2012) reported that the "most significant findings" (from this study) suggest that *higher* levels of equality are associated with less alcohol

In the current context of this equality, the initiation of alcohol use—and the development of alcohol-related problems—are not only occurring among increasing numbers of women, but are beginning at younger and younger ages. Women, who are at particular risk for AUDs, include:

- Women who are in their twenties
- Women who are in their sixties
- Women who are of Alaska Native or American Indian descent
- Women who are poor, particularly those who are homeless
- Women who have PTSD, including that associated with IPV and childhood or adulthood sexual abuse
- Women who have a genetic predisposition for alcoholism (i.e., positive family history of AUDs)
- Women who have histories of child abuse or neglect
- Women who identify as bisexual, lesbian, or trans

(Forcehimes, Venner, & Bogenschutz, 2011; Green & Feinstein, 2012; Pagliaro & Pagliaro, 2000; Spatz Widom, Raskin White, & Czaja, 2007)

Unfortunately, several physiological differences (e.g., *increased* body fat among women; *decreased* alcohol metabolism among women) make women *more* vulnerable than men to both the acute and chronic effects associated with alcohol use, including the development of physical dependence (see earlier related discussion in this chapter)—despite having used less alcohol and using it for a shorter period of time.[44] This accelerated progression to alcohol dependence among women, when compared to men, has been identified as the "telescoping effect" (Clarke, Kim, & White, 2013; Diehl, Croissant, & Batra, 2007; Greenfield, Back, & Lawson, 2010; Keyes, Martins, & Blanco, 2010; Stewart, 2009; Zilberman, Tavares, & el-Guebaly, 2003). For example, as noted by Hernandez-Avila, Rounsaville, and Kranzler (2004, p. 265):

> Alcohol-dependent women progress faster from onset of alcohol drinking to entry into treatment, experiencing an earlier onset (i.e., "telescoping") of alcohol-related complications.

---

consumption overall" (p. 60). However, it was identified that the study used "multi-level linear and logistic regression models adjusted for individual demographics as well as state-level income inequality, median income, and % Evangelical Protestant/Mormon" (p. 62), which may have biased the reported results.

[44] For example, Randall, Roberts, and Del Boca (1999), based on an analysis of data from 419 women enrolled in *Project MATCH*—a multisite alcohol treatment matching study, found that, when compared to men, women, on average: (1) first got drunk at a later age (i.e., 26.6 years versus 22.7 years); experienced first drinking problems at a later age (i.e., 27.5 versus 25.0 years); and (3) exhibited loss of control over drinking at a later age (29.8 versus 27.2 years).

Similarly, as noted by Greenfield, Back, and Lawson (2010, p. 339):

> Compared with men, women experience significantly shorter time intervals between the initiation of alcohol use and the onset of significant alcohol-related problems and treatment entry.

Women drink alcohol primarily to achieve a *disinhibition euphoria*, or *high*. Alcohol also is drunk to: achieve a general sense of well-being; reduce anxiety or stress; decrease sexual or social inhibitions; elevate mood; forget problems; cure loneliness; just relax; and prevent or self-manage the alcohol withdrawal syndrome. An effective psychodepressant, alcohol also is used for the perpetration of robberies and other drug-facilitated crimes. In fact, alcohol is the most common sedative-hypnotic involved in sexual assaults, including date rapes. There are nine, well-defined patterns, or levels, of personal use of alcohol (and other drugs and substances of abuse). Each of these levels are briefly presented and discussed. (For additional detailed discussion, see Chapter 8, *Preventing and Treating Women's Drug and Substance Abuse*.)

Nonuse, Initial Use, and Social Use

Nonuse is the first level and characterizes young girls, adolescent girls, and women who have *never* tried an alcoholic beverage. Of the 20% of women who do *not* consume alcohol, approximately one-half state that they do so for religious reasons (e.g., Church of Jesus Christ of Latter-Day Saints [Mormons], Muslims [Religion of Islam], Seventh Day Adventists).[45]

Initial use characterizes the first taste of alcohol (e.g., a sip of beer offered by a parent; a swig of whiskey shared with a playmate; a taste of a fancy martini offered by a colleague over lunch; a drink of wine offered at a first participation in a religious ceremony; gulping down a *Grande margarita* during an exotic vacation to see what it's like to get drunk [*experimental use*]).

The most common form of personal use is *social use*, which involves the ingestion of alcohol, in the form of beer, wines, and distilled spirits (i.e., whiskey, vodka, liqueurs), in social situations with others (e.g., birthday, holiday, and wedding celebrations; job promotions; graduating from high school or college). The social customs of various cultural groups in the U.S. significantly affect women's drinking at this level. Other factors include:

- Age
- Alcohol availability

[45] Of all of the women in the U.S., those of Asian descent are most likely to report that they were "lifetime abstainers" from alcohol use (i.e., 61%) (Clayton, Brooks, & Kornstein, 2014, pp. 85–86).

- Continental descent (including genetic predisposition for a tolerance to the use of alcohol, e.g., Jewish women), or lack thereof (e.g., sensitivity of Asian women to alcohol as characterized by the common occurrence of the *Asian Flush*)[46]
- Legal restrictions (e.g., drinking age in a particular state; religious prohibition)
- Personal preferences
- Sexual orientation

Among millennial women in the U.S., 56.9% of those who are between 18 and 25 years-of-age, report being "current drinkers," while 50.1% of those who are 26 years-of-age and older, report being "current drinkers" (SAMHSA, 2014, p. 37)—a slight, but significant difference as identified by McHugh, Wigderson, and Greenfield (2014).[47]

Development of Habitual Use, Abuse, and Compulsive Use

In the U.S., alcohol use generally begins at or before, 13 years-of-age—the age reported by most women at which time they consumed their first *non-sip* alcoholic drink (Alcohol Use USA, 2010). Once alcohol consumption begins, it generally continues throughout a woman's life characterized by a level of use without serious problems (i.e., social use, habitual use). However, for many women whose use is associated with characteristic patterns of abuse and compulsive use—except for those who can control their alcohol use or completely discontinue their alcohol use (i.e., *controlled use* and *resumed nonuse*, respectively) primarily for religious or health reasons—suffer increasingly harmful effects that for some may be fatal. A history of childhood, adolescent, and/or adult sexual abuse/assault has been *highly* correlated with women's alcohol use (Parkhill, Norris, & Davi, 2014), particularly among bisexual and lesbian women (Gilmore, Koo, & Nguyen, 2014; Pagliaro & Pagliaro, 2012).

Overall, approximately one in five women in the U.S. report significant harm, at some time during their lives, that was associated with their alcohol use (Pagliaro & Pagliaro, 2009, 2012).

---

[46] The *Asian Flush* also is known as the *Asian Flush Syndrome* or the *Oriental Flushing Syndrome*. The characteristic flushing, or blushing, of the skin associated with drinking alcohol, usually involves the face, neck, and shoulders. It is caused by the accumulation of *acetaldehyde* in the blood stream associated with a deficiency of *acetaldehyde dehydrogenase*—the enzyme primarily responsible for the metabolism of acetaldehyde in the body. This genetically controlled, or inherited, deficiency is particularly common among people of Asian descent—thus, the name, Asian Flush (Crabb, Edenberg, & Bosron, 1989; Xiao, Weiner, & Crabb, 1996). (Also, see earlier discussion in the Women's Basic Pharmacology section, *Pharmacokinetics*, "Metabolism and Elimination.")

[47] Reported current alcohol use was noted to decrease significantly (i.e., to 9.4%) among pregnant women, aged 15 to 44 years (SAMHSA, 2014).

> The prevalence of alcohol use disorders in women is approximately 4.9% in the past year and 19.5% lifetime.
>
> *(McHugh, Wigderson, & Greenfield, 2014, p. 177)*

Harmful patterns of alcohol use are particularly prevalent among young adults. For example, it has been estimated that *annually* on college/university campuses across the U.S., alcohol use has been *directly* associated with: 1,400 student deaths; 500,000 unintentional injuries; and 600,000 physical assaults (including rape) (Hingson, Heeren, & Zakocs, 2002). Younger women consume more alcohol than their older cohorts. They also suffer from significantly *higher* rates of AUDs—rates that also *exceed* the reported rates of AUDs for men who drink (Epstein, Fischer-Elber, & Al-Otaiba, 2007).[48]

Popular Notion: While men in college/university fraternities are extensively involved in excessive alcohol use, women in related sororities are not.

NOT TRUE. Consider, for example, the following reports of sorority *hazing* activities:

> About the hazing she experienced while pledging Kappa Kappa Gamma ... It's come to be almost expected that there's drinking involved in Greek Life, but the ritual takes things to a new—and incredibly dangerous—level. The woman, who didn't share her name—describes a ritual where pledges were put in the back seat of a car, made to chug alcoholic punch (each pledge got her own, huge 64 oz. bottle), given several vodka shots, and then forced out of the car. Did the pledge make her way back to safety? Well, she wouldn't know—she only remembers waking up in the ICU unit...
>
> *(Ava, 2015, pp. 11–12)*

Or consider the following related report:

> Forced to answer trivia questions with her pledging sisters, and if she got an answer wrong, do a shot of straight vodka. Reckless, but not unheard of for college students, right? However, if the pledges got more than a certain number wrong, in place of a bit of vodka, their "sisters" gave them four other options—a sharpie, a knife, a hammer, and sex toys.
>
> *(Ava, 2015, p. 16)*

---

48 Since the early 1980s, alcohol abuse has been an increasingly significant problem for women of *all* ages across the U.S., including rural women (Boyd, 2003).

Perhaps *not* surprisingly,[49] college/university students are *more* likely to engage in harmful patterns of drinking than are women of the same age who do *not* attend college/university (e.g., O'Malley & Johnston, 2002).[50] Over 30% of four-year college/university students sampled in the U.S., reported harmful patterns of alcohol use (e.g., alcohol-related academic problems; drinking in hazardous situations, such as drinking and driving) (Knight, Wechsler, & Kuo, 2002). As identified by Presley, Meilman, and Leichliter (2002), rates of excessive alcohol use are *highest* at U.S. colleges/universities:

1. In which, fraternities and sororities play a dominant social role
2. Where athletic events and campus sports are held in particularly *high* esteem
3. That are in the northeast region of the U.S.

It also has long been noted that the incidence of harmful drinking is significantly *higher* among bisexual and lesbian women than among other women (Drabble, Midanik, & Trocki, 2005; Green & Feinstein, 2012; Hughes & Wilsnack, 1997; Hyde, Comfort, & McManus, 2009). Contributing to this pattern of alcohol abuse is the historical observation that bisexual and lesbian women have traditionally used bars as their main gathering places for meeting, as well as socializing with, other bisexual and lesbian women (Pagliaro & Pagliaro, *Clinical Patient Data Files*).

Consistent with these observations, in terms of alcohol abuse and associated alcohol use disorder (AUD), a preponderance of current research data support the observation that, among *all* women, bisexual women had the *highest* incidence—followed by lesbians (Green & Feinstein, 2012; Kerr, Ding, & Burke, 2015; Kerr, Ding, & Chaya, 2014).[51] In addition, among female state prison inmates, drug and substance dependence is extremely prevalent and often higher than that reported for male inmates (Fazel, Bains, & Doll, 2006; Pagliaro & Pagliaro, *Clinical Patient Data Files*). Proctor (2012) found that alcohol dependence (30.2%) was the *highest* of all drug dependences reported for female inmates.

Alcohol and Caffeinated Energy Drinks

Energy drinks are non-alcoholic beverages (e.g., Red Bull®, RevItUp®, and Rock Star®) that are heavily laden with caffeine (see related discussion in Chapter 4, *Women's Caffeine and Nicotine Abuse*). Throughout the first 2 decades of the new

[49] But certainly, disappointingly, particularly to us as a pair of life-long, university academics.

[50] Several factors appear to affect the number of underage drinkers (younger than 21 years-of-age) on college/university campuses. These factors include, in *decreasing* order: (1) drinking beer; (2) residing in a fraternity or sorority; (3) having easy access to alcohol; and (4) being able to obtain alcohol at *lower* prices (Wechsler, Kuo, & Lee, 2000). Interestingly, beer consumption has overtaken wine consumption among women during the new millennium (Pagliaro & Pagliaro, *Clinical Patient Data Files*).

[51] Although this observation is confounded by the common practice of combining data from bisexual and lesbian women in many reported studies (Hughes & Eliason, 2002).

millennium, these beverages have become increasingly attractive to young women, including college/university students, who drink them to: stay awake; increase energy to "party" and have fun; "cram" for a final examination; or finish a term paper (Nordt, Vilke, & Clark, 2012; Pagliaro & Pagliaro, 2009, 2012).

As noted, many young adults generally assume that the *psychostimulant* actions of caffeine can "balance out" the *psychodepressant* actions of alcohol and, consequently, they can drink as much alcohol as they want without becoming drunk. However, the cognitive and psychomotor impairment associated with increasing BACs (see Table 2.1) are *not* reduced by the caffeine consumed in energy drinks (Ferreira, de Mello, & Pompeia, 2006; Ferreira, de Mello, & Rossi, 2004)—even though these young adults generally incorrectly perceive themselves as being significantly "less intoxicated" than they are (Marczinski & Fillmore, 2006).

Malinauskas, Aeby, and Overton (2007) found that over 50% of U.S. college/university students reported regularly consuming energy drinks. They also found that almost half of these young adults reported commonly consuming three or more energy drinks, together with alcoholic drinks, while "partying." Miller (2008) found that the association between energy drink consumption and aggression, insomnia, and other related problems behaviors among undergraduate college/university students in the U.S. was particularly significant for students of European continental descent, but *not* for those of African continental descent.

College students also use energy drinks to increase the amount of alcohol they consume during a drinking episode without becoming "overly intoxicated." As noted by Marczinski (2011), "to get drunk and reduce sedation compared to alcohol alone" (p. 3232). As we have previously noted in several other venues, what is achieved with a "caffeinated drunk" is simply a "wide-awake drunk." Instead of falling asleep, or "passing out," with a BAC of 0.25 to 0.30, these young adults remain awake and, consequently, can engage in harmful and often hazardous behaviors (e.g., accidental falls; drunk driving; physical assault) that can result in increased personal harm to self and others. (See Table 2.2 and previous related discussion in the section, *Pharmacology*, "Undesired, or Harmful, Effects and Toxicities.")

Binge Drinking

Binge drinking has been highly correlated with acute impairment and related harmful consequences (Pagliaro & Pagliaro, 2012). The incidence of binge drinking episodes has increased significantly over the past 2 decades and appears to be continuing to increase across the U.S., particularly among young adult women—as well as men (Naimi, Lipscomb, & Brewer, 2003; Pagliaro & Pagliaro, 2009). As noted by the U.S. Surgeon General:

> In 2015 … over 66 million people (nearly a quarter of the adult and adolescent population) reported binge drinking in the past month.
>
> *(U.S. Department of Health and Human Services, 2016, p. ES-1)*

> The *highest* observed rates of binge drinking in the U.S. is reported for the Northern states along the Canadian border (except Washington state) and the states of Alaska and Hawaii—as well as the District of Columbia.
>
> *(Sacks, Gonzales, & Bouchery, 2015, p. e73)*

In addition, as noted by the CDC:

> Binge drinking was responsible for more than half of the estimated 79,000 deaths and two thirds of the estimated 2.3 million years of potential life lost as a result of excessive drinking each year in the United States during 2001–2005.
>
> *(CDC, 2010, p. 1274)*

For women, binge drinking is traditionally defined as consuming *4 or more* alcoholic drinks in a row during a drinking episode. For men, it is defined as consuming *5* or more alcoholic drinks in a row during a drinking episode (see earlier discussion in the *Pharmacology* section, "Pharmacokinetics" (Metabolism and Elimination). This pattern of alcohol abuse is *highly* correlated with a rapid *increase* in BACs and associated impairments that are often related to significant adverse health consequences (Pagliaro & Pagliaro, 2009, 2012). For women, as well as for men, binge drinking is generally defined as a drinking episode during which the amount of alcohol that is consumed is equivalent to the amount of alcohol that is necessary to achieve minimally, on average, a BAC of approximately 0.08 gram % (i.e., 80 mg per 100 ml)—the legal level of alcohol intoxication in the U.S. (NIAAA, National Institute on Alcohol Abuse and Alcoholism, 2004).

Paul, Grubaugh, and Frueh (2011) found that 15% of the participants in their large nationally representative sample of more than 300,000 adults living in the U.S., were binge drinkers. The incidence of binge drinking is generally more common among:

1. Men when compared to women[52]
2. Younger adults when compared to older adults
3. Adults with at least some college education when compared to adults with only high school education
4. Adults with *higher* median incomes when compared to adults with *lower* median incomes

(CDC, 2009, 2010; Paul, Grubaugh, & Frueh, 2011)

---

[52] For example, a U.S. national survey found that: "among persons aged 26 or older ... the rate of binge drinking for males was approximately twice the rate for females (30.7 vs. 14.7 percent)" (SAMHSA, 2014, p. 37). However, this effect is *not* consistently noted and is subject to both significant temporal and sampling effects. For example, Keyes, Li, and Hasin (2011) found that for adults in the U.S. (but not in Australia or Western Europe):

> Women in younger cohorts are at especially high risk for heavy episodic drinking and alcohol disorders.
>
> *(p. 2101)*

However, both the highest number of drinks consumed (i.e., *intensity*) and the number of drinks consumed (i.e., *frequency*) in the U.S. were *highest* among adults, across *all* 50 states, for adults who: (1) were 65 years-of-age or older; and (2) did *not* graduate from high school (Kanny, Liu, & Brewer, 2013).

> More than 38 million U.S. adults binge drink about 4 times a month, and the largest number of drinks per binge is, on average, 8.
>
> *(CDC, 2012b, p. 1)*

In addition, as found by McHugh, Wigderson, & Greenfield (2014):

> Binge drinking among young women has increased … Currently one out of every eight U.S. women (nearly 14 million) binge drink approximately 3 times each month with an average of 6 drinks per binge.
>
> *(p. 177)*

As previously noted, binge drinking episodes for adults *increased* significantly over the past 2 decades and appear to continue to *increase* across the U.S., particularly among young adults (Courtney & Polich, 2009; Grucza, Norberg, & Bierut, 2009; Pagliaro & Pagliaro, 2009, 2012). Grucza, Norberg, and Bierut (2009), in their study of binge drinking, found the highest rates for young adults, 21 to 23 years-of-age (i.e., 38.6% for young women and 58% for young men). Overall, women of European descent have generally been found to have the highest reported incidence of binge drinking in the past year (i.e., approximately 30%). However, as identified by Clayton, Brooks, and Kornstein (2014):

> Rates of binge drinking differed significantly by ethnic groups. Among Asian women, Koreans (29 percent) were more likely to engage in binge drinking in the past year than were Chinese (5 percent) … Among Hispanic women, more than half (51 percent) of South Americans reported binge drinking in the past year compared with 22 percent of Mexicans and 14 percent of Central Americans.
>
> *(p. 87)*

It also has long been noted that binge drinking is significantly *higher* among young women who are bisexual or lesbian (Drabble, Midanik, & Trocki, 2005; Hughes & Wilsnack, 1997; Hyde, Comfort, & McManus, 2009). As reported by Centers for Disease Control and Prevention (2012a), in the U.S., binge drinkers, who are:

1. 18 to 34 years-of-age, comprise the largest group of adults who binge drink
2. 65 years-of-age, or older, "binge drink" most often

3. Of African continental descent or Hispanic descent, have the *highest* average number of drinks per binge drinking episode (i.e., *more* than 8 drinks)

In addition, Stahre, Brewer, and Fonseca (2009) found that over 40% of U.S. active-duty military personnel reported binge drinking within the past month. On average, these military personnel were involved in approximately 30 episodes of binge drinking per person per year.

In another study focusing on alcohol use among military personnel, Brown, Bray, and Hartzell (2010) found that enlisted women and men were significantly more likely to engage in *heavy* or binge drinking (and to experience alcohol-related harmful effects and associated problems) than were their officers. As a growing number of women in the military participate in active combat duty roles, it is expected that the percentage of women military personnel with significant harmful patterns of alcohol use (e.g., binge drinking) and related "problems" will increase significantly (Pagliaro & Pagliaro, *Clinical Patient Data Files*).

Bisexual and Lesbian Women

Bisexual and lesbian women comprise another group of women who have relatively *high* rates of binge drinking and AUDs—regardless of age and continental or other descent (Pagliaro & Pagliaro, *Clinical Patient Data Files*). This group of women[53] has been identified as sharing the following characteristics, when compared to heterosexual women who drink:

- *Higher* incidence of binge drinking, heavy drinking, and other problem drinking behaviors
- *Higher* rates of alcohol-related problems
- *Higher* rates of binge drinking
- *Higher* rates of attendance in bars, clubs, and house parties for drinking purposes
- *Higher* risk for AUDs and SUDs
- *Lower* rates of alcohol abstinence
- *Lower* rates of decline in binge drinking, heavy drinking, and other problem drinking in relation to increasing age
- *More* likely to seek formal treatment for AUDs

Unfortunately, our analysis and reflective synthesis of these data have led us to the conclusion that contrary to the admonition and celebration of some women

[53] In regard to alcohol use and AUDs research, data from bisexual and lesbian women in the U.S. have been generally collapsed into one group in order to increase subject numbers for appropriate statistical analyses (e.g., to meet specific test assumptions), even though they very likely display significant differences. Acknowledging this factor, we present these data as reported in the published literature.

regarding the freedom to "drink like men," the reckless drinking of alcohol is something *not* to be proud of nor to actively emulate. The consequences of "drinking like men" offers several harmful consequences for women across the lifespan, as presented and documented throughout this chapter, including many that are unique to women (e.g., FAS/FASD; ineffective and inconsistent mothering). As noted by Delker, Brown, and Hasin (2016), in their review of women's alcohol use across the U.S.—citing data from Keyes, Grant, and Hasin (2008) and Keyes, Martins, and Blanco (2010):

> As Western social norms continue to shift away from traditional gender roles that see women only as homemakers and mothers, women report greater lifetime largest number of drinks consumed in one sitting and greater frequency of binge drinking, than they did in earlier surveys, leading to a closing of the gender gap not only in consumption but also in alcohol-related consequences.
>
> *(p. 12)*

References[54,55,56]

Abbey, A. (2011). Alcohol's role in sexual violence perpetration: Theoretical explanations, existing evidence, and future directions. *Drug and Alcohol Review*, 30(5), 481–489. doi:10.1111/j.1465-3362.2011.00296.x

Abel, E. L. (1995, July–August). An update on incidence of FAS: FAS is not an equal opportunity birth defect. *Neurotoxicology and Teratology*, 17(4), 437–443.

Abel, E. L., & Sokol, R. J. (1987). Incidence of fetal alcohol syndrome and economic impact of FAS-related anomalies. *Drug and Alcohol Dependence*, 19(1), 51–70.

Abel, E. L., & Sokol, R. J. (1991). A revised conservative estimate of the incidence of FAS and its economic impact. *Alcoholism, Clinical and Experimental Research*, 15(3), 514–524.

Afifi, T. O., Henriksen, C. A., & Asmundson, G. J. (2012). Victimization and perpetration of intimate partner violence and substance use disorders in a nationally representative sample. *Journal of Nervous and Mental Disease*, 200(8), 684–691. doi:10.1097/NMD.0b013e3182613f64

Alcohol Use USA. (2010, January 6). *Alcohol use USA*. Retrieved from Alcohol and Drug Guide: www.alcohol-and-drug-guide.com/alcohol-use-usa.html

54 As per publisher style, only the first three authors are listed for each reference.

55 Several times the number of references listed were found, obtained, and analyzed by the authors during the preparation of this chapter. However, only the references that were cited at least once in the body of the text are included in the list. Major reasons for not citing other references, include that they: (1) did not provide any additional unique data; (2) were not well researched or written (i.e., were evaluated as not being valid or reliable); (3) were based predominantly, or exclusively, on animal studies; (4) provided usage statistics from outside the U.S.; and/or (5) were redundant with, or not as recent as, the already cited references.

56 The reference citation, "Pagliaro & Pagliaro, *Clinical Patient Data Files*," refers to unpublished data collected, with permission, over the last 50 years by the authors, in the formal course of their professional academic roles as clinician scientists and professors—by permission from their patients, research subjects, and students, from the 1970s to date.

Aronson, K. (2003). Alcohol: A recently identified risk factor for breast cancer. *CMAJ, Canadian Medical Journal*, 168(9), 1147–1148.

Asante, K. O., & Nelms-Matzke, J. (1985). *Report on the Survey of Children with Chronic Handicaps and FAS in the Yukon and Northwest British Columbia*. Terrace, BC: Mills Municipal Hospital.

Ava. (2015, July 29). 13 of the most terrifying sorority hazing stories. *TheTalko.com*, pp. 1–50. Retrieved November 18, 2016, from www.thetalko.com/1

Avalos, L. A., Roberts, S. C., & Kaskutas, L. A. (2014). Volume and type of alcohol during early pregnancy and the risk of miscarriage. *Substance Use & Misuse*, 49(11), 1437–1445. doi:10.3109/10826084

Bada, H. S., Das, A., & Bauer, C. R. (2007). Impact of prenatal cocaine exposure on child behavior problems through school age. *Pediatrics*, 119, e348–e359.

Bailey, R. K., Patel, T. C., & Avenido, J. (2011). Suicide: Current trends. *Journal of the National Medical Association*, 103(7), 614–617.

Baraona, E., Abittan, C. S., & Dohmen, K. (2001). Gender differences in pharmacokinetics of alcohol. *Alcoholism: Clinical and Experimental Research*, 25(4), 502–507.

Bertrand, J. (2009). Interventions for children with fetal alcohol spectrum disorders (FASDs): Overview of findings for five innovative research projects. *Research in Developmental Disabilities*, 30(5), 986–1006.

Bertucci, V., & Krafchik, B. R. (1994, June). What syndrome is this? Fetal alcohol syndrome. *Pediatric Dermatology*, 11(2), 178–180.

Bickel, W. K., Moody, L., & Mueller, E. T. (2013). Executive dysfunction among alcohol- and cocaine-dependent women. *American Psychological Association 2013 Convention Presentation*.

Boyd, M. R. (2003). Vulnerability to alcohol and other drug disorders in rural women. *Archives of Psychiatric Nursing*, 17(1), 33–41.

Brooks, P. J., & Zakhari, S. (2013). Moderate alcohol consumption and breast cancer in women: From epidemiology to mechanisms and interventions. *Alcoholism: Clinical and Experimental Research*, 37(1), 23–30. doi:10.1111/j.1530-0277.2012.01888.x

Brown, J. M., Bray, R. M., & Hartzell, M. C. (2010). A comparison of alcohol use and related problems among women and men in the military. *Military Medicine*, 175(2), 101–107. Retrieved July 16, 2014

Butchart, A., Poznyak, V., & Bellis, M. (2006). Child maltreatment and alcohol. *WHO Facts On…*, pp. 1–11. Geneva, Switzerland: World Health Organization. Retrieved October 10, 2016, from www.who.int/violence_injury_prevention/publications/violence/en/index/html

Cao, Y., Willett, W. C., & Rimm, E. B. (2015, August 18). Light to moderate intake of alcohol, drinking patterns, and risk of cancer: Results from two prospective US cohort studies. *BMJ*. doi:10.1136/bmj.h4238

Carpentier, M. (2015, July 7). *When drugs are used to coerce sex, it's rape. Even if you're Bill Cosby*. Retrieved January 2, 2016, from The Guardian, pp. 1–3: www.theguardian.com/comentisfree/2015/jul/07/bill-cosby-drugs-coerced-sex-rape-allegations

Caruso, K., & ten Bensel, R. (1993). Fetal alcohol syndrome and fetal alcohol effects. The University of Minnesota experience. *Minnesota Medicine*, 76(4), 25–29.

CDC, Centers for Disease Control and Prevention. (2002, May 24). Fetal alcohol syndrome—Alaska, Arizona, Colorado, and New York, 1995–1997. *MMWR: Morbidity and Mortality Weekly Report*, 51(20), 433–435.

CDC, Centers for Disease Control and Prevention. (2003, July 18). Fetal alcohol syndrome—South Africa, 2001. *MMWR: Morbidity and Mortality Weekly Report*, 52(28), 660–662.

CDC, Centers for Disease Control and Prevention. (2004). Alcohol-attributable deaths and years of potential life lost—United States, 2001. *MMWR, Morbidity and Mortality Weekly Report*, 53(37), 866–870.

CDC, Centers for Disease Control and Prevention. (2009). Sociodemographic differences in binge drinking among adults—14 States, 2004. *MMWR, Morbidity and Mortality Weekly Report*, 58(12), 301–304.

CDC, Centers for Disease Control and Prevention. (2010). Vital signs: Binge drinking among high school students and adults—United States 2009. *MMWR, Morbidity and Mortality Weekly Report*, 59(39), 1274–1279.

CDC, Centers for Disease Control and Prevention. (2012a, July 20). Alcohol use and binge drinking among women of childbearing age—United States, 2006–2010. *MMWR, Morbidity and Mortality Weekly Report*, 61(28), 534–538.

CDC, Centers for Disease Control and Prevention. (2012b). *Underlying cause of death, 1999–2008 results form*. Retrieved from CDC.gov, pp. 1–9: https://wonder.cdc.gov/cmf-icd10-archive2008.html

CDC, Centers for Disease Control and Prevention. (2016, March 7). *Fact Sheets—Excessive alcohol use and risks to women's health*. Retrieved from CDC, Centers for Disease Control and Prevention: Division of Population Health: www.cdc.gov/NCCDPHP/dph/

Chasnoff, I. J., Wells, A. M., & King, L. (2015). Misdiagnosis and missed diagnoses in foster and adopted children with prenatal alcohol exposure. *Pediatrics*, 135(2), 264–270.

Chavez, G. F., Cordero, J. F., & Becerra, J. E. (1988, July). Leading major congenital malformations among minority groups in the United States, 1981–1986. *MMWR. CDC Surveillance Summaries*, 37(3), 17–24.

Child Welfare Information Gateway. (2014). *Parental substance use and the child welfare system*, pp. 1–13. Washington, DC: U.S. Department of Health and Human Services, Children's Bureau.

Chudley, A. E., Conry, J., & Cook, J. L. (2005). Fetal alcohol spectrum disorder: Canadian guidelines for diagnosis. *CMAJ, Canadian Medical Association Journal*, 172(5 Supplement), S1–S21.

Clarke, N., Kim, S.-Y., & White, H. R. (2013). Associations between alcohol use and alcohol-related negative consequences among black and white college men and women. *Journal of Studies on Alcohol and Drugs*, 74, 521–531.

Clarren, S. K., & Smith, D. W. (1978, May 11). The fetal alcohol syndrome. *The New England Journal of Medicine*, 298(19), 1063–1067. doi:10.1056/NEJM197805112981906

Clayton, J. A., Brooks, C. E., & Kornstein, S. G. (2014, October). *Women of color health data book* (4th ed.). NIH Publication No. 14-4247. Bethesda, MD: National Institutes of Health, Office of Research on Women's Health.

Connors, N. A., Bradley, R. H., & Whiteside Mansell, L. (2003). Children of mothers with serious substance abuse problems: An accumulation of risks. *The American Journal of Drug and Alcohol Abuse*, 29(4), 743–758. doi:10.1081/ADA-120026258

Cook, J. L., Green, C. R., & Lilley, C. M. (2016, February 16). Fetal alcohol spectrum disorder: A guideline for diagnosis across the lifespan. *CMAJ: Canadian Medical Association Journal*, 188(3), 191–197.

Courtney, K. E., & Polich, J. (2009). Binge drinking in young adults: Data, definitions, and determinants. *Psychological Bulletin*, 135(1), 142–156.

Crabb, D. W., Edenberg, H. J., & Bosron, W. F. (1989). Genotypes for aldehyde dehydrogenase deficiency and alcohol sensitivity. The inactive ALDH2(2) allele is dominant. *Journal of Clinical Investigation*, 83(1), 314–316.

Crunelle, C. L., Yegles, M., & van Nuijs, A. L. (2014, January 1). Hair ethyl glucuronide levels as a marker for alcohol use and abuse: A review of the current state of the art. *Drug and Alcohol Dependence*, 134, 1–11. doi:10.1016/j.drugalcdep.2013.10.008

Delker, E., Brown, Q., & Hasin, D. S. (2016). Alcohol consumption in demographic subpopulations: An epidemiologic overview. *Alcohol Research: Current Reviews*, 38(1), 7–15.

Denny, C. H., Tsai, J., & Floyd, R. L. (2009). Alcohol use among pregnant and non-pregnant women of childbearing age: United States, 1991–2005. *Morbidity and Mortality Weekly Report*, 58(19), pp. 529–532.

Devries, K. M., Child, J. C., & Bacchus, L. J. (2014). Intimate partner violence victimization and alcohol consumption in women: A systematic review and meta-analysis. *Addiction*, 109(3), 379–391. doi:10.1111/add.12393

Diehl, A., Croissant, B., & Batra, A. (2007). Alcoholism in women: Is it different in onset and outcome compared to men? *European Archives of Psychiatry and Clinical Neuroscience*, 257(6), 344–351. doi:10.1007/s00406-007-0737-z

Douzgou, S., Breen, C., & Crow, Y. J. (2012). Diagnosing fetal alcohol syndrome: New insights from newer genetic technologies. *Archives of Disease in Childhood*, 97(9), 812–817.

Drabble, L., Midanik, L. T., & Trocki, K. (2005). Reports of alcohol consumption and alcohol-related problems among homosexual, bisexual and heterosexual respondents: Results from the 2000 National Alcohol Survey. *Journal of Studies on Alcohol*, 66(1), 111–120.

DUI/DWI Laws (2010). pp. 1–8: www.drunk-driving.com/dui-dwi-laws

Duimstra, C., Johnson, D., & Kutsch, C. (1993, March–April). A fetal alcohol syndrome surveillance pilot project in American Indian communities in the Northern Plains. *Public Health Reports*, 108(2), 225–229.

Egeland, G. M., Perham-Hester, K. A., & Gessner, B. D. (1998). Fetal alcohol syndrome in Alaska, 1977 through 1992: An administrative prevalence derived from multiple data sources. *American Journal of Public Health*, 88(5), 781–786.

Epstein, E. E., Fischer-Elber, K., & Al-Otaiba, Z. (2007). Women, aging, and alcohol use disorders. *Journal of Women & Aging*, 19(1–2), 31–48.

Ethen, M. K., Ramadhani, T. A., & Scheurle, A. E. (2009). Alcohol consumption by women before and during pregnancy. *Maternal and Child Health Journal*, 13(2), 274–285.

Eustace, L. W., Kang, D. H., & Coombs, D. (2003). Fetal alcohol syndrome: A growing concern for health care professionals. *Journal of Obstetric, Gynecologic, & Neonatal Nursing*, 32(2), 215–221.

Fazel, S., Bains, P., & Doll, H. (2006). Substance abuse and dependence in prisoners: A systematic review. *Addiction*, 101(2), 181–191.

Feigelson, H. S., Jonas, C. R., & Robertson, A. S. (2003). Alcohol, folate, methionine, and risk of incident breast cancer in the American Cancer Society Cancer Prevention Study II Nutrition Cohort. *Cancer Epidemiology, Biomarkers, & Prevention*, 12(2), 161–164.

Ferreira, S. E., de Mello, M. T., & Pompeia, S. (2006). Effects of energy drink ingestion on alcohol intoxication. *Alcoholism: Clinical and Experimental Research*, 30(4), 598–605.

Ferreira, S. E., de Mello, M. T., & Rossi, M. V. (2004). Does an energy drink modify the effects of alcohol in a maximal effort test? *Alcoholism: Clinical and Experimental Research*, 28(9), 1408–1412.

Fitzpatrick, J. P., Latimer, J., & Carter, M. (2015). Prevalence of fetal alcohol syndrome in a population-based sample of children living in remote Australia: The Lililwan Project. *Journal of Paediatrics and Child Health*, 51(4), 450–457. doi:10.1111/jpc.12814

Floyd, R. L., Weber, M. K., & Denny , C. (2009). Prevention of fetal alcohol spectrum disorders. *Developmental Disabilities Research Reviews*, 15(3), 193–199. doi:10.1002/ddrr.75

Forcehimes, A. A., Venner, K. L., & Bogenschutz, M. P. (2011). American Indian methamphetamine and other drug use in the southwestern United States. *Cultural Diversity & Ethnic Minority Psychology*, 17(4), 366–376. doi:10.1037/a0025431

Fox, D. J., Pettygrove, S., & Cunniff, C. (2015, January 30). Fetal alcohol syndrome among children aged 7–9 years—Arizona, Colorado, and New York, 2010. *MMWR: Morbidity and Mortality Weekly Report*, 64(3), 54–57.

Freud, S. (1930/1989). *Civilization and its discontents.* New York, NY: Norton.

Frisk, A. (2016, July 7). *Alcoholic mother who hosted naked twister party with teen daughter won't face jail.* Retrieved July 11, 2016, from Globalnews.ca, p. 1: http://globalnews.ca/news/2809582/alcoholic-mother-who-hosted-naked-twister-party-with-teen-daughter-wont-face-jail/

Gardiner, A. S., Gutierrez, H. L., & Luo, L. (2016). Alcohol use during pregnancy is associated with specific alterations in microRNA levels in maternal serum. *Alcoholism: Clinical and Experimental Research*, 40(4), 826–837. doi:10.1111/acer.13026

George, W. H., Davis, K. C., & Masters, N. T. (2014). Sexual victimization, alcohol intoxication, sexual-emotional responding, and sexual risk in heavy episodic drinking. *Archives of Sexual Behavior*, 43(4), 645–658. doi:10.1007/s10508-013-0143-8

Gilmore, A. K., Koo, K. H., & Nguyen, H. V. (2014). Sexual assault, drinking norms, and drinking behavior among a national sample of lesbian and bisexual women. *Addictive Behaviors*, 39(3), 630–636. doi:10.1016/j.addbeh.2013.11.015

Gilmore, A. K., Stappenbeck, C. A., & Lewis, M. A. (2015). Sexual assault history and its association with the use of drinking protective behavioral strategies among college women. *Journal of Studies on Alcohol and Drugs*, 76(3), 459–464.

Ginsburg, K. A., Blacker, C. M., & Abel, E. L. (1991). Fetal alcohol exposure and adverse pregnancy outcomes. *Contributions to Gynecology and Obstetrics*, 18, 115–129.

Glaser, G. (2013, June 21). *Why she drinks: Women and alcohol abuse.* Retrieved October 27, 2016, from WSJ, The Wall Street Journal, pp. 1–5: www.wsj.com/articles/SB10001424127887323893504578555270434071876

Green, K. E., & Feinstein, B. A. (2012). Substance use in lesbian, gay, and bisexual populations: An update on empirical research and implications for treatment. *Psychology of Addictive Behaviors*, 26(2), 265–278. doi:10.1037/a0025424

Greenfield, S. F., Back, S. E., & Lawson, K. (2010). Substance abuse in women. *Psychiatric Clinics of North America*, 33(2), 339–355. doi:10.1016/j.psc.2010.01.004

Grucza, R. A., Norberg, K. E., & Bierut, L. J. (2009). Binge drinking among youth and young adults in the United States: 1979–2006. *Journal of the American Academy of Child & Adolescent Psychiatry*, 48(7), 692–702.

Habbick, B. F., Nanson, J. L., & Snyder, R. E. (1996, May–June). Foetal alcohol syndrome in Saskatchewan: Unchanged incidence in a 20-year period. *Canadian Journal of Public Health*, 87(3), 204–207.

Hannan, S. M., Orcutt, H. K., & Miron, L. R. (2015, June 30). Childhood sexual abuse and later alcohol-related problems: Investigating the roles of revictimization, PTSD, and drinking motivations among college women. *Journal of Interpersonal Violence* [Epub ahead of print]. Retrieved March 6, 2016, from www.ncbi.nlm.nih.gov/pubmed doi: 10.1177/0886260515591276

Hanson, J. D., Winberg, A., & Elliott, A. (2012). Development of a media campaign on fetal alcohol disorders for Northern Plains American Indian communities. *Health Promotion Practice*, 13(6), 842–847. doi:10.1177/1524839911404232

Harris, K. R., & Bucens, I. K. (2003, September–October). Prevalence of fetal alcohol syndrome in the Top End of the Northern Territory. *Journal of Paediatrics and Child Health*, 39(7), 528–533.

Harris, S. R., Osborn, J. A., & Weinberg, J. (1993). Effects of prenatal alcohol exposure on neuromotor and cognitive development during early childhood: A series of case reports. *Physical Therapy*, 73(9), 608–617.

Hasin, D. S., Stinson, F. S., & Ogburn, E. (2007). Prevalence, correlates, disability, and comorbidity of DSM-IV alcohol abuse and dependence in the United States: Results from the National Epidemiologic Survey on Alcohol and Related Conditions. *Archives of General Psychiatry*, 64(7), 830–842.

Hernandez-Avila, C. A., Rounsaville, B. J., & Kranzler, H. R. (2004). Opioid-, cannabis-, and alcohol-dependent women show more rapid progression to substance abuse treatment. *Drug and Alcohol Dependence*, 74(3), 265–272.

Hill, P. M., Hegemier, S., & Tennyson, L. M. (1989, Fall). The fetal alcohol syndrome: A multihandicapped child. *Neurotoxicology*, 10(3), 585–595.

Hilton, M. (2014). APIS: The NIAAA alcohol policy information system. *Alcohol Research: Current Reviews*, 35(2), 184–185.

Hingson, R. W., Heeren, T., & Zakocs, R. C. (2002). Magnitude of alcohol-related mortality and morbidity among U.S. college students ages 18–24. *Journal of Studies on Alcohol*, 63(2), 136–144.

Howland, J., Rohsenow, D. J., & Allensworth-Davies, D. (2008). The incidence and severity of hangover the morning after moderate alcohol intoxication. *Addiction*, 103(5), 758–765.

Howland, J., Rohsenow, D. J., & Edwards, E. M. (2008). Are some drinkers resistant to hangover? A literature review. *Current Drug Abuse Reviews*, 1(1), 42–46.

Hughes, T. L., & Eliason, M. (2002, Spring). Substance use and abuse in lesbian, gay, bisexual and transgender populations. *The Journal of Primary Prevention*, 22(3), 263–298. doi:0278-095X/02/0300-0263/0

Hughes, T. L., Johnson, T., & Wilsnack, S. C. (2001). Sexual assault and alcohol abuse: A comparison of lesbians and heterosexual women. *Journal of Substance Abuse*, 13(4), 515–532.

Hughes, T. L., Szalacha, L. A., & Johnson, T. P. (2010). Sexual victimization and hazardous drinking among heterosexual and sexual minority women. *Addictive Behaviors*, 35(12), 1152–1156. doi:10.1016/j.addbeh.2010.07.004

Hughes, T. L., & Wilsnack, S. C. (1997). Use of alcohol among lesbians: Research and clinical implications. *American Journal of Orthopsychiatry*, 67(1), 20–36.

Hyde, Z., Comfort, J., & McManus, A. (2009, September). Alcohol, tobacco and illicit drug use amongst same-sex attracted women: Results from the Western Australian Lesbian and Bisexual Women's Health and Well-Being Survey. *BioMed Central Public Health*, 9, 317.

Ikonomidou, C., Bittigau, P., & Koch, C. (2001). Neurotransmitters and apoptosis in the developing brain. *Biochemical Pharmacology*, 62(4), 401–405.

Jefferies, J. L., & Towbin, J. A. (2010). Dilated cardiomyopathy. *The Lancet*, 375(9716), 752–762.

Jones, A. W., & Harding, P. (2013). Driving under the influence with blood alcohol concentrations over 0.4 g%. *Forensic Science International*, 231(1–3), 349–353. doi:10.1016/j.forsciint.2013.06.010

Jones, C. M., Paulozzi, L. J., & Mack, K. A. (2014). Alcohol involvement in opioid pain reliever and benzodiazepine drug abuse-related emergency department visits and drug-related deaths—United States, 2010. *MMWR, Morbidity and Mortality Weekly Report*, 63(40), 881–885.

Joya, X., Friguls, B., & Ortigosa, S. (2012). Determination of maternal-fetal biomarkers of prenatal exposure to ethanol: A review. *Journal of Pharmaceutical and Biomedical Analysis*, 69, 209–222. doi:10.1016/j.jpba.2012.01.006

Kanny, D., Liu, Y., & Brewer, R. D. (2013, November 22). Binge drinking—United States, 2011. *Morbidity and Mortality Weekly Report (MMWR)*, 62(3), 77–80.

Karp, R. J., Qazi, Q., & Hittleman, J. (1993). Fetal alcohol syndrome. In R. J. Karp (Ed.), *Malnourished children in the United States: Caught in the cycle of poverty* (pp. 101–108). New York, NY: Springer.

Kerr, D., Ding, K., & Burke, A. (2015). An alcohol, tobacco, and other drug use comparison of lesbian, bisexual, and heterosexual undergraduate women. *Substance Use & Misuse*, 50(3), 340–349. doi:10.3109/10826084.2014.980954

Kerr, D. L., Ding, K., & Chaya, J. (2014). Substance use of lesbian, gay, bisexual and heterosexual college students. *American Journal of Health Behavior*, 38(6), 951–962. doi:10.5993/AJHB.38.6.17

Keyes, K. M., Grant, B. F., & Hasin, D. S. (2008). Evidence for a closing gender gap in alcohol use, abuse, and dependence in the United States population. *Drug and Alcohol Dependence*, 93(1–2), 21–29.

Keyes, K. M., Li, G., & Hasin, D. S. (2011). Birth cohort effects and gender differences in alcohol epidemiology: A review and synthesis. *Alcohol Clinical and Experimental Research*, 35(12), 2101–2112. doi:10.1111/j.1530-0277.2011.01562.x

Keyes, K. M., Martins, S. S., & Blanco, C. (2010). Telescoping and gender differences in alcohol dependence: New evidence from two national surveys. *American Journal of Psychiatry*, 167(8), 969–976. doi:10.1176/appi.ajp.2009.09081161.

Khan, B. A., Robinson, R. F., & Smith, J. J. (2013, August 5). Prenatal alcohol exposure among Alaska Native/American Indian infants. *International Journal of Circumpolar Health*, 72. doi:10.3402/ijch.v72i0.20973

Knight, J. R., Wechsler, H., & Kuo, M. (2002). Alcohol abuse and dependence among U.S. college students. *Journal of Studies on Alcohol*, 63(3), 263–270.

Kvigne, V. L., Randall, B., & Simanton, E. G. (2012). Blood alcohol levels for American Indian mothers and newborns. *Pediatrics*, 130(4), e1015–e1018. doi:10.1542/peds.2011-1400

Lee, W. K., & Regan, T. J. (2002). Alcoholic cardiomyopathy: Is it dose-dependent? *Congestive Heart Failure*, 8(6), 303–306.

Ling, J., Stephens, R., & Heffernan, T. M. (2010). Cognitive and psychomotor performance during alcohol hangover. *Current Drug Abuse Reviews*, 3(2), 80–87.

Liu, Y., Colditz, G. A., & Rosner, B. (2013). Alcohol intake between menarche and first pregnancy: A prospective study of breast cancer risk. *Journal of the National Cancer Institute*, 105(20), 1571–1578. doi:10.1093/jnci/djt213

Liu, Y., Nguyen, N., & Colditz, G. A. (2015). Links between alcohol consumption and breast cancer: A look at the evidence. *Women's Health (London, England)*, 11(1), 65–77. doi:10.2217/whe.14.62

Madea, B., & MuBhoff, F. (2009). Knock-out drugs: Their prevalence, modes of action, and means of detection. *Deutsches Azteblatt International*, 106(20), 341–347.

Malcom, R. J. (2003). GABA systems, benzodiazepines, and substance dependence. *The Journal of Clinical Psychiatry*, 64(3 Supplement), 36–40.

Malinauskas, B. M., Aeby, V. G., & Overton, R. F. (2007). A survey of energy drink consumption patterns among college students. *Nutrition Journal*, 6, 35.

Mancinelli, R., Vitali, M., & Ceccanti, M. (2009). Women, alcohol and the environment: An update and perspectives in neuroscience. *Functional Neurology*, 24(2), 77–81.

Marchetta, C. M., Denny, C. H., & Floyd, R. L. (2012, July 20). Alcohol use and binge drinking among women of childbearing age—United States, 2006–2010. *MMWR, Morbidity and Mortality Weekly Report*, 61(28), 534–538.

Marczinski, C. A. (2011). Alcohol mixed with energy drinks: Consumption patterns and motivations for use in U.S. college students. *International Journal of Environmental Research and Public Health*, 8(8), 3232–3245.

Marczinski, C. A. (2014). Combined alcohol and energy drink use: Hedonistic motives, adenosine, and alcohol dependence. *Alcoholism: Clinical and Experimental Research*, 38(7), 1822–1825. doi:10.1111/acer.12493

Marczinski, C. A., & Fillmore, M. T. (2006). Clubgoers and their trendy cocktails: Implications of mixing caffeine into alcohol on information processing and subjective reports of intoxication. *Experimental and Clinical Psychopharmacology*, 14(4), 450–458.

Martin, S. L., Beaumont, J. L., & Kupper, L. L. (2003). Substance use before and during pregnancy: Links to intimate partner violence. *The American Journal of Drug and Alcohol Abuse*, 29(3), 599–617.

May, P. A. (1991). Fetal alcohol effects among North American Indians: Evidence and implications for society. *Alcohol, Health and Research World*, 15(3), 239–248.

May, P. A., Baete, A., & Russo, J. (2014). Prevalence and characteristics of fetal alcohol spectrum disorders. *Pediatrics*, 134(5), 855–866. doi:10.1542/peds.20123-3319

May, P. A., Blankenship, J., & Marais, A. S. (2013). Approaching the prevalence of the full spectrum of fetal alcohol spectrum disorders in a South African population-based study. *Alcoholism: Clinical and Experimental Research*, 37(5), 818–830. doi:10.1111/acer.12033

May, P. A., de Vries, M. M., & Marais, A. S. (2016, February 1). The continuum of fetal alcohol spectrum disorders in four rural communities in South Africa: Prevalence and characteristics. *Drug and Alcohol Dependence*, 159, 207–218. doi:10.1016/j.drugalcdep.2015.12.023

May, P. A., Fiorentino, D., & Coriale, G. (2011). Prevalence of children with severe fetal alcohol spectrum disorders in communities near Rome, Italy: New estimated rates are higher than previous estimates. *International Journal of Environmental Research and Public Health*, 8(6), 2331–2351. doi:10.3390/ijerph8062331

May, P. A., & Gossage, J. P. (2001). Estimating the prevalence of fetal alcohol syndrome. A summary. *Alcohol Research & Health*, 25(3), 159–167.

May, P. A., Gossage, J. P., & Kalberg, W. O. (2009). Prevalence and epidemiologic characteristics of FASD from various research methods with an emphasis on recent in-school studies. *Developmental Disabilities Research Reviews*, 15(3), 176–192. doi:10.1002/ddrr.68

May, P. A., Gossage, J. P., & Marais, A. S. (2007, May 11). The epidemiology of fetal alcohol syndrome and partial FAS in a South African community. *Drug and Alcohol Dependence*, 88(2–3), 259–271. doi:10.1016/j.drugalcdep.2006.11.007

May, P. A., Hymbaugh, K. J., & Aase, J. M. (1983, Winter). Epidemiology of fetal alcohol syndrome among American Indians of the Southwest. *Social Biology*, 30(4), 374–387.

May, P. A., Keaster, C., & Bozeman, R. (2015, October 1). Prevalence and characteristics of fetal alcohol syndrome and partial fetal alcohol syndrome in a Rocky Mountain Region City. *Drug and Alcohol Dependence*, 155, 118–127. doi:10.1016/j.drugalcdep.20125.08.006

McCauley, J. L., Calhoun, K. S., & Gidycz, C. A. (2010). Binge drinking and rape: A prospective examination of college women with a history of previous sexual victimization. *Journal of Interpersonal Violence*, 25(9), 1655–1668. doi:10.1177/0886260509354580

McCutcheon, V. V., Agrawal, A., & Heath, A. C. (2011). Functioning of alcohol use disorder criteria among men and women with arrests for driving under the influence of alcohol. *Alcoholism: Clinical and Experimental Research*, 35(11), 1985–1993. doi:10.1111/j.1530-0277.2011.01550.x

McHugh, R. K., Wigderson, S., & Greenfield, S. F. (2014). Epidemiology of substance use in reproductive-age women. *Obstetrics and Gynecology Clinics of North America*, 41(2), 177–189. doi:10.1016/j.ogc.2014.02.001

McKetin, R., Coen, A., & Kaye, S. (2015). A comprehensive review of the effects of mixing caffeinated energy drinks with alcohol. *Drug and Alcohol Dependence*, 151, 15–30. doi:10.1016/j.drugalcdep.2015.01.047

McKinney, A. (2010). A review of the next day effects of alcohol on subjective mood ratings. *Current Drug Abuse Reviews*, 3(2), 88–91.

Mengel, M. B., Searight, H. R., & Cook, K. (2006). Preventing alcohol-exposed pregnancies. *The Journal of the American Board of Family Medicine*, 19(5), 494–505.

Michaelson, J. (2015, July 27). *Quaaludes, Cosby's alleged rape drugs of choice, were somehow even scarier than you think.* Retrieved from The Daily Beast, pp. 1–3: www.thedailybeast.com/quaaludes-cosbys-alleged-rape-drugs-of-choice-were-somehow-even-scarier-than-you-think

Miller, K. E. (2008). Energy drinks, race, and problem behaviors among college students. *The Journal of Adolescent Health*, 43(5), 490–497.

Mizoue, T., Tanaka, K., & Tsuji, I. (2006, July 26). Alcohol drinking and colorectal cancer risk: An evaluation based on a systemic review of epidemiologic evidence among the Japanese population. *Japanese Journal of Clinical Oncology*, 1–16. doi:10.1093/jjco/hy1069

Montag, A. (2016). Fetal alcohol-spectrum disorders: Identifying at-risk mothers. *International Journal of Women's Health*, 8, 311–323.

Mouilso, E. R., Fischer, S., & Calhoun, K. S. (2012). A prospective study of sexual assault and alcohol use among first-year college women. *Violence and Victims*, 27(1), 78–94.

Naimi, T. S., Lipscomb, L. E., & Brewer, R. D. (2003). Binge drinking in the preconception period and the risk of unintended pregnancy: Implications for women and their children. *Pediatrics*, 111(5, Part 2), 1136–1141.

Naimi, T. S., Nelson, D. E., & Brewer, R. D. (2009). Driving after binge drinking. *American Journal of Preventive Medicine*, 37(4), 314–320.

NIAAA, National Institute on Alcohol Abuse and Alcoholism. (2004). NIAAA Council approves definition of binge drinking. *NIAAA Newsletter*, 3, 3.

Nordt, S. P., Vilke, G. M., & Clark, R. F. (2012). Energy drink use and adverse effects among emergency department patients. *Journal of Community Health*, 37(5), 976–981. doi:10.1007/s10900-012-9549-9

Olney, J. W., Wozniak, D. F., & Jevtovic-Todorovic, V. (2002). Drug-induced apoptotic neurodegeneration in the developing brain. *Brain Pathology*, 12(4), 488–498.

O'Malley, P. M., & Johnston, L. D. (2002, March). Epidemiology of alcohol and other drug use among American college students. *Journal of Studies on Alcohol* (14 Supplement), 23–39.

Pagliaro, A. M. (1986). Pharmacologic aspects of nursing: A historical overview. In A. M. Pagliaro, & L. A. Pagliaro (Eds.), *Pharmacologic aspects of nursing* (pp. 3–29). St. Louis, MO: C. V. Mosby.

Pagliaro, A. M., & Pagliaro, L. A. (1995). Abusable psychotropic use among children and adolescents. In L. A. Pagliaro, & A. M. Pagliaro (Eds.), *Problems in pediatric drug therapy* (3rd ed., pp. 507–540). Hamilton, IL: Drug Intelligence.

Pagliaro, A. M., & Pagliaro, L. A. (1996). *Substance use among children and adolescents.* New York, NY: John Wiley & Sons.

Pagliaro, A. M., & Pagliaro, L. A. (1997). Teratogenic effects of in utero exposure to alcohol and other abusable psychotropics. In P. Budetti, & M. Haack (Eds.), *Drug-dependent mothers and their children: Issues in public policy and public health* (pp. 31–63). New York, NY: Springer.

Pagliaro, A. M., & Pagliaro, L. A. (2000). *Substance use among women: A reference and research guide.* Philadelphia, PA: Brunner/Mazel.

Pagliaro, A. M., & Pagliaro, L. A. (2003). Alcohol and other drug use during pregnancy: Effects on the developing fetus, neonate, and infant. In R. Saitz (Ed.), *Principles of addiction medicine* (3rd ed.). Washington, DC: American Society of Addiction Medicine.

Pagliaro, L. A., & Benet, L. Z. (1975). Critical compilation of terminal half-lives, percent excreted unchanged, and changes of half-life in renal and hepatic dysfunction for studies in humans with references. *Journal of Pharmacokinetics and Biopharmaceutics*, 3, 333–383.

Pagliaro, L. A., & Levin, R. (Eds.). (1979). *Problems in pediatric drug therapy.* Bethesda, MD: Drug Intelligence Publications.

Pagliaro, L. A., & Pagliaro, A. M. (Eds.). (1987). *Problems in pediatric drug therapy* (2nd ed.). Hamilton, IL: Drug Intelligence Publications.

Pagliaro, L. A., & Pagliaro, A. M. (1992). Alcohol metabolism. *CMAJ: Canadian Medical Association Journal*, 146(12), 2141.

Pagliaro, L. A., & Pagliaro, A. M. (Eds.). (2002). *Problems in pediatric drug therapy* (4th ed.). Washington, DC: American Pharmaceutical Association.

Pagliaro, L. A., & Pagliaro, A. M. (2009). *Pagliaros' comprehensive guide to drugs and substances of abuse* (2nd ed.). Washington, DC: American Pharmacists Association.

Pagliaro, L. A., & Pagliaro, A. M. (2012). *Handbook of child and adolescent drug and substance abuse.* Hoboken, NJ: Wiley & Sons.

Parkhill, M. R., Norris, J., & Davi, K. C. (2014). The role of alcohol use during sexual situations in the relationship between sexual revictimization and women's intentions to engage in unprotected sex. *Violence and Victims*, 29(3), 492–505.

Paul, L. A., Grubaugh, A. L., & Frueh, B. C. (2011). Associations between binge and heavy drinking and health behaviors in a nationally representative sample. *Addictive Behaviors*, 36(12), 1240–1245.

Pedersen, A., Johansen, C., & Gronbaek, M. (2003). Relations between amount and type of alcohol and colon and rectal cancer in a Danish population based cohort study. *Gut*, 52(6), 861–867.

Pelucchi, C., Tramacere, I., & Boffetta, P. (2011). Alcohol consumption and cancer risk. *Nutrition and Cancer*, 63(7), 983–990. doi:10.1080/01635581.2011.596642

Peoples, R. W., Li, C., & Weight, F. F. (1996). Lipid versus protein theories of alcohol action in the nervous system. *Annual Review of Pharmacology and Toxicology*, 36, 185–201.

Petkovic, G., & Barisic, I. (2013). Prevalence of fetal alcohol syndrome and maternal characteristics in a sample of school children from a rural province of Croatia. *International*

Journal of Environmental Research and Public Health, 10(4), 1547–1561. doi:10.3390/ijerph10041547

Piano, M. R. (2002). Alcohol cardiomyopathy: Incidence, clinical characteristics, and pathophysiology. *Chest*, 121(5), 1638–1650.

Piasecki, T. M., Robertson, B. M., & Epler, A. (2010). Hangover and risk for alcohol use disorders: Existing evidence and potential mechanisms. *Current Drug Abuse Reviews*, 3(2), 92–102.

Pragst, F., & Yegles, M. (2008). Determination of fatty acid ethyl esters (FAEE) and ethyl glucuronide (EtG) in hair: A promising way for retrospective detection of alcohol abuse during pregnancy? *Therapeutic Drug Monitoring*, 30(2), 255–263. doi:10.1097/FTD.0b013e318167d602

Prat, G., Adan, A., & Perez-Pamies, M. (2008). Neurocognitive effects of alcohol hangover. *Addictive Behaviors*, 33(1), 15–23. doi:10.1016/jaddbeh.2007.05.002

Pregnancy and alcohol: Limitations on criminal prosecution. (2015, January 1). Retrieved March 3, 2016, from APIS-Alcohol Policy Information System, pp. 1–4: http://alcoholpolicy.niaaa.nih.gov/alcohol_and_pregnancy_limitations_on_criminal_prosecution.html

Presley, C. A., Meilman, P. W., & Leichliter, J. S. (2002). College factors that influence drinking. *Journal of Studies on Alcohol* (Supplement 14), S82–S90.

Proctor, S. L. (2012). Substance use disorder prevalence among female state prison inmates. *American Journal of Drug and Alcohol Abuse*, 38(4), 278–285. doi:10.3109/00952990.2012.668596

Randall, C. L., Roberts, J. S., & Del Boca, F. K. (1999). Telescoping of landmark events associated with drinking: A gender comparison. *Journal of Studies on Alcohol*, 60(2), 252–260.

Rehm, J., Taylor, B., & Mohopatra, S. (2010). Alcohol as a risk factor for liver cirrhosis: A systematic review and meta-analysis. *Drug and Alcohol Review*, 29(4), 437–445.

Roberts, S. C. (2012). Macro-level gender equality and alcohol consumption: A multilevel analysis across U.S. states. *Social Science & Medicine*, 75(1), 60–68. doi:10.1016/j.socscimed.2012.02.017

Robertson, A. A., Liew, H., & Gardner, S. (2011, July). An evaluation of the narrowing gender gap in DUI arrests. *Accident Analysis & Prevention*, 43(4), 1414–1420. doi:10.1016/j.aap.2011.02.017

Robinson, G. C., Conry, J. L., & Conry, R. F. (1987, August 1). Clinical profile and prevalence of fetal alcohol syndrome in an isolated community in British Columbia. *CMAJ: Canadian Medical Association Journal*, 137(3), 203–207.

Roeggla, G., Roeggla, H., & Roeggla, M. (1995). Effect of alcohol on acute ventilatory adaptation to mild hypoxia at moderate altitude. *Annals of Internal Medicine*, 122(12), 925–927.

Rojmahamongkol, P., Cheema-Hasan, A., & Weitzman, C. (2015, April). Do pediatricians recognize fetal alcohol spectrum disorders in children with developmental and behavioral problems? *Journal of Developmental & Behavioral Pediatrics*, 36(3), 197–202.

Rosett, H. L., Weiner, L., & Lee, A. (1983). Patterns of alcohol consumption and fetal development. *Obstetrics and Gynecology*, 61(5), 539–546.

Rothman, E. F., McNaughton Reyes, R. L., & Johnson, R. M. (2012). Does the alcohol make them do it? Dating violence perpetration and drinking among youth. *Epidemiologic Reviews*, 34(1), 103–119.

Sacks, J. J., Gonzales, K. R., & Bouchery, E. E. (2015). 2010 national and state costs of excessive alcohol consumption. *American Journal of Preventive Medicine*, 49(5), e73–e79.

Sahn, S. A., Lakshminarayan, S., & Pierson, D. J. (1975). Effect of ethanol on the ventilatory responses to oxygen and carbon dioxide in man. *Clinical Science and Molecular Medicine*, 49(1), 33–38.

Sales, J. M., Brown, J. L., & Vissman, A. T. (2012). The association between alcohol use and sexual risk behaviors among African American women across three developmental periods: A review. *Current Drug Abuse Review*, 5(2), 117–128.

SAMHSA, Substance Abuse and Mental Health Services Administration. (2014). *Results from the 2013 Survey on Drug Use and Health: Summary of National Findings, NSDUH Series H-48, HHS Publication No. (SMA) 14–4863.* Rockville, MD: Substance Abuse and Mental Health Services Administration.

Sampson, P. D., Streissguth, A. P., & Bookstein, F. L. (1997). Incidence of fetal alcohol syndrome and prevalence of alcohol-related neurodevelopmental disorder. *Teratology*, 56(5), 317–326. doi:10.1002/(SICI)1096–9926(199711)56:5<317::AID-TERA5>3.0XO:2-U

Schmidt, L. A. (2014). The equal right to drink. *Drug and Alcohol Review*, 33(6), 581–587. doi:10.1111/dar.12215

Schwartz, J. (2008). Gender differences in drunk driving prevalence rates and trends: A 20-year assessment using multiple sources of evidence. *Addictive Behaviors*, 33(9), 1217–1222. doi:10.1016/j.addbeh.2008.03.014

Schwartz, J., & Davaran, A. (2013). Enforcement following 0.08% BAC law change: Sex-specific consequences of changing arrest practices? *Addictive Behaviors*, 38(10), 2506–2512. doi:10.10165/j.addbeh.2013.04.004

Scoccianti, C., Lauby-Secretan, B., & Bello, P. Y. (2014). Female breast cancer and alcohol consumption: A review of the literature. *American Journal of Preventive Medicine*, 46(3 Supplement 1), S16–S25. doi:10.1016/j.amepre.2013.10.031

Shorey, R. C., Moore, T. M., & McNulty, J. K. (2016). Do alcohol and marijuana increase the risk for female dating violence victimization? A prospective daily diary investigation. *Psychology of Violence*, 6(4), 509–519.

Slattery, M. L., Wolff, R. K., & Herrick, J. S. (2010). Alcohol consumption and rectal tumor mutations and epigenetic changes. *Diseases of the Colon & Rectum*, 53(8), 1182–1189. doi:10.1007/DCR.0b013e3181d325db

Smith, C. M., & Barnes, G. M. (1983). Signs and symptoms of hangover: Prevalence and relationship to alcohol use in a general adult population. *Drug and Alcohol Dependence*, 11(3–4), 249–269.

Smith, P. H., Homish, G. G., & Leonard, K. E. (2012). Intimate partner violence and specific substance use disorders: Findings from the National Epidemiologic Survey on Alcohol and Related Conditions. *Psychology of Addictive Behaviors*, 26(2), 236–245. doi:10.1037/a0024855

Smitherman, C. H. (1994). The lasting impact of fetal alcohol syndrome and fetal alcohol effect on children and adolescents. *Journal of Pediatric Health Care*, 8, 121–126.

Sokol, R. J., & Clarren, S. K. (1989). Guidelines for use of terminology describing the impact of prenatal alcohol on the offspring. *Alcoholism: Clinical and Experimental Research*, 13(4), 597–598.

Sood, B., Delaney-Black, V., & Covington, C. (2001). Prenatal alcohol exposure and childhood behavior at age 6 and 7 years: I. dose-response effect. *Pediatrics*, 108, E34.

Spatz Widom, C. S., Raskin White, S., & Czaja, S. J. (2007). Long-term effects of child abuse and neglect on alcohol use and excessive drinking in middle adulthood. *Journal of Studies on Alcohol and Drugs*, 68(3), 317–326.

Spohr, H. L., Willms, J., & Steinhausen, H. C. (1993). Prenatal alcohol exposure and long-term developmental consequences. *The Lancet*, 341(8850), 907–910.

Spohr, H. L., Willms, J., & Steinhausen, H. C. (2007). Fetal Alcohol Spectrum Disorders in young adulthood. *Journal of Pediatrics*, 150(2), 175–179.

Square, D. (1997, July 1). Fetal alcohol syndrome epidemic on Manitoba reserve. *CMAJ: Canadian Medical Association Journal*, 157(1), 59–60.

Stahre, M. A., Brewer, R. D., & Fonseca, V. P. (2009). Binge drinking among U.S. active-duty military personnel. *American Journal of Preventive Medicine*, 36(3), 208–217.

Stewart, S. H. (2009). Women, girls, and alcohol. In K. T. Brady (Ed.), *Women and addiction: A comprehensive handbook* (pp. 341–359). New York, NY: Guilford.

Streissguth, A. P., Randels, S. P., & Smith, D. F. (1991). A test-retest study of intelligence in patients with fetal alcohol syndrome: Implications for care. *Journal of the American Academy of Child & Adolescent Psychiatry*, 30(4), 584–587. doi:10.1097/00004583-199107000-00009

Stuart, G. L., Meehan, J. C., & Moore, T. M. (2006). Examining a conceptual framework of intimate partner violence in men and women arrested for domestic violence. *Journal of Studies on Alcohol*, 67(1), 102–112.

Stuart, G. L., Moore, T. M., & Ramsey, S. E. (2004). Hazardous drinking and relationship violence perpetration and victimization in women arrested for domestic violence. *Journal of Studies on Alcohol*, 65(1), 46–53.

Stuart, G. L., Temple, J. R., & Follansbee, K. W. (2008). The role of drug use in a conceptual model of intimate partner violence in men and women arrested for domestic violence. *Psychology of Addictive Behaviors*, 22(1), 12–24. doi:10.1037/0893-164X.22.1.12

Sung, J. (2016, August 26). *Baby covered in vomit bathed by cops after being found in backseat of drunk driver.* Retrieved August 26, 2016, from http://globalnews.ca/news/2905718/baby-covered-in-vomit-bathed-by-cops-after-being-found-in-backseat-of-drunk-driver/

Tan, C. H., Denny, C. H., & Cheal, N. E. (2015, September 25). Alcohol use and binge drinking among women of childbearing age—United States, 2011–2013. *Morbidity and Mortality Weekly Report (MMWR)*, 64(37), 1042–1046.

Testa, M., Hoffman, J. H., & Livingston, J. A. (2010). Alcohol and sexual risk behaviors as mediators of the sexual victimization-revictimization relationship. *Journal of Consulting and Clinical Psychology*, 78, 249–259.

Thanh, N. X., Jonsson, E., & Salmon, A. (2014). Incidence and prevalence of fetal alcohol spectrum disorder by sex and age group in Alberta, Canada. *Journal of Population Therapeutics and Clinical Pharmacology*, 21(3), e395–e404.

Thomas, S., Cannon, C., & French, J. (2015). The effects of state alcohol and pregnancy policies on women's health and healthy pregnancies. *Journal of Women, Politics & Policy*, 36, 68–94.

Timko, C., Moos, B. S., & Moos, R. H. (2009). Gender differences in 16-year trends in assault- and police-related problems due to drinking. *Addictive Behaviors*, 34(9), 744–750. doi:10.1016/j.addbeh.2009.04.013

U.S. Department of Health and Human Services, Office of the Surgeon General. (2016). *Facing addiction in America: The Surgeon General's report on alcohol, drugs, and health, executive summary.* Washington, DC: Health and Human Services.

Ullman, S. E., & Sigurvinsdottir, R. (2015). Intimate partner violence and drinking among victims of adult sexual assault. *Journal of Aggression, Maltreatment, & Trauma*, 24(2), 117–130. doi:10.1080/10926771.2015.996312

Wang, C., Xue, H., & Wang, Q. (2014). Effect of drinking on all-cause mortality in women compared to men: A meta-analysis. *Journal of Women's Health (Larchmont, New York)*, 23(5), 373–381. doi:10.1089/jwh.2013.4414

Wechsler, H., Kuo, M., & Lee, H. (2000). Environmental correlates of underage alcohol use and related problems of college students. *American Journal of Preventive Medicine*, 19(1), 24–29.

White, C., Lindsey, S., & Vincente, C. (1981). Alcohol increases sleep apnea and oxygen desaturation in asymptomatic men. *The American Journal of Medicine*, 71(2), 240–245.

Williams, R. J., Odaibo, F. S., & McGee, J. M. (1999, May–June). Incidence of fetal alcohol syndrome in northeastern Manitoba. *Canadian Journal of Public Health*, 90(3), 192–194.

Wilsnack, S. C., Wilsnack, R., & Wolfgang Kantor, L. (2013). Focus on: Women and the costs of alcohol use. *Alcohol Research: Current Reviews*, 219–228.

Wu, S., Li, W. Q., & Qureshi, A. A. (2015). Alcohol consumption and risk of cutaneous basal cell carcinoma in women and men: 3 prospective cohort studies. *American Journal of Clinical Nutrition*, 102(5), 1158–1166. doi:10.3945/ajcn.115.115196

Xiao, Q., Weiner, H., & Crabb, D. W. (1996). The mutation in the mitochondrial aldehyde dehydrogenase (ALDH2) gene responsible for alcohol-induced flushing increases turnover of the enzyme tetramers in a dominant fashion. *Journal of Clinical Investigation*, 98(9), 2027–2032.

Yonker, J. E., Nilsson, L. G., & Herlitz, A. (2005). Sex differences in spatial visualization and episodic memory as a function of alcohol consumption. *Alcohol and Alcoholism*, 40(3), 201–207.

Yost, D. A. (1996). Alcohol withdrawal syndrome. *American Family Physician*, 54(2), 657–664.

Zakhari, S., & Hoek, J. B. (2015). Alcohol and breast cancer: Reconciling epidemiological and molecular data. *Advances in Experimental Medicine and Biology*, 815, 7–39. doi:10.1007/978-3-319-09614-8_2

Zheng, Y. L., Lian, F., & Shi, Q. (2015). Alcohol intake and associated risk of major cardiovascular outcomes in women compared with men: A systematic review and meta-analysis of prospective observational studies. *BMC Public Health*, 15, 773. doi:10.1186/s12889-015-2081-y

Zilberman, M., Tavares, H., & el-Guebaly, N. (2003). Gender similarities and differences: The prevalence and course of alcohol- and other substance-related disorders. *Journal of Addictive Diseases*, 22(4), 61–74. doi:10.1300/j069v22n04_06

3

WOMEN'S PRESCRIPTION SEDATIVE-HYPNOTIC ABUSE

A *sedative* drug reduces response to *all* sensory input by *mildly* depressing the CNS. A *hypnotic* drug causes a state of natural sleep by *moderately* depressing the CNS. A *sedative-hypnotic* drug causes dose-dependent sedation, sleep, or coma, depending on its increasing *dosage* and corresponding blood and brain concentrations. Pharmacologically, virtually, *all* the drugs discussed in this chapter are classified as "sedative-hypnotics." However, some of the sedative-hypnotics discussed in this chapter, may also be classified as "anti-anxiety drugs," "anticonvulsants," or "muscle relaxants" because they were developed and marketed by a pharmaceutical company and approved by the FDA for a particular indication for use. To avoid confusion, we clearly identify these classes of sedative-hypnotics when they are discussed in this chapter.

The focus of this chapter is on *two* major classes of prescription sedative-hypnotics that have been commonly abused by women in the U.S. during the new millennium—*benzodiazepines* and *z-drugs* (Table 3.1). Two *miscellaneous* sedative-hypnotic drugs also are presented and discussed, *suvorexant* (Belsomra®) and *gamma-hydroxybutyrate* (GHB). (For a detailed discussion of alcohol—the *most* commonly used, *non-prescription*, sedative-hypnotic among women—see Chapter 2, *Women's Alcohol Abuse*.)[1]

We first present and discuss the benzodiazepines, followed by the z-drugs, and conclude with the two miscellaneous sedative-hypnotics. For each of these classes of sedative-hypnotics, we give attention to their pharmacology—*pharmacodynamics*,

[1] Other *prescription* sedative-hypnotics, including the barbiturates and other miscellaneous sedative-hypnotics that were more commonly used and abused by women in the U.S. during the last century, are *not* discussed in this chapter. For related detailed information and discussion, see Pagliaro and Pagliaro (2009).

TABLE 3.1 Prescription Sedative-Hypnotics: Benzodiazepines, Z-Drugs, Suvorexant, and GHB

Prescription Sedative-Hypnotics		
Generic Name	*Brand/Trade Names®*[a]	*Common Street Names*[b]
Benzodiazepines		
Alprazolam	Xanax®	Coffins; Footballs; Four Bars: Xannies
Bromazepam	Lectopam®	—
Chlordiazepoxide	Librium®	Gone Time; Goofies; Libs; Libbies
Clonazepam	Klonopin®; Rivotril®	Clo; Klondike Bars; Klonnies; Klons
Clorazepate	Tranxene®	—
Diazepam	Valium®	Blues; Mother's Little Helper; Vs
Estazolam	ProSom®	—
Flunitrazepam	Rohypnol®	Forget Me Pill; Mexican Valium; Papas; Roofies; Wolfies
Flurazepam	Dalmane®	—
Lorazepam	Ativan®	Zzz
Midazolam	Versed®	—
Nitrazepam	Mogadon®	Dons; Moggies
Oxazepam	Serax®	—
Quazepam	Doral®	—
Temazepam	Restoril®	Green Devils; Knockouts; No-Gos; Temmies
Triazolam	Halcion®	Halcyon; Halcyon Daze
Z-Drugs		
Eszopiclone	Lunesta®	—
Zaleplon	Starnoc®; Sonata®	—
Zolpidem	Ambien®; Lunata®	Nappien; Tic-Tacs
Zopiclone	Imovane®; Rhovane®	Vane; Z-Drug; Zoppies
Miscellaneous Sedative-Hypnotics		
Suvorexant	Belsomra®	—
Gamma-hydroxybutyrate (GHB)[c]	Xyrem®	Easy Lay; Georgia Home Boy, GHB; Grievous Bodily Harm; Soap

[a] Examples of common brand/trade names are provided, when available.

[b] *Partial* list. Examples of three to five of the *most* common street names are provided, when available. See Pagliaro and Pagliaro (2009) for a complete listing of the drugs and substances of abuse and their common street names.

[c] Medically referred to by its alternative generic name—*sodium oxybate*.

or mechanism of action; *pharmacokinetics*, or absorption, distribution, metabolism, and excretion; and undesired, or harmful, effects and toxicities. We conclude the chapter with an analysis and reflective synthesis of women's medical and personal use and abuse of the prescription sedative-hypnotics, during the new millennium, in the U.S.

Benzodiazepines

The benzodiazepine molecule was *synthesized* in the 1950s as a pharmacotherapeutic alternative to the barbiturates (i.e., derivatives of barbituric acid) that had dominated the sedative-hypnotic market for the previous 100 years. Over the last 60 years more than 2,000 *different* benzodiazepine derivatives were developed. The benzodiazepines were widely advertised and marketed as being the *safest* drugs available for managing anxiety and insomnia because, in comparison to the barbiturates, they possess a significantly *higher* therapeutic index. For these reasons, and because the benzodiazepines were found to be relatively safe and effective for use in clinical practice—they became the *most* widely medically-prescribed and *abused* sedative-hypnotics in the U.S., as well as the rest of the world. Although the benzodiazepines continue to be widely abused for their desired *sedative* and *hypnotic* actions, their use is now being increasingly replaced by the more recently developed *z-drugs*. In fact, the *z-drugs* have now become the *most* medically-prescribed and abused sedative-hypnotics in the U.S. (See the later section, *Z-Drugs*.)[2]

Pharmacology

The benzodiazepines and their active metabolites generally share similar sedative and hypnotic actions with no one benzodiazepine being significantly superior to the others.[3] However, some women may react differently to various benzodiazepines, particularly regarding associated undesired, or harmful, effects and toxicities (see later discussion). This variability in women's individual response may, in large part, be due to the *placebo effect*.[4] These effects and toxicities are discussed in

---

[2] Although the use of the z-drugs has gained in popularity during the new millennium (see later discussion), there are *no* current available data that support their significant superiority in terms of clinical efficacy and safety over the benzodiazepines.

[3] However, the benzodiazepines do significantly differ regarding their anticonvulsant actions. Generally, only clonazepam (Rivotril®), clorazepate (Tranxene®), diazepam (Valium®), and lorazepam (Ativan®) are used to pharmacologically manage seizure disorders. Clonazepam is probably more appropriately classified primarily as an anticonvulsant rather than as a sedative-hypnotic because of its pharmacologic actions and primary medical use.

[4] The placebo effect is a psychological mechanism of drug action that applies to *all* drugs, whether pharmacologically active (e.g., prescription analgesic) or not (e.g., sugar tablet; normal saline injection). Placebo and other drug actions are *not* mutually exclusive. In fact, they generally occur together with the use of most drugs (e.g., headache relief within seconds after swallowing an aspirin tablet with a glassful of water). Only the percentage of response due to the placebo effect differs from

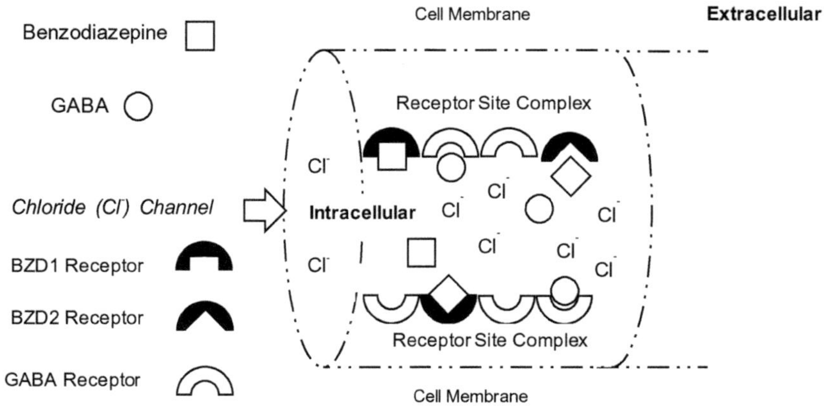

FIGURE 3.1 Mechanism of Benzodiazepine Action

the following sections, along with other related basic pharmacological principles and concepts. We begin with the *pharmacodynamics* of the benzodiazepines—their mechanism of psychodepressant action.

Pharmacodynamics: Mechanism of Action

Although the benzodiazepines have been commercially available since the late 1950s, the precise sites and specific mechanisms of their sedative and hypnotic actions are *not* completely understood. It is thought that the benzodiazepines act in the CNS along with gamma-aminobutyric acid (GABA) to *inhibit* neurotransmission, particularly in the cerebral cortex and the limbic system, including the amygdala and the thalamus. A GABA receptor complex has been identified at which the benzodiazepines appear to enhance GABA-mediated chloride influx through chloride ion channels (see Figure 3.1).

In the absence of GABA, the benzodiazepines appear to be *unable* to open the chloride channels and elicit their sedative and hypnotic actions. Although it has been clearly demonstrated that the benzodiazepines have a high affinity for binding at the GABA receptor complex,[5] it has *not* yet been proved that this action directly, and *solely*, is responsible for their observed pharmacologic actions in humans. It also has been suggested that, at least for women between menarche and menopause, progesterone may have some direct agonistic action at the $GABA_A$

woman to woman and drug to drug based largely on several variables that are related to the patient, prescriber, drug, and clinical context of use.

[5] Endogenous ligands for the benzodiazepine-binding site (i.e., the "brain's Valium") are known as *endozepines* and consist of a group, or family, of neuropeptides. The major identified ligands in this family include: (1) nonpeptidic endozepines; (2) oleamides; and (3) diazepam-binding inhibitor (Farzampour, Reimer, & Huguenard, 2015).

receptor that may enhance the actions of the benzodiazepines and, thus, contribute to women's benzodiazepine abuse (Babalonis, Lile, & Martin, 2011a, 2011b).

Pharmacokinetics: Absorption, Distribution, Metabolism, and Excretion

The basic *pharmacokinetics* of the benzodiazepines—the processes of *absorption, distribution, metabolism,* and *excretion*—are described and discussed with, whenever possible, attention to women's biology. We begin with *absorption.*

Absorption. The benzodiazepines are generally well-absorbed after oral ingestion. Although food can sometimes delay the *rate* of absorption, it does not generally affect the *extent* of absorption. For example, diazepam (Valium®) is virtually completely absorbed after oral ingestion and can achieve peak blood concentrations within 1 to 2 hours. After intravenous (IV) injection,[6] peak blood concentrations are achieved within 15 minutes. After intramuscular (IM) injection,[7] peak blood concentrations usually occur within 2 hours.

Distribution. The benzodiazepines are highly bound to plasma proteins (e.g., albumin) and are widely distributed throughout body tissues. However, the benzodiazepines and their metabolites readily cross the blood-brain and the placental "barriers." They also are excreted in breast milk.

Metabolism and Excretion. Most of the benzodiazepines are mainly metabolized in the liver by the *hepatic microsomal enzyme system.* Therefore, liver disease or dysfunction (e.g., cirrhosis of the liver; hepatitis) can *slow* benzodiazepine metabolism and, consequently, increase toxicity. Some benzodiazepines, including *flurazepam* (Dalmane®), undergo *extensive* first-pass hepatic metabolism.[8] Other benzodiazepines, such as: *lorazepam* (Ativan®), *oxazepam* (Serax®), and *temazepam* (Restoril®) are metabolized primarily by urinary conjugation to *more* water-soluble (i.e., *polar*) glucuronide derivatives that are, subsequently, excreted in the urine.

---

6 Absorption is immediate and, by definition, 100% following *intravenous* injection.

7 Following *intramuscular* injection, absorption may be erratic (increased or decreased or quickened or slowed) depending on blood flow to the specific muscle site.

8 Following *oral* ingestion, a drug is first transported to the liver by way of the portal vein system before being released into the general systemic circulation. As it passes through the liver, some, or occasionally most, is metabolized to a less active or completely inactive form (the amount/percentage metabolized, on this single pass through the liver, is commonly referred to as the hepatic extraction ratio). This entire process is called first-pass hepatic metabolism, or the "first-pass effect." The first-pass effect does *not* occur when drugs or substances of abuse are administered by other common routes that allow them to immediately enter the circulatory system, such as: buccal and sublingual placement in the cheek and under the tongue, respectively; intramuscular, intravenous, and subcutaneous injection; pulmonary inhalation; rectal insertion; and transdermal and transmucosal delivery.

It is important for health and social care providers to recognize that benzodiazepine metabolism rates may be *slowed* among some women, making these women *more* predisposed to toxicity. For example, women who have *severe* liver disease (e.g., alcoholic cirrhosis of the liver; hepatitis, including that associated with intravenous drug use), particularly if they are older and have age-related changes in liver function, may metabolize benzodiazepines *more* slowly.

The benzodiazepines can have *slow*, *intermediate*, or *rapid* elimination profiles. Benzodiazepines that have *slow* elimination profiles are those that produce *active metabolites*, either from: (1) *parent drugs*, or *compounds*; or (2) *inactive pro-drugs*.

The benzodiazepines that have *slow* elimination profiles include:

- *Active parent drugs, or compounds*
  - Chlordiazepoxide (Librium®)
  - Diazepam (Valium®)
  - Flurazepam (Dalmane®)
- *Inactive pro-drugs*
  - Clorazepate (Tranxene®)
  - Halazepam (Paxipam®)
  - Prazepam (Centrax®)

The benzodiazepines that have *intermediate* elimination profiles include:

- Alprazolam (Xanax®)
- Clonazepam (Rivotril®)
- Lorazepam (Ativan®)
- Oxazepam (Serax®)
- Temazepam (Restoril®)

Finally, the benzodiazepines that have *rapid* elimination profiles include:

- Midazolam (Versed®)
- Triazolam (Halcion®)

Undesired, or Harmful, Effects and Toxicities

As noted earlier in this chapter, the benzodiazepines have a relatively *high* therapeutic index. Even so, several undesired, or harmful, effects and toxicities have been associated with their abuse. These effects can generally be classified as either *acute* or *chronic* effects.

Acute Effects. Acute effects include: blurred vision; diplopia; dizziness; drowsiness (somnolence); muscle weakness; psychomotor impairment; slurred speech; and speech impairment related to a weakening of the tongue muscle (dysarthria).

They also include amnesias, particularly anterograde amnesia,[9] and other memory impairments, such as those affecting long-term, explicit (e.g., episodic) and implicit (e.g., procedural) memory, and short-term (e.g., active) memory.

These acute harmful effects often occur together (e.g., blurred vision, cognitive impairment, confusion, and dizziness). Consequently, they contribute to a *higher* risk for: (1) falling down a flight of stairs and suffering a serious head injury or fractured hip);[10] and (2) being involved in motor vehicle crashes (MVCs) (e.g., Pagliaro & Pagliaro, 1983; van Strien, Koek, & van Marum, 2013).[11] Thus, health and social care professionals are reminded to:

- Remain consciously aware of the direct pharmacologic actions of the benzodiazepines (and z-drugs—see later section, *Z-drugs*) that may contribute to fatal injuries
- Take appropriate precautions to minimize the risk for fatal injuries, particularly for older women (e.g., initiate pharmacotherapy with a dosage that is one-half of the usual recommended starting dosage for younger women, and slowly increase the dosage with careful monitoring)
- Remind women, particularly older women, who medically use benzodiazepines, to avoid concurrent use of other sedative-hypnotics, including alcohol

Other acute harmful effects include aggression and violent behavior. Generally considered to be idiosyncratic personality effects, these effects are, more likely,

---

9 *Anterograde* amnesia is the primary memory impairment generally associated with the use of the benzodiazepines. This type of amnesia causes a loss of memory for events that occur *after* the benzodiazepine was used. This action of the benzodiazepines is used both therapeutically (e.g., to provide amnesia of surgical events for patients requiring surgery) and criminally (e.g., to facilitate crimes including robbery and *date rape*—see later *Sexual Assault* section). In some contexts of use, the benzodiazepine-related memory impairment resembles *alcoholic blackouts* (see Chapter 2, *Women's Alcohol Abuse*, for further discussion).

10 Given the well-documented propensity of accidental injuries among older women, and men—both in the U.S. and worldwide prior to and over the new millennium (Pagliaro & Pagliaro, 1983; Stevens, Mack, & Paulozzi, 2008)—it is imperative that health and social care professionals increase their awareness of this serious, and often fatal problem. For example, as reported by Binder (2002), "about 39,000 women and men aged 65 years-of-age and older die each year in the U.S. from injuries—the top three causes of which being falls, those related to motor vehicle crashes, and suicide" (p. iv2). Recognizing that 15,802 women and men, 65 years-of-age or older, died from fall injuries in 2005, and that the number of those seeking outpatient treatment for minor or moderate fall injuries was *unknown*, Stevens, Mack, and Paulozzi (2008), further investigated the problem. They found that, "approximately 5.8 million (15.9%)" women and men, 65 years-of-age or older, "reported falling at least once during the preceding three months, and 1.8 million (31.3%) of those who fell sustained an injury that resulted in a doctor visit or restricted activity for at least one day" (p. 345).

11 The combined cognitive and psychomotor impairment, which is directly related to benzodiazepine use, has been associated with a significant *increase* in both the risk and responsibility for MVCs (Dassanayake, Michie, & Carter, 2011), particularly among older women (Meuleners, Duke, & Lee, 2011).

a *consequence* of benzodiazepine-induced disinhibition among women who have pre-existing aggressive and hostile tendencies or personalities (Pagliaro & Pagliaro, *Clinical Patient Data Files*). (Also, see related discussion in the later section, *Physical and Psychological Dependence*, "Fatalities.")

Chronic Effects. Regular, long-term use of the benzodiazepines is associated with: apathy; decreased impulse control;[12] diminished sleep quality;[13] emotional instability; lethargy; memory impairment; mental depression; and rebound anxiety.[14] They also are associated with physical and psychological dependence characterized by tolerance, craving, and the benzodiazepine withdrawal syndrome (see following section, *Physical and Psychological Dependence*).

These chronic undesired, or harmful, effects and toxicities are generally *increased* among women who have:

- Alcoholism
- Chronic obstructive pulmonary, or lung, disease (COPD), including asthma, bronchitis, and emphysema
- Liver disease (e.g., cirrhosis of the liver; hepatitis) or an age-related change in liver function
- Personality disorders, such as borderline personality disorder

In addition, women, who daily abuse benzodiazepines for months or years, may experience a small, but *permanent* and significant, *decrease* in attention, concentration, and other cognitive abilities. These effects on cognitive function appear to be *more* pronounced among older women (Barker, Greenwood, & Jackson, 2003). Older women also appear to be *more* susceptible to the effects of benzodiazepines on memory function, including having a greater risk for anterograde amnesia (Pagliaro & Pagliaro, 2009). Increased risk of Alzheimer's disease also has been suggested among older women who have abused benzodiazepines for 10 years or longer (Koyama, Steinman, & Ensrud, 2013). However, at this point, although a correlational association between chronic benzodiazepine abuse and Alzheimer's disease has been clearly established, it is *not* yet clear whether this relationship is causal (Billioti de Gage, Moride, & Ducruet, 2014).

Other Effects. Other effects associated with women's benzodiazepine abuse, include: fatalities; sexual assault; and, if used during pregnancy, *teratogenesis*. These and other related effects are discussed in the following sections.

---

12 *Impulsivity* (i.e., decreased impulse control) appears to be *higher* among prison inmates, particularly women, who are lifetime users of the benzodiazepines (Bernstein, McSheffrey, & van den Berg, 2015).

13 A *decrease* in sleep quality appears to be related to the development of signs and symptoms of mental depression among chronic benzodiazepine abusers (Bourgeois, Elseviers, & Van Bortel, 2014b).

14 *Rebound anxiety* occurs when the regular, long-term (over 30 days) use of a sedative-hypnotic is abruptly discontinued. The anxiety that was initially being treated returns, but at a much greater degree.

FATALITIES. Potentially fatal harmful effects and toxicities have been associated with the combination of benzodiazepines and other drugs and substances of abuse, particularly, *alcohol*. (Also, see Chapter 2, *Women's Alcohol Abuse*.) The sedative-hypnotic actions of the benzodiazepines are *potentiated* by the actions of other psychodepressants (e.g., alcohol; opiate analgesics). In fact, the concomitant use of benzodiazepines and alcohol has resulted in several deaths due to associated respiratory depression (Pagliaro & Pagliaro, 2009; Tanaka, 2002). (Also, see later section, "Overdosage.") Many of these deaths resulted from deliberate, or intentional, suicide attempts that resulted in *completed* suicides. Health and social care professionals should be aware that the risk for suicide attempts among women who abuse benzodiazepines is significantly *higher* for women who regularly use *higher* dosages of the benzodiazepines and *concurrently* have other mental disorders, including:

- Alcohol use disorder (AUD)
- Borderline personality disorder (BPD)
- Substance use disorder (SUD)
- Major depressive disorder (MDD)

(Bellivier, Yon, & Luquiens, 2011; Lekka, Paschalis, & Beratis, 2002; Pagliaro & Pagliaro, Clinical Patient Data Files; *Voaklander, Rowe, & Dryden, 2008)*

SEXUAL ASSAULT. Over the last 3 decades, the benzodiazepines, *alone*, or in combination with alcohol and other drugs and substances of abuse, frequently have been used to perpetrate sexual assaults (Dowd, Strong, & Janicak, 2002; Pagliaro & Pagliaro, 2009).

Popular Notion: The victims of drug-facilitated sexual assault are almost always young or middle-aged women.

NOT TRUE. Adolescent girls, as well as older women—particularly those who are institutionalized in long-term care facilities—also are victims of drug-facilitated sexual assaults (Burgess, Dowdell, & Prentky, 2000; Pagliaro & Pagliaro, *Clinical Patient Data Files;* Ramsey-Klawsnik, 2004; Teaster & Roberto, 2003).

Illicitly used in this context, the benzodiazepines, and other sedative-hypnotics—*z-drugs*, particularly zolpidem (Ambien®), and gamma-hydroxybutyrate (GHB)[15]

[15] GHB ("Great Hormone at Bedtime"; "Grievous Bodily Harm"; "Salty Water") is a naturally occurring cerebral inhibitory neurotransmitter. It acts as both a precursor and a metabolite of gamma-aminobutyric acid (GABA). GHB was first synthesized about 50 years ago, and because of its: (1) ability to produce a disinhibitory euphoria, or *high*; (2) physical-chemical qualities (i.e., being

(see later comprehensive discussions of z-drugs and GHB in this chapter)—are referred to as:

- Acquaintance rape drugs
- Drug-assisted rape/sexual assault drugs
- Date rape drugs (the *most* commonly used term)

(NIDA, 2008; Pagliaro & Pagliaro, 2009)

The use of the date rape drugs is estimated to occur in up to 50% of all rapes in the U.S. (Madea & MuBhoff, 2009; Pagliaro & Pagliaro, 2009). Unfortunately, the use of the benzodiazepines as a means for perpetrating a sexual assault appears to be increasing. In fact, *flunitrazepam* (Rohypnol®)—Forget Me Drug, Mexican Valium, *Papas*, or Roofie—is the benzodiazepine that is *most* often involved in cases of date rape, being simply slipped into the victim's beverage, without her (or his) knowledge, to induce drowsiness or sleep to facilitate the sexual assault. Benzodiazepines also induce anterograde amnesia, which allows the perpetrator to avoid prosecution (e.g., Goulle & Anger, 2004; Pagliaro & Pagliaro, *Clinical Patient Data Files*) by preventing the victim from:

1. Clearly remembering details of the assault
2. Identifying the perpetrator
3. Testifying under oath, in a court of law, that consent was *not* given for the sexual contact or that other related events did or did *not* occur

In addition, it has been increasingly reported, over the new millennium, that young women orally ingest flunitrazepam (Rohypnol®) with an alcoholic beverage in a conscious and deliberate attempt to *decrease* their sexual inhibitions when *clubbing* or attending house parties and raves. In this context, sexual predators commonly take the opportunity to encourage the use of additional alcohol, benzodiazepines, or other drugs and substances of abuse, including psychodelics (e.g., MDMA, or "Ecstasy"), to facilitate the perpetration of the sexual assault (Pagliaro & Pagliaro, *Clinical Patient Data Files*).

Although flunitrazepam is *not* legally produced in the U.S., it is widely available for direct, illicit purchase and, *legally* available in Europe and Mexico; it also is easily purchased from vendors over the Internet (Pagliaro & Pagliaro, 2009).

Coincident with the increasing percentage of women in the U.S. military during the new millennium, is the *increasing* incidence of substance use disorders (SUDs) among woman veterans (Cucciare, Simpson, & Hoggatt, 2013; Pagliaro & Pagliaro, *Clinical Patient Data Files*). These SUDs, particularly those that involve the abuse of prescription sedative-hypnotics, are associated with a *significant* risk

---

colorless, odorless, and readily soluble in alcohol—although producing a distinctly "salty" taste); and (3) associated anterograde amnesia; it is widely used to perpetrate date rape.

for sexual assault (i.e., "unwanted sexual contact") among U.S. active duty service women (Stahlman, Javanbakht, & Cochran, 2015).

Pregnancy, Lactation, and Mothering. The use of selected benzodiazepines during pregnancy has been associated with *teratogenic effects* (i.e., birth defects). For example, the use of diazepam (Valium®) during pregnancy, even at usual prescribed dosages, has resulted in cleft lip and cleft palate among some neonates whose mothers were medically prescribed diazepam for the management of their epilepsy. Craniofacial cleft also was reported involving the newborn baby of a mother who ingested 580 mg of diazepam in a single dose on the 43rd day of pregnancy (Pagliaro & Pagliaro, 2002).

The increased teratogenic risk associated with the use of anticonvulsants/antiepileptics during pregnancy has long been well-documented (Pagliaro & Levin, 1979). However, it has been found to be *highest* among pregnant women who received benzodiazepine monotherapy for the medical management of epilepsy (Deck, Nadkarni, & Montouris, 2015). Even when teratogenic effects (i.e., major physical abnormalities) have *not* been documented (e.g., Wikner & Kallen, 2011), the use of the benzodiazepines during pregnancy has often been associated with higher rates of preterm birth, low birth weight, and or small for gestational age neonates/infants (Okun, Ebert, & Saini, 2015).

Maternal use of the benzodiazepines during labor may result in neonatal sedation and respiratory depression. The benzodiazepines cross the placental barrier and can achieve fetal blood concentrations that are equal to, or *higher*, than maternal blood concentrations. Regular, long-term abuse of the benzodiazepines by women during pregnancy or near term may result in fetal benzodiazepine physical dependence and, at birth, the *neonatal benzodiazepine withdrawal syndrome*, characterized by:

- Drowsiness
- Poor muscle tone
- Poor sucking behavior
- Low *Apgar* scores
- Respiratory depression
- Tremor

Interestingly, but not surprising, Lind, Petersen, and Lederer (2015), in a large study of the *neonatal abstinence syndrome* (NAS) associated with women's opiate analgesic abuse, found that over 40% of the mothers of affected neonates also reported benzodiazepine use during pregnancy. Thus, health and social care professionals must be ever vigilant when assessing and diagnosing pregnant women who most likely have used more than one psychotropic drug or substance of abuse during their pregnancies.

The benzodiazepines also are excreted in breast milk in concentrations that may be sufficient to cause sedation and potential benzodiazepine physical dependence among breast-fed neonates and infants. In addition, if regular, long-term maternal benzodiazepine abuse or breast-feeding is abruptly discontinued, the breast-fed neonate or infant is at risk for the benzodiazepine withdrawal syndrome. Maternal benzodiazepine abuse also has been *indirectly* associated with such major harmful effects as poor maternal-infant bonding, infant physical abuse and neglect, and infant/toddler *failure to thrive*.[16]

Physical and Psychological Dependence. Regarding *abuse potential*, the benzodiazepines have a *low to moderate* potential for physical dependence and a *moderate to high* potential for psychological dependence (Pagliaro & Pagliaro, 2009; Weaver, 2015). It has been long recognized that—at both *lower* and *higher* dosages—*psychological* dependence can develop with the regular, long-term use of the benzodiazepines.

> Plagued by anxiety and depression, Kelly McMillan unwittingly developed a dependency on the very meds [i.e., clonazepam; Klonopin®] that were supposed to help her.
>
> *(McMillan, 2014, p. 1)*

However, during the 1960s through the 1980s, it was generally thought that *physical* dependence, in the strictest sense, did *not* occur. Available data now indicate that the regular, long-term use of the benzodiazepines, even within therapeutic dosage ranges, can lead to a *true physical dependence* (i.e., *addiction*) in a significant *minority* of people (Pagliaro & Pagliaro, 2009), particularly women who have a past personal or family history of alcoholism. In addition, as noted by Evans and Levin (2002), women were at *greater* risk for both physical and psychological benzodiazepine dependence, if they also consumed *moderate to heavy* amounts of alcohol.

Some general indicators of benzodiazepine physical and psychological dependence, include:

- Regular use of a benzodiazepine for longer than 30 days
- An expressed *craving*, or a desire, for the benzodiazepine
- A need to *increase* the dosage of the benzodiazepine in order to achieve, or maintain, the desired effect(s)[17]

---

[16] *Failure to Thrive* (FTT) is a condition in which neonates and young infants and toddlers stop meeting developmental goals for growth (i.e., length, height, and weight gain) along with those for emotional and social development even with the adequate provision of clinical attention and nutrients. *Regression*, or the tendency to lose developmental progress that has recently been made, also occurs. FTT has been characterized as a form of infant *anaclitic depression* (Masten & O'Connor, 1989; Singer, Song, & Hill, 1990).

[17] A generally prototypical, related indictor is a pattern of *increasing* requests for early refills of benzodiazepine prescriptions (Pagliaro & Pagliaro, *Clinical Patient Data Files*).

- Characteristic signs and symptoms of the benzodiazepine withdrawal syndrome when the use of the benzodiazepine is abruptly discontinued for *any* reason, such as:
  - Inability to renew a prescription
  - Lack of funds to buy more of the drug
  - Inability to ingest dosages because of illness, including nausea or vomiting

(Also, see the later section, *Benzodiazepine Withdrawal Syndrome*.)

As noted by Canham, Gallo, and Simoni-Wastila (2014, p. 873):

> 35% of persons who take benzodiazepines regularly for four weeks or longer will develop dependence; after 4 to 6 months of daily use, the majority of users will develop dependence.

TOLERANCE. Tolerance to the actions of the benzodiazepines—the need to use more of the drug more frequently in an effort to achieve desired actions—develops within 4 months of initial, daily use—regardless of the dosage range (i.e., low or high) or if medically prescribed or not. However, the rate of the development of tolerance varies both among women and from benzodiazepine to benzodiazepine. Generally, tolerance develops more quickly to the hypnotic (i.e., sleep-inducing) effects of the benzodiazepines than to the anxiolytic (anxiety-reducing) effects.

BENZODIAZEPINE WITHDRAWAL SYNDROME. The characteristic signs and symptoms of the *benzodiazepine withdrawal syndrome* are widely documented in the context of the abrupt discontinuation of regular, long-term benzodiazepine use (e.g., Bateson, 2002).[18] Usually, *mild to moderate* in intensity, the signs and symptoms of the benzodiazepine withdrawal syndrome may include:

- Anxiety
- Convulsions
- Insomnia
- Irritability
- Nervousness
- Shaking
- Sweating
- Tension

[18] Interestingly, the signs and symptoms of the benzodiazepine withdrawal syndrome also have been noted with the discontinuation of concurrent pharmacotherapy that inhibits the cytochrome P450 isoenzymes responsible for the metabolism of the benzodiazepines. This action allows the benzodiazepines to be more quickly metabolized and, consequently, eliminated from the body more rapidly (Ninan, 2001).

These characteristic signs and symptoms, which are essentially the *opposite* of the *desired* effects of the benzodiazepines, are more likely to occur with:

1. *Short-acting* benzodiazepines (e.g., alprazolam, Xanax®; lorazepam, Ativan®; triazolam, Halcion®)[19]
2. *Higher* dosages of benzodiazepines
3. Regular, daily use of benzodiazepines for *4* months, or longer
4. Abrupt discontinuation of benzodiazepines after regular, daily use

Generally, the benzodiazepine withdrawal syndrome can be avoided, or at least minimized, by gradually *decreasing* the dosage. It is often handled *cold-turkey* — without medical care or drug therapy—even among long-term nursing home patients (Bourgeois, Elseviers, & Van Bortel, 2014a). It also can be medically managed with the substitution of an equivalent dose of a *long-acting* benzodiazepine (e.g., diazepam [Valium®]) that is gradually reduced over a period of 2 to 3 weeks (Pagliaro & Pagliaro, 2009).[20] (Also, see related discussion in Chapter 8, *Preventing and Treating Women's Drug and Substance Abuse.*)

Overdosage

Among new millennial women in the U.S., a significant number of overdosages and ER visits have been associated with a combination of a benzodiazepine (primarily alprazolam, Xanax®) and an opiate analgesic (primarily, oxycodone, Oxycontin®) (Preidt, 2014; Sharp & Melnik, 2015). Poisonings among women of reproductive age involving benzodiazepines increased during the first decade of the new millennium. Among this cohort of women, intentional poisoning (e.g., involving a deliberate suicide attempt) was *highest* among women between 15 and 24 years-of-age (Cox, Kuo, & Jamieson, 2011).

Signs and symptoms of benzodiazepine overdosage, include: coma, confusion, diminished reflexes, drowsiness (somnolence), and incoordination. Respiratory

[19] Short-acting benzodiazepines are more likely to produce insomnia when they are abruptly discontinued than are long-acting benzodiazepines. Their short action also may contribute to their continued use. Long-acting benzodiazepines are less likely to produce insomnia, or the other symptoms of withdrawal, when they are discontinued probably because of their longer half-life of elimination. It is generally thought that the longer half-life of elimination may provide a "built-in" *tapering-off* effect.

[20] Some clinicians and researchers (e.g., Hood, Norman, & Hince, 2014) suggest the use of a low dose "infusion" of the benzodiazepine antagonist, *flumazenil*, to treat benzodiazepine withdrawal. We have found insufficient data to support the efficacy of this pharmacotherapeutic intervention. Consequently, we do *not* recommend this suggestion for flumazenil use. (See Chapter 8, *Preventing and Treating Women's Drug and Substance Abuse.*) In addition, others (e.g., Lin, 2014) have advocated the use of acetylcholinesterase inhibitors (e.g., donepezil, rivastigmine)—for the rapid detoxification of benzodiazepine (or z-drug) dependence. As we also noted regarding the suggested use of flumazenil in this context, insufficient supportive data are available for us to recommend this pharmacotherapeutic use of the acetylcholinesterase inhibitors.

arrest occurs more commonly with *short-acting* benzodiazepines (e.g., alprazolam [Xanax®], midazolam [Versed®], and triazolam [Halcion®]).

Benzodiazepine overdosage is *not* usually fatal because the benzodiazepines have a *high* therapeutic index, or $LD_{50.}$[21] (Also, see related earlier discussion, *Fatalities.*) Regardless, benzodiazepine overdosage requires emergency medical support of body systems, with attention to increasing benzodiazepine elimination. The benzodiazepine antagonist, *flumazenil* (Anexate®, Romazicon®), may be required. However, some caution is warranted because flumazenil antagonism may precipitate the benzodiazepine withdrawal syndrome among women who are physically dependent on the benzodiazepines. Health and social care professionals also should recognize that flumazenil is a relatively short-acting competitive inhibitor of benzodiazepine receptor activity with a half-life of elimination of approximately 1 hour (Pagliaro & Pagliaro, 1999, 2009). This observation is clinically significant because it explains why overdosages with long-acting benzodiazepines often require subsequent additional doses of flumazenil.

In addition, as noted earlier, benzodiazepine overdosage frequently involves the concomitant use of other psychodepressants (e.g., alcohol; barbiturates; opiate analgesics) (Jones, Paulozzi, & Mack, 2014) that are *not* amenable to the antagonist effects of flumazenil (Pagliaro & Pagliaro, 2009; Sharp & Melnik, 2015). For example, a popular combination of psychodepressants used among women in Texas since the beginning of the new millennium, consists of: the benzodiazepine, *alprazolam*, a miscellaneous sedative-hypnotic from the miscellaneous subgroup, *carisoprodol*; and the opiate analgesic, *hydrocodone* (Forrester, 2011). As noted by the FDA, overall "overdose deaths that involved both opioid analgesic and benzodiazepines [increased significantly] in the U.S. from 2004 to 2011" (Jones & McAninch, 2015, p. 493).

It is important to remember that alcohol is involved in a significant number of opiate analgesic and benzodiazepine-related ED visits and drug-related deaths (Jones, Paulozzi, & Mack, 2014, p. 881). In fact, the total number of deaths associated with benzodiazepine use among women has had an approximately *fourfold* increase during 2001 (i.e., approximately 800 deaths) to 2014 (i.e., approximately 3,000 deaths) (NIDA, 2015).

Women's Medical and Personal Benzodiazepine Use and Abuse

The benzodiazepines are approved for several medical conditions, including:

- Anxiety disorders, including panic attacks (e.g., alprazolam, Xanax®)
- Insomnia (e.g., oxazepam, Serax®)
- Lower back pain (e.g., diazepam, Valium®, as a muscle relaxant)

[21] The LD_{50} is the symbol or abbreviation for the *median* lethal dose, or the dose that would be fatal for one-half of the population. It is more often associated with toxicology testing with population samples of laboratory animals (e.g., Sprague Dawley albino rats).

- Management of seizures associated with the alcohol withdrawal syndrome (i.e., long-acting benzodiazepines, such as diazepam, Valium®)
- Pre-medication for medical procedures or surgical adjunct to anesthesia (e.g., lorazepam, Ativan®; midazolam, Versed®)[22]
- Seizure disorders (e.g., clonazepam, Rivotril®; diazepam, Valium®)

(Holbrook, Crowther, & Lotter, 1999; Pagliaro & Pagliaro, 2009)

Since the benzodiazepines were synthesized, they have been medically and personally abused by women particularly for their *anxiolytic* and *hypnotic* actions. This section presents an overview of women's medical and personal abuse of this sedative-hypnotic.

Women's Medical Benzodiazepine Use/Abuse

The first benzodiazepine, *chlordiazepoxide* (Librium®), was synthesized in the early 1950s by Leo Sternbach (1908–2005), a chemist working in New Jersey at a branch of the Swiss pharmaceutical company, Hoffmann-La Roche. However, its potential use was *not* immediately recognized and it sat on a shelf in the laboratory for several years until, by accident, and with the help of a laboratory assistant, Sternbach discovered its efficacy as a sedative-hypnotic.

Subsequently, chlordiazepoxide was marketed as an effective sedative-hypnotic *without* abuse potential.[23] It was an immediate marketing success. By 1963, a *chemical sister*, diazepam (Valium®) joined the market and, over the following decade, more than two dozen additional chemical cousins were synthesized, developed, and marketed. (For further related discussion, see Pagliaro & Pagliaro, 2004, 2009.)

In the song, *Mother's Little Helper*, by the Rolling Stones (1966), the songwriters, Mick Jagger and Keith Richards, comment on the use of "a little yellow pill"[24] by mothers. According to the lyrics, although the mother is "not really ill" she requires that pill to "calm her down" and "get her through her busy day." Around the time of the song's release, that pill was extensively over-prescribed by physicians to a wide variety of patients—mostly women. That "yellow pill" served as a "shelter" for the mother in the song, which she regularly relies upon to help ease her stress and anxiety (i.e., "to calm her down"). Consequently, she pleads with her physician, "Doctor please, some more of these."

---

[22] Lorazepam and midazolam are used as *pre-medications* to both: (1) decrease anxiety among patients undergoing surgery; and (2) to produce *anterograde amnesia*, or the loss of memory of the event, so that patients do not later recall potentially stressful or distressing surgical experiences.

[23] Chlordiazepoxide (Librium®) is *not* alone in this false claim. Throughout the modern history of pharmaceutical synthesis and marketing of various drugs, it seems that whenever a new *psychotropic*—particularly, one with *psychodepressant actions*—was developed (e.g., heroin; pentazocine [Talwin®]; zoplicone [Imovane®]), it was marketed as *non-habit forming*. In fact, heroin was specifically marketed during the late 19th century as a *cure* for *morphinism* (morphine addiction)—see Chapter 1, *Women's Opiate Analgesic Abuse*.

[24] The "little yellow pill" is, of course, a 5-mg tablet of diazepam (Valium®).

The use of the benzodiazepines peaked, worldwide, during the late-1970s. Concerns regarding an *over-medicated society* increased and resulted in a re-evaluation of the prescribing practices of physicians. Thus, the use of the benzodiazepines, and the other sedative-hypnotics, generally declined. However, the benzodiazepines continued to be widely prescribed in the U.S.[25] and throughout the world, particularly for *women* (Cloos & Ferreira, 2009; Pagliaro & Pagliaro, 2009). In fact, regardless of age, *women* are prescribed more *psychodepressants* than men and they also receive more prescriptions per year for benzodiazepines.[26]

Benzodiazepines also are often medically prescribed for veterans to manage posttraumatic stress disorder (PTSD), particularly: woman veterans; veterans living in rural areas; and veterans of European or American Indian descent (Bernardy, Lund, & Alexander, 2014). This indication increased steadily through the first and second decades of the new millennium (Hawkins, Malte, & Imel, 2012), probably due to the:

1. Ever *growing* numbers of veterans with PTSD returning from conflicts in the Middle East (i.e., wars in Afghanistan and Iraq)
2. Woeful inability of the Veterans Administration (VA) hospital system to adequately treat these veterans (Pagliaro & Pagliaro, *Clinical Patient Data Files*)

For example, Bernardy, Lund, and Alexander (2013), in their study, which utilized national administrative VA data from 1999 to 2009 to evaluate gender differences in prescribing among veterans diagnosed with PTSD, found that:

> The most notable gender discrepancy was observed for benzodiazepines where prescriptions decreased for men (36.7% in 1999 to 29.8% in 2009) but steadily increased for women from 33.4% to 38.3% … Prescribing frequency for benzodiazepines showed a marked gender difference with a steady increase for women despite guideline recommendations against use and a decrease for men.
>
> *(p. S542)*

---

[25] For example, in 2008, according to the CDC, the *most* prescribed benzodiazepine in the U.S. was alprazolam (Xanax®) (Cai, Crane, & Poneleit, 2010).

[26] As noted by Bepko (1989/1991), 25 years ago, women were at *higher* risk than men for the development of problems related to benzodiazepine and other drug use because women:

> … are twice as likely to abuse tranquillizers and sedatives and are consequently at greater risk for accidental overdose. It is hypothesized that while men are more likely to abuse illicit drugs … women suffer more from poly-drug use because they are routinely tranquillized and sedated by doctors. Symptoms of addiction in women are frequently misdiagnosed as *depression, hysteria*, or, as a local doctor termed one patient's problem, *husbanditis*.
>
> *(p. 416)*

In addition, women, as well as men, are *twice* as likely to receive a medical prescription for a benzodiazepine if they are:

- Chronically ill
- 65 years-of-age, or older
- Institutionalized[27]

Women with Chronic Illness. Up to 70% of benzodiazepine prescriptions are for chronic, non-psychiatric conditions that include GI, genitourinary, and other chronic conditions. For example, the benzodiazepines are commonly prescribed for the symptomatic relief of the signs and symptoms associated with gastric ulcers, menstrual disorders and menopause, and nervousness—in many cases, without attempting to treat the underlying cause of the condition.

As illustrated in an "all too common story" shared by a woman, who struggled with prescription benzodiazepine abuse, it usually begins with a legitimate prescription for a legitimate medical disorder, such as *chronic insomnia*:[28]

> I saw Dr. Dave four times in six months. At each visit, he would listen to my despair about my recurrent insomnia, restate his belief that I'd eventually recover my hormonal sensibilities and double my benzodiazepine dose. My third and fourth visits were a mere month apart. Dr. Dave offered 4 mg of Ativan at the second visit, with three refills. One month later, he suggested that I try hopping over to Xanax occasionally for a different benzo visit and wrote me a prescription for 2 mg of Xanax with three refills. At my last visit, six months after the first, he wrote two brief lines of clinical notes: "Patient requiring 4–5 mg of Ativan to sleep so will write prescription for 6 mg to cover this. Five refills."
>
> *(Bond, 2012, p. 5)*

---

[27] Certain factors have been identified that correlate with the medical over-prescription of the benzodiazepines for these groups. These "physician factors" include: (1) being a general practitioner; (2) being in solo practice; (3) having a large patient load; and (4) the number of years practicing since medical school (Chambers, White, & Lindquist, 1983). It is interesting to note that, although this study was published over 30 years ago, available data (e.g., Lilja & Larsson, 1994; Pagliaro & Pagliaro, *Clinical Patient Data Files*) suggest that the *same* factors correlate with medical over-prescription, today. For example, Amos, Keith, and Del Canale (2015) found that the major characteristics of general medical practitioners that are associated with inappropriate prescribing for older women are: (1) older age; (2) male gender; and (3) solo practice. Data also suggest that sedative-hypnotics, including the benzodiazepines, are still inappropriately prescribed for what has been pejoratively referred to as, "crowd control," particularly in residential and extended care facilities.

[28] In addition to the factors identified in the previous footnote that significantly contribute to the inappropriate, over-prescription of benzodiazepines for women, we would add the often, manipulative—although often generally extremely effective—behaviors of women, who request prescriptions (or refills), in order to maintain their illicit abuse of their benzodiazepines (Pagliaro & Pagliaro, *Clinical Patient Data Files*).

Women 65 Years-of-Age and Older. Over the last 60 years, in the U.S., older adults have received approximately *twice* as many prescriptions per year as matched groups of younger adults (Pagliaro & Pagliaro, 1983, 2009). Of these prescriptions, the single most commonly prescribed group of drugs was the *benzodiazepines* (Pagliaro & Pagliaro, 1992, 2009; Widlitz & Marin, 2002).[29] The benzodiazepines have been among the most widely prescribed drugs in the world and, of all the benzodiazepines, diazepam (Valium®) has been the *most* frequently prescribed (Pagliaro & Pagliaro, 2004). Even during the new millennium, women in the U.S. routinely receive approximately twice the number of prescriptions for benzodiazepines than men and that number nearly doubles for older women when compared to younger women (Olfson, King, & Schoenbaum, 2015).

Women in Institutional Care. Women, as well as men, who are old, mentally ill, or mentally retarded,[30] and who are living in institutional long-term care, or residing in nursing homes or facilities for assisted care, are often prescribed benzodiazepines at *2 to 4 times* the rate used by women and men who are *not* in institutional care (Conn & Madan, 2006; Gallagher, Barry, & O'Mahony, 2007; Garcia-Gollarte, Baleriola-Julvez, & Ferrero-Lopez, 2012; Pagliaro & Pagliaro, 1983; Pagliaro & Pagliaro, *Clinical Patient Data Files*).

The overuse of the benzodiazepines has been related, in large part, to the advertisements in professional medical journals that some drug companies use to persuade prescribers that all institutionalized people require chemical control (e.g., to decrease aggressive and other unwanted behavior, such as wandering; to increase conformity regarding basic needs; to decrease staff workload). In this regard, several studies and reports (e.g., Pisani, Bramley, & Vest, 2013) have noted that *higher* dosages of psychodepressants, including the benzodiazepines, are administered, particularly to older patients during evening nursing shifts when compared to other nursing shifts. In addition, women incarcerated in prisons have been found to be 3 times more likely to be using benzodiazepine sedative-hypnotics than are their male counterparts.

---

29 The major concern about this significantly higher use of benzodiazepines by elderly people is related to the fact that, consequently, they are *4* times more likely to suffer an *adverse drug reaction* (i.e., undesired, or harmful, effect or toxicity) than are younger adults (Pagliaro & Pagliaro, 1983). These adverse drug reactions often involve a fall (MacReady & Barclay, 2009) and a related bone fracture(s) (van der Hooft, Schoofs, & Ziere, 2008) often within the first two weeks following the initiation of benzodiazepine use (Wagner, Zhang, & Soumerai, 2006).

30 This term is used in place of more *politically correct* terms, but scientifically inaccurate—terms such as mentally challenged or mentally capable—because it is the correct medical and psychological term for this condition. Terms such as mentally challenged are so broad and inclusive that they are virtually meaningless (i.e., *all* humans, at some time or other, in various contexts, are mentally challenged to some degree).

<u>Popular Notion</u>: Drugs and substances of abuse, including the benzodiazepines and z-drugs, do *not* cause physical dependence when medically prescribed by a physician for an active and appropriate clinical condition.

NOT TRUE. Whether this is good or bad medical practice depends upon the context of medical practice and the analysis of individual cases—which, we leave to others. However, "mis-prescription" has long been widely associated with a *false* and dangerous belief that the drugs and substances of abuse are *not* addicting when they are prescribed by a physician.

> [Benzodiazepine abuse] is *not* characteristically an iatrogenic condition and should *not* be regarded as a substantial risk for benzodiazepine therapy.
>
> *(Woods, Katz, & Winger, 1988, p. 3476)*

This false belief has significantly contributed to the *iatrogenic* (i.e., physician-caused) physical and psychological dependence on the benzodiazepines of literally millions of people worldwide over the past 6 decades (Pagliaro & Pagliaro, 2009). This false belief is based on a poor understanding of the pharmacology of the benzodiazepines (and other drugs and substances of abuse). As expressed by a psychiatrist, who published a review article on the benzodiazepines:

> It is important to distinguish between addiction to and normal physical dependence on benzodiazepines … Due to the chronic nature of anxiety, long-term low-dose benzodiazepine treatment may be necessary for some patients; this continuation of treatment should not be considered abuse or addiction.
>
> *(O'Brien, 2005, p. 28)*[31]

We call attention to this view of addiction because it also concerns the prescription of other drugs and substances of abuse (e.g., opiate analgesics, see Chapter 1, *Women's Opiate Analgesic Abuse*). Health and social care professionals should be

[31] This view has become *enshrined* by psychiatrists in the 5th, and latest, edition of the classification scheme for mental disorders, the *Diagnostic and Statistical Manual for Mental Disorders* (DSM-5):

> According to Charles O'Brien, Chair of the Substance-related Disorders Work Group, the term dependence is misleading because it is often confused with addiction, when in fact the tolerance and withdrawal patients experience are normal responses … So, we're eliminating that bad terminology.
>
> *(Cassels, 2010, p. 2)*

Perhaps this issue is just a matter of *semantics* (i.e., the study of the meaning of words and phrases). However, we would like to remind readers of the extremely relevant words of William Shakespeare (1564–1616) in *Romeo and Juliet*, written in 1594: *What's in a name? That which we call a rose by any other name would smell as sweet.* (See additional related discussion in Chapter 1, *Women's Opiate Analgesic Abuse*.)

aware of this situation and use this knowledge in the context of their own practices, particularly when working with women whose abuse of a drug or substance of abuse may be related, at least initially, to an *iatrogenic* cause. Additionally, health and social care professionals also need to be aware of this situation so that they can actively contribute to its prevention.

Unfortunately, many women who are regular, long-term benzodiazepine abusers, particularly older women, steadfastly deny their dependence on benzodiazepines and, instead, view their benzodiazepine abuse as simply the continuous use of a needed prescription drug, such as the chronic, continued use of anti-hypertensives for the management of high blood pressure or diabetic medications to control diabetes (Canham, Gallo, & Simoni-Wastila, 2014; Pagliaro & Pagliaro, *Clinical Patient Data Files*).

For example, as noted by McMillan (2014, p. 2), concerning her own story of benzodiazepine dependence:

> I sometimes took a few more pills than prescribed, on nights when I couldn't sleep or days when I felt particularly anxious. I never took Klonopin® [clonazepam] to get high; I took it "as needed," as the label said to.

Two other groups of women for whom benzodiazepines have been over-prescribed, are women of American Indian descent and those of Alaska Native descent. These women not only obtain their benzodiazepines, in large part, from *inappropriate prescriptions* (Pagliaro & Pagliaro, 2009; Wardman, Khan, & el-Guebaly, 2002), but also from using the benzodiazepines that have been prescribed for their family members and friends who *intentionally* share them to relieve similar conditions. This pattern of use also can occur when the benzodiazepines are taken, without permission, from family members and friends for whom the drug was prescribed and are either used *to get high*, traded for other drugs and substances of abuse, or sold for cash (e.g., when a granddaughter steals her grandmother's prescriptions from her purse or medicine cabinet). (Also, see the following section *Women's Personal Benzodiazepine Use/Abuse.*)

The *over-prescribing* and *misprescribing* of the benzodiazepines by physicians *decreased* significantly during the first 2 decades of the new millennium. However, the benzodiazepines continue to be among the *most* widely over-prescribed and *misprescribed* drugs in the world, particularly among older women and men (Sweeney, Laoire, & Linehan, 2015), including the prescription for many "non-mental" disorders among women such as: burning mouth syndrome; colonoscopy; COPD; endoscopy; fibromyalgia; menopause; menstrual disorders; and pelvic floor dysfunction (Childers, Williams, & Sonnenberg, 2015; Crisp, Vaccaro, & Estanol, 2013; Garewal, Powell, & Milan, 2012; Halvorsen & Martinussen, 2015; Ko, Kim, & Lee, 2012; Pinto, Sollecito, & DeRossi, 2003; Skaer, 2014).[32]

---

[32] Obviously, the prescription of benzodiazepines for women with these conditions may be appropriate depending upon the clinical context of use (i.e., the individual woman and the related clinical factors).

The benzodiazepines are increasingly obtained by women for personal abuse by *double-doctoring* (i.e., "doctor shopping") and through purchase from illicit dealers and available internet sources (Pagliaro & Pagliaro, 2009; Worley, Hall, & Hall, 2012). The benzodiazepines, particularly alprazolam (Xanax®), clonazepam (Rivotril®), diazepam (Valium®), and lorazepam (Ativan®), account for most of these reports. In addition, up to one-third of women who seek assistance/treatment for cocaine or opiate analgesic dependence, also have issues with benzodiazepine abuse.

> The estimated number of ED visits involving nonmedical use of benzodiazepines increased from 143,500 in 2004 to 271,700 in 2008 (i.e., 89%).[33]
>
> *(Centers for Disease Control and Prevention, 2010, p. 706)*

Women's Personal Benzodiazepine Use/Abuse

Although the overall personal abuse of the benzodiazepines has significantly decreased from the *highs* observed during the end of the last century, their use continues to be significant as indicated by reports from both addiction treatment centers and hospital emergency departments across the U.S. (Forrester, 2006; O'Brien, 2008).

During the new millennium, the benzodiazepines continued to be personally abused by women, young and old alike. Young women often abuse benzodiazepines to *fully* enjoy the dance and night club scenes (Kurtz, Surratt, & Levi-Minzi, 2011),[34] while, older women often abuse benzodiazepines because they feel socially *isolated* and *lonely* (Canham, 2015; Canham, Gallo, & Simoni-Wastila, 2014). They also continue to be personally abused by women for several other reasons that are *not* so different from those shared by women during the past century, including to:

- Achieve an alcohol-like *disinhibitory* euphoria, or *high*
- Cope with anxiety and stress (e.g., mothering and child-rearing; caring for older parent(s); managing family finances; home, job, and other responsibilities while balancing spousal/partner responsibilities)
- Facilitate the perpetration of crimes, including robbery and sexual assault, or *date rape*
- "Get a good night's sleep" (i.e., manage fatigue related to everyday demands, problems, and worries)
- Prevent, or self-manage, the *benzodiazepine withdrawal syndrome*

---

[33] N.B. The associated rates of benzodiazepine-related emergency department visits in 2008 were significantly *higher* for women when compared to men.

[34] These young adult women (i.e., 18 to 29 years-of-age), in the context of the club scene featuring electronic dance music, reportedly have "the highest rates of benzodiazepine misuse in the United States" (Kurtz, Buttram, and Surratt, 2017, p. 39).

In addition, during the new millennium, women, who are primarily in their late twenties—of all continental descents and sociocultural norms (e.g., whether living independently or with their parents; whether having dropped out of high school or with some college education)—routinely *co-abuse* alcohol, cannabis, cocaine, and 3,4-methylenedioxymethamphetamine (MDMA, "Ecstasy") with their benzodiazepines. These young women also share one other major variable, which has *not* been significantly identified among other cohorts of women, *sexual victimization before they were 18 years-of-age*.

The exact significance of this pattern of victimization is confounded by the observations during the new millennium that: (1) sexual victimization is steadily becoming a "norm"[35] in the U.S.; and (2) young women routinely, and on their own volition, co-abuse benzodiazepines and other drugs and substances of abuse reportedly to *decrease* their own sexual inhibitions in order to "party" in "risky" contexts that may readily place them at higher risk for sexual victimization (Pagliaro & Pagliaro, *Clinical Patient Data Files*).[36]

We now turn to the *z-drugs*.

Z-Drugs

The *z-drugs* are currently the *most* frequently medically prescribed sedative-hypnotic in the U.S. This subgroup of the prescription sedative-hypnotics includes *four* major drugs that are abused by women during the new millennium: (1) *zaleplon* (Sonata®); (2) *zolpidem* (Ambien®); (3) *zopiclone* (Imovane®); and (4) *eszopiclone* (Lunesta®).[37]

Pharmacology

The z-drugs have a relatively *rapid* onset (i.e., they reduce sleep latency, or the time it takes to fall asleep after going to bed) and short duration of hypnotic actions. Consequently, they generally are associated with minimal "next day," or so-called "hangover effects." Although their chemical structures are different from the basic benzodiazepine molecular structure, they have a virtually identical spectrum of pharmacological actions—primarily, because they elicit their effects by means of binding to the benzodiazepine receptors.

---

[35] "Norm" is used here in the statistical sense and does not, in any manner, signify or indicate our acceptance or validation of this immoral and illegal behavior.

[36] These factors are frequently discussed in the context of public media reviews of *high*-profile cases of sexual assault.

[37] Eszopiclone is an isomer of zopiclone. An *isomer* is a closely related chemical that has the exact *same* molecular formula, but a *different* physical structure (e.g., one drug may be *dextro*, or "right-handed," and the other drug may be *levo*, or "left-handed"). Health and social care professionals should be aware that a *difference* in physical structure may result in a *difference* in actions, particularly when the site of action is a drug receptor site.

Zaleplon (Sonata®) shares many features with the benzodiazepine, *triazolam* (Halcion®), and another z-drug, *zolpidem* (Ambien®). Zolpidem is a short-acting z-drug and is available in tablet form for oral ingestion. It also is the *most* widely prescribed sedative-hypnotic in the U.S. and, although its pharmacological actions are like the benzodiazepines, it is chemically distinct. *Zopiclone* (Imovane®), also a short-acting z-drug, shares a virtually identical spectrum of pharmacological action with the benzodiazepines.

Zoplicone became commercially available in Europe in 1986 and in the United States in 2005. Currently, it is one of the most widely used sedative-hypnotics in the U.S., and throughout the world. Its levorotatory isomer, eszopiclone (*Lunesta*®) also is available. Eszopiclone was approved in Europe in 1992 and later approved for use in the U.S. in 2004. The tablet forms of both drugs are generally orally ingested by women, often with an alcoholic beverage to enhance euphoric or stress-reducing actions.

Pharmacodynamics: Mechanism of Action

The z-drugs are *not* benzodiazepines. However, current data suggest that *all* the z-drugs act at the benzodiazepine receptor. Specifically, the z-drugs appear to act at the benzodiazepine recognition site of the $GABA_A$ receptor complex, particularly the omega-1 receptor at its alpha subunit. Working together with the inhibitory neurotransmitter $GABA_A$, they appear to *potentiate* the GABA-evoked chloride current (see Figure 3.1). A noted placebo effect also appears to play a significant part in their action to produce sleep among women and men, who have insomnia, or other sleep disorders (Huedo-Medina, Kirsch, & Middlemass, 2012).

Pharmacokinetics: Absorption, Distribution, Metabolism, and Excretion

The z-drugs are rapidly absorbed following oral ingestion and achieve peak blood concentrations and related effects within 1 to 2 hours. However, absorption is delayed when zolpidem is ingested with food. The half-life of elimination for the z-drugs usually ranges from 1 to 5 hours. Typically, less than 5% of an oral dosage is excreted in unchanged form in the urine. Thus, renal impairment, including that associated with normal aging, does not usually affect their: (1) dosing, or half-life of elimination; (2) possible accumulation in the body; or (3) occurrence of undesired, or harmful, effects and toxicities. The z-drugs are extensively metabolized in the liver by the hepatic microsomal (isoenzyme) system, particularly CYP3A4.[38] Consequently, their metabolism may be reduced for women

[38] In addition, CYP3A4 is involved in the metabolism of various benzodiazepines (e.g., alprazolam [Xanax®], midazolam [Versed®], and triazolam [Halcion®]). CYP3A4 is significantly *inhibited* by the selective serotonin re-uptake inhibitors (SSRIs)—fluoxetine (Prozac®), fluvoxamine (Luvox®), and sertraline (Zoloft®). It also may be inhibited by the ingestion of grapefruit juice. The

who have liver disease (e.g., alcoholic cirrhosis of the liver; drug-induced hepatitis) or age-related liver dysfunction, which generally occurs among women who are 65 years-of-age or older.

In the following sections, we consider the pharmacokinetics of each of the z-drugs, beginning with zaleplon.

Zaleplon (Sonata®). Zaleplon is rapidly absorbed following oral ingestion and achieves peak blood concentrations within 1 hour. However, because of its *extensive* first-pass hepatic metabolism, its oral bioavailability is limited (i.e., F = 0.3). *Extensively* metabolized to several inactive metabolites by the aldehyde oxidase enzyme and the hepatic microsomal enzyme, CYP3A4, less than 1% of zaleplon is excreted in unchanged form in the urine. The half-life of elimination is approximately 1 hour (Gunja, 2013a) and, because of its short half-life of elimination, zaleplon is associated with *fewer* residual "hangover" effects (Drover, 2004).

Healthcare professionals are reminded that, as with other z-drugs, *renal* impairment does *not* affect dosing, half-life of elimination, potential accumulation in the body, or associated undesired, or harmful, effects and toxicities. However, *hepatic* impairment can significantly affect the blood concentration of zaleplon and all of the other z-drugs.

Zolpidem (Ambien®). Zolpidem is rapidly and moderately well-absorbed after oral ingestion. It achieves peak blood concentrations within 1.5 hours. However, ingesting zolpidem with food delays and decreases its absorption. Zolpidem is approximately 92% bound to plasma proteins and has an apparent volume of distribution of 0.7 L/kg. It is metabolized extensively in the liver and its metabolites are primarily excreted in the urine. Less than 1% of zolpidem is excreted in unchanged form in the urine.

Metabolism is dependent on the mixed cytochrome P450 isoenzymes, particularly the hepatic isoenzyme, CYP3A4, but also involves CYP2C9 and CYP1A2 (Gunja, 2013a). The mean elimination half-life is 2.5 hours (range, 1.5 to 4.5 hours). The half-life of elimination may be prolonged in women with hepatic dysfunction, but is *not* significantly affected by renal dysfunction.

Zolpidem clearance is significantly lower in women when compared to men. Thus, the incidence of undesired, or harmful, effects and toxicities (e.g., dizziness; drowsiness; "hangover" effects; memory impairment) is *increased* among women, particularly *older* women (Cubata, Landowski, & Wichowicz, 2007). These effects may contribute to falls, resultant hip fractures, and other injuries among this population group (Frey, Ortega, & Wiseman, 2011).

In response, the FDA required pharmaceutical manufacturers of zolpidem to *lower* the recommended dosage for women, particularly among older women, to *reduce* "hangover" effects and associated falls and/or impaired driving ability

---

consequence of this "inhibition" of CYP3A4 is a significant increase in the blood concentrations of the z-drugs and the benzodiazepines—without any changes in their dosages.

(Booth, Behring, & Cantor, 2016; FDA, 2013a, 2013b). In addition, a *lower* dosage sublingual formulation of zolpidem (i.e., 1.75 mg Intermezzo® sublingual tablet) was approved for women with insomnia due to middle-of-the-night awakenings. It produces effects within 20 minutes of sublingual placement. These effects peak within 40 minutes and usually fully dissipate within 5 hours (i.e., within the time frame of approximately 2 half-lives of elimination).

Zopiclone (Imovane®). Zopiclone is rapidly and well-absorbed following oral ingestion (F = 0.70) and reaches peak blood concentrations in approximately 2 hours. However, the ingestion of foods that are *high* in fat content may *delay* reaching peak blood concentrations and associated psychodepressant actions. Zopiclone is weakly bound to plasma proteins (i.e., approximately 50%) and has an apparent volume of distribution of approximately 120 L. It is extensively metabolized in the liver, principally by the hepatic isoenzymes CYP3A4 and CYP2E1, to several metabolites, particularly zopiclone-N-oxide (inactive) and N-desmethylzopiclone (active). Only 5% of zopiclone is excreted in unchanged form in the urine. Zopiclone has a mean elimination half-life of approximately 5 hours (range, 4 to 7 hours). Its longer half-life, in comparison to other z-drugs, may contribute to its greater efficacy in terms of maintaining a full night's sleep with fewer "wake-up" periods (Drover, 2004), but may also contribute to residual "hangover" effects in the morning upon awakening.

Undesired, or Harmful, Effects and Toxicities

The spectrum of undesired, or harmful, effects and toxicities associated with the z-drugs appears to be similar to those associated with the benzodiazepines (Gunja, 2013b). In this regard, the z-drugs have been associated with both *acute* and *chronic* toxicities, including physical and psychological dependence. These undesired, or harmful, effects and toxicities are summarized in the following sections. The noted incidence and severity of these effects and toxicities are significantly *increased* by the concomitant use of additional sedative-hypnotics (e.g., alcohol; benzodiazepines). For example, the concomitant use of a z-drug and a benzodiazepine significantly increases the risk for falls and associated hip fractures among older women (Hines & Murphy, 2011). (Also, see earlier discussion in the section, *Benzodiazepines*, "Acute Effects.")

Acute Toxicities. Zaleplon (Sonata®) has been associated with such *acute* toxicities, as: ataxia; cognitive and memory impairment; dizziness, or light-headedness; falls; postural instability; and psychomotor impairment. *Zolpidem* (Ambien®) has been associated with several similar *acute* toxicities, including: anterograde amnesia; ataxia, or postural sway; blurred vision; cognitive impairment; confusion, and impaired judgment; constipation; delirium; dizziness, or light-headedness; dry mouth; dyspepsia; falls; hallucinations (i.e., *visual*, particularly with extremely *high* dosages); "hangover" effects; headaches; increased appetite; memory impairment;

nausea; nightmares; psychomotor impairment; red eyes; ringing in the ears (*tinnitus*); sleep driving; sleepwalking; somnolence; tremors; and weakness (Holm & Goa, 2000).

Zopiclone (Imovane®) also is associated with several *acute* toxicities. These toxicities include: anterograde amnesia; anxiety; bitter, metallic taste in the mouth; cognitive impairment; confusion; constipation; daytime fatigue; dizziness; dyspepsia; dry mouth; falls; "hangover" effects, including grogginess and cognitive impairment upon awakening; headache; loss of strength, or weakness (i.e., *asthenia*); memory impairment; postural instability; psychomotor impairment; and somnolence.

Chronic Toxicities. The major chronic toxicity associated with *zaleplon* (Sonata®) is mental depression. Reportedly, the regular, long-term use of *zolpidem* (Ambien®) by older women *doubles* their risk for hip fracture because of accidents and falls associated with its CNS depressant actions (Chang, Chen, & Tsai, 2011; Finkle, Der, & Greenland, 2011; Gunja, 2013a; Wang, Bohn, & Glynn, 2001).

The *major* chronic toxicity associated with *zopiclone* (Imovane®) is mental depression. *Eszopiclone* (Lunesta®) shares a similar profile of undesired, or harmful, effects and toxicities with its levorotatory isomer, zopiclone. Both zopiclone and eszopiclone have been associated with increased reports of extended hangover effects lasting over 11 hours and resultant impaired driving skills. As a result, in 2014 the FDA recommended the discontinuation of the 3-mg evening dosage and reduction of the starting dosage to 1 mg (Abramowicz, 2014).

Physical and Psychological Dependence. Regular, long-term abuse of zaleplon (Sonata®) is associated with a *low* potential for physical dependence and a *low* to *moderate* potential for psychological dependence. Based on its similarity to the benzodiazepines, a zaleplon (Sonata®) withdrawal syndrome is expected to occur with regular, long-term abuse. However, it has *not* yet been confirmed in human studies or clinical reports.

The regular, long-term abuse of zolpidem (Ambien®) has been associated with the development of *low to moderate* physical dependence and *moderate* psychological dependence. In a study evaluating dependence among long-term users of either zolpidem or zopiclone, Yen, Yen, and Ko (2015) found that: (1) zolpidem users reported *more* severe dependence than did zopiclone users; and (2) severe dependence, which was reported, was significantly correlated with reports of severe mental depression.

A zolpidem withdrawal syndrome has been associated with the abrupt discontinuation of its regular, long-term use. Like the benzodiazepine withdrawal syndrome (see earlier section, *Benzodiazepines*, "Benzodiazepine Withdrawal Syndrome"), the zolpidem withdrawal syndrome is characterized, in severe cases, by seizures and drug-induced psychosis (Hypnotic dependence, 2001; Pagliaro & Pagliaro, 2009). The standard 7-day diazepam (Valium®) withdrawal program, which utilizes tapering diazepam doses, has been used to successfully manage the zolpidem withdrawal syndrome. (Also, see later section, *Pregnancy and Lactation*.)

The regular long-term use of zopiclone (Imovane®) has been associated with *low* potential for physical dependence and *low to moderate* potential for psychological dependence. However, healthcare providers are reminded that individual differences in drug response may occur and *any* woman can be an exception to the general expected effects of a drug or substance of abuse. For example, consider the reported case of a 31-year-old woman of European descent, and a history of anorexia nervosa, who came to abuse zopiclone:

> Zopiclone was described as "her best friend" and, like alcohol, it gave her confidence, relaxed her and enhanced her self-esteem. She said that she was ultra-possessive about her supply and would not be separated from it, keeping it with her at all times. During the 13 years of using there had only been one relatively short period of abstinence, which occurred six years ago, when she was in the hospital for an alcohol and zopiclone detoxification. However, this ended with the recurrence of the anorexia and she was prescribed zopiclone to help her sleep.
>
> *(Morinan & Keaney, 2010, p. 2)*

A *zopiclone* (Imovane®) withdrawal syndrome, like the alcohol and benzodiazepine withdrawal syndromes, has been observed upon abrupt discontinuation of its regular, long-term medical or personal abuse (Cimolai, 2007; Pagliaro & Pagliaro, 2009). This withdrawal syndrome is characterized by agitation, anxiety, confusion, delirium, hallucinations, headache, irritability, nightmares, palpitations, rebound anxiety, rebound insomnia, seizures (rare), tachycardia, and tremor.

Regular, long-term abuse of zopiclone (Imovane®) should be gradually discontinued to avoid the occurrence of this syndrome. *Eszopiclone* (Lunesta®), the levorotatory isomer (see earlier discussion) of zopiclone, can produce a similar withdrawal syndrome.

Pregnancy and Lactation. Various adverse pregnancy outcomes (e.g., increased rate of preterm births; low birth weight and/or small for gestational age among neonates/infants) have been reported to be *higher* among women who received zolpidem (Ambien®) for the management of insomnia during pregnancy when compared to women who did not (Wang, Lin, & Lin, 2010). Based on reported data of thousands of live births among mothers, who used various z-drugs during pregnancy, it appears, overall, that the use of z-drugs by women during pregnancy is *not* related to teratogenesis—in terms of major congenital malformations. However, zolpidem has been demonstrated to cross the placenta. Consequently, cautious use is indicated for women who are pregnant (Pagliaro & Pagliaro, 2009).

Overdosage

Overdosages involving the z-drugs generally include such signs and symptoms as: ataxia, or postural sway; confusion; dizziness; hypotension; lethargy; muscular incoordination; psychomotor impairment; respiratory depression; or somnolence. *Zolpidem* overdosage is also associated with contracted pupils[39] and respiratory depression.

Impaired consciousness that ranges from drowsiness to light coma also can occur in cases of severe overdosage. However, overdosages involving the z-drugs are *rarely* fatal because of their pharmacological similarity to the benzodiazepines—*except* in the context of poly-drug overdosage (Gunja, 2013a). It is important for health and social care professionals to remember that the concurrent use of a z-drug with other psychodepressants, including alcohol, can significantly *increase* the risk for overdosage, including *fatal* overdosage (Zosel, Osterberg, & Mycyk, 2011). Fatalities also can be associated with the risky behavior that can accompany z-drug abuse (Pagliaro & Pagliaro, 2009). For example, driving under the influence (DUI) of z-drugs and *sleep driving* (i.e., *sleep-deprived* or *drowsy driving*), associated with excessive dosages, also can have fatal consequences (Pressman, 2011).

Overdosages involving *zolpidem* require emergency medical support of body systems, with attention to: (1) maintaining adequate respiratory function; and (2) increasing *zolpidem* elimination. There is *no* known antidote. However, the benzodiazepine antagonist, *flumazenil* (Anexate®, Romazicon®), reportedly is of some benefit in the management of *zolpidem* overdosage. Caution is required because the use of flumazenil may precipitate a benzodiazepine-like withdrawal syndrome among women who are physically dependent on *zolpidem*.

Both *zopiclone* (Imovane®) and *eszopiclone* (Lunesta®) overdosages are generally *not* life-threatening when the overdosage involves either *zopiclone* or *eszopiclone*, alone. Associated signs and symptoms include: ataxia; coma; confusion; somnolence; hallucinations; hypotension; hypoxia; lethargy; respiratory depression; slurred speech; tachycardia; and vomiting (Forrester, 2009). Overdosages involving *zopiclone* or *eszopiclone* require emergency medical support of body systems, with attention to maintaining cardiac and respiratory function. The benzodiazepine antagonist *flumazenil* (Anexate®; Romazicon®) may be of assistance (Gunja, 2013b). However, caution is required because the use of flumazenil may precipitate an alcohol- or benzodiazepine-like withdrawal syndrome among women who are physically dependent on *zopiclone* or *eszopiclone*. In addition, overdosages involving a deliberate suicide attempt often involve the ingestion of additional drugs and substances of abuse (Forrester, 2007).[40]

---

[39] Contracted pupils, or *miosis*, is also a common feature of opiate analgesic abuse and overdosage (see Chapter 1, *Women's Opiate Analgesic Abuse*, "Overdosage" section).

[40] In *all* cases of overdosage that *potentially*, or *actually*, involve a suicide attempt, we strongly urge clinicians to formally recommend and properly encourage follow-up with an appropriate clinical psychologist or psychiatrist.

Women's Medical and Personal Z-Drug Use and Abuse

The z-drugs, used for 10 to 25 years in Asia and Europe before being introduced into the U.S., are legally produced by pharmaceutical manufacturers in capsule or tablet forms for oral ingestion. Since the beginning of the new millennium, their medical abuse *increased* significantly as did their attraction for women across the lifespan. The z-drugs are now prescribed and abused *more* than any other prescription sedative-hypnotic in the U.S.

Zolpidem (Ambien®) was introduced into clinical practice in the U.S. in 1983 as a *sleeping aid* that had *little risk* for physical or psychological dependence. However, its use for the short-term symptomatic medical management of insomnia has now been associated with *both* physical and psychological dependence—particularly, when prescribed and used in *higher* dosages or for *longer* periods of time than recommended.

The z-drugs continue to be prescribed for the short-term symptomatic management of sleep disorders, including insomnia. Unfortunately, since the beginning of the new millennium prescribers have largely ignored the well-known and well-documented pharmacotherapeutic limitations and precautions associated with their use. For example, as noted in the review, *Prescrire International*:

> Loss of efficacy can occur after a few weeks of treatment with zolpidem and zopiclone.
>
> *(Hypnotic dependence, 2001, p. 15)*

Despite these warnings, and the admonitions and lamentations of concerned clinicians and researchers, including ourselves, many prescribers continue to inappropriately prescribe z-drugs to women, particularly older women, on a regular, long-term basis. This inappropriate pharmacotherapy results in suboptimal therapeutic outcomes, and gives rise to unnecessary undesired, or harmful, effects and toxicities, including falls and physical and psychological dependence.

In extended care and other facilities, the z-drugs also are widely *misused* for the behavioral management of older women, including "troublesome patients or residents." (Also, see previous related discussion.)

Women's Medical Z-Drug Use/Abuse

As national attention increasingly focused on the: (1) medical abuse of benzodiazepines during the second decade of the new millennium; and (2) efforts to realize positive change were enacted, a major unanticipated outcome regarding the restriction of benzodiazepine Medicare coverage for older women and men, was identified. As increasing numbers of older Medicare members lost their coverage for benzodiazepines, most of these older members, particularly women, simply switched to z-drugs (Chen & Kreling, 2014). This situation is particularly distressing because alternative approaches are available. As noted by Conn and Madan (2006), in their review of the "use of sleep-promoting medications in nursing home residents," "nonpharmacological interventions for insomnia are underutilized in many clinical settings despite evidence that they are often highly effective" (p. 271).

Women's Personal Z-Drug Use/Abuse

In the U.S., women personally abuse the z-drugs for their psychodepressant actions—to achieve an *alcohol-like disinhibitory euphoria*, or *high*, and to reduce anxiety or stress. They also abuse them to prevent or self-manage specific z-drug withdrawal syndromes. Generally obtained by women of all ages by medical prescription, they also are *illegally* obtained on-the-street or from internet vendors. Women often ingest oral capsules and tablets with a glassful of wine, or other alcoholic beverage, to *increase* the associated euphoria and other desired psychodepressant effects.

Healthcare professionals need to be aware that screening for z-drug abuse is *not* generally undertaken in drug treatment programs. Thus, z-drugs may be used by women enrolled in these programs without the knowledge of staff members. The z-drugs also are used in the perpetration of drug-facilitated crimes (e.g., robbery; sexual assault, or *date rape*) being given to intended victims without the victim's knowledge. In the following section, we consider more specific patterns of women's abuse of the z-drugs, beginning with *zaleplon*.

Zaleplon (Sonata®). Women's personal abuse of zaleplon in the U.S. almost always begins with a medical prescription to treat their insomnia. Although generally prescribed for "short-term use only," they typically continue to use their zaleplon well beyond the prescribed time frame (see earlier related discussion in this section). They may also increase their daily prescribed dosages 5 to 10 times (or more) than what was originally prescribed. Ranging in age from 20 to 80 years-of-age, women who abuse zaleplon typically also concomitantly abuse other drugs and substances of abuse, including alcohol. While most of these women orally ingest their capsules and tablets, many young women choose to empty their capsules, or pulverize their tablets, and *snort*, the fine powder in a manner similar to snorting cocaine, heroin, or other drugs and substances of abuse.

Zolpidem (Ambien®). Known on the street as "Nappien" or "Tic-Tacs," zolpidem is personally abused by women to achieve an alcohol-like disinhibitory euphoria, or *high*, and hallucinations, or visual illusions. The tablet is usually crushed and intranasally snorted. Rarely, it is "cooked"—dissolved in a warm liquid, cooled, and intravenously injected (Pagliaro & Pagliaro, *Clinical Patient Data Files*). In the U.S., most women who abuse zolpidem are of European descent and are between 20 and 40 years-of-age. Initially prescribed by their physicians to manage anxiety or sleep disorders, these women use *higher* dosages than prescribed for *longer* periods of time than recommended. As physical dependence develops, regular, long-term abusers of zolpidem may also use it to prevent or self-manage the zolpidem withdrawal syndrome. This behavior is exemplified in a case report that reflects women's global abuse of zolpidem during the new millennium:

> A 39 years old female … diagnosed as a case of primary insomnia and started on zolpidem 10 mg at bed time. Over the next few weeks she had gradually increased the dose as she found the prescribed dose to be having no significant effect … she was taking about 120 mg/day of zolpidem in 2–3 divided doses. She had made several attempts in the past to reduce the dose but failed due to the resulting anxiety, restlessness, tremulousness and disturbed sleep.
>
> *(Pardal, Praksh, & Konwar, 2011, p. 388)*

Zolpidem also has been purposely given to women, without their knowledge, to perpetrate *drug-facilitated crimes* (e.g., robbery; sexual assault, including date rape). Zolpidem's relatively *short* half-life of elimination, and its pattern of prescription use for older women receiving nursing and other personal care services in their own homes, and extended care, or other institutional care settings, contribute to this risk. For example, as noted by Kintz, Villain, and Dumestre-Toulet (2005), zolpidem is commonly administered at night to older women "to help them sleep" or "to provide crowd control" for the night staff. It also is commonly used to sexually assault older, institutionalized women. Unfortunately, because of the zolpidem-induced occurrence of anterograde amnesia among victims and because zolpidem is generally not detected in most routine drug screens, suspected perpetrators are rarely charged and, for those who are, convictions are rarely obtained due to a lack of evidence (Carter, 2011).

Miscellaneous Sedative-Hypnotics[41]

Suvorexant (Belsomra®) is the *newest* miscellaneous prescription sedative-hypnotic abused by women in the U.S. Women also abuse the *illicitly* obtained miscellaneous prescription sedative-hypnotic, gamma-hydroxybutyrate (GHB). The pharmacology of these two sedative-hypnotic drugs is presented and briefly discussed

[41] Other miscellaneous sedative-hypnotics—which may be obtained via the Internet and used by some millennial women—generally have long histories of women's medical and personal use and abuse that extend over the past 50 to 150 years. These sedative-hypnotics include the: barbiturates, chloral hydrate, ethchlorvynol, meprobamate, and methaqualone. For detailed information regarding these miscellaneous sedative-hypnotics, readers are referred to Pagliaro & Pagliaro (2004, 2009).

in the following sections. Although limited information is available for women's suvorexant use and abuse over the new millennium, due primarily to its relatively recent availability, data regarding women's use and abuse of GHB, which has been used/abused for a longer period of time, is much more extensive and detailed.

Suvorexant

Suvorexant (Belsomra®), the *newest* prescription sedative-hypnotic in the U.S., was introduced into clinical practice in 2014 (Jacobson, Callander, & Hoyer, 2014). As a prototype for a new subgroup of sedative-hypnotics known as *dual orexin receptor antagonists*, or *DORAs* (Owen, 2016), it can facilitate both the *onset* and *duration* of sleep. As such, suvorexant has been found, when compared to a placebo, to be efficacious for the treatment of insomnia, demonstrating improved: (1) "subjective total sleep time"; (2) "wake after sleep onset"; and (3) "latency to persistent sleep" (Patel, Aspesi, & Evoy, 2015, p. 477).

Pharmacology

Pharmacodynamics: Mechanism of Action. Orexin (hypocretin) is a "wakefulness-promoting" neuropeptide that acts in the signaling control of vigilance and sleep/wake states (Reddy, Puvvada, & Kommisetti, 2015; Winrow & Renger, 2014). As such, it is a master regulator of the sleep-wake cycle, with: (1) *high* activity of the orexin cells in the lateral hypothalamus (LH) during the wake cycle; and (2) almost *no* activity during the sleep cycle (Hoyer & Jacobson, 2013). Suvorexant (Belsomra®) acts as an active *dual* orexin-1 receptor and orexin-2 receptor *antagonist* (Yang, 2014). Neurons in the LH produce orexin A and orexin B, which bind to orexin receptors 1 and 2 (i.e., OX_1R and OX_2R) eliciting the desired physiologic response (i.e., wakefulness) (Hopkins, 2012). Blocking of the orexin receptors results in the promotion of sleep. The onset of action, following the oral ingestion of suvorexant, is approximately 30 to 60 minutes.

Pharmacokinetics: Absorption, Distribution, Metabolism, and Excretion. Due to the relatively recent introduction of suvorexant, little published research is available regarding its pharmacokinetics. This area of clinical research requires attention, particularly in relation to women's pharmacology and patterns of use and abuse.

Summary pharmacokinetic data indicate that suvorexant is well-absorbed following oral ingestion with action occurring approximately 1 hour later. Suvorexant is *highly* protein bound (i.e., 99.5%) and has a total volume of distribution of approximately 106 liters. Suvorexant is metabolized primarily in the liver. Its metabolism is mediated by the cytochrome P450 CYP3A4 hepatic enzyme. Suvorexant is predominantly excreted in the form of inactive metabolites in the feces. However, a small amount of inactive metabolites undergo renal excretion. The half-life of elimination is approximately 12 hours (range, 8 to 19 hours) (Bennett, Bray, & Neville, 2014; Cui, Cabalu, & Yee, 2016; Dubey, Handu, & Mediratta, 2015). In addition, several specific pharmacokinetic research outcomes have been identified by Dailey (2015), including:

- Absorption and, consequently, latency time from administration to sleep, may be *delayed* when suvorexant is ingested with food or meals
- Blood suvorexant concentrations at steady state are approximately 15% higher among older adults in comparison to younger adults
- Obese women, when compared to non-obese men of similar body weight, have blood suvorexant concentrations that are 1.5-fold higher
- Blood suvorexant concentrations are *not* affected by *renal* impairment (i.e., *renal* excretion of unchanged suvorexant is *not* significant)
- The half-life of elimination of suvorexant among *healthy* adults is approximately 14.7 hours
- The half-life of elimination for suvorexant is increased to 19.1 hours among adults with *hepatic* impairment

As specified in the official prescription package insert from Merck & Company:

> Belsomra® is not recommended for use with strong CYP3A *inhibitors* (e.g., carbamazepine, ketoconazole, nefazodone, phenytoin, rifampin, saquinavir).
>
> *(Merck, 2016, p. 3)*

Undesired, or Harmful, Effects and Toxicities. A relatively *new* drug and drug class of the sedative-hypnotics, there are limited available data regarding the undesired, or harmful, effects and toxicities associated with the clinical use of suvorexant, particularly for women. However, the incidence and severity of undesired, or harmful, effects and toxicities, as expected, *increase* with *increasing* dosages. In addition, as noted in the FDA-approved "package insert" produced by Merck & Company in 2016, obese women are at particular risk for experiencing undesired, or harmful, effects and toxicities (Merck, 2016). For example:

> At doses of 15 mg or 20 mg, the incidence of somnolence was higher in females (8%) than in males (3%). The incidence of headache, abnormal dreams, dry mouth, cough, and upper respiratory tract infection occurrence in women was at least twice that in men.
>
> *(Merck, 2016, p. 2)*

The most frequently encountered undesired effects associated with FDA recommended dosages of suvorexant, are daytime drowsiness, or somnolence, and headache (Hopkins, 2012). Other reported undesired effects include: abnormal dreams; aggressive behavior; amnesia; anxiety; cataplexy (mild); confusion; cough;

dizziness; hallucinations (hypnagogic and hypnopompic); "hangover" effects; impaired driving skills; mental depression; muscle weakness; nightmares/bizarre dreams; respiratory impairment; sleep paralysis; sleep driving; sleep walking; suicide ideation; and a weak feeling in the legs (Jacobson, Callander, & Hoyer, 2014; Merck, 2016; Norman & Anderson, 2016).

PHYSICAL AND PSYCHOLOGICAL DEPENDENCE. Little significant data are available regarding the abuse potential of suvorexant.[42] However, the FDA classified it as a controlled substance (C-IV). Based on clinical trials, suvorexant also was identified, in a National Drug Monograph, as having human abuse potential similar to that for the z-drug, zolpidem (Dailey, 2015; Schoedel, Sun, & Sellers, 2016). Merck, the manufacturer of suvorexant (Belsomra®) in the U.S., noted in their prescribing information that "in clinical trials, there was no evidence of physical dependence" (Merck, 2016, p. 1).

PREGNANCY AND LACTATION. The effects of the use of suvorexant by women who are pregnant or breast-feeding is currently unknown. Caution is indicated.

Overdosage. The incidence and severity of the signs and symptoms of suvorexant overdosage increase both with: (1) *increased* dosage; and (2) concurrent use with alcohol or other psychodepressants. Additional data are *not* currently available.

Gamma-Hydroxybutyrate (GHB)

Gamma-hydroxybutyrate is unique among all the sedative-hypnotics because it occurs *naturally* in the human body as both a *precursor* and a *metabolite* of GABA. As such it is an *endogenous CNS inhibitory neurotransmitter*. GHB is available as an oral solution by its generic, prescription name, *sodium oxybate* (Xyrem®). *Illicit* GHB,[43] in both oral solutions and powder, is produced, imported, distributed, and sold across the U.S. Women commonly add GHB oral solution to a bottle of water prior to their attendance at a rave so that they can slowly "swig it" through the night.[44] Colorless, and virtually tasteless,[45] it also may be mixed into an alcoholic drink at a party or dance club to increase sexual arousal and experiences—or to

[42] Historically-derived experience with all other clinically effective sedative-hypnotics suggests that *all* bear some degree of risk for physical and psychological dependence. In addition, data regarding related DORAs, which are not yet on the market (e.g., almorexant), indicate that this pharmacological class of prescription sedative-hypnotics carry this risk. For example, Cruz, Hoever, and Chakraborty (2014) found that, in a randomized, crossover placebo controlled study, experimental subjects reported significant subjective measures of abuse potential (e.g., "drug liking") for almorexant.

[43] GHB is known on the street by many different names. Some of the trendiest and most commonly used street names, include: "Easy Lay"; "G"; "Gamma-Oh"; "Georgia Home Boy"; "Great Hormones at Bedtime"; "Grievous Bodily Harm"; "Liquid G"; "OxySleep"; "Salty Water"; and "Soap."

[44] Sold at raves, a single dose of GHB oral solution is often referred to as a "swig."

[45] However, when dissolved in water, GHB imparts a distinctly *salty* taste to the water.

facilitate date rape. In these contexts, it also can be secretly added to a woman's drink when left unattended or mixed into a large punch bowl to *liven up* the party.

Pharmacology

Pharmacodynamics: Mechanism of Action. The exact mechanism by which GHB produces its sedative-hypnotic actions has *not* been determined. However, the following *four* actions have been revealed and *confirmed* by empirical research, and may contribute, in various ways, to GHB's sedative-hypnotic mechanism(s) of action:

1. GHB binds to its own endogenous receptors in the CNS, predominantly in the basal ganglia and hippocampus
2. GHB appears to enhance the inhibitory actions that are modulated by the $GABA_B$ receptors
3. GHB acts both pre-synaptically and post-synaptically to modulate the activity of other neurotransmitters in the CNS
4. GHB pre-synaptically inhibits the release of dopamine into the synaptic cleft, resulting in an accumulation of dopamine in the pre-synaptic neuron

Pharmacokinetics: Absorption, Distribution, Metabolism, and Excretion. GHB is rapidly, but incompletely, absorbed from the GI tract. Oral availability is relatively low (F = 0.25) with peak plasma levels obtained approximately 30 minutes after oral ingestion. Oral ingestion with a high-fat meal significantly delays and reduces absorption. Metabolism, primarily by GHB dehydrogenase and the Krebs cycle, provides the major elimination pathway for GHB. Less than 5% is excreted in unchanged form in the urine. The half-life of elimination for GHB is approximately 30 minutes and effects may persist for 3 to 6 hours. GHB appears to follow dose-dependent, or *nonlinear*, pharmacokinetics.

Undesired, or Harmful, Effects and Toxicities. The use of GHB has been associated with several common undesired, or harmful, effects and toxicities, both *acute* and *chronic*. These effects also include physical and psychological dependence, those associated with pregnancy and lactation, and overdosage.

ACUTE AND CHRONIC EFFECTS. Acute effects include: amnesia; apnea; ataxia; bradycardia; cognitive impairment; coma; confusion; diaphoresis; diarrhea; dyspepsia; dizziness; enuresis; headache; hypotension; nausea; respiratory depression (associated with higher dosages); sleep (deep); slurred speech; somnolence; vomiting; and weakness.[46] Chronic effects associated with the regular, long-term use of GHB

---

[46] Interestingly, some researchers (e.g., Zvosec & Smith, 2005) have noted *non-sedative* effects (e.g., agitation; bizarre or self-injurious behavior; combativeness) in association with GHB toxicity. These noted signs and symptoms appear to be quite similar to those occasionally associated with

include: menstrual cycle irregularities; physical dependence (low); psychological dependence (moderate); somnambulism; and tinnitus.

PHYSICAL AND PSYCHOLOGICAL DEPENDENCE. Generally, GHB is associated with a *low* risk for physical dependence and moderate risk for psychological dependence. However, concern has been raised concerning the possible underreporting of GHB abuse (Brennan & Van Hout, 2014). A specific GHB withdrawal syndrome has been reported and likened, in both nature and significance, to the ethanol/alcohol withdrawal syndrome (Mason & Kerns, 2002). Signs and symptoms of the GHB withdrawal syndrome include: agitation;[47] anxiety; autonomic nervous system excitation, or instability; delirium; diaphoresis, heavy or profuse; hallucinations; hypertension; insomnia; nystagmus, psychosis; rhabdomyolysis; seizures; tachycardia; and tremor.

The GHB withdrawal syndrome may begin within 1 hour of the last use of GHB among women who are regular, long-term abusers, and last for up to 15 days. It may be potentially life-threatening and is often quite resistant to medical management with benzodiazepines, such as diazepam (Valium®) or lorazepam (Ativan®). In cases of *severe* GHB withdrawal, a barbiturate may be more effective. The GHB withdrawal syndrome, because it is potentially life-threatening, should always be considered a medical emergency that requires prompt and appropriate referral for emergency medical management (Brunt, Van Amsterdam, & van den Brink, 2014).

Overdosage. Gamma-hydroxybutyrate overdosage is relatively common (Miotto, Darakjian, & Basch, 2001) and may be fatal (Zvosec, Smith, & Porrata, 2011). However, fatalities are *rare* and are usually associated with poly-drug and substance abuse (Knudsen, Jonsson, & Abrahamsson, 2010). Alcohol, heroin, and MDMA are the other drugs and substances of abuse that are most often involved in GHB overdosage.[48] Women who have overdosed usually present to the emergency department in an unconscious state, often in a coma. Other presenting signs and symptoms of overdosage may include: agitation; blurred vision; bradycardia; confusion; delirium; diaphoresis (heavy or profuse); headache; hypothermia; loss of bladder and bowel control; muscle jerks or twitches (myoclonic movements);

---

phencyclidine (PCP) use (see Chapter 6, *Women's Psychodelic Abuse*). Upon reflection, we would most likely ascribe the noted "non-sedative" effects to be due to: (1) concurrent use of GHB with another psychotropic, such as a psychostimulant (e.g., methamphetamine, see Chapter 5, *Women's Amphetamine and Cocaine Abuse*) or PCP; (2) exacerbation of an underlying personality-predisposition in association with a GHB-induced decrease in cognitively-mediated measures of "social control"; or (3) the GHB withdrawal syndrome (see additional discussion in the next section, *Physical and Psychological Dependence*).

47 May be quite severe and require appropriate physical or chemical restraint (or both) to prevent injury to self or others.

48 Deaths associated with GHB overdosage, when they do occur, are generally secondary to respiratory failure.

muscle weakness; psychomotor impairment; respiratory impairment; seizures; and vomiting. Death may occur because of cardiorespiratory depression (Busardo & Jones, 2015).

> ...responded to a report of a woman that had collapsed after having taken GHB ... found the woman passed out in the bathroom. By the time emergency personnel arrived, two more people were in medical distress, after also taking GHB.
>
> *(Judd, 2014, p. 1)*

> One teenager said three friends were having a bad reaction to the GHB. When officers arrived, they found a 19-year-old man and a 15-year-old girl unresponsive and a 17-year-old girl who was semi-conscious.
>
> *(Judd, 2015, p. 1)*

> A 44-year-old woman died from a possible overdose of GHB ... transported to the hospital in full cardiac arrest and later died.
>
> *(Suter, 2015, p. 1)*

GHB overdosage should always be treated as a medical emergency with immediate referral for assistance, as needed. With proper recognition and care, particularly with attention to cardiac and respiratory support,[49] complete recovery generally occurs within 6 to 8 hours, without *sequelae*, or any "after" effect of the overdosage (Mason & Kerns, 2002). There is *no* known antidote for GHB overdosage.

Women's Medical and Personal GHB Use and Abuse

Gamma-hydroxybutyrate (GHB) has had a relatively short, but interesting history being first synthesized over 140 years ago in 1874 by the Russian chemist, Alexander Zaytsev (1841–1910). Surprisingly, it was not used until the 1960s when the French physician, Henri Laborit (1914–1995), began to study its use as an anesthetic and a sedative-hypnotic with human patients. By the 1980s, GHB became widely available in health food stores and was promoted and used as a nutritional supplement, primarily by body builders.

Because of a growing incidence of use for its sedative-hypnotic actions, which often resulted in toxicity and death, the FDA banned the non-prescription, or over-the-counter sale, of GHB for human consumption in the U.S. However, by this time the effects of GHB had become well-known. Through the 1990s, its use as a date rape drug increased significantly (Marinetti & Montgomery, 2010).

---

[49] Interestingly, in a 3-year retrospective analysis of data from two major inner city emergency departments (EDs), Dietze, Horyniak, and Agius (2014) found that, in cases of uncomplicated GHB-related coma, conservative airway management—without the use of intubation—was associated with *shorter* length of stay in the ED.

In response, the *Hillory J. Farias and Samantha Reid Date Rape Drug Prohibition Act* was passed and signed into law in 2000. This Act placed GHB on *Schedule I* of the Controlled Substances Act, prohibiting its prescription or legal sale in the U.S. (Placement of, 2000).

Women's Medical GHB Use/Abuse. In 2002, the FDA approved the prescription use of GHB for the medical management of narcolepsy (excessive day-time sleepiness with "sleep attacks") in patients who experience episodes of cataplexy (a sudden loss of muscle tone and strength, which commonly occurs with narcolepsy). To protect the public, GHB, when used in this medical context, is referred to as, and prescribed by, the alternate generic name, sodium oxybate (Xyrem®).[50]

Women's Personal GHB Use/Abuse. GHB is generally used/abused by women in the U.S. to achieve various desired effects, including:

1. Alcohol-like disinhibitory euphoria, or *high* (without the hangover effect associated with alcohol or other sedative-hypnotics)[51]
2. Improved body build (used as a nutritional supplement)
3. Enhanced sexual experience[52,53]
4. Increased sociability
5. Means to prevent/self-manage the alcohol withdrawal syndrome
6. Relaxation

---

50 GHB also has been used in Europe to treat the alcohol withdrawal syndrome. It is being reviewed for similar clinical use in the U.S. In this clinical context of use, GHB pharmacotherapy has been demonstrated to be equivalent, or superior, to benzodiazepines or placebo in several studies (e.g., Caputo, Skala, & Mirijello, 2014; Keating, 2014; Leone, Vigna-Taglianti, & Avanzi, 2010; Skala, Caputo, & Mirijello, 2014). However, several researchers (e.g., Keating, 2014) have voiced concern that the use of GHB among women "with alcohol dependence and borderline personality disorder or who are in remission from heroin or cocaine addiction" may be unsuitable because of an *increased* risk for GHB abuse (p. 63).

51 As shared by a 20-year-old woman who commonly uses GHB in a social context—similar to alcohol:

> I sort of look at it on the same level as having a drink. Often times it affects me for a shorter period of time and I don't have any hangover the next day, it doesn't make me feel crappy ... get great sleep.
>
> (*Barker, Harris, & Dyer, 2007, p. 123*)

52 Kapitany-Foveny, Mervo, and Corazza (2015), in a study of 60 *recreational* GHB users, found that this particular "reason for use" included: (1) increased sexual arousal; (2) more intense attraction toward their partners; and (3) increased openness to having sexual intercourse with strangers.

53 As noted by a 30-year-old woman who deliberately uses (i.e., self-administers) GHB to enhance, or facilitate, sexual activity:

> G feels to me like it has the qualities of teaching you how to open up to people and have less inhibitions naturally and also sexually, you can open up, it's to me the best. It is the most perfect drug for sexual interaction, the best sexual function, the best sexual function, the best.
>
> (*Barker, Harris, & Dyer, 2007, p. 120*)

GHB also is purposely administered to others secretly (i.e., without their knowledge) in the context of perpetrating a drug-facilitated crime (e.g., robbery; sexual assault, including date rape).[54]

Because of the relative difficulty associated with obtaining and diverting prescription GHB (i.e., sodium oxybate, Xyrem®) for abuse, women generally obtain their GHB by purchase: (1) over the Internet; or (2) from street dealers, who offer, in addition to GHB, readily available precursors of GHB, *γ-butyrolactone* (GBL) and *1,4-butanediol* (BD). Once ingested, both GBL and BD are rapidly converted (t ½ = 1 minute) to GHB (Busardo & Jones, 2015). Regardless of source, women who abuse GHB commonly consume it multiple times throughout the day until their supply is depleted and they are unable to obtain any additional GHB or GBL or BD (Miotto, Darakjian, & Basch, 2001; Pagliaro & Pagliaro, *Clinical Patient Data Files*).

References[55,56,57]

Abramowicz, M. (2014). Lowering the dose of Lunesta. *The Medical Letter on Drugs and Therapeutics*, 56(1444), 48.

Amos, T. B., Keith, S. W., & Del Canale, S. (2015). Inappropriate prescribing in a large community-dwelling older population: A focus on prevalence and how it relates to patient and physician characteristics. *Journal of Clinical Pharmacology and Therapeutics*, 40(1), 7–13. doi:10.1111/jcpt.12212

Babalonis, S., Lile, J. A., & Martin, C. A. (2011a). Physiological doses of progesterone potentiate the effects of triazolam in healthy, premenopausal women. *Psychopharmacology (Berl)*, 215(3), 429–439. doi:10.1007/s00213-011-2206-7

Babalonis, S., Lile, J. A., & Martin, C. A. (2011b). Progesterone effects on the discriminative stimulus, subjective and performance effects of triazolam in healthy, premenopausal women. *Behavioural Pharmacology*, 22(5–6), 441–449. doi:10.1097/FBP.0b013e328349fc02

Barker, J. C., Harris, S. L., & Dyer, J. E. (2007, June). Experiences of gamma hydroxybutyrate (GHB) ingestion: A focus group study. *Journal of Psychoactive Drugs*, 39(2), 115–129.

[54] Generally used in combination with alcohol for this purpose. Intended victims lose their ability to fend off their assailant and, because of GHB-induced amnesia, become unreliable witnesses if charges are brought against the assailant.

[55] As per publisher style, only the first three authors are listed for each reference.

[56] Several times the number of references listed were found, obtained, and analyzed by the authors during the preparation of this chapter. However, only the references that were cited at least once in the body of the text are included in the list. Major reasons for *not* citing other references, include that they: (1) did *not* provide any additional unique data; (2) were *not* well researched or written (i.e., were evaluated as *not* being valid or reliable); (3) were based predominantly, or exclusively, on animal studies; (4) provided usage statistics from outside the U.S.; and/or (5) were redundant with, or *not* as recent as, the already cited references.

[57] The reference citation, "Pagliaro & Pagliaro, *Clinical Patient Data Files*," refers to unpublished data collected, with permission, over the last 50 years by the authors, in the formal course of their professional academic roles as clinician scientists and professors—by permission from their patients, research subjects, and students, from the 1970s to date.

Barker, M. J., Greenwood, K. M., & Jackson, M. (2003). Cognitive effects of benzodiazepine use: A review. *Australian Psychologist*, 38, 202–213.

Bateson, A. N. (2002). Basic pharmacologic mechanisms involved in benzodiazepine tolerance and withdrawal. *Current Pharmaceutical Design*, 8(1), 5–21.

Bellivier, F., Yon, L., & Luquiens, A. (2011). Suicidal attempts in bipolar disorder: Results from an observational study (EMBLEM). *Bipolar Disorders*, 13(4), 377–386.

Bennett, R., Bray, D., & Neville, M. W. (2014). Suvorexant, a dual orexin receptor antagonist for the management of insomnia. *Pharmacy and Therapeutics*, 39(4), 264–266.

Bepko, C. (1989/1991). Disorders of power: Women and addiction in the family. In M. McGoldrick, C. M. Anderson, & F. Walsh (Eds.), *Women in families: A framework for family therapy* (pp. 406–426). New York, NY: W. W. Norton.

Bernardy, N. C., Lund, B. C., & Alexander, B. (2013). Gender differences in prescribing among veterans diagnosed with posttraumatic stress disorder. *Journal of General Internal Medicine*, 28(Supplement 2), S542–S548. doi:10.1007/s11606-012-2260-9

Bernardy, N. C., Lund, B. C., & Alexander, B. (2014). Increased polysedative use in veterans with posttraumatic stress disorder. *Pain Medicine*, 15(7), 1083–1090. doi:10.1111/pme.12321

Bernstein, M. H., McSheffrey, S. N., & van den Berg, J. J. (2015, March). The association between impulsivity and alcohol/drug use among prison inmates. *Addictive Behaviors*, 42, 140–143. doi:10.1016/j.addbeh.2014.11.016

Billioti de Gage, S., Moride, Y., & Ducruet, T. (2014). Benzodiazepine use and risk of Alzheimer's disease: Case-control study. *BMJ*, 349, 1–10. doi:10.1136/bmj.g5205

Binder, S. (2002, December). Injuries among older adults: The challenge of optimizing safety and minimizing unintended consequences. *Injury Prevention*, 8(Supplement 4), iv2–iv4.

Bond, M. (2012, September 26). *Killer brain candy: One woman's odyssey through benzodiazepine addiction and withdrawal or how chicken little got her head crushed*. Retrieved October 5, 2016, from www.melissaabond.com, pp. 1–10: www.madinamerica.com/2012/killer-brain-candy-one-womans-odyssey-through-benzodiazepine-addiction-and-withdrawal-or-how-chicken-little-got-her-head-crushed/

Booth, J. N., Behring, M., & Cantor, R. S. (2016). Zolpidem use and motor vehicle collisions in older drivers. *Sleep Medicine*, 20, 98–102. doi:10.1016/j.sleep.2015.12.004

Bourgeois, J., Elseviers, M. M., & Van Bortel, L. (2014a). Feasibility of discontinuing chronic benzodiazepine use in nursing home residents: A pilot study. *European Journal of Pharmacology*, 70(10), 1251–1260. doi:10.1007/s00228-014-1725-7

Bourgeois, J., Elseviers, M. M., & Van Bortel, L. (2014b). One-year evolution of sleep quality in older users of benzodiapines: A longitudinal cohort study in Belgian nursing home residents. *Drugs and Aging*, 31(9), 677–682. doi:10.1007/s40266-014-0203-3

Brennan, R., & Van Hout, M. C. (2014). Gamma-hydroxybutyrate (GHB): A scoping review of pharmacology, toxicology, motives for use, and user groups. *Journal of Psychoactive Drugs*, 46(3), 243–251. doi:10.1080/02791072.2014.921746

Brunt, T. M., Van Amsterdam, J. G., & van den Brink, W. (2014). GHB, GBL and 1,4-BD addiction. *Current Pharmaceutical Design*, 20(25), 4076–4085.

Burgess, A., Dowdell, E., & Prentky, R. (2000). Sexual abuse of nursing home residents. *Journal of Psychosocial Nursing*, 38(6), 10–18.

Busardo, F. P., & Jones, A. W. (2015). GHB pharmacology and toxicology: Acute intoxication, concentrations in blood and urine in forensic cases and treatment of the withdrawal syndrome. *Current Neuropharmacology*, 13(1), 47–70. doi:10.2174/1570159X13666141210215423

Cai, M. S., Crane, E., & Poneleit, K. (2010). Emergency department visits involving nonmedical use of selected prescription drugs—United States, 2004–2008. *MMWR, Morbidity and Mortality Weekly Reports*, 59(23), 705–709.

Canham, S. L. (2015). What's loneliness got to do with it? Older women who use benzodiazepines. *Australasian Journal of Ageing*, 34(1), E7–E12. doi:10.1111/ajag.12133

Canham, S. L., Gallo, J., & Simoni-Wastila, L. (2014). Perceptions of benzodiazepine dependence among women age 65 and older. *Journal of Gerontology and Social Work*, 57(8), 872–888. doi:10.1080/01634372.2014.901470

Caputo, F., Skala, K., & Mirijello, A. (2014). Sodium oxybate in the treatment of alcohol withdrawal syndrome: A randomized double-blind comparative study versus oxazepam. The GATE 1 trial. *CNS Drugs*, 28(8), 743–752. doi:10.1007/s40263-014-0183-1

Carter, L. P. (2011). Potential impact of drug effects, availability, pharmacokinetics, and screening on estimates of drugs implicated in cases of assault. *Drug Testing and Analysis*, 3(9), 586–593.

Cassels, C. (2010, February 10). *APA releases proposed draft of the DSM-5.* Retrieved from Medscape Medical News, pp. 1–4: www.medscape.com/viewarticle/716807?sssdmh=dml.588982&src=nldne&uac=144544HX

Centers for Disease Control and Prevention. (2010). Emergency department visits involving nonmedical use of selected prescription drugs—United States, 2004–2008. *MMWR, Morbidity and Mortality Weekly Report*, 59(23), 705–709.

Chambers, C. D., White, O. Z., & Lindquist, J. H. (1983). Physician attitudes and prescribing practices: A focus on minor tranquilizers. *Journal of Psychoactive Drugs*, 15(1–2), 55–59. doi:10–1080/02791072.1983.10472123

Chang, C. M., Chen, M. J., & Tsai, C. Y. (2011). Medical conditions and medications as risk factors of falls in the inpatient older people: A case-control study. *International Journal of Geriatric Psychiatry*, 26(6), 602–607.

Chen, Y. C., & Kreling, D. H. (2014). The effect of the Medicare Part D benzodiazepine exclusion on the utilization patterns of benzodiazepines and substitute medications. *Research in Social and Administrative Pharmacy*, 10(2), 438–447. doi:10.1016/j.sapharm.2013.06.008

Childers, R. E., Williams, J. L., & Sonnenberg, A. (2015). Practice patterns of sedation for colonoscopy. *Gastrointestinal Endoscopy*, 82(3), 503–511. doi:10.1016/j.gie.2015.01.041

Cimolai, N. (2007). Zopiclone: Is it a pharmacologic agent for abuse? *Canadian Family Physician*, 53(12), 2124–2129.

Cloos, J. M., & Ferreira, V. (2009). Current use of benzodiazepines in anxiety disorders. *Current Opinion in Psychiatry*, 22(1), 90–95.

Conn, D. K., & Madan, R. (2006). Use of sleep-promoting medications in nursing homes residents: Risks versus benefits. *Drugs & Aging*, 23(4), 271–287.

Cox, S., Kuo, C., & Jamieson, D. J. (2011). Poisoning hospitalisations among reproductive-aged women in the USA, 1998–2006. *Injury Prevention*, 17(5), 332–337. doi:10.1136/ip.2010.029793

Crisp, C. C., Vaccaro, C. M., & Estanol, M. V. (2013). Intra-vaginal diazepam for high-tone pelvic floor dysfunction: A randomized placebo-controlled trial. *International Urogynecology Journal*, 24(11), 1915–1923. doi:10.1007/s00192-013-2108-9

Cruz, H. G., Hoever, P., & Chakraborty, B. (2014). Assessment of the abuse liability of a dual orexin receptor antagonist: A crossover study of almorexant and zolpidem in recreational drug users. *CNS Drugs*, 28(4), 361–372. doi:10.1007/s40263-014-0150-x

Cubata, W. J., Landowski, J., & Wichowicz, H. M. (2007). Zolpidem abuse, dependence and withdrawal syndrome: Sex as susceptibility factor for adverse effects. *BJCP, British Journal of Clinical Pharmacology*, 65(3), 444–445.

Cucciare, M. A., Simpson, T., & Hoggatt, K. J. (2013). Substance use among women veterans: Epidemiology to evidence-based treatment. *Journal of Addictive Diseases*, 32(2), 119–139. doi:10.1080/10559887.2013.795465

Cui, D., Cabalu, T., & Yee, K. L. (2016). In vitro and in vivo characterisation of the metabolism and disposition of suvorexant in humans. *Xenobiotica*, 46(10), 882–895. doi:10.3109/00498254.2015.1129565

Dailey, J. H. (2015, October). *Suvorexant (Belsomra) National Drug Monograph*. Retrieved June 11, 2016, from VA BPM Services Drug Monographs, pp. 1–14: www.pbm.va.gov

Dassanayake, T., Michie, P., & Carter, G. (2011). Effects of benzodiazepines, antidepressants and opioids on driving: A systematic review and meta-analysis of epidemiological and experimental evidence. *Drug Safety*, 34(2), 125–156. doi:10.2165/11539050-000000000-00000

Deck, G. M., Nadkarni, N., & Montouris, G. D. (2015). Congenital malformations in infants exposed to antiepileptic medications in utero at Boston Medical Center from 2003 to 2010. *Epilepsy & Behavior*, 51, 166–169. doi:10.1016/j.yebeh.2015.07.001

Dietze, P., Horyniak, D., & Agius, P. (2014). Effect of intubation for gamma-hydroxybutyric acid overdose on emergency department length of stay and hospital admission. *Academic Emergency Medicine*, 21(11), 1226–1231. doi:10.1111/acem.12516

Dowd, S. M., Strong, M. J., & Janicak, P. G. (2002). The behavioral and cognitive effects of two benzodiazepines associated with drug-facilitated sexual assault. *Journal of Forensic Sciences*, 47(5), 1101–1107.

Drover, D. R. (2004). Comparative pharmacokinetics and pharmacodynamics of short-acting hypnosedatives: Zaleplon, zolpidem and zopiclone. *Clinical Pharmacokinetics*, 43(4), 227–238.

Dubey, A. K., Handu, S. S., & Mediratta, P. K. (2015, April–June). Suvorexant: The first orexin receptor antagonist to treat insomnia. *Journal of Pharmacology & Therapeutics*, 6(2), 118–121. doi:10.4103/0976-500X.155496

Evans, F. M., & Levin, F. R. (2002). The effects of alprazolam and buspirone in light and moderate female social drinkers. *Behavioural Pharmacology*, 13(5–6), 427–439.

Farzampour, Z., Reimer, R. J., & Huguenard, J. (2015). Endozepines. *Advances in Pharmacology*, 72, 147–164. doi:10.1016/bs.apha.2014.10.005

FDA. (2013a, May 14). *FDA drug safety communication: FDA approves new label changes and dosing for zolpidem products and a recommendation to avoid driving the day after using Ambien CR*. Retrieved October 5, 2016, from FDA Drug Safety Communication: www.fda.gov/Drugs/DrugSafety/ucm352085.htm

FDA. (2013b, January 13). *FDA safety communication: Risk of next-morning impairment after use of insomnia drugs; FDA requires lower recommended doses for certain drugs containing zolpidem (Ambien, Ambien CR, Edluar, and Zolpimist)*. Retrieved October 5, 2016, from FDA Drug Safety Communication: www.fda.gov/Drugs/DrugSafety/ucm334033.htm

Finkle, W. D., Der, J. S., & Greenland, S. (2011). Risk of fractures requiring hospitalization after an initial prescription for zolpidem, alprazolam, lorazepam, or diazepam in older adults. *Journal of the American Geriatrics Society*, 59(10), 1883–1890.

Forrester, M. B. (2006). Flunitrazepam abuse and malicious use in Texas, 1998–2003. *Substance Use & Misuse*, 41(3), 427–439.

Forrester, M. B. (2007). Eszopiclone ingestions reported to Texas poison control centers, 2005–2006. *Human & Experimental Toxicology*, 26(10), 795–800.

Forrester, M. B. (2009). Immediate- and controlled-release zolpidem ingestions reported to Texas poison centers. *Human & Experimental Toxicology*, 28(8), 505–509. doi:10.1177/0960327109106971

Forrester, M. B. (2011). Ingestions of hydrocodone, carisoprodol, and alprazolam in combination reported to Texas poison centers. *Journal of Addictive Diseases*, 30(2), 110–115. doi:10.1080/10550887.2011.554778

Frey, D., Ortega, J. D., & Wiseman, C. (2011). Influence of zolpidem and sleep inertia on balance and cognition during nighttime awakening: A randomized placebo-controlled trial. *Journal of the American Geriatrics Society*, 59(1), 73–81.

Gallagher, P., Barry, P., & O'Mahony, D. (2007). Inappropriate prescribing in the elderly. *Journal of Clinical Pharmacy and Therapeutics*, 32(2), 113–121.

Garcia-Gollarte, F., Baleriola-Julvez, J., & Ferrero-Lopez, I. (2012). Inappropriate drug prescription at nursing home admission. *Journal of the American Medical Directors Association*, 83.e9–83.e15.

Garewal, D., Powell, S., & Milan, S. J. (2012, June 13). Sedative techniques for endoscopic retrograde cholangiopancreatography. *The Cochrane Database of Systematic Reviews*, 6, CD007274. doi:10.1002/14651858.CD007274.pub2

Goulle, J. P., & Anger, J. P. (2004). Drug facilitated robbery or sexual assault: Problems associated with amnesia. *Therapeutic Drug Monitoring*, 26(2), 206–210.

Gunja, N. (2013a). The clinical and forensic toxicology of z-drugs. *Journal of Medical Toxicology*, 9, 155–162. doi:10.1007/s13181-013-0292-0

Gunja, N. (2013b). In the Zzz Zone: The effects of Z-drugs on human performance and driving. *Journal of Medicine and Toxicology*, 9, 163–171. doi:10.1007/s13181-013-0294-y

Halvorsen, T., & Martinussen, P. E. (2015). Benzodiazepine use in COPD: Empirical evidence from Norway. *International Journal of Chronic Obstructive Pulmonary Disease*, 10, 1695–1702. doi:10.2147/COPD.S83107

Hawkins, E. J., Malte, C. A., & Imel, Z. E. (2012). Prevalence and trends of benzodiazepine use among Veteran Affairs patients with posttraumatic stress disorder, 2003–2010. *Drug and Alcohol Dependence*, 124(1–2), 154–161. doi:10.1016/j.drugalcdep.2012.01.003

Hines, L. E., & Murphy, J. E. (2011). Potentially harmful drug-drug interactions in the elderly: A review. *The American Journal of Geriatric Pharmacotherapy*, 9(6), 364–377.

Holbrook, A. M., Crowther, R., & Lotter, A. (1999). Meta-analysis of benzodiazepine use in the treatment of acute alcohol withdrawal. *CMAJ, Canadian Medical Association Journal*, 169(5), 649–655.

Holm, K. J., & Goa, K. L. (2000). Zolpidem: An update of its pharmacology, therapeutic efficacy and tolerability in the treatment of insomnia. *Drugs*, 59(4), 865–889.

Hood, S. D., Norman, A., & Hince, D. A. (2014). Benzodiazepine dependence and its treatment with low dose flumazenil. *British Journal of Clinical Pharmacology*, 77(2), 285–294. doi:10.1111/bcp.12023

Hopkins, C. R. (2012). ACS chemical neuroscience molecule spotlight on suvorexant. *ACS Chemical Neuroscience*, 3, 647–648. doi:10.1021/cn300086a

Hoyer, D., & Jacobson, L. H. (2013). Orexin in sleep, addiction and more: Is the perfect insomnia drug at hand? *Neuropeptides*, 47(6), 477–488. doi:10.1016/j.npep.2013.10.009

Huedo-Medina, T. B., Kirsch, I., & Middlemass, J. (2012). Effectiveness of non-benzodiazepine hypnotics in treatment of adult insomnia: Meta-analysis of data submitted to the Food and Drug Administration. *BMJ*, 345, 1–13. doi:10.1136/bmj.e8343

Hypnotic dependence: Zolpidem and zopiclone too. (2001, February). *Prescrire International*, 10(51), 15.

Jacobson, L. H., Callander, G. E., & Hoyer, D. (2014). Suvorexant for the treatment of insomnia. *Expert Review of Clinical Pharmacology*, 7(6), 711–730. doi:10.1586/17512433.2014.966813

Jones, C. M., & McAninch, J. K. (2015). Emergency department visits and overdose deaths from combined use of opioids and benzodiazepines. *American Journal of Preventive Medicine*, 49(4), 493–501.

Jones, C. M., Paulozzi, L. J., & Mack, K. A. (2014). Alcohol involvement in opioid pain reliever and benzodiazepine drug abuse—Related emergency department visits and drug-related deaths—United States, 2010. *Morbidity and Mortality Weekly Report (MMWR)*, 63(40), 881–885.

Judd, A. (2014, October 27). 3 people rushed to hospital after intentionally taking "date rape" drug, GHB. *Global News Online*. Shaw Media. Retrieved November 1, 2016, from http://globalnews.ca/news/1638045/3-people-rushed-to-hospital-after-intentionally-taking-date-rape-drug-ghb/

Judd, A. (2015, June 22). 3 Abbotsford teens in serious condition after overdosing on GHB. *Global News Online*. Shaw Media. Retrieved November 1, 2016, from http://globalnews.ca/news/2068211/3-abbotsford-teens-in-serious-condition-after-overdosing-on-ghb/

Kapitany-Foveny, M., Mervo, B., & Corazza, O. (2015). Enhancing sexual desire and experience: An investigation of the sexual correlates of gamma-hydroxybutyrate (GHB) use. *Human Psychopharmacology*, 30(4), 276–284. doi:10.1002/hup.2491

Keating, G. M. (2014). Sodium oxybate: A review of its use in alcohol withdrawal syndrome and in the maintenance of abstinence in alcohol dependence. *Clinical Drug Investigation*, 34(1), 63–80. doi:10.1007/s40261-013-0158-x

Kintz, P., Villain, M., & Dumestre-Toulet, V. (2005). Drug-facilitated sexual assault and analytical toxicology: The role of LC-MS/MS A case involving zolpidem. *Journal of Clinical Forensic Medicine*, 12(1), 36–41.

Knudsen, K., Jonsson, U., & Abrahamsson, J. (2010). Twenty-three deaths with gamma-hydroxybutyrate overdose in western Sweden between 2000 and 2007. *Acta Anaesthesiologica Scandinavica*, 54(8), 987–992.

Ko, J. Y., Kim, M. J., & Lee, S. G. (2012, November–December). Outcome predictors affecting the efficacy of clonazepam therapy for the management of burning mouth syndrome (BMS). *Archives of Gerontology and Geriatrics*, 55(3), 755–761. doi:10.1016/j.archger.2011.10.001

Koyama, A., Steinman, M., & Ensrud, K. (2013). Ten-year trajectory of potentially inappropriate medications in very old women: Importance of cognitive status. *Journal of the American Geriatric Society*, 61(2), 258–263. doi:10.1111/jgs.12093

Kurtz, S. P., Buttram, M. E., & Surratt, H. L. (2017). Benzodiazepine dependence among young adult participants in the club scene who use drugs. *Journal of Psychoactive Drugs*, 49(1), 39–46. doi: 10.1080/02791072.2016.1269978

Kurtz, S. P., Surratt, H. L., & Levi-Minzi, M. A. (2011). Benzodiazepine dependence among multidrug users in the club scene. *Drug and Alcohol Dependence*, 119(1–2), 99–105. doi:10.1016/j,drugalcdep.2011.05.036

Lekka, N. P., Paschalis, C., & Beratis, S. (2002). Suicide attempts in high-dose benzodiazepine users. *Comprehensive Psychiatry*, 43(6), 438–442.

Leone, M. A., Vigna-Taglianti, F., & Avanzi, G. (2010, February 17). Gamma-hydroxybutyrate (GHB) for treatment of alcohol withdrawal and prevention of relapses. *Cochrane Database of Systematic Reviews* (2), CD006266. doi:10.1002/14651858.CD006266.pub2

Lilja, J., & Larsson, S. (1994). Social pharmacology: Unresolved critical issues. *International Journal of the Addictions*, 29(13), 1647–1737.

Lin, S. K. (2014, July). Rapid detoxification of benzodiazepine or Z-drugs dependence using acetylcholinesterase inhibitors. *Medical Hypotheses*, 83(1), 108–110. doi:10.1016/j.mehy.2014.03.032

Lind, J. N., Petersen, E. E., & Lederer, P. A. (2015). Infant and maternal characteristics in neonatal abstinence syndrome—Selected hospitals in Florida, 2010–2011. *MMWR, Morbidity and Mortality Weekly Report*, 64(8), 213–216.

MacReady, N., & Barclay, L. (2009). Psychotropic medications associated with falls in elderly people. *Archives of Internal Medicine*, 169, 1952–1960.

Madea, B., & MuBhoff, F. (2009). Knock-out drugs: Their prevalence, modes of action, and means of detection. *Deutsches Azteblatt International*, 106(20), 341–347.

Marinetti, L., & Montgomery, M. A. (2010). The use of GHB to facilitate sexual assault. *Forensic Science Review*, 22(1), 41–59.

Mason, P. E., & Kerns 2nd, W. P. (2002). Gamma hydroxybutyric acid (GHB) intoxication. *Academic Emergency Medicine*, 9(7), 730–739.

Masten, A. S., & O'Connor, M. J. (1989). Vulnerability, stress, and resilience in the early development of a high risk child. *Journal of the American Academy of Child & Adolescent Psychiatry*, 28(2), 274–278.

McMillan, K. (2014, April 25). The truth about prescription pills: One writer's story of anxiety and addiction. *Vogue Magazine*. Retrieved August 15, 2015, from www.vogue.com/contributor/kelley-mcmillan/

Merck & Company. (2016). *Dependence: Safety and tolerability of Belsomra*, 1–3. Merck & Company. Retrieved November 27, 2016, from www.merckconnect.com/belsomra/safety-and-toleravbility-dependence.html?hcpUser=yes

Meuleners, L. B., Duke, J., & Lee, A. H. (2011). Psychoactive medications and crash involvement requiring hospitalization for older drivers: A population-based study. *Journal of the American Geriatrics Society*, 59(9), 1575–1580. doi:10.1111/j.1532-5415.2011.03561.x

Miotto, K., Darakjian, J., & Basch, J. (2001). Gamma-hydroxybutyric acid: Patterns of use, effects and withdrawal. *The American Journal on Addictions*, 10(3), 232–241.

Morinan, A., & Keaney, F. (2010). Long-term misuse of zopiclone in an alcohol dependent woman with a history of anorexia nervosa: A case report. *Journal of Medical Case Reports*, 4(1), 1–5.

NIDA, National Institute on Drug Abuse. (2008, August). *Club drugs (GHB, ketamine, and Rohypnol)*. Retrieved from NIDA InfoFacts, pp. 1–3.

NIDA, National Institute on Drug Abuse. (2015, December). *Overdose death rates*. Retrieved February 21, 2016, from National Institute on Drug Abuse (NIDA), pp. 1–7: www.drugabuse.gov/related-topics/trends-statistics/overdose-death-rates

Ninan, P. T. (2001). Pharmacokinetically induced benzodiazepine withdrawal. *Psychopharmacology Bulletin*, 35(4), 94–100.

Norman, J. L., & Anderson, S. L. (2016). Novel class of medications, orexin receptor antagonists, in the treatment of insomnia—critical appraisal of suvorexant. *Nature and Science of Sleep*, 8, 239–247.

O'Brien, C. P. (2005). Benzodiazepine use, abuse, and dependence. *Journal of Clinical Psychiatry*, 66(Supplement 2), 28–33.

O'Brien, M. P. (2008, June). Epidemiological trends in drug abuse. *Proceedings of the Community Epidemiology Work Group. Volume 1: highlights and executive summary*. Bethesda, MD: National Institute on Drug Abuse, U.S. Department of Health and Human Services.

Okun, M. L., Ebert, R., & Saini, B. (2015). A review of sleep-promoting medications used in pregnancy. *American Journal of Obstetrics and Gynecology*, 212(4), 428–441. doi:10.1016/j.ajog.2014.10.1106

Olfson, M., King, M., & Schoenbaum, M. (2015). Benzodiazepine use in the United States. *JAMA Psychiatry*, 72(2), 136–142. doi:10.1001/jamapsychiatry.2014.1763

Owen, R. T. (2016). Suvorexant: Efficacy and safety profile of a dual orexin receptor antagonist in treating insomnia. *Drugs of Today (Barcelona, Spain)*, 52(1), 29–40. doi:10.1358/dot.2016.52.1.2439940

Pagliaro, L. A., & Levin, R. H. (Eds.). (1979). *Problems in pediatric drug therapy* (1st ed.). Hamilton, IL: Drug Intelligence Publications.

Pagliaro, L. A., & Pagliaro, A. M. (Eds.). (1983). *Pharmacologic aspects of aging.* St. Louis, MO: CV Mosby.

Pagliaro, L. A., & Pagliaro, A. M. (1992). Phenomenon of drug and substance abuse among the elderly, part 1: An overview. *Journal of Pharmacy Technology*, 8, 65–73.

Pagliaro, L. A., & Pagliaro, A. M. (1999). *PPDR: Psychologists' psychotropic drug reference.* Philadelphia, PA: Brunner/Mazel.

Pagliaro, L. A., & Pagliaro, A. M. (Eds.). (2002). *Problems in pediatric drug therapy* (4th ed.). Washington, DC: American Pharmaceutical Association.

Pagliaro, L. A., & Pagliaro, A. M. (2004). *Pagliaros' comprehensive guide to drugs and substances of abuse* (1st ed.). Washington, DC: American Pharmacists Association.

Pagliaro, L. A., & Pagliaro, A. M. (2009). *Pagliaros' comprehensive guide to drugs and substances of abuse* (2nd ed.). Washington, DC: American Pharmacists Association.

Pagliaro, L. A., & Pagliaro, A. M. (2012). *Handbook of child and adolescent drug and substance abuse: Pharmacological, developmental, and clinical considerations.* Hoboken, NJ: John Wiley & Sons.

Pardal, P. K., Praksh, J., & Konwar, R. (2011, October). Zolpidem dependence. *Delhi Psychiatry Journal*, 14(2), 388–389.

Patel, K. V., Aspesi, A. V., & Evoy, K. E. (2015). Suvorexant: A dual orexin receptor antagonist for the treatment of sleep onset and sleep maintenance insomnia. *Annals of Pharmacotherapy*, 49(4), 477–483. doi:10.1177/1060028015570467

Pinto, A., Sollecito, T. P., & DeRossi, S. S. (2003). Burning mouth syndrome. A retrospective analysis of clinical characteristics and treatment outcomes. *The New York State Dental Journal*, 69(3), 18–24.

Pisani, M. A., Bramley, K., & Vest, M. T. (2013). Patterns of opiate, benzodiazepine, and antipsychotic drug dosing in older patients in a medical intensive care unit. *American Journal of Critical Care*, 22(5), e62–69. doi:10.4037/ajcc2013835

Placement of gamma-butyrolactone in List I of the Controlled Substances Act (21 U.S.C. 802934). Drug Enforcement Administration, Justice. Final rule. (2000, April 24). *Fed Regist, 65*(79), 21645–21647.

Preidt, R. (2014, May 22). *Sharp rise in ER visits tied to abuse of sedative, study finds.* Retrieved June 28, 2014, from U.S. News and World Report, pp. 1–2: https://consumer.healthday.com/mental-health-information-25/addiction-news-5/sharp-rise-in-er-visits-tied-to-abuse-of-sedative-study-finds-688047.html

Pressman, M. R. (2011). Sleep driving: Sleepwalking variant or misuse of z-drugs? *Sleep Medicine Review*, 15(5), 285–292. doi:10.1016/j.smrv.2010.12.004

Ramsey-Klawsnik, H. (2004). Elder sexual abuse perpetrated by residents in care settings. *Victimization of the Elderly and Disabled*, 6(6), 81, 93–95.

Reddy, A., Puvvada, S. C., & Kommisetti, S. (2015). Suvorexant: Something new for sleep? *Acta Neuropsychiatrica*, 27(1), 53–55. doi:10.1017/neu.2014.31

Schoedel, K. A., Sun, H., & Sellers, D. M. (2016, August). Assessment of the abuse potential of the orexin receptor antagonist, suvorexant, compared with zolpidem in a randomized crossover study. *Journal of Clinical Psychopharmacology*, 36(4), 314–323. doi:10.1097/JCP.0000000000000516

Sharp, M. J., & Melnik, T. A. (2015, April 17). Poisoning deaths involving opioid analgesics—New York State, 2003–2013. *MMWR, Morbidity and Mortality Weekly Report*, 64(14), 377–380.

Singer, L. T., Song, L. Y., & Hill, B. P. (1990). Stress and depression in mothers of failure-to-thrive children. *Journal of Pediatric Psychology*, 15(6), 711–720.

Skaer, T. L. (2014). Fibromyalgia: Disease synopsis, medication cost effectiveness and economic burden. *Pharmacoeconomics*, 32(5), 457–466. doi:10.1007/s40273-014-0137-y

Skala, K., Caputo, F., & Mirijello, A. (2014). Sodium oxybate in the treatment of alcohol dependence: From the alcohol withdrawal syndrome to the alcohol relapse prevention. *Expert Opinion on Pharmacotherapy*, 15(2), 245–257. doi:10.1517/14656566.2014.863278

Stahlman, S., Javanbakht, M., & Cochran, S. (2015). Mental health and substance use factors associated with unwanted sexual contact among U.S. active duty service women. *Journal of Traumatic Stress*, 28(3), 167–173. doi:10.1002/jts.22009

Stevens, J. A., Mack, K. A., & Paulozzi, L. J. (2008). Self-reported falls and fall-related injuries among persons aged 65 or greater—United States, 2006. *Journal of Safety Research*, 39(3), 345–349. doi:10.1016/j.jsr.2008.05.002

Suter, L. (2015, July 12). Woman dies of possible GHB overdose in Venice. *ABC7.com*. ABC News. Retrieved November 1, 2016, from htpp://abc7.com/news/woman-dies-of-possible-ghb-overdose-in-venice/845829/

Sweeney, J., Laoire, F. O., & Linehan, G. (2015). A review of potentially inappropriate prescribing in over 65's in Livinghealth Clinic. *IMJ, Irish Medical Journal*, 108(6), 180–181.

Tanaka, E. (2002). Toxicological interactions between alcohol and benzodiazepines. *Journal of Toxicology. Clinical Toxicology* , 40(1), 69–75.

Teaster, P., & Roberto, K. (2003). Sexual abuse of older women living in nursing homes. *Journal of Gerontological Social Work*, 40(4), 105–119.

van der Hooft, C. S., Schoofs, M. W., & Ziere, G. (2008). Inappropriate benzodiazepine use in older adults and the risk of fracture. *British Journal of Clinical Pharmacology*, 66(2), 276–282.

van Strien, A. M., Koek, H. L., & van Marum, R. J. (2013). Psychotropic medications, including short acting benzodiazepines, strongly increase the frequency of falls in elderly. *Maturitas*, 74(4), 357–362. doi:10.1016/j.maturitas.2013.01.004

Voaklander, D. C., Rowe, B. H., & Dryden, D. M. (2008). Medical illness, medication use and suicide in seniors: A population-based case-control study. *Journal of Epidemiology & Community Health*, 62(2), 138–146.

Wagner, A. K., Zhang, F., & Soumerai, S. B. (2006). Benzodiazepine use and hip fractures in the elderly: Who is at greatest risk? *Archives of Internal Medicine*, 164(14), 1567–1572.

Wang, L. H., Lin, H. C., & Lin, C. C. (2010). Increased risk of adverse pregnancy outcomes in women receiving zolpidem during pregnancy. *Clinical Pharmacology & Therapeutics*, 88(3), 369–374. doi:10.1038/clpt.2010.97

Wang, P. S., Bohn, R. L., & Glynn, R. J. (2001). Zolpidem use and hip fractures in older people. *Journal of the American Geriatrics Society*, 49(12), 1685–1690.

Wardman, D., Khan, N., & el-Guebaly, N. (2002). Prescription medication use among an aboriginal population accessing addiction treatment. *Canadian Journal of Psychiatry*, 355–360.

Weaver, M. F. (2015). Prescription sedative misuse and abuse. *Yale Journal of Biology and Medicine*, 88, 247–256.

Widlitz, M., & Marin, D. B. (2002). Substance abuse in older adults. An overview. *Geriatrics*, 57(12), 29–34, 37.

Wikner, B. N., & Kallen, B. (2011). Are hypnotic benzodiazepine receptor agonists teratogenic in humans? *Journal of Clinical Psychopharmacology*, 31(3), 356–359. doi:10.1097/JCP.0b013e3182197055

Winrow, C. J., & Renger, J. J. (2014). Discovery and development of orexin receptor antagonists as therapeutics for insomnia. *British Journal of Pharmacology*, 171(2), 283–293. doi:10.1111/bph.12261

Woods, J. H., Katz, J. L., & Winger, G. (1988). Use and abuse of benzodiazepines. Issues relevant to prescribing. *JAMA, Journal of the American Medical Association*, 260(23), 3476–3480.

Worley, J., Hall, J., & Hall, J. (2012). Doctor shopping: A concept analysis. *Research & Theory for Nursing Practice*, 26(4), 262–278.

Yang, L. P. (2014). Suvorexant: First global approval. *Drugs*, 74(15), 1817–1822. doi:10.1007/s40265-014-0294-5

Yen, C. F., Yen, C. N., & Ko, C. H. (2015). Correlates of dependence and beliefs about the use of hypnotics among zolpidem and zopiclone users. *Substance Use & Misuse*, 50(3), 350–357. doi:10.3109/10826084.2014.980955

Zosel, A., Osterberg, E. C., & Mycyk, M. B. (2011). Zolpidem misuse with other medications or alcohol frequently results in intensive care unit admission. *American Journal of Therapeutics*, 18(4), 305–308.

Zvosec, D. L., & Smith, S. W. (2005, May). Agitation is common in gamma-hydroxybutyrate toxicity. *The American Journal of Emergency Medicine*, 23(3), 316–320.

Zvosec, D. L., Smith, S. W., & Porrata, T. (2011). Case series of 226 y-hydroxybutyrate-associated deaths: Lethal toxicity and trauma. *The American Journal of Emergency Medicine*, 29(3), 319–332. doi:10.1016/j.ajem.2009.11.008

4

WOMEN'S CAFFEINE AND NICOTINE ABUSE

Caffeine and nicotine are *natural* psychostimulants that are abused by women in the U.S. to: "achieve a sense of well-being;" "increase alertness and attention;" "keep going;" "lose, or maintain, desired body weight;" and "relax."[1] Legally available for personal use, women have often used these two psychostimulants together—a cup of coffee and a cigarette before going to work, during a break, or after a meal. Both caffeine and nicotine have interesting pharmacology and patterns of personal use among women of all ages. Thus, we present and discuss them together in this chapter. We begin with *caffeine*.

Caffeine

Approximately 90% of women in the U.S. use caffeine on a regular, daily basis. These women, generally, consider caffeine to be relatively harmless. However, caffeine is a *major* drug and substance of abuse and, like other drugs and substances of abuse, its use is associated with several undesired, or harmful, effects and toxicities, including physical and psychological dependence. Although most health and social care providers seldom encounter women whose *major* presenting problem is caffeine addiction, they often encounter women who socially use, habitually use, abuse, or compulsively use caffeine, which is readily available from many popular sources.

---

[1] For an overview and discussion of two other psychostimulants that are commonly abused by women in the U.S., see Chapter 5, *Women's Amphetamine and Cocaine Abuse*.

Popular Sources of Caffeine

Over 97% of the daily caffeine intake among women during the new millennium is by the ingestion of caffeine-containing beverages (Chen, Bell, & Browne, 2014; Mitchell, Knight, & Hockenberry, 2014; Somogyi, 2010). These beverages, traditionally include: coffee, tea, and cocoa, as well as caffeinated, carbonated drinks (i.e., colas). Also, popular among new millennial women are energy drinks and energy shots, which are often mixed into alcoholic beverages. Other sources include more recently developed caffeine delivery systems and products (see Table 4.1).

Coffee, Tea, and Cocoa

Caffeine, in the form of coffee (e.g., Java, Joe), is ingested worldwide by millions of women every morning upon awakening to "get them going," and during work breaks throughout the day, to "keep them going." For many, coffee also is ingested throughout the evening—to complete an enjoyable dinner, relax from a hectic day, or to keep awake during a night shift, to watch "movies till dawn," or to "party all night." Ground and dripped from a favorite coffee maker, "perked" on the stove, push-buttoned from a single-cup coffee pod, French-pressed from a Bodum®, stirred into a hot cup of water, selected from a long list on the wall of coffee delights—Americano, cappuccino, espresso, and latte—or hurriedly grabbed from a drive-thru window—caffeine is the number one drug for many women. In addition to various coffees, caffeine also comes in a variety of black, china, Earl Grey, orange pekoe, green, and jasmine teas.

Although caffeine is found in over 60 different plants, the major natural sources of the caffeine that is used by women in the U.S. are generally obtained from the:

- Beans of two species of coffee, *Coffea arabica* and *Coffea robusta*
- Leaves of one species of tea, *Camellia sinensis*
- Beans of *Theobroma cacao*, from which cocoa is obtained and chocolate is made

Coffea arabica, which is native to Ethiopia, is now widely grown in Brazil and Colombia. *Coffea robusta*, which is native to Saudi Arabia, also is currently widely grown in Brazil, as well as Africa and Indonesia. The caffeine content in a cup of coffee (generally, 65 to 150 mg) depends on: (1) the type of coffee bean selected; and (2) its method of roasting. For example, *Arabica* coffee generally contains *less* caffeine than the *Robusta* variety and *dark-roast* coffee generally contains *less* caffeine than *light-roast* coffee.[2]

[2] The roasting process *reduces* caffeine content (Somogyi, 2010). On average, roasted coffee beans contain between 1% and 3% caffeine.

TABLE 4.1 Average Caffeine Content of Selected Beverages, Foods, and Other Products[a,b]

Beverages, Foods, & Other Products	*Caffeine Content[c,d] (Average)*
Beverages	
Ammo®	171 mg per 1 ounce
AMP® energy drink	75 mg per 8.4 ounces
Chocolate milk	1 to 2 mg per ounce
Coffee, decaffeinated[e]	3 to 12 mg per 8 ounces
Coffee, Dunkin Donuts® regular brewed	206 mg per 16 ounces
Coffee, Einstein Bros.® espresso	75 mg per 1 ounce
Coffee, Einstein Bros.® regular brewed	300 mg per 16 ounces
Coffee, espresso	30 to 90 mg per 1 ounces
Coffee, instant	60 to 100 mg per 8 ounces
Coffee, regular brewed	80 to 200 mg per 8 ounces
Coffee, Starbucks® brewed	320 mg per 16 ounces, *Grande* cup
Coffee, Starbucks® brewed house blend	260 mg per 16 ounces
Coffee, Starbucks® espresso	75 mg per 1 ounce
Coffee, Starbucks® espresso decaffeinated	4 mg per 1 ounce
Cola drinks	30 to 50 mg per 12 ounces[f]
Enviga® energy drink	100 mg per 12 ounces
Fanta® soda	0 mg per 12 ounces
Frappuccino, Starbucks®	115 mg per 9.5 ounces
Fresca®	0 mg per 12 ounces
Fuel Cell®	180 mg per 2 ounces
Full Throttle® energy drink	144 mg per 16 ounces
Hot cocoa	3 to 13 mg per 8 ounces
Jolt®	71.2 mg per 12 ounces
Latte (vanilla), Starbucks®	150 mg per 16 ounces
Monster® energy drink	160 mg per 16 ounces
Morning Spark® energy drink	200 mg per *ready-mix* packet
Mountain Dew MDX®	71 mg per 12 ounces
Mug Root Beer®	0 mg per 12 ounces
No Name® (formerly, Cocaine®)	280 mg per 8.4 ounces
NOS® energy drink[g]	125 mg per 16 ounces
NOS Powershot®	125 mg per 2 ounces
Powershot®	100 mg per 1 ounce
Red Bull® energy drink	80 mg per 8.3 ounces
Rock Star® energy drink[h]	160 mg per 16 ounces
Rip It® energy drink	100 mg per 8 ounces
SoBe Adrenaline Rush® energy drink	79 mg per 8.3 ounces
SoBe Essential Energy® energy drink	48 mg per 8 ounces
SoBe No Fear® energy drink	174 mg per 16 ounces
Spike Shooter® energy drink	300 mg per 8.4 ounces
Sprite® soda	0 mg per 12 ounces
Tea, Arizona® black iced	32 mg per 16 ounces
Tea, Arizona® green iced	15 mg per 16 ounces
Tea, black brewed	40 to 120 mg per 8 ounces

TABLE 4.1 *(cont.)*

Beverages, Foods, & Other Products	*Caffeine Content[c,d] (Average)*
Tea, black decaffeinated	2 to 10 mg per 8 ounces
Tea, green	30 to 60 mg per 8 ounces
Tea, herbal	0 mg per 8 ounces
Tea, iced	70 mg per 12 ounces
Tea, iced Lipton® Brisk Lemon	7 mg per 12 ounces
Tea, iced Nestea®	26 mg per 12 ounces
Tea, Snapple® flavored	42 mg per 16 ounces
Tea, Snapple® plain unsweetened	18 mg per 16 ounces
Vault® soft drink	71 mg per 12 ounces
Water Joe® bottled water	60 mg per 16.9 ounces
Whoop Ass® energy drink	50 mg per 8.3 ounces
7-Up®	0 mg per 12 ounces
Foods	
Bakers® Chocolate	26 mg per 1 ounce
Ben & Jerry's Coffee Buzz® Ice Cream	72 mg per 8 ounces
Ben & Jerry's Coffee-flavored Ice Cream	68 mg per 8 ounces
Ben & Jerry's Coffee Health Bar Crunch®	84 mg per 8-ounce bar
Butterfinger Buzz® candy bar	80 mg per bar
Buzz Bites Chocolate Chews®	100 mg per 1 piece, or *chew*
Chocolate candy bar (dark)	19 mg per 1 ounce
Chocolate candy bar (milk)	7 mg per 1 ounce
Chocolate (dark, semi-sweet)	20 mg per 1 ounce
Chocolate-flavored syrup	4 mg per 1 ounce
Dannon® Coffee Yogurt	36 mg per 6-ounce tube
Hagen-Dazs® Coffee Frozen Yogurt	58 mg per 8 ounces
Hagen-Dazs® Coffee Ice Cream	58 mg per 8 ounces
Hershey's Chocolate Kisses®	1 mg per piece, or *kiss*®
Hershey's® cocoa powder	66 mg per 1 ounce
Hershey's Special Dark® chocolate bar	31 mg per bar (1.45 ounces)
Hershey's® unsweetened baking chocolate	30 mg per 1 ounce
Morning Spark Oatmeal® cereal	80 mg per individual serving packet
NRG Phoenix Fury® potato chips	350 mg per 3.5 ounces' bag
Perky Jerky®	150 mg per 1 ounce
Raging Bull® candy	80 mg per 1 piece
Snickers Charged® candy bar	60 mg per 1.83 ounces' bar
Starbucks® Coffee Ice Cream	60 mg per 8 ounces
Other Products	
AMP® energy gum	40 mg per 1 piece
Black Black® gum	5 mg per 1 piece
Blitz® energy gum	55 mg per 1 piece
Foosh® mints	100 mg per 1 mint
Go Fast! ® energy gum	100 mg per 1 piece
Jolt® gum	33 mg per 1 piece
Revive® mints	85 mg per 1 mint

TABLE 4.1 *(cont.)*

Beverages, Foods, & Other Products	*Caffeine Content[c,d] (Average)*
Rock Star® energy gum	40 mg per 1 piece
Stay Alert® gum	100 mg per 1 piece
Think® gum	10 mg per 1 piece

[a] Nutritional supplements are *not* included in this list because they are not primarily used to achieve psychostimulant effects (e.g., to achieve feelings of euphoria or *to get high*). Generally, they are primarily used for body building, to *improve* physical physique, and to *increase* athletic performance (i.e., they are used as an *ergogenic aid*). However, readers are reminded that adolescent girls and young women, in particular, are among the largest group of users of *caffeine-containing* nutritional supplements. The use of these multi-ingredient products, which, in addition to caffeine, often contain a variety of vitamins, minerals, proteins, and ephedrine, can significantly contribute to the user's total daily caffeine consumption and, consequently, to the occurrence of caffeine toxicity.

[b] For comparison, the following are some common non-prescription products that contain caffeine: Anacin®, extra strength, 32 mg per tablet; Excedrin®, extra strength, 65 mg per tablet; No Doz®, maximum strength, 200 mg per tablet; and Vivarin®, 200 mg per tablet.

[c] The *average* amount of caffeine content is listed with the typical beverage serving size.

[d] Source: Pagliaro & Pagliaro, 2009; product websites.

[e] When coffee beans are decaffeinated by the typical *Swiss water process*, approximately 98% of the natural caffeine is removed.

[f] The FDA limit for caffeine added to cola drinks is 71 mg per 12 ounces.

[g] NOS is advertised as being able to provide the same *boost* to the user's performance as nitrous oxide gives to motor vehicle performance.

[h] Rock Star + Vodka® contains 30 mg of caffeine and 6.9% alcohol per 16 ounces. Generally, across North America, distillers are forbidden by law to directly add caffeine to alcoholic beverages. However, when the source of the caffeine is a natural product, such as *guarana* or *yerbe mate*—as is the case for Rock Star + Vodka®—then it is permitted. (For further related discussion, also see Chapter 2, *Women's Alcohol Abuse*.)

Camellia sinensis, a tea bush native to China and India, continues to be grown primarily in these two countries. Black tea, green tea, oolong, white tea, and yellow tea all come from the leaves of the *Camellia sinensis* plant. Fresh tea leaves contain approximately 4% caffeine and the average cup of tea contains approximately 20 to 80 mg per cup. The differences in color and flavor of these teas are due to their methods of processing and the associated chemical reaction (i.e., oxidation). Indian teas (i.e., *Assam* and *Darjeeling*) also are made from *Camellia sinensis*, but from a different variety of the plant. Although tea is the most widely consumed prepared beverage in the world, more women and men in the U.S. drink coffee.

Coffee and tea grow best in the "coffee bean belt," the area within 1,000 miles of the equator, or the band that encircles the earth between the Tropic of Capricorn and the Tropic of Cancer. The well-known *Kona* coffee, grown on coffee plantations in the Hawaiian Islands, particularly the big island of Oahu, is the *only* coffee grown in the U.S. Most teas, sold in cans of loose tea leaves or packages of tea bags, are composed of various tea blends. Scents and flavorings also may be added to improve taste and to distinguish one brand or type of tea from another. For example, *Earl Grey* tea contains oil of bergamot, while *Jasmine* tea contains jasmine flowers or jasmine oil.

Theobroma cocoa, which is native to South America, now grows in several parts of the world, although South America continues to be the primary source of cocoa beans. Cocoa is commonly ingested by women in chocolate candy, cakes, ice cream, and hot chocolate. (Also, see Table 4.1. *Common Daily Sources of Caffeine in the U.S.*)[3] In addition to cocoa, women in the U.S. also ingest caffeine in the form of *caffeinated beverages*.

Caffeinated Beverages

There are four major caffeinated beverages that are consumed by women in the U.S.: (1) carbonated colas; (2) energy drinks; (3) energy shots; and (4) caffeinated alcoholic beverages. These caffeinated beverages contain considerable amounts of caffeine (see Table 4.1) because they are made with:

- Caffeine-containing extracts of the nuts of the *Cola acuminata* (i.e., guru nuts that are traditionally chewed by indigenous peoples of the Sudan for their psychostimulant effects)
- Guarana, which naturally contains higher concentrations of caffeine than found in cocoa, coffee, kola, or tea
- Additional caffeine that is added during their production

Carbonated Colas. Carbonated colas are non-alcoholic, sweetened (with sugar or artificial sweeteners) beverages to which caffeine has been added or included as a natural derivative of the ingredients used in the preparation of the cola beverage. Carbonated colas typically contain approximately 40 mg of caffeine per 12 ounces of beverage.[4]

---

[3] The generally *mild* psychostimulant effect associated with cocoa is primarily due to its *low* level of caffeine (i.e., 11 to 15 mg in a typical 1-ounce chocolate bar). Other methylxanthines (i.e., theobromine and theophylline) found in cocoa also may contribute to the observed psychostimulation associated with the ingestion of chocolate.

[4] It is interesting that carbonated cola drinks were initially referred to as "soft drinks" to differentiate them from those that contained *high* percentages of alcohol (i.e., "hard liquor"). During the late 19th and early 20th centuries, the original carbonated cola drink produced in the U.S., *Coca-Cola*®, contained *cocaine* as its active psychostimulant until it was replaced by *caffeine* in 1903 (Pagliaro & Pagliaro, 2004).

Energy Drinks and Shots. Like carbonated colas, *energy drinks* are sweetened or unsweetened, non-alcoholic beverages to which caffeine, vitamins, and various herbs (e.g., guarana; taurine) are added to improve alertness and physical performance—to provide additional "energy."[5] Energy drinks typically contain approximately 200 mg of caffeine per 12 ounces of beverage. *Energy shots* are *concentrated* versions of energy drinks and typically contain approximately 200 mg of caffeine per 2 ounces of beverage.

Caffeinated Alcoholic Beverages. Caffeinated alcoholic beverages are alcoholic beverages to which *significant* amounts of caffeine have been added. The caffeine can be added: (1) during commercial production (e.g., Four Loko®; Joose®; Moonshot®);[6] (2) by a bartender while mixing a cocktail (e.g., vodka Red Bull®);[7] or (3) by the drinker, herself (e.g., mixing a shot of Jagermeister® in a pint glass filled with an energy drink to create a "Jagerbomb"). When compared to the use of caffeine or alcoholic beverages alone, women's use of caffeinated alcoholic beverages potentially *increases* the risk for: alcohol dependence; binge drinking;[8] impaired driving; risky sexual behavior; and sexual assault (Marczinski, 2015; Marczinski & Fillmore, 2014).

Despite these concerns, young women, who choose to drink caffeinated alcoholic beverages (i.e., alcohol mixed with energy drinks), do so because they generally endorse the explanation that, "the experience of drinking alcohol appears to be more rewarding when combined with energy drinks" (Marczinski, 2015, p. 96). Specifically, these women reported that the ingestion of caffeinated alcoholic beverages "increased stimulation and alertness, offset fatigue from drinking, and facilitated drinking" (McKetin, Coen, & Kaye, 2015, p. 15). The reported "stimulation and alertness" associated with the ingestion of caffeinated alcoholic beverages was primarily limited to altered perceptions or interpretations (Marczinski, Fillmore, & Bardgett, 2011; Marczinski, Fillmore, & Henges, 2012). (For additional related discussion, see Chapter 2, *Women's Alcohol Abuse*.)

---

[5] A significant number of medical students, both women and men, have reported favorable attitudes toward the use of cognitive performance enhancing drugs, including, "high caffeine products" (Kudlow, Naylor, & Xie, 2013, p. 360).

[6] In November 2010, the FDA expressed concerns about the safety of these products and the commercial preparations were subsequently removed from the U.S. market.

[7] The standard caffeinated alcohol cocktail contains a favorite energy drink/shot mixed with a favorite variety of vodka (Pagliaro & Pagliaro, *Clinical Patient Data Files*).

[8] Interestingly, Watson, Sweeney, and Louis (2014) identified that binge drinkers and caffeinated alcoholic beverage consumers both reported *higher* and *similar* measures of *sensation-seeking* and *drinking-induced disinhibition* behaviors—suggesting the potential interaction of certain personality traits and the use of major classes of psychotropic drugs and substances of abuse (i.e., in this example, psychodepressants that suppress conscious fear of known consequences of behavior [e.g., STD infection, pregnancy, getting into fights] and psychostimulants that encourage such behaviors).

Popular Notion: When you drink energy drinks, you can drink *all* the alcohol you want *without* getting drunk.

NOT TRUE. Although caffeine, as a psychostimulant, can *reduce* some of the psychodepressant actions associated with low blood alcohol concentrations (BACs) (see Chapter 2, *Women's Alcohol Abuse*), as the BAC *increases*, the *only* thing that caffeine can do is to create a "wide-awake drunk" (O'Brien, McCoy, & Rhodes, 2008; Pagliaro & Pagliaro, *Clinical Patient Data Files*).

The mental impairment associated with the ingestion of alcohol (e.g., diminished judgment and problem solving) are *unaffected* by any caffeine that may be ingested. Thus, women who believe the popular notion, and practice it, are cautioned that as a "wide-awake drunk" they are *more* likely to engage in hazardous behavior (e.g., drunk driving; physical assault; unsafe sex) that may cause harm to themselves and to others (Bigard, 2010; Cleary, Levine, & Hoffman, 2012; Pagliaro & Pagliaro, 2012).

Undesired, or harmful, effects and toxicities have been reported by approximately one-third of *caffeinated beverage* (e.g., energy drink; energy shot) drinkers. Those associated with blood caffeine concentrations include: chest pain; dyspepsia; headache; heart palpitations; insomnia; and jitteriness. Additional effects include: accidents and related injuries; motor vehicle crashes; and seizures, which are *more* likely related to the concomitant use of other psychostimulants (i.e., cocaine; methamphetamine) or alcohol (Jackson, Cotter, & Merchant, 2013; Mora-Rodriguez & Pallares, 2014; Nordt, Vilke, & Clark, 2012).

In addition, adolescent girls and young women who are regular, long-term drinkers of alcohol in combination with caffeinated energy drinks, are at significantly *greater* risk for becoming physically dependent on alcohol than those who drink only alcohol (Arria, Caldeira, & Kasperski, 2011).

Other "Specialized" Caffeine Sources

Three more recent products have been marketed for the convenient oral, inhalable, and intranasal delivery of caffeine for personal use:

1. *AeroShot*®, an orally ingested product that was initially advertised as an "inhalable" product
2. *SurgeStix*®, an inhalable product
3. *TurboSnort*®, an intranasal spray

AeroShot®, *Surge Stix*®, and *Turbo Snort*® were *not* developed as drug delivery systems. Thus, their production, in the U.S., did *not* require the submission of new drug application (NDA) data to the Food and Drug Administration (FDA) prior to marketing. Because of this "loophole," related pharmacokinetic data, such as the effect of the associated methods of administration (i.e., oral ingestion; pulmonary inhalation; or intranasal insufflation) on the absorption of caffeine, are *not* available. However, to help to assure that health and social care professionals are aware of these products and their use, the information, which is available, is briefly discussed in the following sections.

Aeroshot® Energy. To make it easier and faster to obtain a *caffeine fix*, Dave Edwards, a professor at Harvard University, invented *AeroShot® Energy*. *AeroShot® Energy*, which was released for commercial sale early in 2012, is a small canister about the size and shape of a tube of lipstick. It contains 100 mg of caffeine combined with a mixture of B vitamins.

Popular Notion: *AeroShot® Energy* is an *inhalable* form of caffeine.

NOT TRUE. This popular notion started with the name of the U.S. company that produces *AeroShot®—Breathable Foods, Inc.*

The confusion that developed regarding the product's method of use necessitated a warning letter form the FDA (2012) expressing its concerns over both: (1) labeling; and (2) safety issues. Specific *concerns* were that *AeroShot®*:

- "Should be inhaled"
- "Is not intended for people under 12" (which implies that it is okay, or safe, to use for tweens, adolescents, and adults)
- Might possibly be used "in combination with alcohol"

(FDA, 2012; Jalonick, 2012; Roosevelt, 2012)

Each single-use canister delivers up to six shots, or puffs, of a fine, lime-flavored and calorie-free powder form of caffeine. Users place one end of the canister in the mouth and take a puff (i.e., draw in a breath) that causes the release and delivery of the fine powder into the mouth, where it dissolves in the saliva and is swallowed and absorbed into the blood stream (Aubrey, 2012).

Thus, although promoted in the literature and perceived by most users as a product used by pulmonary inhalation, *AeroShot® Energy* is *not* delivered to the lungs for absorption. Rather, it is delivered to the inner mouth, or oral cavity, primarily to the tongue, where it dissolves with the saliva and is swallowed, along with the vitamins that are also contained in the product. Subsequently, the caffeine, as well as the vitamins, are absorbed in the GI tract in much the same ways as orally ingested caffeine-containing foods, beverages, and candies. Once dissolved in the saliva, the caffeine also may be transmucosally absorbed from the mucous membranes of the mouth, including the inner cheeks (i.e., buccal absorption). *AeroShot® Energy* is primarily marketed in and around college campuses in both convenience and campus stores as a novel, convenient, and readily available source of "breathable energy, any time, any place" (Aubrey, 2012).

SurgeStix®. Although *AeroShot® Energy* does *not* deliver caffeine by pulmonary inhalation to the lungs for absorption, another non-prescription, or over-the-counter, product does—*SurgeStix®*. Designed, produced, and marketed to resemble tobacco cigarettes, a *SurgeStix®* delivers caffeine to the lungs in much the same way as tobacco cigarettes deliver nicotine. Created and marketed primarily with adolescents and young adults in mind, we expect that the use of this product also will be attractive to children for whom use may prove particularly problematic. As noted by the *SurgeStix®* website advertisement retrieved from www.thinkgeek.com (2012, March, p. 1):

> You don't actually light *SurgeStix®*, that's too 1990, instead you bend them (like a glow stick) until you hear a snap. This will send the caffeine solution flowing into the filter-looking end. Wait five seconds for the "filter" to absorb the solution. You will notice a slight temperature increase as the solution reacts with the harmless chemicals in the "filter" which causes the caffeine to vaporize. Then, take a drag. Each "puff" will suck roughly 18 mg of caffeine into your lungs (and right into your bloodstream!) With about 10 "tokes" per *SurgeStix®*, you'll get 180 mg of caffeine in just a few breaths. That's more caffeine than a really strong cup of coffee just by breathing. Ouch.

TurboSnort®. A "caffeine energy nasal spray," *TurboSnort®* contains caffeine in the form of "caffeinated herbs" and an amino acid complex. Like *AeroShot®* and similar energy products, this product—to avoid related FDA regulations and testing (e.g., the need to provide pharmacokinetic data)—claims to be a *nutritional* product, as opposed to a *drug* product.

The delivery device for *TurboSnort®* resembles many similar nasal pump devices that are used to deliver both prescription and non-prescription (i.e., over-the-counter) drugs to the nasal cavity. Data provided on the product labeling and website, state that:

> *TurboSnort®* delivers 1 mg of caffeine per metered [dose] spray … There are approximately 223 metered sprays per bottle.
>
> *(About TurboSnort, 2014, p. 1)*

Pharmacology

Caffeine, a *methylxanthine*, is a mild, natural psychostimulant. Chemically known as 1,3,7-trimethylxanthine, it was identified by the German analytical chemist,

Friedrich Ferdinand Runge (1795–1867), who first isolated it from the coffee bean in 1819. The cerebral cortex is the part of the CNS that is most sensitive to the *dose-dependent* actions of caffeine. Thus, it is affected first, followed next by the medulla oblongata, or brain stem. The spinal cord is affected last, and only after extremely *high* dosages of caffeine are ingested (see later section, *Undesired, or Harmful, Effects and Toxicities*). In addition to the CNS, caffeine also affects other body systems, particularly the cardiopulmonary system.

Desired Effects on the CNS and Other Body Systems

The ingestion of caffeine produces such desired CNS effects as: *increased* mental alertness; a faster, more clear flow of thoughts; and wakefulness *without* disrupting coordinated intellectual or psychomotor performance (e.g., prevention or amelioration of decreased reaction times due to fatigue [van Duinen, Lorist, & Zijdewind, 2005]). Consequently, unlike most other drugs and substances of abuse, caffeine, as well as other psychostimulants (e.g., nicotine), when used at specific dosages and under specific conditions, *improves* performance on vigilance tasks (Smith, 2002).

For example, in one of the few studies of its kind, Sharwood, Elkington, and Meuleners (2013) evaluated the use of caffeine by over 1,000 long-distance commercial truck drivers (both women and men) and its relationship to crashes that were attended by police. Forty-three percent of the commercial drivers consumed caffeine products "for the express purpose of staying awake" (p. 1). When compared to drivers who did *not* use caffeine to stay awake, the caffeine-consuming drivers "had a 63% reduced likelihood of crashing."

Caffeine also sustains intellectual effort, such as studying for a test or final examination; with the ingestion of as little as 100 to 200 mg of caffeine, or 1 to 2 cups of coffee.[9] Caffeine facilitates learning primarily by improving attention, particularly among women, at both extremes of the age continuum, who are tired, sleepy, or otherwise in a less than optimal state of alertness (Lorist & Tops, 2003; Nehlig, 2010; Pagliaro & Pagliaro, 2012). At *low* caffeine dosages, restlessness also commonly occurs because the cerebral cortex is affected by smaller amounts of caffeine than are required to excite the brain stem (Brice & Smith, 2002). As a potentially related corollary, and consistent with reported data, the CNS stimulation produced by caffeine may *lower* suicide risk (Lucas, O'Reilly, & Pan, 2014).

In addition to its psychostimulant actions on the CNS, caffeine also affects cardiovascular and pulmonary systems, and indirectly, other systems. *Cardiovascular effects* include: (1) marginal *increase* in heart rate; (2) *increased* cardiac contractility; and (3) increased blood pressure, particularly diastolic pressure. Together, these three effects *increase* cardiac output. Caffeine also produces dilation of the coronary arteries and,

[9] Hence, also the rationale for the development and use of traditional non-prescription, solid oral dosage forms of caffeine (e.g., 200 mg NoDoz® caplets, Stay Awake® tablets) that have been available and used for over 50 years as aids to *increase* alertness and *forestall* sleep.

thus, *increases* in the amount of oxygen that is delivered to the heart muscle, or myocardium. These effects result in an *increase* in cardiac work capacity, or performance. By increasing cardiac performance, caffeine *increases* renal blood flow and causes a mild diuretic effect. In addition, caffeine *constricts* cerebral blood vessels that results in *decreased* blood flow to the brain. Thus, caffeine provides relief for both hypertensive, and certain migraine, headaches—conditions for which caffeine is medically used.

Caffeine also stimulates the respiratory center in the lower brain stem, or medulla oblongata, particularly in response to functional changes in the body associated with disease or injury (e.g., respiratory depression associated with opiate analgesic overdosage). Caffeine appears to *increase* the sensitivity of the respiratory center in the medulla to the stimulant action of carbon dioxide. This action, in turn, *increases* the volume of air that is inhaled or exhaled in one minute. Caffeine also affects the smooth muscles of the bronchi causing *mild* bronchodilation that makes breathing easier and facilitates air exchange.

Pharmacodynamics: Mechanism of Action

Caffeine produces psychostimulant actions by *competitively* binding to adenosine receptor sites (see Figure 4.1). These receptor *sites* are found in many body organs, but are particularly found in the brain where adenosine functions as an *inhibitory* neurotransmitter that promotes sedation. As an inhibitory neurotransmitter, it *prevents*: (1) synaptic transmission; and (2) release of other neurotransmitters, particularly dopamine. Caffeine does *not* have its own receptor sites. However, being similar to adenosine in chemical structure, it binds to adenosine receptor *site* subtypes, specifically subtypes A1 and A2a. Acting as an *adenosine antagonist*, it blocks adenosine's inhibitory actions (Pagliaro & Pagliaro, 2009). Consequently, within 30 minutes of ingesting a low to moderate dosage of caffeine, the following desired excitatory effects are produced and can last for approximately 3 hours:

1. *Heightened alertness*, because of increased CNS neuron activity and transmission
2. *A sense of well-being, or mild euphoria*, because of the increased release of dopamine

Ergogenic Actions. The use of caffeine has long been thought to produce energy and endurance and to *increase* work output—thus, contributing to the establishment of the now traditional "coffee break" that, in the U.S., is inculcated at specific times during the day in almost every work setting. Several possible mechanisms have been proposed to explain these *ergogenic* effects (e.g., Beedie, 2010; Davis & Green, 2009), including the ability of caffeine to:

- Antagonize adenosine-mediated pain perception and sleep induction
- Enhance muscle metabolism by increasing the availability of free fatty acids
- Increase epinephrine concentrations in the blood plasma

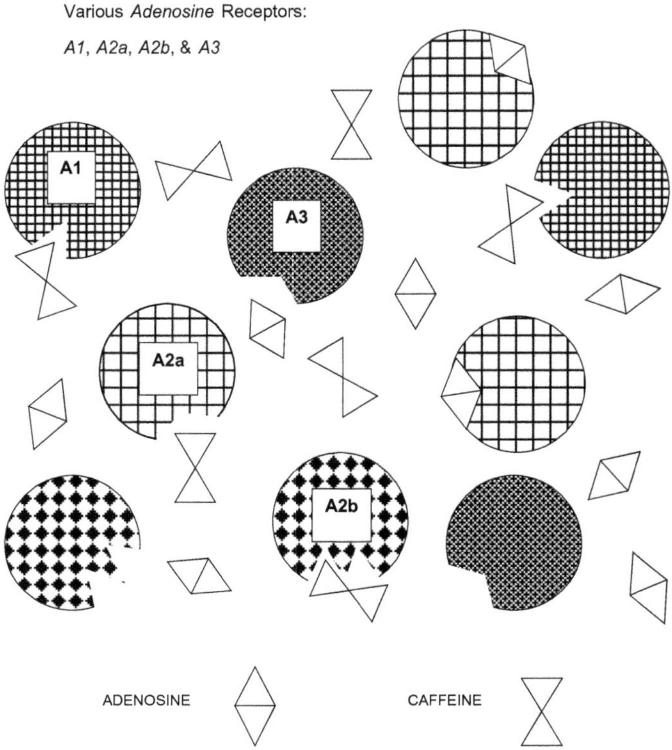

FIGURE 4.1 Caffeine: Mechanism of Psychostimulant Action

Lower dosages of caffeine also enhance athletic performance by releasing *more* calcium in muscles allowing them to contract and relax more efficiently (Tarnopolsky, 2008). In addition, it *inhibits* an enzyme that ordinarily breaks down cyclic *adenosine monophosphate* (cyclic AMP) to its *inactive end product*. The *increased* intracellular glucose production makes more energy available to allow *higher* rates of cellular activity. Thus, the use of caffeine can enable the athlete to train at greater power output and can increase the speed required for running races (Graham, 2001).

Because of its ergonomic actions, caffeine was classified by the International Olympic Committee (IOC) as a *doping agent* (Keisler & Armsey, 2006). However, it continues to be widely used by athletes, particularly body builders and weight lifters, and several studies have demonstrated significant performance gains associated with caffeine use. For example, Lara, Gonzalez-Millan, and Salinero (2014) found that the ingestion of an energy drink equivalent to 3 mg of caffeine/kg body weight by 18 women soccer players resulted in significant *increases* in their: (1) total running distance; (2) number of sprints/bouts; and (3) running distance covered over 18 km/hr.

Conversely, other researchers have *not* demonstrated reported significant performance gains. For example, Astorino, Matera, and Basinger (2012) found *no* significant ergogenic benefit in repeated sprint performance among women athletes when one serving of Red Bull® was administered at a dosage of 1.3 mg of caffeine/kg body weight. However, examining these two studies, it is obvious that the differences in caffeine dosage reported in each study may explain the differences reported in their respective findings. As well, other researchers also have postulated different reasons for the observed differences (i.e., inconsistencies) in caffeine-related ergonomic studies. For example, the ergonomic effects of caffeine have been explained, at least in part, as a *placebo effect* (Duncan, Lyons, & Hankey, 2009).

Pharmacokinetics: Absorption, Distribution, Metabolism, and Excretion

Caffeine, in its various forms and products, is usually orally ingested. However, within the last decade, several novel caffeine delivery systems and products have been developed. These alternative methods of caffeine use may affect the rate and extent of caffeine absorption, distribution, metabolism, and excretion (see earlier section, *Other Caffeine Products*).

Absorption. Caffeine is well-absorbed (i.e., 75% to 90%) from the GI tract following oral ingestion. Peak plasma concentrations generally occur within 45 to 90 minutes.

Distribution. Caffeine is distributed to *all* body tissues following absorption with an apparent volume of distribution of 0.6 L/kg. It readily crosses the blood-brain barrier and the human placenta. (Also, see later section, *Undesired, or Harmful, Effects and Toxicities*, "Pregnancy and Lactation.")

Metabolism. Caffeine is extensively metabolized in the liver by the cytochrome P450 oxidase enzyme system, particularly by the CYP1A2 isoenzyme. It has three major *active* metabolites (i.e., *paraxanthine*, *theobromine*, and *theophylline*).[10]

Excretion. The mean half-life of elimination for caffeine is 5 hours. That means that, if a woman drinks a Starbucks® Grande brewed coffee containing 320 mg of caffeine in the morning on the way to work, half of the caffeine ingested from that beverage (in this case, 160 mg of caffeine) will still be working in her body at lunchtime. This half-life of elimination is the reason why consuming caffeine in the evening (i.e., up to 5 hours before retiring to bed) can, for many women, result in one of the most common *undesired* pharmacological effects of caffeine—*insomnia*.

[10] Women who possess a variant genotype for the CYP1A2 have a slowed rate of caffeine metabolism. Consequently, they may be at *increased* risk for caffeine-induced toxicity such as hypertension and myocardial infarction (Meredith, Juliano, & Hughes, 2013). (Also, see following section, *Undesired, or Harmful, Effects and Toxicities.*)

The half-life of elimination may be *increased* by several factors including age-related changes in liver function. In fact, many older women will share that they do *not* drink coffee with dinner anymore, or after 5 pm when out with friends, because they will be "awake all night" (Pagliaro & Pagliaro, *Clinical Patient Data Files*). In addition, severe liver disease (e.g., alcoholic cirrhosis; hepatitis C) can *increase* caffeine's half-life of elimination up to 100 hours. The half-life of caffeine also may be increased from 5 hours to 10 hours among women who are pregnant or who are using oral contraceptives. However, nicotine tobacco smoking can significantly *decrease* caffeine's half-life of elimination by *increasing* the production of the hepatic isoenzyme, CYP1A2 (Zevin & Benowitz, 1999).

Less than 2% of ingested caffeine is excreted in unchanged form in the urine. The *active* metabolites of caffeine are further metabolized and are also excreted in the urine.

Undesired, or Harmful, Effects and Toxicities

The undesired, or harmful, effects and toxicities associated with caffeine use are primarily dose-related (i.e., mild to moderate use; moderate to high use; very high to extremely high use; and overdosage). They also involve different body systems (e.g., CNS; cardiopulmonary system; urinary system). Women's use of caffeine also has been associated with birth defects, cancers, and other medical conditions (e.g., osteoporosis), as well as physical and psychological dependence. These are presented in the following sections.

Relatively Minor and More Serious Effects. Low to moderate caffeine use is associated with relatively *minor* undesired effects that are generally related to its actions as a psychostimulant. These effects include:

- *Excitement*
- *Insomnia*, particularly when caffeine beverages are ingested later in the day or prior to retiring for bed in the evening
- *Nervousness or restlessness* (i.e., *the jitters*), particularly at the end of a busy work day during which caffeine beverages were ingested throughout the day

Also included are *diuresis*, *flushed face*, and *GI disturbance*.

While low to moderate daily caffeine use (i.e., the ingestion of less than 400 mg per day) is usually *not* associated with any significant harmful effects or toxicities in healthy women (Nawrot, Jordon, & Eastwood, 2003), more serious toxicities are associated with *higher* daily dosages, including: *caffeinism*; *cancer*; *cardiovascular effects*; *mental disorders*; and *osteoporosis*. Each of these more serious effects are discussed in the following sections.

CAFFEINISM. Intense caffeine stimulation, or *caffeinism*, is usually associated with the regular, long-term use of *large amounts* of caffeine. For example, the ingestion of:

- *12 or more cups of coffee a day* (1.5 grams of caffeine) can cause *intense* psychostimulation characterized by: agitation, anxiety, cardiac dysrhythmias, heart palpitations, hyperventilation, irritability, tachycardia, and tremors.
- *20 to 50 cups of coffee a day* (i.e., 2 to 5 grams) can excite the spinal cord causing *increased* stimulation of the spinal reflexes.
- *100 cups of coffee a day, or more* (i.e., *over* 10 grams), can cause convulsions and death. Although fatalities are probably unlikely because of the large amounts of coffee, or other common caffeine-containing beverages (e.g., cola, tea), that need to be ingested, the availability and use of energy drinks and other more recently produced *high* caffeine content products (e.g., bars), increase the risk.

CANCER. Hypothetical concerns regarding the relationship between caffeine use among women and various cancers (e.g., breast, colon, rectal, or endometrial cancer) have been widely studied for several decades with the result of *no* definitive consensus among findings. The preponderance of available data (e.g., Dik, Bueno-de-Mesquita, & Van Oijen, 2014; Ganmaa, Willett, & Feskanich, 2008; Gierach, Freedman, & Andaya, 2012; Oh, Sandin, & Strom, 2015; Yang, Crowe, & Cairns, 2015) indicate that proposed relationships, if they exist, are *tenuous* at best and any noted correlations are probably best accounted for by genetic and/or environmental variables. For example, as identified by Jiang, Wu, and Jiang (2013), in their meta-analysis of 37 published articles, "coffee/caffeine might be weakly associated with breast cancer risk for postmenopausal women, and the association for BRCA1 mutation carriers deserves further investigation" (p. 620).

CARDIOVASCULAR EFFECTS. The ingestion of *low to moderate* amounts of caffeine does *not* appear to *increase* the risk for heart problems even among women with pre-existing heart disease (Klatsky, Hasan, & Armstrong, 2011; Pelchovitz & Goldberger, 2011). As found by Rhee, Qin, and Hedlin (2016), in their large prospective study of the possible relationships between coffee (and total caffeine intake) and the incidence of hypertension among postmenopausal women: "coffee and caffeine are *not* risk factors for hypertension in postmenopausal women" (p. 210).

However, *high* daily caffeine use, usually in the form of the ingestion of coffee, may cause various cardiac toxicities including: cardiac dysrhythmias; heart palpitations; and tachycardia. Atrial tachycardia, or supraventricular tachycardia, has been associated with the ingestion of various amounts of caffeine from several caffeine-containing sources, including: candy; coffee; cola drinks; and tea. For women who are at risk (i.e., those with pre-existing heart disease, including dysrhythmias), *low* dosages of caffeine may be sufficient to cause the effects. However, in most reported cases, the caffeine dosages are *high* (e.g., *more* than a pot of coffee daily) (Kinugawa, Kurita, & Nohara, 2011; Pagliaro & Pagliaro, *Clinical Patient Data Files*).

During the past decade, the use of caffeinated energy drinks and energy shots (see earlier sections, *Carbonated Colas* and *Energy Drinks and Shots*) among adults has resulted in increased cases of atrial fibrillation. This condition can adversely affect the normal working of the heart and, if not medically treated, can progress to the lower chambers of the heart causing ventricular fibrillation and death.

Reported cases also have been increasing among adolescent girls without previous significant history of heart disease (Di Rocco, During, & Morelli, 2011). While the overwhelming majority of cases of caffeine-induced cardiac toxicity spontaneously return to normal when acute ingestion of caffeine is discontinued, caffeine-induced cardiac toxicity, on occasion, may be *fatal* (Artin, Singh, & Richeh, 2010; Mostofsky, Schlaug, & Mukamal, 2010).

> Fourteen-year-old Anais Founier downed two 24-ounce Monster energy drinks … the Maryland teenager went into cardiac arrest [and died] … Anais and her family knew she had a common heart condition called mitral valve prolapse, which caused one of the heart's valves to malfunction.
>
> *(TODAY, 2012, p. 1)*

As noted by the SAMHSA (2011), regarding ED visits that involved caffeinated energy drinks between 2005 and 2009:

- Visits *increased* tenfold to over 13,000 visits annually in the U.S.[11]
- 52% of the visits (i.e., over half) by young adults, 18 to 25 years-of-age (36% women, 64% men), also involved other drugs and substances of abuse that, for women, were more likely to be pharmaceuticals, and for men, alcohol
- 67% of visits were for undesired, or harmful, effects and toxicities that did *not* involve other drugs or substances of abuse

Additionally, the SAMHSA (2014a) reported that:

- 1 in 10 energy drink-related emergency department visits resulted in hospitalization

As reported by Cleary, Levine, and Hoffman (2012) in a case series study of 11 emergency department visits for alcohol intoxication associated with the use of the caffeinated alcoholic beverage, *Four Loko*®:

> All arrived by emergency medical services (EMS) … patients were found in high-risk settings, with altered mental status on subway tracks, in public buildings, or parks after dark…
>
> *(p. 67)*

[11] This trend has continued into the second decade of the new millennium. As noted by Mattson (2013), using data from the Drug Abuse Warning Network (DAWN):

> The estimated number of ED visits involving energy drinks doubled from 10,068 visits in 2007 to 20,783 visits in 2011.
>
> *(p. 1)*

In addition, the oily lipid components of coffee contain both *cafestol* and *kahweol*. These components appear to raise serum cholesterol levels, which increase the risk for the blockage of blood vessels and heart damage, including stroke (i.e., cerebral vascular accidents) and heart attack (i.e., myocardial infarction) (Butt & Sultan, 2011). This risk would be particularly significant among women who both:

1. Have familial hypercholesterolemia
2. Regularly consume large amounts of coffee daily

MENTAL DISORDERS. Using data obtained from 2,270 women participants in the *Virginia Adult Twin Study of Psychiatric and Substance Use Disorders*, Bergin and Kendler (2012) identified significant correlations between women's genetic constitution, mental disorder (i.e., anorexia nervosa, bulimia nervosa, generalized anxiety disorder, or major depressive disorder) and caffeine use, particularly regarding *tolerance* and *withdrawal*. It is relevant to note that caffeine and nicotine (e.g., a cup of coffee and a tobacco cigarette) are two of the most commonly abused drugs and substances of abuse by women who have a contemporaneous diagnosis (see Chapter 7, *Identifying Women's Contemporaneous Diagnoses*).

OSTEOPOROSIS. Osteoporosis is a chronic condition in which bone mass (i.e., weight and strength) is reduced. In the U.S., approximately 1 in 3 women who are postmenopausal have osteoporosis. Caffeine, as well as alcohol and nicotine (in tobacco smoke), *increases* the risk of osteoporosis by *increasing* the amount of calcium excreted in the urine. The daily equivalent of 4, or more, regular cups of coffee per day (i.e., daily caffeine intake of 320 mg per day, or more) significantly *increases* the risk of developing osteoporosis, and associated bone fractures, and related sequelae. It has been suggested that this risk may be ameliorated by increasing calcium intake (e.g., adding milk to a cup of coffee) (Barrett-Connor, Chang, & Edelstein, 1994).

In the U.S., the risk for osteoporosis is *highest* among women, particularly *older* women, who:

1. Are of Asian or European descent
2. Are thin, or small-framed
3. Are postmenopausal
4. Drink alcohol in excess
5. Ingest 320 mg, or more, of caffeine daily
6. Have low sun exposure resulting in low levels of vitamin D
7. Have low levels of daily physical activity
8. Have low calcium intake
9. Have high sodium intake
10. Smoke tobacco cigarettes

These *ten* factors, compiled from the findings of several researchers (e.g., Body, Bergmann, & Boonen, 2011; Hallstrom, Wolk, & Glynn, 2006; Hansen, Folsom, & Kushi, 2000), likely account for *most* of the variation reported in the findings of studies examining the relationship between coffee (caffeine) consumption and osteoporosis. Contrary findings also have been reported, for example: "No association was found between calcium and caffeine intake and bone mass" (Hallstrom, Wolk, & Glynn, 2006, p. 1055); "High coffee consumption was associated with a small reduction in bone density that did not translate into an increased risk of fracture" (Hallstrom, Byberg, & Glynn, 2013, p. 898); and "No association was found between calcium and caffeine intake and bone mass" (Harter, Busnello, & Dibi, 2013, p. 315). Other likely significant factors, including genetic differences and caffeine dosage, also may contribute to the observed variance in these reported results.

Physical and Psychological Dependence. The regular, long-term use of caffeine is associated with both physical and psychological dependence.[12] In regard to the former, both the development of tolerance to the desired effects of caffeine and a caffeine withdrawal syndrome have been identified. Regarding the latter, craving is the primary characteristics of psychological dependence (Pagliaro & Pagliaro, 2009).

Popular Notion: Caffeine is *not* like the other drugs and substances of abuse because it is primarily a *nutrient.*

NOT TRUE, on *both* counts.

First, caffeine is exactly like the other drugs and substances of abuse because it meets the general criteria required for this classification:

- Caffeine is primarily used for its major psychotropic actions (i.e., psychostimulation)
- Regular, long-term use of caffeine is associated with both physical and psychological dependence

Second, caffeine, although commonly found in several popular beverages, foods, candies, and gums is *not* a nutrient and does *not* provide the body with any elements necessary for metabolism.

[12] A study of 94 regular caffeine users, who identified as being physically or psychologically dependent upon caffeine and who sought treatment, reported a daily caffeine consumption range of 120 mg to 2,667 mg (mean, 548 mg; median, 388 mg) (Juliano, Evatt, & Richards, 2012).

TOLERANCE. The regular, long-term use of *lower* dosages of caffeine is associated with the development of a *lower* degree of tolerance, particularly to its psychostimulant actions (Watson, Deary, & Kerr, 2002). Correspondingly, the regular, long-term use of *higher* dosages of caffeine is associated with a *higher* degree of tolerance.

CAFFEINE WITHDRAWAL SYNDROME. The regular, long-term use of *moderate* amounts of caffeine (e.g., approximately 5 or more 6-ounce cups of caffeinated coffee daily) may result in the caffeine withdrawal syndrome that occurs when caffeine use is abruptly discontinued (Addicott, 2014; Juliano & Griffiths, 2004). The caffeine withdrawal syndrome is characterized by:

- Anxiety
- Drowsiness
- Depressed mood, or dysphoria
- Fatigue (marked)
- Headaches
- Impaired concentration
- Irritability
- Muscle pain and stiffness
- Nausea
- Weakness

(Dews, O'Brien, & Bergman, 2002)

These signs and symptoms are generally *mild* and short-lived beginning within 12 to 24 hours after the last use of caffeine and peaking between 24 and 48 hours after onset. They last for up to a week.

The caffeine withdrawal syndrome is promptly relieved by the ingestion of caffeine (Pagliaro & Pagliaro, 2009). In the past, women who had relatively *mild* dose-related signs and symptoms of caffeine withdrawal, tended to manage them with a cup of coffee "first thing in the morning" and periodically throughout the day while at home or work. However, more recently, the caffeine concentrations now available in many beverages, foods, and other products contain several times the amount of caffeine that similar serving sizes contained at the turn of the century. These sources of caffeine, particularly the more recently developed dosage forms (e.g., Blast® caffeine powder and various energy shots) contain such *high* amounts of caffeine per serving that they can produce *high* enough blood caffeine concentrations to result in a pronounced caffeine withdrawal syndrome if regular, long-term use is abruptly discontinued.

In fact, in the past, these blood caffeine levels would require women to drink 50 cups of coffee a day. Thus, health and social care professionals may be confronted with a new population of women who require assistance with the prevention and management of harmful patterns of caffeine use. In this regard, they also need to be aware that, like other drugs and substances of abuse, genetic and other factors may affect both the incidence and severity of the caffeine withdrawal syndrome experienced by new millennial women. They also are reminded that when trying to "cut down" or "quit" their use of caffeine, individual and novel treatment approaches may be required because of the following factors:

- Different signs and symptoms of caffeine withdrawal (e.g., dose-related moderate to severe effects; prolonged withdrawal period)
- Multiple-drug and substance abuse withdrawal syndromes that may be concomitant (e.g., caffeine, nicotine, and alcohol) with each other
- Substance use disorders or other mental disorders that would affect positive treatment outcomes. For example, women who have specific mental disorders (i.e., anorexia nervosa; anxiety disorders; major depressive disorder; panic disorder) have a significantly *high* correlation with caffeine tolerance and withdrawal (i.e., possess shared genetic liability—see earlier related discussion) (Bergin & Kendler, 2012)
- Several *unsuccessful* attempts to decrease or totally discontinue caffeine use (i.e., several attempts to maintain *resumed nonuse* with several returns to *relapsed use*) (Juliano, Evatt, & Richards, 2012)
- Cost of fifty dollars per week, or more, for caffeinated beverages, foods, or other caffeine products
- Persistent dyspepsia or gastric ulcer disease that are aggravated by the continued use of caffeine (Juliano, Evatt, & Richards, 2012; Pagliaro & Pagliaro, *Clinical Patient Data Files*)

Pregnancy and Lactation. Caffeine has been associated with birth defects, or teratogenesis, among certain animal species. However, it has *not* been associated with physical birth defects among neonates whose mothers used caffeine during pregnancy (Brent, Christian, & Diener, 2011; Browne, Hoyt, & Feldkamp, 2011; Christian & Brent, 2001; Pagliaro & Pagliaro, 2012). The *only* apparent fetotoxic effect associated with maternal caffeine use during pregnancy is a low birth weight (i.e., intrauterine growth restriction) among neonates born to mothers who daily ingested 3 cups of coffee (300 mg of caffeine), or more (Bracken, Triche, & Belanger, 2003; Nawrot, Jordan, & Eastwood, 2003; Pagliaro & Pagliaro, 2002; Rhee, Kim, & Kim, 2015).

In addition, a comprehensive meta-analysis of published data, 1966 to 2010, found *no* significant association between the ingestion of caffeine during pregnancy and the risk of miscarriage or preterm birth. In contrast, a large Danish study found that caffeine ingestion during the *first* trimester of pregnancy was associated with an increased risk for spontaneous abortion (Hahn, Wise, & Rothman, 2015). The authors noted that the size of the relationship effect was *small* and that it was *not* linear. However, a meta-analysis of 26 related studies published during the same year found that "consumption of caffeine and coffee during pregnancy seems to increase the risk for pregnancy loss" (Li, Zhao, & Song, 2015, p. 116).

To reduce any associated risk, however small, for preterm birth or low birth weight among neonates, study guidelines suggest that the use of caffeine during pregnancy be limited to approximately *2* cups of coffee per day (i.e., less than 200 mg per day) (Food Standards Agency, 2008; Rubin, 2008).[13] (See Table 4.1: *Average Caffeine Content of Selected Beverages, Foods, and Other Products.*) A positive trend in the U.S. appears to be that, in comparison to other adult groups, several studies (e.g., Somogyi, 2010) have reported *lower* coffee consumption and, consequently, *lower* daily ingestion of caffeine among women of childbearing age. As noted by Chen, Bell, and Browne (2014), in their large retrospective review of pregnant women in the U.S. from 1997 to 2007:

> Most mothers stopped or decreased their caffeinated beverage consumption during pregnancy.
>
> *(p. 2446)*

Women's Medical and Personal Caffeine Use and Abuse

Women's medical and personal use and abuse of caffeine are discussed in the following sections. We begin with women's medical caffeine use/abuse.

Women's Medical Caffeine Use/Abuse

Caffeine is used as a medical respiratory stimulant. For example, caffeine (generally in the form of caffeine citrate) is therapeutically indicated for the treatment of neonates who are diagnosed with *apnea of prematurity*, a respiratory condition characterized by a temporary cessation of breathing among babies who are born earlier than their estimated date of birth (Aranda, Beharry, & Valencia, 2010; Lemke, 2002).

Classic pharmacologic studies of caffeine published during the first half of the 20th century confirmed the stimulant actions that have been associated with caffeine use, including an elevated mood, decreased fatigue, and increased capacity for work. These studies also revealed that methylxanthines, such as caffeine, possess other important pharmacologic properties. These properties were exploited for many years in a variety of therapeutic applications that are now being generally treated with more specific and effective pharmacotherapy. However, more recent research (e.g., Biessels, 2010; Butt & Sultan, 2011; Lucas, Mirzaei, & Pan, 2011; Patil, Lavie, & O'Keefe, 2011) is currently focused on the potential use of caffeine for the prevention of several medical conditions, including:

- Diabetes mellitus
- Mental depression

---

13 If the mother has a history of miscarriage, we would recommend total abstinence from coffee and other foods and beverages that are *high* in caffeine content until after delivery.

- Parkinsonism (i.e., Parkinson's disease)
- Pre-senile dementia (i.e., Alzheimer's disease)

For example, the regular, long-term use of *moderate to high* amounts of caffeinated coffee (i.e., 4 to 8 cups of coffee daily) appears to *decrease* the risk for Type II diabetes mellitus. Apparently, the higher the consumption of caffeinated coffee on a regular daily basis, the *lower* the risk for developing Type II diabetes mellitus (Campos & Baylin, 2007; Loopstra-Masters, Liese, & Haffner, 2011; Salazar-Martinez, Willett, & Ascherio, 2004; van Dam & Hu, 2005).

However, other researchers have reported that caffeine does *not* appear to act alone in lowering the risk for diabetes mellitus (van Dieren, Uiterwaal, & van der Schouw, 2009). In fact, several other factors appear to be involved, particularly:

- *Weight loss.* The consumption of *caffeinated* and *decaffeinated* coffee has been associated with weight loss and a lower incidence of diabetes among moderate coffee drinkers (Greenberg, Boozer, & Geliebter, 2006; Heckman, Weil, & Gonzalez de Mejia, 2010). Because these results were observed for both caffeinated and decaffeinated coffee drinkers, it appears that caffeine, as well as other constituents of coffee, may be involved in weight loss and the resultant protection for diabetes mellitus.
- *Components in coffee other than caffeine.* Components found in coffee other than caffeine (e.g., *chlorogenic acid*; *trigonelline*) may delay or reduce the absorption of body sugar (i.e., glucose) from the intestines, and, thus, be responsible for the associated lower incidence of diabetes among moderate coffee drinkers (Johnston, Clifford, & Morgan, 2003; van Dijk, Olthof, & Meeuse, 2009).

Much remains to be learned about the complex relationship between caffeine and diabetes, including the effects of the:

- Amount of caffeine consumed on a regular basis (*low*, *moderate*, or *high*)
- Gender of the caffeine user
- Source of the caffeine (e.g., caffeine capsule or tablet; cup of caffeinated coffee)
- Type of diabetes mellitus (i.e., gestational, Type I, or Type II)
- Weight loss associated with caffeine use

While the nature of the relationship between coffee consumption and diabetes is still tenuous and, most likely, multifactorial, a more recent study has shed some additional light on this issue. Doo, Morimoto, and Steinbrecher (2014), in a large Hawaiian study of over 75,000 women and men of various continental descents, found that the daily consumption of 3 or more cups of *caffeinated* coffee was associated with a *lower* risk of diabetes among *women* of *all* continental descents, but *not* for men.

Women's Personal Caffeine Use/Abuse

Popular Notion: Caffeine has little or no abuse liability.

NOT TRUE.

Several specific terms have been used as diagnostic labels to denote caffeine's physical and psychological dependence. These terms include, for example:

- Caffeine dependence syndrome (ICD-10)
- Caffeine use disorder (DSM-V)
- Substance use disorder (DSM-IV)

However, there is consensus that caffeine possesses abuse liability like all the other drugs and substances of abuse (Budney, Lee, & Juliano, 2015; Meredith, Juliano, & Hughes, 2013; Pagliaro & Pagliaro, 2009; Striley, Griffiths, & Cottler, 2011).

The use and abuse of caffeine among women in the U.S., particularly millennial women, depend on several factors, including age, religion, and other factors. For example, 30-year-old women consume approximately half the number of cups of coffee per day as 60-year-old women (Mitchell, Knight, & Hockenberry, 2014; Somogyi, 2010). Other women do *not* drink coffee or use other caffeine containing foods and beverages at all. For example, because of religious dictates, Mormon women generally do *not* drink, or otherwise use, caffeine, while Muslim women use it extensively. In addition, as noted in a previous section, women of childbearing age generally drink *less* coffee than any other group of women (Somogyi, 2010).

At end of the first decade of the new millennium, it was identified that women ingested approximately 300 mg of caffeine per day (Somogyi, 2010). More recently, Fulgoni, Keast, and Liegerman (2015) placed the daily amount of caffeine by women in the U.S. as being closer to 200 mg/day. The sources of caffeine have generally remained the same, and include:

- Coffee, 50%
- Tea, 31%
- Chocolate, 7%
- Cola beverages, 7%
- Energy drinks/shots, 2% to 3%[14]

---

[14] Overall, it is estimated that approximately 2% to 3% of American adults regularly consume energy drinks and that for those caffeine users, the daily intake of caffeine is closer to *465 mg* (Somogyi, 2010).

It is estimated that, in the U.S., approximately 90% of women and men, 18 years-of-age and older, ingest caffeine products daily with men, on average, consuming one-third *more* than women. Mitchell, Knight, and Hockenberry (2014) also found that men, on average, consumed *more* milligrams (mgs) of caffeine daily in comparison to women. However, after adjusting for body weight (i.e., mg/kg), the daily ingestion of caffeine was *higher* for women. Regardless, for *all* groups of women, *coffee* is the *major* contributor to daily caffeine use for several reasons, including:

- "It gives you a feeling of well-being"
- "It makes you relax"
- "It helps you to think"
- "It keeps you going"

(Fulgoni, Keast, & Lieberman, 2015; Lieberman, Stavinoha, & McGraw, 2012)

In addition, as with all drugs and substances of abuse, *expectancies* play a major role in the initiation and continuation of use. Huntley and Juliano (2012), who developed the *Caffeine Expectancy Questionnaire*, found that:

> The frequency and quantity of caffeine use were associated with greater expectancies for withdrawal/dependence, energy/work enhancement, appetite suppression, social/mood enhancement, and physical performance enhancement and lower expectancies for anxiety/negative physical effects and sleep disturbance. Caffeine expectancies predicted various caffeine-associated features of substance dependence (e.g., use despite harm, withdrawal incidence and severity, perceived difficulty stopping use, tolerance). Expectancies for caffeine consumed via coffee were stronger than for caffeine consumed via soft drinks or tea.
>
> *(p. 592)*

Popular Notion: Women drink coffee primarily to "calm down" and "relax." NOT TRUE.

Generally, women who state that they drink coffee "to calm down and relax" are, in fact, most likely drinking coffee to relieve the common signs and symptoms of the caffeine withdrawal syndrome (see earlier section, *Physical and Psychological Dependence*, "Caffeine Withdrawal Syndrome"). In fact, among women who are regular, long-term coffee drinkers, this statement signifies that they are probably physically dependent on caffeine and that their attempts "to calm down and relax" are an attempt to manage the signs and symptoms of caffeine withdrawal (i.e., because caffeine is a psychostimulant, it is counter-intuitive to think that it would "calm users down").

The *exact* number of *women* in the U.S. who are: (1) coffee drinkers or other caffeine users; and (2) physically dependent on caffeine is unknown. However, it is estimated to be in the range of 10% to 30% of women.

Over the last 2 decades, caffeinated energy drinks, primarily, and other related foods and products, have become increasingly popular sources of caffeine among young women. These products are attractive to young women because of their:

1. Relatively *high* caffeine content when compared to common traditional sources (e.g., coffee; colas; tea)
2. Marketing and advertising campaigns that specifically target young women with promises of relief of fatigue and improved athletic and sexual performance *(Oddy & O'Sullivan, 2009; Pagliaro & Pagliaro, 2009)*

In fact, the sale and use of energy drinks, alone, increased over 500% from 2002 to 2006 (Reissig, Strain, & Griffiths, 2009).[15] Currently approximately one-third of the annual U.S. energy drink market share is controlled by Red Bull® (Somogyi, 2010). Another contributing factor associated with the popularity of energy drinks is related to the notion that caffeinated alcoholic beverages, or combining caffeine with beverage alcohol, enable women, as well as men, to drink for longer periods of time (Attwood, Rogers, & Ataya, 2012). (Also, see related discussion in Chapter 2, *Women's Alcohol Abuse*.)

We now turn to women's use and abuse of *nicotine*.

Nicotine

Nicotine is a widely available and relatively *safe* psychostimulant that is commonly used by women in the U.S. for a variety of reasons including its ability to: produce feelings of well-being; enhance attention; lose, or maintain body weight; or "to have smaller babies that are easier to deliver" (Pagliaro & Pagliaro, *Clinical Patient Data Files*). However, its general method of use, *tobacco cigarette smoking*, has been identified as the *largest* single cause of premature death worldwide and is estimated to kill more than 5 million people each year. Although nicotine is only *one* of approximately 4,000 chemicals found in tobacco smoke, and is *less* toxic than *most* of the other chemicals, it is the *only* chemical responsible for the development of physical and psychological dependence.

---

[15] The use of caffeinated energy drinks has become so ubiquitous that it is added to U.S. army rations to help maintain cognitive performance among soldiers, women and men alike (Lieberman, Stavinoha, & McGraw, 2012).

Pharmacology

Nicotine is a *natural* occurring liquid alkaloid that was *first* isolated from the leaves of the tobacco plant (*Nicotiana tabacum*) by two German students at the university of Heidelberg—Wilhelm Heinrich Posselt (1806–1877) and Karl Ludwig Reimann (1804–1872). Finding the pure chemical salt form of nicotine bitter to the taste, they considered it to be a poison (Pagliaro & Pagliaro, 2004).[16] Nicotine was later correctly identified as a *psychostimulant*. A tobacco cigarette usually contains 1% to 2% nicotine.

After smoking 1 to 2 cigarettes, there is a significant *increase* in the plasma concentration of neurotransmitters, particularly *noradrenaline* and *glutamate*, in specific areas of the central nervous, cardiovascular, pulmonary, and other body systems. In the central nervous system (CNS), nicotine stimulates the *cerebral cortex*, where it causes *increased* cognitive activity,[17] followed by *depression*. It also stimulates the *ventral tegmental area* (VTA), where it causes the release of dopamine and further stimulates the release of the amino acid, glutamate. These actions trigger additional dopamine release in the *limbic system* causing feelings of euphoria (Zickler, 2003).

Cardiovascular effects associated with nicotine use include tachycardia, vasoconstriction, and, consequently, increased blood pressure associated with nicotine's stimulation of *sympathetic ganglia* and the *adrenal medulla* and its activation of aortic and carotid chemoreceptors. Muscular-skeletal system effects on motor neurons lead to a marked *reduction* in muscle tone and associated feelings of relaxation, which are often reported by tobacco smokers. Nicotine, in addition to *decreasing* deep-tendon reflexes, also typically causes an *increase* in hand tremor, an alerting pattern on the electroencephalogram (EEG), and a *decrease* in the muscle tone of some skeletal muscles (e.g., *rectus femoris* muscles of the thighs). These effects are thought to involve the stimulation of the Renshaw cells in the spinal cord.

Pharmacodynamics: Mechanism of Action

Nicotine's psychostimulant action is *dose-dependent*. At *lower* dosages, nicotine acts as an *agonist* and *stimulates* the autonomic ganglia. At *higher* dosages, it acts like an *antagonist* and *blocks* autonomic ganglia (Heeschen, Weis, & Aicher, 2002; Kimura, Ushiyama, & Fujii, 2003). Interestingly, for women who are regular, long-term nicotine users, agonistic actions may vary according to their degree of nicotine *tolerance*.

---

[16] Nicotine use is hazardous to humans (e.g., Rogers, Denk, & Wax, 2004) (see later section, *Undesired, or Harmful, Effects and Toxicities*). Although it has been used as an insecticide, this use of nicotine has now been largely replaced by a related and more potent class of insecticides, the *neonicotinoids* (Tomizawa & Casida, 2005, 2009).

[17] These CNS actions are associated with the observed attention-enhancing effects of nicotine (Hahn, 2015).

Nicotine exerts its psychostimulant actions by stimulating *nicotinic acetylcholine (cholinergic) receptors* (nAChRs). The nAChRs are *ligand-gated* ion channels, or "pores" in cell plasma membranes, that open and close when stimulated.[18] Nicotine rapidly *increases* the cellular permeability of nAChRs to sodium (Na^+) and calcium (Ca^{++}) ions resulting in their depolarization and resultant excitation. For nAChR subunit combinations located at skeletal neuromuscular junctions (e.g., α1-ε-α1-β1-δ), depolarization primarily affects muscle tone by producing muscular contraction. For nAChR combinations located at synapses between neurons in the CNS (e.g., α4-β2-α4-β2-β2), associated depolarization and excitation primarily produce: arousal; enhanced cognitive functioning, including learning and memory; and reward.

There are *five* types of structurally diverse subunits of nAChRs: (1) *alpha* (α); (2) *beta* (β); (3) *delta* (δ); (4) *epsilon* (ε); and (5) *gamma* (γ). These subunits are found in *six* different combinations. In the CNS, combinations of *α* subunits and *β* subunits appear to be particularly relevant to the achievement of both the *desired* and *undesired* actions of nicotine (Figure 4.2). For example, the α4 and β2 subunits appear to contribute to the *euphoria* associated with nicotine use, whereas the α3, α5, and β3 subunits appear to be responsible for determining both the *risk* for, and *severity* of, nicotine physical dependence (Whitten, 2009).

Subunits in autonomic ganglia also affect depolarization and firing of postganglionic neurons and, in the adrenal medulla, affect the secretion of catecholamines, because of the opening of cation channels and the influx of calcium ions through the depolarized membrane pores of the nAChRs (Araki, Suemaru, & Gomita, 2002).

Thought to be genetically influenced, the response of the nAChRs to nicotine helps to explain various patterns of women's nicotine use, including the development of physical and psychological dependence and the signs and symptoms of the nicotine withdrawal syndrome that occurs when regular, long-term nicotine use is abruptly discontinued.[19] For example, *collectively*, "the protective effects of progesterone on *craving* in nicotine-dependent women may be mediated through its *inhibitory* effect on β2-nAChR function" (Moran-Santa Maria, Flanagan, & Brady, 2014, p. 5). However, *individually*, women "inherit different forms of half a dozen genes that dictate the features of the brain receptor to which nicotine binds" (Whitten (2009, p. 1).

Pharmacokinetics: Absorption, Distribution, Metabolism, and Excretion

Absorption and Distribution. An average tobacco cigarette, when smoked, delivers *only* about 1 mg of nicotine because approximately 90% of the nicotine is destroyed

[18] A ligand binds, or attaches, to a chemical—in this case, acetylcholine or nicotine—to elicit an action.

[19] More recent research (e.g., Gamaleddin, Trigo, & Gueye, 2015) suggests a significant role of endocannabinoids and the associated CB_1 receptors in modulating the effects of nicotine—both reinforcing effects and those involved with nicotine withdrawal. (See Chapter 6, *Women's Psychodelic Abuse*, for additional related discussion of the endocannabinoids and their receptors.)

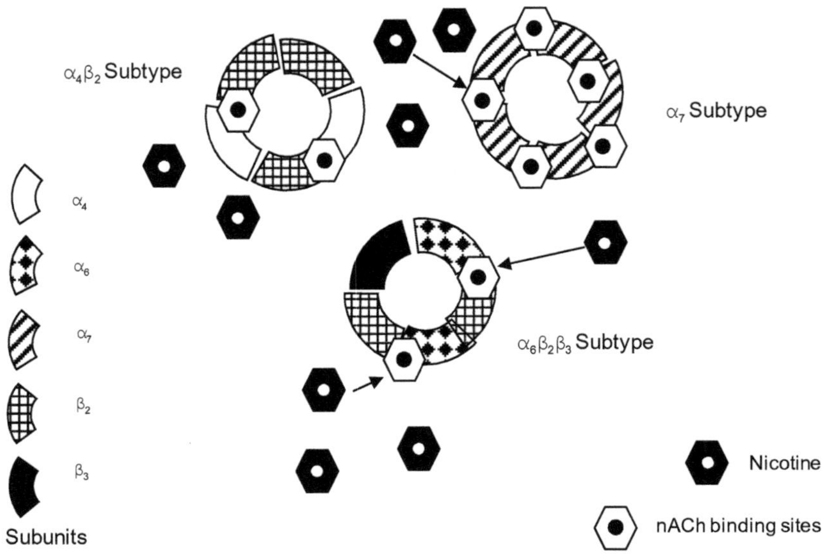

FIGURE 4.2 Nicotine: Mechanism of Psychostimulant Action

by *pyrolysis*. Regardless, women who smoke tobacco cigarettes can achieve relatively *high* blood nicotine concentrations because the *pulmonary* absorption of nicotine is *high* (F = 0.9) due to the relatively large surface area of the lungs and its excellent blood supply. Bioavailability also can be increased several-fold by the actual smoking techniques used by women who smoke tobacco cigarettes. For example, they can:

1. Increase the number of puffs on a cigarette
2. Inhale the smoke more deeply into the lungs
3. Hold the inhaled smoke in the lungs for a longer period of time before exhaling it

If nicotine was *swallowed*, its absorption into the blood stream would be *low* (i.e., F = 0.3, or approximately 30%). It also would undergo *first-pass hepatic metabolism* (see following section) resulting in *rapid* and *extensive* inactivation. However, if chewed and held in the mouth before being spat out, as occurs with chewing tobacco or nicotine chewing gum, *buccal* absorption from the inner cheeks of the mouth is *rapid*. It also *avoids* first-pass hepatic metabolism. For example, when chewed, buccally absorbed nicotine chewing gum formulations (e.g., Nicorette®) can achieve blood nicotine concentrations that approximate that obtained by smoking a regular tobacco cigarette (i.e., 90%). However, the nicotine in chewing gum products, which is bound to an ion-exchange resin, is *only* released by chewing. Thus, the amount of nicotine released from the chewing gum, and the resultant blood nicotine concentrations that are achieved, are related to the *rate* and *vigor* of chewing. There also are nicotine buccal absorption spray products and lozenges that are available for women who want to *quit* tobacco smoking (see Chapter 8, *Preventing and Treating Women's Drug and Substance Abuse*). Once absorbed, nicotine is only *slightly* bound to plasma proteins (i.e., less than 5%). The volume of distribution is approximately 2 to 3 L/kg.

Metabolism. Nicotine is primarily metabolized in the liver by the hepatic microsomal enzyme CYP2A6 to its *inactive* metabolite, *cotinine*. Cotinine is subsequently metabolized to 3-hydroxycotinine. The hepatic clearance rate of nicotine is approximately 1.2 L/minute, which means that the liver is very efficient at clearing and, hence, removing nicotine from the blood stream. However, nicotine clearance is *highly* correlated with age, sex, and continental descent. This inter-individual variability is primarily due to the genetic polymorphism of CYP2A6 and contributes to the observed differences in: (a) patterns of tobacco cigarette smoking; (b) nicotine physical and psychological dependence; and (c) quitting tobacco smoking success (Tanner, Chenoweth, & Tyndale, 2015). Over 20 different metabolites of nicotine have been identified. These metabolites are *less* pharmacologically active than their parent drug, nicotine.

The mean half-life of elimination for nicotine is 2 hours. This means that women who are regular, long-term smokers of tobacco cigarettes will need to "light-up," on average, at least every 2 hours in order to maintain blood nicotine concentrations that are needed to avoid signs and symptoms of the nicotine withdrawal syndrome (see related discussion in the later section, *Undesired, or Harmful, Effects and Toxicities*, Physical and Psychological Dependence, "Nicotine Withdrawal Syndrome").

Excretion. Nicotine and its metabolites are *rapidly* excreted in the urine (approximately 10% to 15% in *unchanged* form). Affected by urinary pH, nicotine excretion is *decreased* in alkaline urine (i.e., urine pH above 7.4), and *increased* in acidic urine (i.e., urine pH below 7.4). In fact, the acidification of the urine to *below* a pH of 5 can result in up to 30% of a dosage of nicotine being excreted in the urine in *unchanged* form.

Undesired, or Harmful, Effects and Toxicities

Tobacco use is the leading preventable cause of disease, disability, and death in the United States. According to the Centers for Disease Control and Prevention (CDC), cigarette smoking results in more than 480,000 premature deaths in the United States each year—about 1 in every 5 U.S. deaths—and … for every one person who dies from smoking, about 30 more suffer from at least one serious tobacco-related illness (NIDA, 2016, p. 1).

The major undesired, or harmful, effects and toxicities associated with *nicotine* are related to its:

1. *Direct* effects on the CNS and other body systems, which can be *acute or chronic, mild or severe*, or, *rarely* fatal
2. *Indirect* effects associated with its method of use, particularly tobacco cigarette smoking

As noted by Carter, Abnet, and Feskanich (2015), "mortality among current smokers is 2 to 3 times as high as that among persons who never smoked" (p. 631).

Direct Effects. Although many of the *acute* psychostimulant effects related to nicotine use are *desired* effects, including euphoria, increased cognitive abilities, and vigilance, the use of nicotine also is associated with such *undesired* effects as: diarrhea; dizziness; edema; flushing; GI cramps; headache; heart palpitations; increased blood pressure, heart rate, and respiratory rate; insomnia; irritability; lightheadedness; nausea; tinnitus; tremors; and vomiting. It also induces the formation of oxygen radicals and reduces the antioxidant capacity of the lungs (Maritz, 2008). With regular, long-term tobacco smoking, these effects generally become increasingly more serious.

Convulsions also can occur if *large* amounts of nicotine are *intentionally* ingested (e.g., in cases of suicide attempts). They also can occur in cases of *unintentional*, or accidental, poisoning (e.g., when a toddler eats a mother's nicotine patch or a curious preschooler ingests a nicotine-containing insecticide). The acute fatal dosage of nicotine for an adult is probably about 60 mg of the base. Signs and symptoms of *acute nicotine poisoning* include:

- abdominal pain
- agitation
- cold sweat
- confusion
- diarrhea
- dizziness
- disturbed hearing and vision
- faintness
- headache
- lethargy
- low blood pressure
- nausea
- pallor
- profuse sweating
- salivation
- tearing, or watery eyes
- vomiting
- weak, irregular pulse

(Also, see later section, *Overdosage.*)

Indirect Effects: Passive Exposure, Secondhand, or Sidestream, Smoke. Tobacco smoke has been associated with premature aging of the skin, increased occurrence of cardiovascular and pulmonary heart disease, and several cancers. In fact, during the first decade of the new millennium, tobacco smoking was identified as the *highest* single preventable cause of illness and disease in the U.S. where it contributes to an estimated 1,500 deaths *every* day.[20] As such, tobacco smoke is identified as the leading cause of preventable and unnecessary deaths adding up to over 500,000 deaths annually with approximately 50,000 of these deaths due to passive exposure (i.e., secondhand, or sidestream, smoke) (Carter, Abnet, & Feskanich, 2015; CDC, 2010; Danaei, Ding, & Mozaffarian, 2009; Pagliaro & Pagliaro, 2009).
As noted by the CDC (2010):

> Secondhand exposure to tobacco smoke causes heart disease and lung cancer in nonsmoking adults and sudden infant death syndrome, acute respiratory infections, middle ear disease, exacerbated asthma, respiratory symptoms, and *decreased* lung function in children.
>
> *(p. 1)*

Passive exposure to tobacco smoke varies among women of different continental descents. For example, the CDC (2015, p. 103), based on an analysis of data for the years 2011–2012, found that approximately 50% of "Black nonsmokers," 25% of "Mexican-American nonsmokers," and 20% of "Non-Hispanic White nonsmokers" were exposed to secondhand smoke.

Most exposure to secondhand smoke occurs in homes and workplaces. However, significant exposure still occurs across the U.S. in various public places, including bars, casinos, and restaurants (CDC, 2016a, p. 1). The CDC goes on to note that:

> Separating smokers form nonsmokers, opening windows, or using air filters does not prevent people from breathing secondhand smoke.
>
> *(2016a, p. 1)*

As further noted in "Ellie's Story":

> Ellie is an active member of the LGBT communities. In her mid-thirties, Ellie was diagnosed with asthma. Ellie never smoked but worked in a bar [in

[20] N.B. The contributions of cigarette smoking to illness and death are often difficult to identify. Consequently, the actual rate of illness and death may be *higher* than what is presented. For example, O'Cleirigh, Valentine, and Pinkston (2015), in their study of people living in the U.S. with HIV, found that the tobacco smoking rate among participants in the study was *triple* that reported for the general population (i.e., 57% versus 19%). They also identified several confounding findings when they compared smokers to non-smokers in their study. Smokers were identified as having: *lower* adherence to anti-AIDS medication regimens; *higher* detectable viral load; *fewer* routine medical visits; *more* recent hospitalization; and *more* concurrent drug and substance abuse, particularly alcohol, cocaine, heroin, and/or marijuana (p. 178). Thus, the total impact of smoking on the health of those women with HIV is significant, but complex, and, thus, extremely difficult to directly quantify.

> her LGBT community] that allowed smoking. Her doctor said her asthma attacks were triggered by secondhand smoke [exposure that occurred while working in the bar]...
>
> *(CDC, 2016b, p. 1)*

IRRITATING AND DAMAGING EFFECTS OF TOBACCO SMOKE. All smoke, regardless of the source, is comprised of colorless gases that contain particulate, or solid, matter. The generally warm gases and particulate matter dispersed in tobacco smoke, irritate and dry the respiratory tract leading to a characteristic dry, non-productive cough (i.e., "smokers cough"). Regular, long-term exposure to tobacco smoke leads to the loss of muscle mass and the development of related respiratory dysfunction even before the development of overt, symptomatic pulmonary toxicity (Degens, Gayan-Ramirez, & van Hees, 2015). In addition, particulate matter that makes its way into the alveolar sacs can get trapped and compromise alveolar function.

OTHER CHEMICALS PRESENT IN TOBACCO SMOKE. The chemicals present in tobacco smoke include: (1) chemicals naturally found in tobacco leaves (e.g., heavy metals, such as arsenic, chromium, and lead); (2) chemicals added during the farming (e.g., insecticides) and curing processes (e.g., menthol flavoring); and (3) chemicals produced by pyrolysis (e.g., carbon dioxide; tar). For example, carbon dioxide can be found in concentrations 200 to 300 times that found in normal room air. The high concentrations of carbon dioxide (i.e., approximately 13%) have been associated with an inflammatory response in pulmonary tissue (Guais, Brand, & Jacquot, 2011; Schwartz, Guais, & Chaumet-Riffaud, 2010). The *two* major classes of carcinogens present in tobacco smoke are: (1) *polycyclic aromatic hydrocarbons* (PAHs), including benzo(a)pyrene, chrysene, and naphthalene;[21] and (2) *nicotine-derived nitrosamines* (NDNs).[22]

CARDIOVASCULAR DISEASES. The association between tobacco smoke and coronary heart disease was identified over 75 years ago, by English, Willius, and Berkson (1940)—cited by Paul (1989). It is now recognized that tobacco smoke is associated with a two to fourfold *increased* risk for coronary heart disease among regular, long-term tobacco smokers—both women and men. Several interrelated factors contribute to the complex cardiovascular toxicity associated with tobacco smoke. As noted by D'Allessandro, Boeckelmann, and Hammwhoner (2012), regarding cardiac dysrhythmias, the:

---

[21] Several studies have found that "flue-cured" tobacco typically can deliver more PAHs than other tobacco types (e.g., Ding, Yan, & Jain, 2006, p. 1133).

[22] *NDNs* also are referred to in the literature as *tobacco-specific nitrosamines* (TSNAs) (Wu, Zhang, & Jain, 2005). Two major TSNAs that are present in tobacco and tobacco smoke are 4-(methylnitrosamino)-1-(3-pyridyl)-1-butanone (NNB) and N^1-nitrosonornicotine (NNN) (Hecht, 2014; Pfeifer, Denissenko, & Olivier, 2002; Vu, Taylor, & Holman, 2015; Wang, Li, & Guo, 2016).

> profibrotic effect of nicotine on myocardial tissue with consequent increased susceptibility to catecholamine might play a role. In addition, other constituents of tobacco smoke, such as carbon monoxide and oxidative stress, are likely to contribute to the generation of cardiac dysrhythmias. Finally, tobacco smoke may induce coronary artery disease and chronic obstructive pulmonary disease, which may cause dysrhythmias independently.
>
> *(p. 297)*

PULMONARY DISEASES. Pulmonary toxicity associated with tobacco smoke among women (i.e., cancer of the lungs, bronchi, and trachea; chronic obstructive pulmonary disease [COPD]) is associated with *three* major factors: (1) *direct irritant and damaging effects of tobacco smoke*; (2) carcinogens present in tobacco and/or produced by the pyrolysis of tobacco leaves and wrapping paper; and (3) other chemicals present in tobacco smoke. In addition, nicotine, itself, induces the formation of oxygen radicals and reduces the antioxidant capacity of the lungs (Henley, Thomas, & Sharapova, 2016; Maritz, 2008).

As noted in "Becky's Story":

> Becky started smoking cigarettes in 1976 as an exchange student when she was living with a host family in Germany … At age 45, Becky was diagnosed with chronic obstructive pulmonary disease (COPD) … Today, Becky needs continuous oxygen to help her breathe…
>
> *(CDC, 2016c, p. 1)*

TOBACCO SMOKE AND LUNG CANCER. Tobacco smoke is clearly associated with an *increased* risk for lung cancer. Of concern is the fact that the overall risk for mortality associated with tobacco smoke is the same for women as it is for men (CDC, 2002). The reason for this statistic includes a "600-percent increase since 1950 in women's death rates for lung cancer, a disease primarily caused by cigarette smoking" (Satcher, 2001). In addition, many women, who do *not* smoke tobacco, are still subjected to, and suffer from, significant exposure to secondhand smoke—primarily from spouses and other family members, or significant others, and occupational exposure (Pagliaro & Pagliaro, *Clinical Patient Data Files*). In fact, over 1 decade ago in a special report, the U.S. Surgeon General identified "that there is no level of risk-free exposure to secondhand smoke" (U.S. Department of Health and Human Services, 2006, p. 1). However, as of December 31, 2015, 18 different states (i.e., Alabama, Alaska, Arkansas, Florida, Idaho, Indiana, Kentucky, Louisiana, Mississippi, Nevada, New Hampshire, Oklahoma, Pennsylvania, South Carolina, Tennessee, Texas, West Virginia, and Wyoming) did *not* prohibit tobacco smoking in bars—a work site that employs a great number of women (Tynan, Holmes, & Promoff, 2016).

As noted in "Rose's Story":

> Rose started smoking at age 13 and continued for many years, smoking two packs a day. Rose developed lung cancer from smoking cigarettes and … had chemotherapy, surgery, radiation, and a painful drainage tube in her left chest … She died in January 2015, at age 60 from cancer caused by smoking.
>
> *(CDC, 2016d, p. 1)*

TOBACCO SMOKE AND OTHER CANCERS. Tobacco smoke also has been associated with cancers of the: breast; cervix; colon; esophagus; head; kidney and renal pelvis; larynx; liver; neck; mouth and oropharynx; ovaries; pancreas; rectum; stomach; and urinary bladder (Beral, Gaitskell, & Hermon, 2012; Henley, Thomas, & Sharapova, 2016; Johnson, 2001; Kuper, Boffetta, & Adami, 2002; Nagata, Mizoue, & Tanaka, 2006; Thun, Henley, & Calle, 2002; Wakai, Inoue, & Mizoue, 2006), and acute myeloid leukemia. For many of these cancers, a direct cause-and-effect relationship with tobacco smoke remains tentative. Research increasingly suggests a significant *genetic* contribution to the relationship between tobacco smoke and cancer. However, this putative relationship is complex and research results have *not* always been consistent (e.g., Fagan, Moolchan, & Pokhrel, 2015). For example, tobacco smokers with *higher* CYP2A6 activity have *higher* rates of nicotine metabolism. Thus, they smoke more extensively and, consequently, are exposed to more carcinogens in tobacco smoke and related greater risk for developing cancer (Derby, Cuthrell, & Caberto, 2008).

We have consistently noted, for *over* 3 decades, that nicotine, *in the form of tobacco smoke*, is unique among all other drugs and substances of abuse in that it has *no* safe level of use. The therapeutic index for tobacco smoke is *zero*. As noted by the World Health Organization (2009):

> There is *no* safe level of exposure to tobacco smoke. All people should be protected from such exposure.
>
> *(p. 14)*

Unfortunately, the use of nicotine in cigarettes, cigars, and pipes continues to be widespread in the U.S. and appears to be *increasing* in certain population groups (e.g., adolescent girls; women in the military; women who have mental disorders) (see later discussion in the section, *Women's Personal Nicotine Use/Abuse*) despite cautions and wide publicity of the harmful effects and toxicities associated with its use.[23]

---

[23] To reduce the toxicity associated with tobacco cigarette smoking, the composition of cigarettes was significantly changed in the U.S. during the last half of the 20th century. As noted by Hoffmann and Hoffmann (1997):

> In the United States the sales-weighted average "tar" and nicotine yields have declined from a *high* of 38 mg *tar* and 2.7 mg *nicotine* in 1954 to 12 mg and 0.95 mg in 1992, respectively.
>
> *(p. 307)*

The serious toxicities associated with tobacco smoke—as well as associated decreased rates of smoking in the U.S.—have been the basis for the increased attention of cigarette manufacturers to the development of *smoke-free* nicotine products. This attention has involved research with various concentrations and flavors utilizing convenient delivery systems that, in general, are both attractive and similar in shape to traditional cigarettes (i.e., electronic cigarettes, or e-cigarettes) (Pagliaro & Pagliaro, 2009). E-cigarettes, which vaporize the nicotine for pulmonary inhalation, were introduced to the U.S. market in 2007. They produced inhalable nicotine vapor without the need to burn tobacco and, consequently, avoid the creation of tobacco smoke (Czogala, Goniewicz, & Fidelus, 2014; Oh & Kacker, 2014; Rom, Pecorelli, & Valacchi, 2015). (See additional discussion in the later section, *E-cigarettes*.)

Physical and Psychological Dependence. Prior to the 1970s, the medical and scientific communities generally agreed that the regular, long-term use of nicotine as a component of tobacco smoke, did *not* cause physical dependence (i.e., *addiction*), but that tobacco smoking could result in *psychological* dependence (i.e., *habituation*). These views were strongly supported by the large tobacco companies and the research that they financially supported (including much university-based research).[24] Over the 1970s and 1980s, scientific data accumulated that increasingly supported a change in view. The regular, long-term use of nicotine was found to cause both physical and psychological dependence. A decade later, Collins (1990, p. 84) summarized the 20th Report of the Surgeon General on the health consequences of smoking, which was entitled *Nicotine Addiction*. The summary, a 500-page comprehensive review of over 1,000 published studies, led to the conclusions that:

1. Tobacco products are associated with the development of physical dependence
2. Nicotine in tobacco products *is* the substance identified as causing the physical dependence
3. Becoming physically dependent on nicotine is a process similar to that observed for heroin and cocaine
4. Physical dependence also occurs with the use of smokeless tobacco products because the same blood nicotine concentrations can be achieved as are achieved with tobacco cigarette smoking

Since the publication of this report in 1990, it has been generally agreed that nicotine is, in fact, the *major* component of tobacco smoke that is responsible for the development of physical dependence related to tobacco products (Benowitz, 1999; Dani & De Biasi, 2001; Pagliaro & Pagliaro, 2009). Based on a sample of

[24] Prior to, and during this period, it was common to have patients and healthcare professionals, particularly nurses, pharmacists, and physicians, smoking cigarettes in healthcare facilities, including offices and hospitals (Pagliaro & Pagliaro, *Clinical Patient Data Files*).

over 30,000 adults drawn from the 2001 to 2002 *National Epidemiological Survey of Alcoholism and Related Conditions* (NESARC), Goodwin, Keyes, and Hasin (2009) found that, although the overall *rate* of cigarette use *declined* significantly between 1964 and 2002, the *rate* of nicotine dependence did *not* decline. In addition, they reported that:

> The group most at risk of nicotine dependence among cigarette users is women in poverty in the most recent birth cohort [i.e., new millennial women], whose risk is substantially higher than that calculated for the overall population.
>
> *(p. 1476)*

In addition, most *hard* science researchers in this area of study (e.g., Vetulani, 2001) agree that the development of physical dependence to nicotine is caused by the release of brain dopamine.[25] The dopamine, subsequently, interacts at neural reward centers in the brain that are primarily located in the limbic system. However, other positivist researchers have suggested that any, or all, of the following four proposed mechanisms could play a major role in the development of physical dependence to nicotine:

1. Nicotine-induced alteration in nAChR synaptic plasticity (e.g., Dani & De Biasi, 2001; Dani, Ji, & Zhou, 2001)
2. Nicotine-induced release of other neurotransmitters and neuromodulators (e.g., Kenny & Markou, 2001)
3. Up-regulation of nAChRs following prolonged exposure to nicotine (e.g., Buisson & Bertrand, 2002)
4. Interaction with, or modification by, the activation of the endogenous cannabinoid receptor, CB_1 (e.g., Gamaleddin, Trigo, & Gueye, 2015)

Regardless of the actual mechanism(s) involved, physical *dependence* is characterized by: (1) the development of *tolerance* with the regular, long-term use of a drug or substance of abuse; and (2) a *withdrawal syndrome* that occurs when the regular, long-term use of a drug or substance of abuse is *abruptly* discontinued and that immediately dissipates when the use of the drug or substance of abuse is resumed. Thus, these two constructs are considered next.

DEVELOPMENT OF TOLERANCE. The regular, long-term use of nicotine in the form of either tobacco smoke from various sources (e.g., cigarettes; cigars) or smokeless tobacco products (e.g., e-cigarettes; pharmaceutical nicotine replacement products; snuff) can result in the development of tolerance as occurs with other drugs and substances of abuse (e.g., alcohol; opiate analgesics). Thus, as women regularly

---

[25] For additional details, also see the earlier section, *Pharmacodynamics: Mechanism of Action.*

use nicotine for desired effects, over time, they need to increase the number of cigarettes they smoke, change the brand of the nicotine product that they use to another that contains higher levels of nicotine, or change the smoking techniques that they use (e.g., increase the number of puffs per cigarette; inhale the tobacco smoke or nicotine vapor more deeply; and hold it in the lungs for a longer period). These changes are made to increase the amount of nicotine absorbed into the systemic circulation for distribution to nicotinic receptors in the brain, and, consequently, to achieve the effects that they desire from nicotine.

Tolerance to the *desired* effects of nicotine (e.g., euphoria; alertness; relaxation) has been well established in humans. Thus, women who smoke tobacco cigarettes, or other sources of nicotine, find that to achieve desired effects over time, they must *increase* the dosage and/or frequency of their nicotine use. Tolerance also develops to most of the undesired effects (e.g., dizziness; nausea; vomiting), but *not* to all. For example, after one or two cigarettes, even a regular, long-term cigarette smoker exhibits an *increase* in blood pressure, pulse rate, and hand tremor. It also has been found that women, who smoke, metabolize nicotine more rapidly than women, who are nonsmokers, but it is likely that tolerance is due primarily to pharmacodynamic changes (e.g., neuroadaptation of nicotine receptors rather than to pharmacokinetic changes). There are conflicting reports on the duration of tolerance. In human smokers, some aspects of tolerance wax and wane repeatedly, thus, the first cigarette of the day produces a much greater cardiovascular and subjective response than subsequent cigarettes through the day. Perhaps, at least in part, because of nonuse withdrawal that occurs overnight.

As previously noted in relation to women's alcohol abuse (also, see Chapter 2, *Women's Alcohol Abuse*), several researchers (e.g., Kinsaul & Copeland, 2013) have reported telescoping in regard to tobacco cigarette smoking and the development of nicotine dependence and other related undesired, or harmful, effects and toxicities. Although, on average, women initiate tobacco smoking at *older* ages than do men, regarding associated negative health consequences, they catch up to men by middle to late adulthood.

NICOTINE WITHDRAWAL SYNDROME. Both central and peripheral groups of nAChRs are involved in mediating the affective and somatic signs and symptoms of nicotine withdrawal. Many women, who use nicotine for its psychostimulant effects, find that after a period of continued use, they are unable to discontinue use without the occurrence of undesired effects. These women often seek professional help (e.g., from a counselor, nurse, pharmacist, physician, or psychologist). However, even with professional help, one-third of these women are unable to discontinue nicotine use for more than a few days, and only 20% to 30% are "nicotine free" 12 months later. Even women who have been advised by a physician or other health professional to discontinue their nicotine use because of serious health concerns (e.g., myocardial infarction; lung cancer), may complain of significant difficulty discontinuing their nicotine use for longer than a few days or weeks.[26]

A nicotine withdrawal syndrome has been clearly identified and appears to be influenced by *both* genetic and environmental factors (McLaughlin, Dani, & De Biasi, 2015). For example, women, who are *faster* metabolizers of nicotine, report *more* frequent and serious signs and symptoms of nicotine withdrawal (Hartz, Short, & Saccone, 2012). Consequently, these women are more likely to *self-medicate* (i.e., "smoke another cigarette") to *immediately* relieve signs and symptoms of withdrawal.

Common signs and symptoms of the nicotine withdrawal syndrome include:

- Anxiety
- Bradycardia
- Fatigue
- Headaches
- Hunger
- Inability to concentrate
- Insomnia
- Irritability
- Lack of energy
- Memory impairment
- Mental depression
- Nightmares
- Restlessness
- Weight gain

These signs and symptoms generally begin within 4 to 24 hours of discontinuing regular, long-term tobacco cigarette smoking or other nicotine use because of nicotine's relatively short half-life of elimination (i.e., approximately 2 hours). To forestall or ameliorate nicotine withdrawal, women, who are physically dependent on nicotine, will generally display various behaviors associated with boosting their blood nicotine levels) (see earlier section, *Pharmacokinetics*):

- Smoking first thing in the morning when they awaken
- Going out in a stormy night to buy a pack of cigarettes when they find they have none in the house
- Taking a "break" as soon as they can during the work day to "take a smoke"

The nicotine withdrawal syndrome may intensify over 2 to 4 days and, then, gradually dissipate over 1 to 3 weeks. The aversive aspects of nicotine withdrawal

[26] For additional information and related discussion, see Chapter 8, *Preventing and Treating Women's Drug and Substance Abuse.*

often contribute to *resumed* nicotine use. Many women attempt to manage nicotine withdrawal by gradually *decreasing* nicotine use by cutting down the number of cigarettes smoked daily and while some may be successful, many others are not. To aid nicotine withdrawal, several pharmacotherapeutic approaches have been developed and approved, including nicotine-containing products, such as NicoDerm® transdermal delivery systems ("patches") and Nicorette® chewing gum and spray products. Non-nicotine containing products, such as bupropion (Zyban®) and varenicline (Chantix®) also are available. (For further related detailed discussion, see Chapter 8, *Preventing and Treating Women's Drug and Substance Abuse*.)

The argument that nicotine is the active substance in tobacco smoke, which is responsible for continued regular use, also is supported by several studies of both *low-yield* nicotine cigarette smokers and *high-yield* nicotine cigarette smokers. For example, cigarette smokers, who use low-yield cigarettes, smoke *more* cigarettes per day than do those who smoke *high*-yield cigarettes. In addition, *brand-switching* studies have reported that when smokers are changed from *high*- to *low*-yield cigarettes, they may unconsciously change their smoking behavior to maintain their blood nicotine concentration by increasing the

1. Number of cigarettes smoked
2. Depth of puffs or rate of puffing
3. Duration of inhalation

An area that requires more study is the individual *differences* in the withdrawal experience reported by women who use nicotine. These experiences have been largely ignored. The assumption is generally made that, for example, a regular, long-term tobacco smoker is physically dependent on tobacco. This assumption may be as *incorrect* as is the assumption that women who drink alcohol daily are physically dependent on alcohol. It may be that some women who smoke tobacco can regularly use nicotine for longer periods of time without becoming physically dependent on nicotine (Pagliaro & Pagliaro, *Clinical Patient Data Files*). In addition, because women who smoke tobacco often use other drugs and substances of abuse (e.g., alcohol; caffeine; marijuana), the synergistic effects of poly-drug and substance use, may play a significant role in the experience of the nicotine withdrawal syndrome.

Pregnancy and Lactation. Approximately 13%, or more than 1 in 8 women in the U.S., report smoking tobacco cigarettes during the last three months of pregnancy (CDC, 2012, p. 1). In this regard, disparity of tobacco smoking rates has been reported among pregnant women in the U.S. of various continental descents. For example, Wright and Tam (2010) found in their study that significantly more women who were Native Hawaiians (21% versus 8%) continued to smoke through pregnancy to within one week of admission for labor. For another example, in a study of 690 pregnant women participants of African (62%) and European (38%)

continental descents at an urban prenatal clinic, De Genna, Goldschmidt, and Day (2016) found that:

1. Rates of chronic smoking and nonsmoking were roughly equivalent (i.e., approximately 33%)
2. Younger pregnant women were more likely to smoke than older pregnant women
3. Pregnant women of European descent were more likely to be chronic smokers
4. Significant co-variants included: educational level, socioeconomic status, and other prenatal drug and substance use

In addition, the CDC evaluated rates of tobacco smoking and cessation among women during the first and second trimesters of pregnancy in 46 states and in the District of Columbia (Mathews, 2016). The data pool accounted for 3,819,113 births and represented 95% of *all* U.S. births in 2014. On average, 20.6% of pregnant women smoked during the first and second trimesters of pregnancy. Regarding smoking cessation during pregnancy, among the 46 states, Dakota had the *highest* cessation rate (i.e., 31.3%) while Kentucky had the *lowest* (i.e., 11.4%). In another study, which examined the course of smoking among pregnant women who also had a concurrent history of other drug and substance abuse, Forray, Gotman, and Kershaw (2014) found that:

> Women were able to discontinue or decrease smoking during pregnancy, but were likely to resume or increase smoking postpartum.
>
> *(p. 749)*

The relationship between maternal use of nicotine during pregnancy and birth defects, or *teratogenesis*, has *not* been well-substantiated. However, smoking tobacco cigarettes has been related to *increased* rates of spontaneous abortion, stillbirth, preterm delivery, neonatal death, and SIDs. It has been hypothesized that the in-utero exposure of the embryo/fetus to nicotine, together with other components of tobacco smoke (e.g., carbon monoxide), can cause vasoconstriction and an associated *decrease in* blood flow to the uterus/placenta that may result in, or contribute to, these toxic effects (Ernst, Moolchan, & Robinson, 2001; Phelan, 2014; Shea & Steiner, 2008). In-utero exposure to nicotine (e.g., in the context of maternal tobacco smoking) may also result in genetic changes that subsequently produce accelerated lung aging and increased susceptibility to the development of obstructive lung disease in the exposed offspring later in life (Maritz & Harding, 2011). A transdisciplinary group, which was formed by the Office of Smoking and Health from the CDC to evaluate "developmental toxicity of nicotine," found that:

> Nicotine contributes critically to adverse effects of gestational tobacco exposure, including reduced pulmonary function, auditory processing defects,

impaired infant cardiorespiratory function, and may contribute to cognitive and behavioral deficits in later life.

(England, Aagaard, & Bloch, 2017, p. 176)

In addition, neonates born to mothers who smoke tobacco cigarettes[27] during pregnancy, have *lower* birth weights (Pagliaro & Pagliaro, 2002, 2012). They also are twice as likely to die during early infancy due to the *Sudden Infant Death Syndrome* (SIDS) (Abbott & Winzer-Serhan, 2012). The SIDS is thought to be related to the infant's exposure to sidestream and environmental tobacco smoke in the home where the mother, father, or other household members and caregivers, smoke tobacco cigarettes.

> Avoid [tobacco] exposure during pregnancy and after birth. Both maternal smoking during pregnancy and smoke in the infant's environment after birth are major risk factors for SIDS.
>
> *(Moon, Darnall, & Goodstein, 2011, p. 1034)*

Regarding *lactation*, nicotine, whether obtained from tobacco cigarette smoking or other methods of use, including e-cigarettes or nicotine replacement products, is excreted in breast milk. Concentrations of nicotine, and its metabolite, cotinine, in breast milk may be as much as 3 times the concentrations present in maternal blood. Breast-fed neonates and infants may display signs and symptoms of nicotine ingestion, including: diarrhea; increased heart rate; restlessness; and vomiting. Adolescent girls and women who are breast-feeding should be advised of the potential risks to their neonates and infants. If tobacco smoking is continued, or if nicotine products are required, breast-feeding should be discontinued.

Overdosage

Overdosage has *not* generally been associated with the regular use of smoking tobacco except when tobacco products are unintentionally ingested by infants and children, or pets. Overdosages associated with nicotine replacement products has been related to simultaneously chewing, or chewing in rapid succession, more

---

27 Although the maternal use of nicotine replacement products may be safer for the embryo/fetus than tobacco smoking (i.e., the fetus is not exposed to additional chemicals that are present in tobacco smoke), the use of nicotine products has been associated, as has tobacco smoking, with spontaneous abortion. Long-term expected pharmacologic actions associated with nicotine may be observed among neonates, including physical dependence and the signs and symptoms of the nicotine withdrawal syndrome. Adolescent girls and women who are pregnant should *not* smoke tobacco and should avoid the use of nicotine replacement products. These products should be used during pregnancy only if the risks to the mother and embryo/fetus or neonate is justified by the risks posed by continued maternal use of nicotine. If nicotine replacement pharmacotherapy is required, pregnant adolescent girls and women should be advised of the potential benefits and possible risks to themselves and their embryo, fetus, or neonate.

than the recommended number of nicotine chewing gum squares. It also has been reported with inadvertent access of young children to transdermal nicotine delivery systems.

Although nicotine has a *low* LD_{50} (i.e., 50 mg to 60 mg of nicotine may be *fatal* for an adult), nicotine related deaths are rare because:

1. When tobacco is *smoked*, *most* (i.e., approximately 90%) of the nicotine is destroyed by pyrolysis (see earlier discussion in the *Absorption* section)
2. When tobacco is *ingested*, the oral bioavailability of nicotine from tobacco products is *low* (i.e., F = 0.3) or 30%. More importantly, nicotine stimulates vomiting as blood nicotine concentrations increase. Thus, tobacco products that are swallowed often are vomited—offering some protection against fatal nicotine overdosages (i.e., the tobacco is removed from the stomach by vomiting, and, consequently, the nicotine is *not* further absorbed into the bloodstream).

The signs and symptoms of *acute* nicotine overdosage can be *mild to moderate*, or *moderate to severe*. *Mild to moderate* signs and symptoms include: abdominal pain; cold sweat; confusion; diarrhea; diaphoresis; dizziness; headache; hearing and vision disturbances; nausea; pallor; salivation (excessive); vomiting; and weakness (marked). *Moderate to severe* signs and symptoms include: breathing difficulty; confusion; circulatory collapse; faintness and prostration; hypotension; rapid, weak, irregular pulse; and terminal convulsions. Death can occur within minutes because of respiratory failure due to paralysis of the muscles of respiration.

There have been incidents of patients simultaneously applying several transdermal delivery systems or swallowing these systems (Pagliaro & Pagliaro, *Clinical Patient Data Files*). Signs and symptoms of overdosage associated with nicotine transdermal and other delivery systems are the same as those associated with other nicotine overdosage. Hypotension, prostration, and respiratory failure may be observed with severe overdosage. Convulsions and death may follow because of peripheral or central respiratory paralysis or, less frequently, cardiac failure. In cases of overdosage, the use of any nicotine product should be discontinued immediately; this includes immediate removal of the transdermal delivery system. After removal of the transdermal system, the skin should be flushed with water. Soap must not be used, because it may increase nicotine absorption from the skin site. Nicotine will continue to be delivered into the blood stream for several hours after removal of the system, because of the depot of nicotine that is formed in the skin as part of the pharmacologic bioavailability of the nicotine transdermal delivery system.

Suspected, or actual, nicotine overdosage requires emergency medical support of body systems, with attention to maintaining adequate respiratory function and increasing nicotine elimination. There is *no* known specific antidote.

Women's Medical and Personal Nicotine Use and Abuse

The following sections highlight and describe women's medical and personal use and abuse of nicotine.

Women's Medical Nicotine Use/Abuse

For most of its history, the pharmacotherapeutic use of nicotine received little medical attention because of its early, and correct, identification as a *poison*. However, during the late 1970s, amidst the accumulation of research data supporting a relationship between tobacco smoking and lung cancer, *nicotine replacement therapy* was medically initiated as an aid to facilitate the cessation of tobacco smoking among both women and men who wanted to "kick-the-habit" (Hyde, Paxton, & Carr, 1982). Nicotine replacement therapy, in its various formulations (e.g., chewing gums, intranasal sprays, oral lozenges, and transdermal delivery systems), continues to be medically used because of its safety and efficacy in regard to reducing the undesired signs and symptoms associated with nicotine withdrawal and enhancing associated successful outcomes regarding "quitting" nicotine use. (Also, see Chapter 8, *Preventing and Treating Women's Drug and Substance Abuse*.)

Both former and active tobacco smoking has been long associated with the occurrence of *Alzheimer's disease* (Chang, Ho, & Wong, 2014; Durazzo, Mattsson, & Weiner, 2014). However, more recently, it has been associated with *improved* attention and memory among patients diagnosed with Alzheimer's disease. Consequently, nicotine is *now* suggested for the possible efficacious medical management of Alzheimer's disease (Appleby & Cummings, 2013; Durazzo, Mattsson, & Weiner, 2014).

Regarding *Parkinson's disease*, extensive pre-clinical research using experimental laboratory animal models and the post-mortem examination of human brains, have revealed a *neuroprotective* effect associated with nicotine—particularly, in the nigrostriatal area of the brain where damage associated with Parkinson's disease is usually expressed (Chang, Ho, & Wong, 2014; Quik, Huang, & Parameswaran, 2009; Quik, Zhang, & McGregor, 2015). In addition, smoking tobacco cigarettes has been associated with a *reduced* risk for developing Parkinson's disease (Thiriez, Villafane, & Grapin, 2011). Research is now evaluating the potential therapeutic use of nicotine in the medical management of Parkinson's disease.

Women's Personal Nicotine Use/Abuse

> <u>Popular Notion</u>: When compared to other women in the U.S., women of American Indian descent generally have *lower* levels of tobacco use because they primarily smoke tobacco as a part of traditional tobacco ceremonies.
>
> NOT TRUE—on both counts. See the following related discussion.

Tobacco smokers *cannot* be generally defined as belonging preferentially to any continental descent, ethnicity, or socioeconomic group. They include approximately one-fourth of the adult population in the U.S.,[28] most of whom began to smoke before they were 14 years-of-age. It is estimated that, every day of the year in the U.S., more than 3,000 children and adolescents—mostly girls—begin to smoke tobacco (Pagliaro & Pagliaro, 2009). In the U.S., of the people who reported use during the previous year:

> Women represented over 40% of users of tobacco products (33 million women).
>
> *(McHugh, Wigderson, & Greenfield, 2014, p. 177)*

Generally, approximately 25% of women, during the new millennium in the U.S., reported past month cigarette use.[29] However, this number *declined* significantly (i.e., to approximately 15%) for women who were pregnant. A further *slight* reduction (i.e., to approximately 13%) occurs as pregnancy progresses to the third trimester (SAMHSA, 2014b).[30] (For further related discussion, see the earlier section, *Undesired, or Harmful, Effects and Toxicities*, "Pregnancy and Lactation.")

---

[28] N.B. Tobacco smoking rates in the U.S. are difficult to fully compare and evaluate because different surveys *define* the sample measures in a variety of ways that generally preclude collapsing or even directly comparing data from various studies. For example, in the often cited 2015 *National Health Interview Survey* (NHIS), which is a nationally representative, in-person survey of the noninstitutionalized adult (i.e., 18 years-of-age or older) U.S. civilian population conducted on behalf of the CDC, "current cigarette smokers" are defined as "adults who smoked 100 or more cigarettes during their lifetime and, at the time of the interview, smoked every day or on some days" (CDC, 2016f, p. 1205). In that study, "current cigarette smoking among U.S. adults [was reported to have] declined from 20.9% in 2005 to 15.1% in 2015" (p. 1205). Although the trend (i.e., decline in cigarette smoking) appears to be accurate and substantiated by (i.e., consistent with) data from other related studies, the magnitude (i.e., as based on reported percentages) is *less* reliable because of the related definition of "cigarette smoking" and the defined characteristics of the samples. In addition, other tobacco use—such as the use of cigars and pipe tobacco—as well as "e-cigarette" use (see later discussion in the section, "E-cigarettes"), were not included. However, in this context, a more recent study, which used data from Wave 1 (i.e., September 2013 through December 2014) of the *Population Assessment of Tobacco and Health (PATH) Study*, and determined prevalence estimates for the use of 12 different forms of tobacco products in the U.S., found that:

> More than a quarter (27.6%) of adults were current users of at least one type of tobacco product in 2013 and 2014 … [In addition,] approximately 40% of tobacco users, adults and youths alike, used multiple tobacco products; cigarettes plus e-cigarettes was the most common combination.
>
> *(Kasza, Ambrose, & Conway, 2017, p. 342)*

[29] Daily tobacco smoking by U.S. women is estimated to be approximately 20% (Agaku, King, & Husten, 2014). However, it is significantly *higher* for women of American Indian descent (e.g., Jamal, King, & Neff, 2016). For example, Forster, Poupart, and Rhodes (2016) found that, among sampled American Indians in the Upper Midwest, the prevalence of tobacco smoking (non-ceremonial) was 55.8% for women.

[30] A small number of pregnant women "keep smoking through pregnancy just because they want to give birth to a smaller baby" (Adams, 2011, p. 1).

In addition, women's nicotine use can be differentiated by:

1. Source of nicotine (i.e., tobacco cigarette versus smokeless tobacco)
2. Geographical location

For example, based on a survey of women in the U.S. by the Centers for Disease Control and Prevention, Nguyen, Marshall, and Brown (2016) reported:

- Rates of cigarette smoking varied from 8.2% in Utah to 25.6% in West Virginia
- Rates of smokeless tobacco use varied from 0.4% in Maryland to 3.4% in Mississippi
- Rates of any cigarette smoking and/or smokeless tobacco use varied from 8.5% in Utah to 25.5% in West Virginia

In the U.S., *most* women who abuse nicotine for alerting, euphoric, and other desired effects, obtain their nicotine by smoking tobacco cigarettes (Hu, Neff, & Agaku, 2016; Pagliaro & Pagliaro, 2000, 2009).[31,32] While a *high* percentage of these women are in the military (Durazzo, Mattsson, & Weiner, 2014), the *highest* percentage of women who abuse nicotine are found among women who have mental disorders, particularly: anxiety disorders;[33] major depressive disorder; and

---

[31] Except for nicotine replacement pharmacotherapy (see Chapter 8, *Preventing and Treating Women's Drug and Substance Abuse*).

[32] A specific reason for smoking tobacco cigarettes (i.e., loss of, or control of, body weight) is almost exclusively reported by women, particularly women in the U.S. of European continental descent in contrast to women of African continental descent (Sanchez-Johnson, Spring, & Kaplan Sommerfeld, 2005). In addition to psychological variables (e.g., oral stimulation associated with smoking tobacco cigarettes) and possible placebo effect for managing stress and other conditions, nicotine, itself, helps to prevent weight gain by *suppressing* the appetite for sweet-tasting foods and increasing energy expenditure, both at rest and during exercise by approximately 10% (Pagliaro & Pagliaro, 2009). As noted by Chiolero, Faeh, and Paccaud (2008):

> Numerous cross-sectional studies indicate that body weight, or body mass index (BMI; kg/m^2), is *lower* in cigarette smokers than in nonsmokers.
>
> *(p. 801)*

Smoking cessation typically results in a weight gain of 7 to 9 pounds within 8 years of ceasing tobacco smoking (Audrain-McGovern & Benowitz, 2011; Sifferlin, 2012). The mechanisms primarily involved in the weight gain include both *decreased* metabolic rate and *increased* caloric intake (i.e., effects clearly associated with nicotine withdrawal, which is associated with effects opposite those of nicotine). Based on their study of smoking cessation among premenopausal women, Ferrara, Kumar, and Nicklas (2001) suggest that an *increase* in adipose tissue lipoprotein lipase (AT-LPL) activity and a *decrease* in lipolysis also significantly contribute to weight gain following smoking cessation.

[33] In a comprehensive review of the relationship between posttraumatic stress disorder (PTSD) and tobacco smoking, Fu, McFall, and Saxon (2007) found that active tobacco smoking was significant (i.e., ranging from 40% to 86%) among those with PTSD.

psychotic disorder (i.e., schizophrenia) (Jessup, Dibble, & Cooper, 2012; Johnson, Ratner, & Malchy, 2010; Morisano, Bacher, & Audrain-McGovern, 2009; Peiper & Rodu, 2013; Ziedonis, Hitsman, & Beckham, 2008). (Also, see Chapter 7, *Identifying Women's Contemporaneous Diagnoses.*) In fact, women who smoke and have mental disorders reportedly have a significantly increased:

1. Risk of experiencing the nicotine withdrawal syndrome
2. Greater difficulty regarding ceasing tobacco smoking even when *highly* motivated to do so (Smith, Homish, & Giovino, 2014).

As noted in "Rebecca's Story":

> Rebecca, age 57, started smoking cigarettes at age 16 … At age 33, Rebecca was diagnosed with depression. She smoked frequently when she felt depressed because she felt smoking might help her cope with her feelings. Rebecca felt ashamed when she smoked, so when she tried to quit and couldn't, she felt even more depressed. "That was just a vicious, vicious cycle," she said…
>
> *(CDC, 2016e, p. 1)*

In their study of a large, convenience sample of women who were tobacco smokers and who also had *contemporaneous diagnoses*,[34] Jessup, Dibble, and Cooper (2012) found that: (1) women of African continental descent; (2) women of American Indian descent; and (3) women who were bisexual reported the *highest* rates of smoking.[35] In a later study of a large sample of undergraduate women and men, who reported daily tobacco cigarette smoking, Buckner and Vinci (2013) found that cigarette smoking was *highly* correlated with social anxiety among women, but *not* men. (Also, see Chapter 7, *Identifying Women's Contemporaneous Diagnoses*, for a related comprehensive discussion and analysis.) In addition, young women living in residential treatment facilities are *more* likely than men to be tobacco smokers (Johnson, Ratner, & Malchy, 2010).

E-Cigarettes. Other current trends among new millennial adolescent girls and women in the U.S. include the use of the *e-cigarette* (*Smoke Stik®*)—an electronic nicotine delivery system (ENDS) that looks like a common tobacco cigarette—making it attractive to traditional cigarette smokers and to new millennial adolescent girls and women in the U.S., who have not yet begun to smoke. However, because there is *no* tobacco to burn, there is *no* odor and *no*, or *very* low, cancer-producing smoke that contains carbon monoxide, tars, and other cancer-causing

34 Having, at the same time, an alcohol use disorder(s) and/or a substance use disorder(s) and/or another mental disorder(s).

35 Hu, Neff, and Agaku (2016) also found that bisexual and lesbian women were *more* likely than other women to report current tobacco use.

chemicals or *carcinogens*, to inhale and to worry about.[36] Typically, the e-cigarettes have several basic components (Brown & Cheng, 2014; Pagliaro & Pagliaro, 2009):

- LED light cover to resemble a burning cigarette and also to indicate that the product is activated
- Rechargeable battery (and external battery charger) in portable models, to provide an energy source so that it can be conveniently used almost anywhere
- Storage unit/space to contain a solution of nicotine (i.e., a refill cartridge)
- Atomizer, or heating element, to vaporize the liquid nicotine[37]
- Flow sensor that controls the amount of nicotine delivered to the atomizer
- Cartridge mouthpiece that is placed between the lips (like a traditional cigarette) to provide a familiar and convenient means for inhaling the vaporized nicotine into the lungs

The liquid nicotine refill cartridges (i.e., e-liquid, e-juice) are available in a number of strengths ranging from 0 mg to 24 mg of nicotine per cartridge.[38] Increasing their attractiveness to women, as well as adolescent girls, they also come in a variety of flavors, including: apple; Boston cream pie; cherry; chocolate; clove; coffee; cola; menthol; pear; peppermint; spearmint; strawberry daiquiri; tobacco; and vanilla.

According to the Centers for Disease Control and Prevention (CDC):

> In 2014, an estimated 3.7% of U.S. adults, including 15.9% of current cigarette smokers and 22% of former cigarette smokers, currently used e-cigarettes every day or some days.
>
> *(Syamial, Jamal, & King, 2016, p. 557)*

In response to the *increasing* use of flavored tobacco products during the first decade of the new millennium, the FDA banned their use in 2009. Many states (e.g., Arizona; Maryland; New Hampshire; New Jersey) also banned the sale of electronic cigarettes to minors. However, these bans may *not* be as effective as anticipated because the e-cigarettes, as well as their liquid nicotine cartridges, are widely available for purchase over the Internet. In addition, although *not* approved

---

[36] Even when concerns are raised and, although, some issues remain unresolved (e.g., the risk posed by products that are *high* in nitrosamines), the general consensus is that "smokeless" tobacco products cause less than 10% of the toxicity associated with an equivalent use of cigarette smoking (Warner & Pollack, 2014).

[37] Propylene glycol and glycerin are generally the major pharmaceutical vehicles for most e-liquid nicotine solutions (Grana, Benowitz, & Glantz, 2014).

[38] More than 500 different brands of e-cigarettes are available over the Internet. Whereas several e-cigarette components, including nicotine solution containing cartridges, are interchangeable among similar products, others are not. Unapproved and inappropriate use of components, which are made for one e-cigarette product, for another product, may subject users to potential harm, including improper delivery of nicotine (i.e., too much or too little) and fires/explosions.

for smoking cessation by the FDA, most sampled users reported using e-cigarettes to help them *decrease* or *quit* their tobacco smoking (Foulds, Veldheer, & Berg, 2011). Healthcare professionals need to be aware that the e-cigarette, because it can deliver as much nicotine as a traditional cigarette, places users at risk for new or continued physical and psychological dependence on nicotine. All of this becomes increasingly significant when one considers that the sale or use of e-cigarettes are projected to increase by over 1,000% (i.e., tenfold) by 2030 (Electronic nicotine delivery systems, 2014).

Some additional, and still largely unresolved concerns accompany the current use of e-cigarettes. These concerns include:

1. Fires and explosions caused by the e-cigarette devices (Roger, Abayon, & Elad, 2016)[39]
2. Irritation of the mouth and throat with a related *dry cough* associated with the aerosolized glycerol and propylene glycol present in the e-cigarette aerosol formulations (Callahan-Lyon, 2014)
3. Toxicity associated with the metal nanoparticles from the vaporizing mechanism (NIDA, 2016)
4. Possible secondhand exposure, particularly to infants and children, of aerosols containing relatively *high* concentrations of nicotine (i.e., *higher* than that found in typical tobacco cigarette smoke) (Callahan-Lyon, 2014)[40]
5. Nicotine physical and psychological dependence associated with e-cigarette use (Schroeder & Hoffman, 2014)
6. Thirdhand exposure to nicotine because of e-cigarette use (Goniewicz & Lee, 2015)[41]

Hookah Use. The hookah, or water pipe, is an ancient smoking device that filters and cools inhaled smoke by drawing it through cold water. Although originally developed in the Middle East to smoke opium and cannabis, particularly hashish, it was quickly adapted to smoke tobacco or mixtures of tobacco and cannabis after tobacco was introduced to the Middle East from the U.S. during the 18th and 19th centuries.

The use of hookahs in the U.S. was relatively uncommon until the hippie days of the 1960s and 1970s. Even then their use was never particularly significant until the beginning of the new millennium when "hookah cafes" began to flourish near college/university campuses across the U.S. together with the

39 Because of this concern, in 2015 the U.S. Department of Transportation banned e-cigarette devices from being packed in checked airline baggage (Roger, Abayon, & Elad, 2016).

40 Because the e-cigarette delivery systems vary from manufacturer to manufacturer (i.e., brand to brand), some contain higher secondhand nicotine concentrations than others.

41 Thirdhand nicotine exposure refers to the nicotine vapor that remains on various surfaces (e.g., floors, tables, walls, windows) in areas where e-cigarette use is significant.

growth of Middle-Eastern communities. The tobacco traditionally smoked in a hookah is called *mu'assel* (maassel) and generally consists of a syrupy mixture of shredded tobacco leaf, flavored molasses or dried fruit, and vegetable glycol, or honey. Typical flavors include: apple; banana; coconut; grape; guava; lemon; licorice; mint; peach; rose; strawberry; and watermelon. In the U.S., the wet, flavored, and sweetened smoking mixture of tobacco is often called *shisha* (Morris, Fiala, & Pawlak, 2012).

Popular Notion: The use of a hookah eliminates virtually *all* the toxicities associated with smoking tobacco cigarettes because the smoke is filtered through water before being inhaled.

NOT TRUE.

Several undesired, or harmful, effects and toxicities are associated with smoking tobacco through a hookah, including:

1. Risk of exposure to harmful chemicals (e.g., carbon monoxide; heavy metals; and tobacco-specific nitrosamines that are *not* filtered out by the water in the hookah (Shihadeh, 2003)
2. Risk of exposure to infectious diseases (e.g., *Helicobacter pylori*; hepatitis; influenza; oral herpes; and tuberculosis) among women, who share the same hookah

In addition, tobacco smoking with a hookah does *not* filter out the nicotine from the smoke. Therefore, smokers are at risk for any nicotine-related toxicity, including physical and psychological dependence (i.e., nicotine *addiction*). Despite these documented toxicities, most young women and men, who smoke tobacco using a hookah, believe it is much safer than smoking tobacco cigarettes (Asfar, Ward, & Eissenberg, 2005; Pagliaro & Pagliaro, *Clinical Patient Data Files*). The *method* of hookah smoking also contributes to other potential toxicities associated with nicotine. For example, hookah smokers puff *more* often, inhale *more* deeply, and smoke for *longer* periods of time during each smoking session.[42] In fact, a typical 1-hour hookah smoking session has been estimated to involve approximately 200 puffs, or 10 times the puffs inhaled when smoking a typical tobacco cigarette (i.e., a typical hookah smoking session is, in this regard, equivalent to smoking approximately 10 filter-tipped tobacco cigarettes) (Hays, 2015; Sathya, 2014).

[42] Methods used for smoking tobacco through a hookah are similar, in many ways, to those used for smoking cannabis with a hookah.

In the U.S., hookah smoking of both tobacco and cannabis, alone or in combination, is relatively common, particularly among young women and men with approximately 20% of high school seniors reporting hookah use within the past year and up to 40% of U.S. college/university students reporting hookah use within the past year (Palamar, Zhou, & Sherman, 2014; Sathya, 2014). Hookah smoking is *highest* among young women and men, 18 to 24 years-of-age and, within this group, particularly those of European descent and Middle-Eastern descent (American Lung Association, 2007).

In response to the steady and rapid *increase* in the use of both e-cigarettes and hookahs for the delivery of nicotine during the new millennium, the FDA extended its full control over the devices in 2016 (U.S. Food and Drug Administration, 2016). Consequently, nationwide tobacco regulations currently extend to *all* tobacco products, including:

- Cigars
- E-cigarettes and their liquid, nicotine solutions
- Hookah tobacco
- Pipe tobacco

(NIDA, 2016)

References[43,44,45]

Abbot, L. C., & Winzer-Serhan, U. H. (2012). Smoking during pregnancy: Lessons learned from epidemiological studies using animal models. *Critical Reviews in Toxicology*, 42(4), 279–303. doi:10.3109/10408444.2012.658506

About Turbo Snort Caffenated Nasal Spray. (2014, December 27). Retrieved December 27, 2016, from Turbo Snort, p. 1: www.turbosnort.com/About_Turbo_Snort.html

Adams, S. (2011, July 7). *Mothers-to-be smoking for smaller babies.* Retrieved March 5, 2016, from Telegraph Media Group, pp. 1–2: www.telegraph.co.uk/news/health/news/8623267/Mothers-to-be-smoking-for-smaller-babies.html

Addicott, M. A. (2014). Caffeine use disorder: A review of the evidence and future implications. *Current Addiction Reports*, 1(3), 186–192. doi:10.1007/s40429-014-0024-9

---

[43] As per publisher style, only the first three authors are listed for each reference.

[44] Several times the number of references listed were found, obtained, and analyzed by the authors during the preparation of this chapter. However, only the references that were cited at least once in the body of the text are included in the list. Major reasons for not citing other references, include that they: (1) did not provide any additional unique data; (2) were not well researched or written (i.e., were evaluated as not being valid or reliable); (3) were based predominantly, or exclusively, on animal studies; (4) provided usage statistics from outside the U.S.; and/or (5) were redundant with, or not as recent as, the already cited references.

[45] The reference citation, "Pagliaro & Pagliaro, *Clinical Patient Data Files*," refers to unpublished data collected, with permission, over the last 50 years by the authors, in the formal course of their professional academic roles as clinician scientists and professors—from their patients, research subjects, and students, from the 1970s to date.

Agaku, I. T., King, B. A., & Husten, C. G. (2014, June 27). Tobacco product use among adults—United States, 2012–2013. *Morbidity and Mortality Weekly Report (MMWR)*, 63(25), 542–547.

American Lung Association. (2007, February). *Tobacco policy trend alert. An emerging deadly trend: Waterpipe tobacco use.* Retrieved June 12, 2016, from lungusa.org, pp. 1–8: www.lungusa.org

Appleby, B. S., & Cummings, J. L. (2013). Discovering new treatments for Alzheimer's disease by repurposing approved medications. *Current Topics in Medicinal Chemistry*, 13(18), 2306–2327.

Araki, H., Suemaru, K., & Gomita, Y. (2002). Neuronal nicotinic receptor and psychiatric disorders: Functional and behavioral effects of nicotine. *The Japanese Journal of Pharmacology*, 88(2), 133–138.

Aranda, J. V., Beharry, K., & Valencia, G. B. (2010). Caffeine impact on neonatal morbidities. *The Journal of Maternal-Fetal & Neonatal Medicine*, 23(Supplement 3), 20–23. doi:10.3109/14767058.2010.517704

Arria, A. M., Caldeira, K. M., & Kasperski, S. J. (2011). Energy drink consumption and increased risk for alcohol dependence. *Alcoholism: Clinical and Experimental Research*, 35(2), 365–375. doi:10.1111/j.1530-0277.2010.01352.x

Artin, B., Singh, M., & Richeh, C. (2010). Caffeine-related atrial fibrillation. *American Journal of Therapeutics*, 17(5), e169–e171. doi:10.1097/MJT.0b013e3181df8cf8

Asfar, T., Ward, K. D., & Eissenberg, T. (2005, February 25). Comparison of patterns of use, beliefs, and attitudes related to waterpipe between beginning and established smokers. *BMC Public Health*, 5, 19.

Astorino, T. A., Matera, A. J., & Basinger, J. (2012). Effects of red bull energy drink on repeated sprint performance in women athletes. *Amino Acids*, 42(5), 1803–1808.

Attwood, A. S., Rogers, P. J., & Ataya, A. F. (2012). Effects of caffeine on alcohol-related changes in behavioural control and perceived intoxication in light caffeine consumers. *Psychopharmacology (Berlin)*, 221(4), 551–560. doi:10.1007/s00213-02112-2601-0

Aubrey, A. (2012, March 7). *Inhalable caffeine maker gets warning letter from FDA.* Retrieved October 6, 2016, from The Salt: NPR: www.npr.org/sections/thesalt/2012/03/07/1481611621/inhalable-caffeine-maker-gets-warning-letter-from-fda

Audrain-McGovern, J., & Benowitz, N. L. (2011). Cigarette smoking, nicotine, and body weight. *Clinical Pharmacology & Therapeutics*, 90(1), 164–168. doi:10.1038/clpt.2011.105

Barrett-Connor, E., Chang, J. C., & Edelstein, S. L. (1994). Coffee-associated osteoporosis offset by daily milk consumption. The Rancho Bernardo Study. *JAMA, Journal of the American Medical Association*, 271(4), 280–283.

Beedie, C. J. (2010). All in the mind? Pain, placebo effect, and ergogenic effect of caffeine in sports performance. *Open Access Journal of Sports Medicine*. 1, 87–94.

Benowitz, N. L. (1999). Biomarkers of environmental tobacco smoke exposure. *Environmental Health Perspectives*, 107(Supplement 2), 349–355.

Beral, V., Gaitskell, K., & Hermon, C. (2012). Ovarian cancer and smoking: Individual participant meta-analysis including 28,114 women with ovarian cancer from 51 epidemiological studies. *The Lancet Oncology*, 13(9), 946–956. doi:10.1016/S1470-2045(12)70322–4

Bergin, J. E., & Kendler, K. S. (2012). Common psychiatric disorders and caffeine use, tolerance, and withdrawal: An examination of shared genetic and environmental effects. *Twin Research and Human Genetics*, 15(4), 473–482. doi:10.1017/thg.2012.25

Biessels, G. J. (2010). Caffeine, diabetes, cognition, and dementia. *Journal of Alzheimer's Disease*, 20(Supplement 1), S143–S150. doi:10.3233/JAD-2010–091228

Bigard, A. X. (2010). Risks of energy drinks in youths. *Archives de Pediatrie*, 17(11), 1625–1631. doi:10.1016/j.arcped.2010.08.001

Body, J., Bergmann, P., & Boonen, S. (2011, March 1). Non-pharmacological management of osteoporosis: A consensus of the Belgian Bone Club. *Osteoporosos International*, 22, 2769–2788. doi:10.1007/s00198-011-1545-x

Bracken, M. B., Triche, E. W., & Belanger, K. (2003). Association of maternal caffeine consumption with decrements in fetal growth. *American Journal of Epidemiology*, 157(5), 456–466.

Brent, R. L., Christian, M. S., & Diener, R. M. (2011). Evaluation of the reproductive and developmental risks of caffeine. *Birth Defects Research. Part B, Developmental and Reproductive Toxicology*, 92(2), 152–187.

Brice, C. F., & Smith, A. P. (2002). Effects of caffeine on mood and performance: A study of realistic consumption. *Psychopharmacology (Berlin)*, 164(2), 188–192. doi:10.1007/s00213-002-1175-2

Brown, C. J., & Cheng, J. M. (2014). Electronic cigarettes: Product characterisation and considerations. *Tobacco Control*, 23(Supplement 2), 4–10. doi:10.1136/tobaccocontrol-2013–051476

Browne, M. L., Hoyt, A. T., & Feldkamp, M. L. (2011). Maternal caffeine intake and risk of selected birth defects in the National Birth Defects Prevention Study. *Birth Defects Research Part A: Clinical and Molecular Teratology*, 91(2), 93–101. doi:10.1002/bdra.20752

Buckner, J. D., & Vinci, C. (2013). Smoking and social anxiety: The roles of gender and smoking motives. *Addictive Behaviors*, 38(8), 2388–2391. doi:10.1016/j.addbeh,2013.03.007

Budney, A. J., Lee, D. C., & Juliano, L. M. (2015). Evaluating the validity of caffeine use disorder. *Current Psychiatry Reports*, 17(9), 74. doi:10.1007/s11920-015-0611-z

Buisson, B., & Bertrand, D. (2002). Nicotine addiction: The possible role of functional upregulation. *Trends in Pharmacological Sciences*, 23(3), 130–136. doi:10.1016/S0165-6147(00)01979-9

Butt, M. S., & Sultan, M. T. (2011). Coffee and its consumption: Benefits and risks. *Critical Reviews in Food Science and Nutrition*, 51(4), 363–373. doi:10.1080/10408390903586412

Callahan-Lyon, P. (2014). Electronic cigarettes: Human health effects. *Tobacco Control*, 23(Supplement 2), 36–40. doi:10.1136/tobaccocontrol-2013–051470

Campos, H., & Baylin, A. (2007). Coffee consumption and risk of type 2 diabetes and heart disease. *Nutrition Reviews*, 65(4), 173–179.

Carter, B. D., Abnet, C. C., & Feskanich, D. (2015). Smoking and mortality—Beyond established causes. *The New England Journal of Medicine*, 372(7), 631–640. doi:10.1056/NEJMsa1407211

CDC, Centers for Disease Control and Prevention. (2002, August 30). Women and smoking: A report of the Surgeon General (executive summary). *MMWR Morbidity and Mortality Weekly Report*, 51(RR12), 1–30.

CDC, Centers for Disease Control and Prevention. (2010). Vital signs: Nonsmokers' exposure to secondhand smoke—United States, 1999–2008. *MMWR Morbidity and Mortality Weekly Report*, 59(35), 1141–1146. Retrieved October 7, 2016, from www.cdc.gov/mmwr/preview/mmwrhtml/mm5935a4.htm

CDC, Centers for Disease Control and Prevention. (2012, January 25). PRAMS and smoking. Division of Reproductive Health, National Center for Chronic Disease Prevention and Health Promotion.

CDC, Centers for Disease Control and Prevention. (2015). Vital signs: Disparities in nonsmokers' exposure to secondhand smoke—United States, 1999–2012. *MMWR Morbidity and Mortality Weekly Report*, 64(4), 103–108. Retrieved from www.cdc.gov/mmwr/preview/mmwrhtml/mm6404a7.htm?s_cid=mm6404a7_w

CDC, Centers for Disease Control and Prevention. (2016a, February 17). Secondhand Smoke (SHS) Facts. *Fact Sheets*. Retrieved from www.cdc.gov/chronicdisease/

CDC, Centers for Disease Control and Prevention. (2016b, October 5). Ellie's Story. 1. Centers for Disease Control and Prevention. Retrieved November 11, 2016, from www.cdc.gov/tobacco/campaign/tips/quit-smoking/index.html?s_cid=OSH_tips_D9317

CDC, Centers for Disease Control and Prevention. (2016c, September 28). Becky's Story. 1. Centers for Disease Control and Prevention. Retrieved November 11, 2016, from www.cdc.gov/tobacco/campaign/tips/quit-smoking/index.html?s_cid=OSH_tips_D9317

CDC, Centers for Disease Control and Prevention. (2016d, October 22). Rose's Story. 1. Retrieved November 11, 2016, from www.cdc.gov/tobacco/campaign/tips/quit-smoking/index.html?s_cid=OSH_tips_D9317

CDC, Centers for Disease Control and Prevention. (2016e, October 12). Rebecca's Story. 1. Centers for Disease Control and Prevention. Retrieved November 11, 2016, from www.cdc.gov/tobacco/campaign/tips/quit-smoking/index.html?s_cid=OSH_tips_D9317

CDC, Centers for Disease Control and Prevention. (2016f, December 30). National Health Interview Survey. CDC/National Center for Health Statistics. Retrieved from www.cdc.gov/nchs/nhis/nhis_listserv.htm

Chang, R. C., Ho, Y. S., & Wong, S. (2014). Neuropathology of cigarette smoking. *Acta Neuropathologica*, 127(1), 53–69. doi:10.1007/s00401-013-1210-x

Chen, L., Bell, E. M., & Browne, M. L. (2014). Exploring maternal patterns of dietary caffeine consumption before conception and during pregnancy. *Maternal and Child Health Journal*, 18(10), 2446–2455. doi:10.1007/s10995-014-1483-2

Chiolero, A., Faeh, D., & Paccaud, F. (2008). Consequences of smoking for body weight, body fat distribution, and insulin resistance. *The American Journal of Clinical Nutrition*, 87(4), 801–809.

Christian, M. S., & Brent, R. L. (2001). Teratogen update: Evaluation of the reproductive and developmental risks of caffeine. *Teratology*, 64(1), 51–78. doi:10.1002/tera.1047

Cleary, K., Levine, D. A., & Hoffman, R. S. (2012). Adolescents and young adults presenting to the emergency department intoxicated from a caffeinated alcoholic beverage: A case series. *Annals of Emergency Medicine*, 59(1), 67–69. doi:10.1016/j.annemergmed.2011.06.015

Collins, A. C. (1990). An analysis of the addiction liability of nicotine. *Advances in Alcohol & Substance Abuse*, 9(1–2), 83–101. Retrieved from www.tandfonline.com/doi/abs/10.1300/J251v09n01_06

Czogala, J., Goniewicz, M. L., & Fidelus, B. (2014). Secondhand exposure to vapors from electronic cigarettes. *Nicotine & Tobacco Research*, 16(6), 655–662. doi:10.1093/ntr/ntt203

D'Alessandro, A., Boeckelmann, I., & Hammwhoner, M. (2012). Nicotine, cigarette smoking and cardiac arrhythmia: An overview. *European Journal of Preventive Cardiology*, 19(3), 297–305.

Danaei, G., Ding, E. L., & Mozaffarian, D. (2009). The preventable causes of death in the United States: Comparative risk assessment of dietary, lifestyle, and metabolic risk factors. *PLoS Medicine*, 6(4), e1000058. doi:10.1371/journal.pmed.1000058

Dani, J. A., & De Biasi, M. (2001). Cellular mechanisms of nicotine addiction. *Pharmacology Biochemistry and Behavior*, 70(4), 439–446.

Dani, J. A., Ji, D., & Zhou, F. M. (2001). Synaptic plasticity and nicotine addiction. *Neuron*, 31(3), 349–352.

Davis, J. K., & Green, J. M. (2009). Caffeine and anaerobic performance: Ergogenic value and mechanisms of action. *Sports Medicine*, 39(10), 813–832. doi:10.2165/11317770-000000000-00000

De Genna, N. M., Goldschmidt, L., & Day, N. L. (2016). Maternal trajectories of cigarette use as a function of maternal age and race. *Addictive Behaviors*, 65, 33–39. doi:10.1016/j.addbeh.2016.09.011

Degens, H., Gayan-Ramirez, G., & van Hees, H. W. (2015). Smoking-induced skeletal muscle dysfunction: From evidence to mechanisms. *American Journal of Respiratory and Critical Care Medicine*, 191(6), 620–625. doi:10.1164/rccm.201410-1830PP

Derby, K. S., Cuthrell, K., & Caberto, C. (2008). Nicotine metabolism in three ethnic/racial groups with different risks of lung cancer. *Cancer Epidemiology, Biomarkers & Prevention*, 17(12), 3526–3535. doi:10.1158/1055-9965.EPI-08-0424

Dews, P. B., O'Brien, C. P., & Bergman, J. (2002). Caffeine: Behavioral effects of withdrawal and related issues. *Food and Chemical Toxicology*, 40(9), 1257–1261.

Di Rocco, J. R., During, A., & Morelli, P. J. (2011). Atrial fibrillation in healthy adolescents after highly caffeinated beverage consumption: Two case reports. *Journal of Medical Case Reports*, 5, 18. doi:10.1186/1752-1947-5-18

Dik, V. K., Bueno-de-Mesquita, H. B., & Van Oijen, M. G. (2014). Coffee and tea consumption, genotype-based CYP1A2 and NAT2 activity and colorectal cancer risk-results from the EPIC cohort study. *International Journal of Cancer*, 135(2), 401–412. doi:10.1002/ijc.28655

Ding, Y. S., Yan, X. J., & Jain, R. B. (2006). Determination of 14 polycyclic aromatic hydrocarbons in mainstream smoke from U.S. brand and non-U.S. brand cigarettes. *Environmental Science & Technology*, 40(4), 1133–1138.

Doo, T., Morimoto, Y., & Steinbrecher, A. (2014). Coffee intake and risk of type 2 diabetes: the Multiethnic Cohort. *Public Health Nutrition*, 17(6), 1328–1336.

Duncan, M. J., Lyons, M., & Hankey, J. (2009). Placebo effects of caffeine on short-term resistance exercise to failure. *International Journal of Sports Physiology and Performance*, 4(2), 244–253.

Durazzo, T. C., Mattsson, N., & Weiner, M. W. (2014). Smoking and increased Alzheimer's disease risk: A review of potential mechanisms. *Alzheimer's & Dementia*, 10(3 Supplement), S122–S145. doi:10.1016/j.jalz.2014.04.009

Electronic nicotine delivery systems. (2014, July 21). *World Health Organization to 6th Session of the Conference of the Parties to the WHO Framework Convention on Tobacco Control*, pp. 2–3. doi:fctc/PDF/cop6/fctc_COP6_10-en.pdf?ua=1

England, L. J., Aagaard, K., & Bloch, M. (2017). Developmental toxicity of nicotine: A transdisciplinary synthesis and implications for emerging tobacco products. *Neuroscience & Biobehavioral Reviews*, 72, 176–189. doi: 10.1016/j.neubiorev.2016.11.013

Ernst, M., Moolchan, E. T., & Robinson, M. L. (2001). Behavioral and neural consequences of prenatal exposure to nicotine. *Journal of the American Academy of Child & Adolescent Psychiatry*, 40(6), 630–641.

Fagan, P., Moolchan, E. T., & Pokhrel, P. (2015). Biomarkers of tobacco smoke exposure in racial/ethnic groups at high risk for lung cancer. *American Journal of Public Health*, 105(6), 1237–1245. doi:10.2105/AJPH.2014.302492

FDA. (2012, March 6). *Press Announcements > FDA issues warning letter to makers of AeroShot "caffeine inhaler."* Retrieved October 5, 2016, from FDA Press Statement: www.fda.gov/NewsEvents/Newsroom/PressAnnouncements/ucm294874.htm

Ferrara, C. M., Kumar, M., & Nicklas, B. (2001). Weight gain and adipose tissue metabolism after smoking cessation in women. *International Journal of Obesity*, 25, 1322–1326.

Food Standards Agency. (2008, November 3). Foods Standards Agency publishes new caffeine advice for pregnant women. *Press Release*. Retrieved from http://tna.europarchive.org/20111116080332/www.food.gov.uk/news/pressreleases/2008/nov/caffeineadvice

Forray, A., Gotman, N., & Kershaw, T. (2014). Perinatal smoking and depression in women with concurrent substance use. *Addictive Behaviors*, 39(4), 749–756. doi:10.1016/j.addbeh.20123.12.008

Forster, J., Poupart, J., & Rhodes, K. (2016). Cigarette smoking among urban American Indian adults—Hennepin and Ramsey counties, Minnesota, 2011. *MMWR, Morbidity and Mortality Weekly Report*, 65(21), 534–537.

Foulds, J., Veldheer, S., & Berg, A. (2011). Electronic cigarettes (e-cigs): Views of aficionados and clinical/public health perspectives. *International Journal of Clinical Practice*, 65(10), 1037–1042. doi:10.1111/j.1742-1241.2011.02751.x

Fu, S. S., McFall, M., & Saxon, A. J. (2007). Post-traumatic stress disorder and smoking: A systemic review. *Nicotine & Tobacco Research*, 9(11), 1071–1084. doi:10.1080/14622200701488418

Fulgoni III, V. L., Keast, D. R., & Lieberman, H. R. (2015). Trends in intake and sources of caffeine in the diets of US adults: 2001–2010. *American Journal of Clinical Nutrition*, 101(5), 1081–1087. doi:10.3945/ajcn.113.080077

Gamaleddin, I. H., Trigo, J. M., & Gueye, A. B. (2015). Role of endogenous cannabinoid system in nicotine addiction: Novel insights. *Frontiers in Psychiatry*, 6(Article 41), 1–2. doi:10.3389/psyt.2015.00041

Ganmaa, D., Willett, W. C., & Feskanich, D. (2008). Coffee, tea, caffeine and risk of breast cancer: a 22-year follow-up. *International Journal of Cancer*, 122(9), 2071–2076. doi:10.1002/ijc.23336

Gierach, G. L., Freedman, N. D., & Andaya, A. (2012). Coffee intake and breast cancer risk in the NIH-AARP diet and health study cohort. *International Journal of Cancer*, 131(2), 452–460. doi:10.1002/ijc.26372

Goniewicz, M. L., & Lee, L. (2015). Electronic cigarettes are a source of thirdhand exposure to nicotine. *Nicotine & Tobacco Research*, 17(2), 256–258. doi:10.1093/ntr/ntu152

Goodwin, R. D., Keyes, K. M., & Hasin, D. S. (2009). Changes in cigarette use and nicotine dependence in the United States: Evidence from the 2001–2002 wave of the National Epidemiologic Survey of Alcoholism and Related Conditions. *American Journal of Public Health*, 99(8), 1471–1477.

Graham, T. E. (2001). Caffeine and exercise: Metabolism, endurance and performance. *Sports Medicine*, 31(11), 785–807.

Grana, R., Benowitz, N., & Glantz, S. A. (2014, May 13). Contemporary reviews in cardiovascular medicine: E-Cigarettes: A scientific review. *Circulation*, 129, 1972–1986. Dallas, TX: American Heart Association. doi:10.116/CIRCULATIONAHA.114007667, p.1978

Greenberg, J. A., Boozer, C. N., & Geliebter, A. (2006). Coffee, diabetes, and weight control. *The American Journal of Clinical Nutrition*, 84(4), 682–693.

Guais, A., Brand, G., & Jacquot, L. (2011). Toxicity of carbon dioxide: A review. *Chemical Research in Toxicology*, 24(12), 2061–2070. doi:10.1021/tx200220r

Hahn, B. (2015). Nicotinic receptors and attention. *Current Topics in Behavioral Neurosciences*, 23, 103–135. doi:10.1007/978-3-319-13665-3_5

Hahn, K. A., Wise, L. A., & Rothman, K. J. (2015). Caffeine and caffeinated beverage consumption and risk of spontaneous abortion. *Human Reproduction*, 30(5), 1246–1255. doi:10.1093/humrep/dev063

Hallstrom, H., Byberg, L., & Glynn, A. (2013). Long-term coffee consumption in relation to fracture risk and bone mineral density in women. *American Journal of Epidemiology*, 178(6), 898–909. doi:10.1093/aje/kwt062

Hallstrom, H., Wolk, A., & Glynn, A. (2006). Coffee, tea and caffeine consumption in relation to osteoporotic fracture risk in a cohort of Swedish women. *Osteoporosis International*, 17(7), 1055–1064.

Hansen, S. A., Folsom, A. R., & Kushi, L. H. (2000). Association of fractures with caffeine and alcohol in postmenopausal women: The Iowa Women's Health Study. *Public Health Nutrition*, 3(3), 253–261.

Harter, D. L., Busnello, F. M., & Dibi, R. P. (2013). Association between low bone mass and calcium and caffeine intake among perimenopausal women in Southern Brazil: Cross-sectional study. *Sao Paulo Medical Journal*, 131(5), 315–322. doi:10.1590/1516-3180.2013.1315428

Hartz, S. M., Short, S. E., & Saccone, N. L. (2012). Increased genetic vulnerability to smoking at CHRNA5 in early-onset smokers. *Archives of General Psychiatry*, 69(8), 854–860. doi:10.1001/archgenpsychiatry.2012.124

Hays, J. T. (2015, June 17). *Is hookah smoking safer than cigarette smoking?* Retrieved April 13, 2016, from Mayo Clinic, pp.1–3: www.mayoclinic.org/healthy-lifestyle/quit-smoking/expert-answers/hookah/faq-20057920?p=1

Hecht, S. S. (2014). It is time to regulate carcinogenic tobacco-specific nitrosamines in cigarette tobacco. *Cancer Prevention Research*, 7(7), 639–647. doi:10.1158/1940–6207.CAPR-14-0095

Heckman, M. A., Weil, J., & Gonzalez de Mejia, E. (2010). Caffeine (1,3,7-trimethylxanthine) in foods: A comprehensive review on consumption, functionality, safety, and regulatory matters. *Journal of Food Science*, 75(3), R77-R87. doi:10.1111/j.1750-3841.2010.01561.x

Heeschen, C., Weis, M., & Aicher, A. (2002). A novel angiogenic pathway mediated by non-neuronal nicotinic acetylcholine receptors. *Journal of Clinical Investigation*, 110(4), 527–536. doi:10.1172/JCI14676

Henley, S. J., Thomas, C. C., & Sharapova, S. R. (2016). Vital signs: Disparities in tobacco-related cancer incidence and mortality—United States, 2004–2013. *MMWR Morbidity and Mortality Weekly Report*, 65, 1212–1218. Retrieved from http://dx.doi.org/10.15585/mmwr.mm6544a3

Hoffmann, D., & Hoffmann, I. (1997). The changing cigarette, 1950–1995. *Journal of Toxicology and Environmental Health*, 50(4), 307–364.

Hu, S. S., Neff, L., & Agaku, I. T. (2016). Tobacco product use among adults—United States, 2013–2014. *MMWR Morbidity and Mortality Weekly Report*, 65, 685–691. doi:10.15585/mmwr.mm6527a1

Huntley, E. D., & Juliano, L. M. (2012). Caffeine expectancy questionnaire (CaffEQ): Construction, psychometric properties, and associations with caffeine use, caffeine dependence, and other related variables. *Psychological Assessment*, 24(3), 592–607. doi:10.1037/a0026417

Hyde, R. F., Paxton, R., & Carr, T. E. (1982, September 18). Nicotine chewing-gum. *British Medical Journal (Clinical Research Edition)*, 285(6344), 811–812.

Jackson, D. A., Cotter, B. V., & Merchant, R. C. (2013). Behavioral and physiologic adverse effects in adolescent and young adult emergency department patients reporting use of energy drinks and caffeine. *American Academy of Clinical Toxicology*, 51(7), 557–565. doi:10.3109/15563650.2013.820311

Jalonick, M. C. (2012, March 6). *FDA issues warning to inhalable caffeine maker.* Retrieved October 6, 2016, from The San Diego Union-Tribune: www.sandiegouniontribune.com/sdut-fda-issues-warning-to-inhalable-caffeine-maker-2012mar06-story.html

Jamal, A., King, B. A., & Neff, L. J. (2016). Current cigarette smoking among adults—United States, 2005–2015. *MMWR Morbidity and Mortality Weekly Report*, 65, 1205–1211. Retrieved from http://dx.doi.org/1015585/mmwr.mm6544a2

Jessup, M. A., Dibble, S. L., & Cooper, B. A. (2012). Smoking and behavioral health of women. *Journal of Women's Health*, 21(7), 783–791. doi:10.1089/jwh.2011.2886

Jiang, W., Wu, Y., & Jiang, X. (2013). Coffee and caffeine intake and breast cancer risk: An updated dose-response meta-analysis of 37 published studies. *Gynecologic Oncology*, 129(3), 620–629. doi:10.1016/j.ygyno.2013.03.014

Johnson, J. L., Ratner, P. A., & Malchy, L. A. (2010). Gender-specific profiles of tobacco use among non-institutionalized people with serious mental illness. *BMC Psychiatry*, 10(101), 1–12. Retrieved from www.biomedcentral.com/1471-244X/10/101

Johnson, K. C. (2001). Re: Passive smoking exposure and female breast cancer mortality. *JNCI, Journal of the National Cancer Institute*, 93(9), 719–720.

Johnston, K. L., Clifford, M. N., & Morgan, L. M. (2003). Coffee acutely modifies gastrointestinal hormone secretion and glucose tolerance in humans: Glycemic effects of chlorogenic acid and caffeine. *The American Journal of Clinical Nutrition*, 78(4), 728–733.

Juliano, L. M., Evatt, D. P., & Richards, P. D. (2012). Characterization of individuals seeking treatment for caffeine dependence. *Psychology of Addictive Behaviors*, 26(4), 948–954. doi:10.1037/a0027246

Juliano, L. M., & Griffiths, R. R. (2004). A critical review of caffeine withdrawal: Empirical validation of symptoms and signs, incidence, severity, and associated features. *Psychopharmacology (Berlin)*, 176, 1–29. doi:10.1007/s00213-004-2000-x

Kasza, K. A., Ambrose, B. K., & Conway, K. P. (2017, January 26). Tobacco-product use by adults and youths in the United States in 2013 and 2014. *The New England Journal of Medicine*, 376, 342–353.

Keisler, B. D., & Armsey 2nd, T. D. (2006). Caffeine as an ergogenic aid. *Current Sports Medicine Reports*, 5(4), 215–219.

Kenny, P. J., & Markou, A. (2001). Neurobiology of the nicotine withdrawal syndrome. *Pharmacology Biochemistry and Behavior*, 70(4), 531–549.

Kimura, R., Ushiyama, N., & Fujii, T. (2003). Nicotine-induced Ca2+ signaling and down-regulation of nicotinic acetylcholine receptor subunit expression in the CEM human leukemic T-cell line. *Life Sciences*, 72(18–19), 2155–2158.

Kinsaul, J. A., & Copeland, A. L. (2013). The role of telescoping in the development of smoking in women. In J. Marich (Ed.), *The psychology of women: Diverse perspectives from the modern world. Psychology of emotions, motivations and actions* (pp. 109–123). Hauppauge, NY: Nova Science.

Kinugawa, T., Kurita, T., & Nohara, R. (2011). A case of atrial tachycardia sensitive to increased caffeine intake. *International Heart Journal*, 52(6), 398–400.

Klatsky, A. L., Hasan, A. S., & Armstrong, M. A. (2011, Summer). Coffee, caffeine, and risk of hospitalization for arrhythmias. *The Permanente Journal*, 15(3), 19–25.

Kudlow, P. A., Naylor, K. T., & Xie, B. (2013). Cognitive enhancement in Canadian medical students. *Journal of Psychoactive Drugs*, 45(4), 360–365.

Kuper, H., Boffetta, P., & Adami, H. O. (2002). Tobacco use and cancer causation: Association by tumour type. *Journal of Internal Medicine*, 252(3), 206–224.

Lara, B., Gonzalez-Millan, C., & Salinero, J. J. (2014). Caffeine-containing energy drink improves physical performance in female soccer players. *Amino Acids*, 46(5), 1385–1392. doi:10.1007/s00726-014-1709-z

Lemke, R. P. (2002). Drug dosing for neonates. In L. A. Pagliaro, & A. M. Pagliaro (Eds.), *Problems in pediatric drug therapy* (4th ed., pp. 531–554). Hamilton, IL: American Pharmaceutical Association.

Li, J., Zhao, H., & Song, J. M. (2015). A meta-analysis of risk of pregnancy loss and caffeine and coffee consumption during pregnancy. *International Journal of Gynaecology & Obstetrics*, 130(2), 116–122. doi:10.1016/j.ijgo.2015.03.033

Lieberman, H. R., Stavinoha, T., & McGraw, S. (2012). Caffeine use among active duty US Army soldiers. *Journal of the Academy of Nutrition and Dietetics*, 112(6), 902–912. doi:10.1016/j.jand.2012.02.001

Loopstra-Masters, R. C., Liese, A. D., & Haffner, S. M. (2011). Associations between the intake of caffeinated and decaffeinated coffee and measures of insulin sensitivity and beta cell function. *Diabetologia*, 54(2), 320–328. doi:10.1007/s00125-010-12957-8

Lorist, M. M., & Tops, M. (2003). Caffeine, fatigue, and cognition. *Brain and Cognition*, 53(1), 82–94.

Lucas, M., Mirzaei, F., & Pan, A. (2011). Coffee, caffeine, and risk of depression among women. *Archives of Internal Medicine*, 171(17), 1571–1578. doi:10.1001/archinternmed.2011.393

Lucas, M., O'Reilly, E. J., & Pan, A. (2014). Coffee, caffeine, and risk of completed suicide: Results from three prospective cohorts of American adults. *World Journal of Biological Psychiatry*, 15(5), 377–386. doi:10.3109/15622975.2013.795243

Marczinski, C. A. (2015). Can energy drinks increase desire for more alcohol? *Advances in Nutrition*, 6(1), 96–101. doi:10.3945/an.114.007393

Marczinski, C. A., & Fillmore, M. T. (2014). Energy drinks mixed with alcohol: What are the risks? *Nutrition Reviews*, 72(1), 98–107. doi:10.1111/nure.12127

Marczinski, C. A., Fillmore, M. T., & Bardgett, M. E. (2011). Effects of energy drinks mixed with alcohol on behavioral control: Risks for college students consuming trendy cocktails. *Alcoholism: Clinical and Experimental Research*, 35(7), 1282–1292. doi:10.1111/j.1530-0277.2011.01464.x

Marczinski, C. A., Fillmore, M. T., & Henges, A. L. (2012). Effects of energy drinks mixed with alcohol on information processing, motor coordination and subjective reports of intoxication. *Experimental and Clinical Psychopharmacology*, 20(2), 129–138. doi:10.1037/a0026136

Maritz, G. S. (2008). Nicotine and lung development. *Birth Defects Research Part C: Embryo Today: Reviews*, 84(1), 45–53. doi:10.1002/bdrc.20116

Maritz, G. S., & Harding, R. (2011). Life-long programming implications of exposure to tobacco smoking and nicotine before and soon after birth: Evidence for altered lung development. *International Journal of Environmental Research and Public Health*, 8(3), 875–898. doi:10.3390/ijerph8030875

Mathews, T. J. (2016, June 10). QuickStats: Smoking cessation during pregnancy—46 States and the District of Columbia. *MMWR, Morbidity and Mortality Weekly Report*, 65(22), 588. doi:10.15585/mmwr.mm6522a6

Mattson, M. E. (2013, January 10). *Update on emergency department visits involving energy drinks: A continuing public health concern.* Retrieved October 6, 2016, from www.ncbi.nlm.gov/pubmed/27606410

McHugh, R. K., Wigderson, S., & Greenfield, S. F. (2014). Epidemiology of substance use in reproductive-age women. *Obstetrics & Gynecology Clinics of North America*, 41(2), 177–189. doi:10.1016/j.ogc.2014.02.001

McKetin, R., Coen, A., & Kaye, S. (2015, June 1). A comprehensive review of the effects of mixing caffeinated energy drinks with alcohol. *Drug and Alcohol Dependence*, 151, 15–30. doi:10.1016/j.drugalcdep.2015.01.047

McLaughlin, I., Dani, J. A., & De Biasi, M. (2015). Nicotine withdrawal. *Current Topics in Behavioral Neurosciences*, 24, 99–123. doi:10.1007/978-3-319-13482-6_4

Meredith, S. E., Juliano, J. L., & Hughes, J. R. (2013). Caffeine use disorder: A comprehensive review and research agenda. *Journal of Caffeine Research*, 3(3), 114–130. doi:10.1089/jcr.20123.0016

Mitchell, D. C., Knight, C. A., & Hockenberry, J. (2014). Beverage caffeine intakes in the U.S. *Food and Clinical Toxicology*, 63, 136–142.

Moon, R. Y., Darnall, R. A., & Goodstein, M. H. (2011). SIDS and other sleep-related infant deaths: Expansion of recommendations for a safe infant sleeping environment. *Pediatrics*, 128(5), 1030–1039. doi:10.1542/peds.2011–2284

Mora-Rodriguez, R., & Pallares, J. G. (2014). Performance outcomes and unwanted side effects associated with energy drinks. *Nutrition Reviews*, 72(Supplement 1), 108–120. doi:10.1111/nure.12132

Moran-Santa Maria, M. M., Flanagan, J., & Brady, K. (2014). Ovarian hormones and drug abuse. *Current Psychiatry Reports*, 16(11), 511. doi: 10.1007/s11920-014-0511-7

Morisano, D., Bacher, I., & Audrain-McGovern, J. (2009). Mechanisms underlying the comorbidity of tobacco use in mental health and addictive disorders. *Canadian Journal of Psychiatry*, 54(6), 356–367.

Morris, D. S., Fiala, S. C., & Pawlak, R. (2012). Opportunities for policy interventions to reduce youth hookah smoking in the United States. *Preventing Chronic Disease*, 9, E165. doi:10.5888/pcd9.120082

Mostofsky, E., Schlaug, G., & Mukamal, K. J. (2010). Coffee and acute ischemic stroke onset: The Stroke Onset Study. *Neurology*, 75(18), 1583–1588. doi:10.1212/WNL.0b013e3181fb443d

Nagata, C., Mizoue, T., & Tanaka, K. (2006). Tobacco smoking and breast cancer risk: An evaluation based on a systematic review of epidemiological evidence among the Japanese population. *Japanese Journal of Clinical Oncology*, 36(6), 387–394. doi:10.1093/jjco/hyl031

Nawrot, P., Jordan, S., & Eastwood, J. (2003). Effects of caffeine on human health. *Food Additives and Contaminants*, 20(1), 1–30. doi:10.1080/0265203021000007840

Nehlig, A. (2010). Is caffeine a cognitive enhancer? *Journal of Alzheimer's Disease*, 20(Supplement 1), S85–S94. doi: 10.3233/JAD-2010-091315

Nguyen, K. H., Marshall, L., & Brown, S. (2016, October 7). State-specific prevalence of current cigarette smoking and smokeless tobacco use among adults—United States, 2014. *MMWR Morbidity and Mortality Weekly Report*, 65(39), 1045–1051.

NIDA, National Institute on Drug Abuse. (2016, May). *Drug facts: Cigarettes and other tobacco products*. Rockville, MD: U.S. Department of Health and Human Services. Retrieved September 8, 2016, from www.drugabuse.gov/publications/drugfacts/cigarettes-other-tobacco-products

Nordt, S. P., Vilke, G. M., & Clark, R. F. (2012). Energy drink use and adverse effects among emergency department patients. *Journal of Community Health*, 37(5), 976–981. doi:10.1007/s10900-012-9549-9

O'Brien, M. C., McCoy, T. P., & Rhodes, S. D. (2008). Caffeinated cocktails: Energy drink consumption, high-risk drinking, and alcohol-related consequences among college students. *Academic Emergency Medicine*, 15(5), 453–460. doi:10.1111/j.1553-2712.2008.00085.x

O'Cleirigh, C., Valentine, S. E., & Pinkston, M. (2015). The unique challenges facing HIV-positive patients who smoke cigarettes: HIV viremia, ART adherence, engagement in HIV care, and concurrent substance use. *AIDS and Behavior*, 19(1), 178–185. doi:10.1007/s10461-014-0762-7

Oddy, W. H., & O'Sullivan, T. A. (2009, December 10). Energy drinks for children and adolescents. *BMJ*, 339, b5268.

Oh, A. Y., & Kacker, A. (2014). Do electronic cigarettes impart a lower potential disease burden than conventional tobacco cigarettes? Review on E-cigarette vapor versus tobacco smoke. *Laryngoscope*, 124(12), 2702–2706. doi:10.1002/lary.24750

Oh, J. K., Sandin, S., & Strom, P. (2015). Prospective study of breast cancer in relation to coffee, tea, and caffeine in Sweden. *International Journal of Cancer*, 137(8), 1979–1989. doi:10.1002/ijc.29569

Pagliaro, A. M., & Pagliaro, L. A. (2000). *Substance use among women: A reference and resource guide.* Philadelphia, PA: Brunner/Mazel.

Pagliaro, L. A., & Pagliaro, A. M. (Eds.). (2002). *Problems in pediatric drug therapy* (4th ed.). Washington, DC: American Pharmaceutical Association.

Pagliaro, L. A., & Pagliaro, A. M. (2004). *Pagliaros' comprehensive guide to drugs and substances of abuse.* Washington, DC: American Pharmacists Association.

Pagliaro, L. A., & Pagliaro, A. M. (2009). *Pagliaros' comprehensive guide to drugs and substances of abuse* (2nd ed.). Washington, DC: American Pharmacists Association.

Pagliaro, L. A., & Pagliaro, A. M. (2012). *Handbook of child and adolescent drug and substance abuse: Pharmacological, developmental, and clinical considerations.* Hoboken, NJ: John Wiley & Sons.

Palamar, J. J., Zhou, S., & Sherman, S. (2014, August). Hookah use among US high school seniors. *Pediatrics*, 134(2), 1–8. doi:10.101542/peds.2014-0538

Patil, H., Lavie, C. J., & O'Keefe, J. H. (2011, November–December). Cuppa joe: Friend or foe? Effects of chronic coffee consumption on cardiovascular and brain health. *Missouri Medicine*, 108(6), 431–438.

Paul, O. (1989, July). Background of the prevention of cardiovascular disease. II. Arteriosclerosis, hypertension, and selected risk factors. *Circulation*, 80(1), 206–214.

Peiper, N., & Rodu, B. (2013). Evidence of sex differences in the relationship between current tobacco use and past-year serious psychological distress: 2005–2008 National Survey on Drug Use and Health. *Social Psychiatry and Psychiatric Epidemiology*, 48(8), 1261–1271. doi:10.1007/s00127-012-0644-0

Pelchovitz, D. J., & Goldberger, J. J. (2011). Caffeine and cardiac arrhythmias: A review of the evidence. *The American Journal of Medicine*, 124(4), 284–289. doi:10.1016/j.amjmed.2010.10.017

Pfeifer, G. P., Denissenko, M. F., & Olivier, M. (2002). Tobacco smoke carcinogens, DNA damage and p53 mutations in smoking-associated cancers. *Oncogene*, 21(48), 7435–7451.

Phelan, S. (2014). Smoking cessation in pregnancy. *Obstetrics and Gynecology Clinics of North America*, 41(2), 255–266. doi:10.1016/j.ogc.2014.02.007

Quik, M., Huang, L. Z., & Parameswaran, N. (2009). Multiple roles for nicotine in Parkinson's disease. *Biochemical Pharmacology*, 78(7), 677–685. doi:10.1016/j.bcp.2009.05.003

Quik, M., Zhang, D., & McGregor, M. (2015). Alpha7 nicotinic receptors as therapeutic targets for Parkinson's disease. *Biochemical Pharmacology*, 97(4), 399–407. doi:10.1016/j.bcp.2015.06.014

Reissig, C. J., Strain, E. C., & Griffiths, R. R. (2009). Caffeinated energy drinks—a growing problem. *Drug and Alcohol Dependence*, 99(1–3), 1–10. doi:10.1016/j.drugalcdep.2008.08.001

Rhee, J. J., Qin, F., & Hedlin, H. K. (2016). Coffee and caffeine consumption and the risk of hypertension in postmenopausal women. *American Journal of Clinical Nutrition*, 103(1), 210–217. doi:10.3945/ajcn.115.120147

Rhee, J., Kim, R., & Kim, Y. (2015). Maternal caffeine consumption during pregnancy and risk of low birth weight: A dose-response meta-analysis of observational studies. *PLoS One*, 10(7), 1–2. doi:10.1371/journal.pone.0132334

Roger, J. M., Abayon, M., & Elad, S. (2016, January 7). Oral tooth trauma and tooth avulsion following explosion of e-cigarette. *Journal of Oral and Maxillofacial Surgery*, 1–2. doi:10.1016/j.joms.2015.12.017

Rogers, A. J., Denk, L. D., & Wax, P. M. (2004). Catastrophic brain injury after nicotine insecticide ingestion. *Journal of Emergency Medicine*, 26(2), 169–172.

Rom, O., Pecorelli, A., & Valacchi, G. (2015, March). Are E-cigarettes a safe and good alternative to cigarette smoking? *Annals of the New York Academy of Sciences*, 1340, 65–74. doi:10.1111/nyas.12609

Roosevelt, M. W. (2012, March 5). Breathable Foods, Inc.—Warning letter. *Inspections, compliance, enforcement, and criminal investigations*. College Park, MD: U.S. Food and Drug Administration. Retrieved October 6, 2016, from www.fda.gov/ICECI/EnforcementActions/WarningLetters/2012/ucm294774.htm

Rubin, R. (2008, January 20). New studies, different outcomes on caffeine, pregnancy. *News: Behavior & Health*. USA Today. Retrieved October 6, 2016, from http://usatoday30.usatoday.com/news/health/2008-01-20-caffeine_N.htm

Salazar-Martinez, E., Willett, W. C., & Ascherio, A. (2004). Coffee consumption and risk for type 2 diabetes mellitus. *Annals of Internal Medicine*, 140(1), 1–8.

SAMHSA, Substance Abuse and Mental Health Services Administration. (2011, November 22). Emergency department visits involving energy drinks. *The DAWN Report*. Rockville, MD: Center for Behavioral Health Statistics and Quality.

SAMHSA, Substance Abuse and Mental Health Services Administration. (2014a, March 13). 1 in 10 energy drink-related emergency department visits results in hospitalization. *The DAWN Report*. Rockville, MD: Center for Behavioral Health Statistics and Quality.

SAMHSA, Substance Abuse and Mental Health Services Administration. (2014b). *Results from the 2013 National Survey on Drug Use and Health: Summary of National Findings, NSDUH Series H-48, HHS Publication No. (SMA) 14–4863*. Rockville, MD.

Sanchez-Johnson, A. P., Spring, B. J., & Kaplan Sommerfeld, B. (2005). Weight concerns and smoking in Black and White female smokers. *Addictive Behaviors*, 30, 601–605. doi:10.1016/j.addbeh.2004.07.007

Satcher, D. (2001, January 1). The unequal burden of cancer. *Cancer*, 91(Supplement 1), 205–207.

Sathya, C. (2014, July 7). *Hookah gains popularity: Nearly 1 in 5 teens have tried*. Retrieved April 13, 2016, from CNN.com: www.cnn.com/2014/07/07/health/hookah-teen-popularity/index.html

Sharwood, L. N., Elkington, J., & Meuleners, L. (2013). Use of caffeinated substances and risk of crashes in long distance drivers of commercial vehicles: Case-control study. *BMJ*, 346, f1140. doi: 10.1136/bmj.f1140

Schroeder, M. J., & Hoffman, A. C. (2014, May 23). Electronic cigarettes and nicotine clinical pharmacology. *Tobacco Control* (Supplement 2), 30–35. doi:10.1136/tobaccocontrol-2013–051469

Schwartz, L., Guais, A., & Chaumet-Riffaud, P. (2010). Carbon dioxide is largely responsible for the acute inflammatory effects of tobacco smoke. *Inhalation Toxicology*, 22(7), 543–551. doi:10.3109/08958370903555909

Shea, A. K., & Steiner, M. (2008). Cigarette smoking during pregnancy. *Nicotine & Tobacco Research*, 10(2), 267–278. doi:10.1080/14622200701825908

Shihadeh, A. (2003, January). Investigation of mainstream smoke aerosol of the argileh water pipe. *Food and Chemical Toxicology*, 41(1), 143–152.

Sifferlin, A. (2012, July 11). *Quiting smoking: You may gain more weight than you think.* Retrieved March 20, 2016, from Time.com: http://healthland.time.com/2012/07/11/how-much-weight-will-you-gain-after-quitting-smoking/

Smith, A. (2002). Effects of caffeine on human behavior. *Food and Chemical Toxicology*, 40(9), 1243–1255.

Smith, P. H., Homish, G. G., & Giovino, G. A. (2014). Cigarette smoking and mental illness: A study of nicotine withdrawal. *American Journal of Public Health*, 104(2), e127–e133. doi:10.2105/AJPH.2013.301502

Somogyi, L. P. (2010). *Caffeine intake by the U.S. population (Subcontract number: 70000073494), pp. 1–85.* Oakridge National Laboratory. Kensington, CA: The Food and Drug Administration.

Striley, L. W., Griffiths, R. R., & Cottler, L. B. (2011). Evaluating dependence criteria for caffeine. *Journal of Caffeine Research*, 1(4), 219–225. doi:10.1089/caf.2011.0029

SurgeStix—Inhalable caffeine stix. (2012, March). Retrieved December 27, 2016, from ThinkGeek, pp. 1–2: www.thinkgreek.com/stuff/41/surgestix.shtml

Syamial, S. G., Jamal, A., & King, B. A. (2016, June 10). Electronic cigarette use among working adults—United States, 2014. *MMWR, Morbidity & Mortality Weekly Report*, 65(22), 557–561. doi:10.15585/mmwr.mm6522a1

Tanner, J. A., Chenoweth, M. J., & Tyndale, R. F. (2015). Pharmacogenetics of nicotine and associated smoking behaviors. *Current Topics in Behavioral Neurosciences*, 23, 37–86. doi:10.1007/978-3-319-13665-3_3

Tarnopolsky, M. A. (2008). Effect of caffeine on the neuromuscular system—potential as an ergogenic aid. *Applied Physiology, Nutrition, and Metabolism*, 33(6), 1284–1289. doi:10.1139/H08-121

Thiriez, C., Villafane, G., & Grapin, F. (2011). Can nicotine be used medicinally in Parkinson's disease? *Expert Review of Clinical Pharmacology*, 4(4), 429–436. doi:10.1586/ecp.11.27

Thun, M. J., Henley, S. J., & Calle, E. E. (2002, October 21). Tobacco use and cancer: An epidemiologic perspective for geneticists. *Oncogene*, 21(48), 7307–7325. doi:10.1038/sj.onc.1205807

TODAY. (2012, March 21). *Teen girl dies of "caffeine toxicity" after downing 2 energy drinks.* Retrieved December 27, 2016, from Today.com, pp. 1–2: www.today.com/health/teen-girl-dies-caffeine-toxicity-after-downing-2-energy-drinks-506441

Tomizawa, M., & Casida, J. E. (2005). Neonicotinoid insecticide toxicology: Mechanisms of selective action. *Annual Review of Pharmacology and Toxicology*, 45, 247–268.

Tomizawa, M., & Casida, J. E. (2009). Molecular recognition of neonicotinoid insecticides: The determinants of life or death. *Accounts of Chemical Research*, 42(2), 260–269. doi:10.1021/ar800131p

Tynan, M. A., Holmes, C. B., & Promoff, G. (2016). State and local comprehensive smoke-free laws for worksites, restaurants, and bars—United States, 2015. *MMWR Morbidity and Mortality Weekly Report*, 65, 623–626.

U.S. Department of Health & Human Services. (2006). *The health consequences of involuntary exposure to tobacco smoke: A report of the Surgeon General.* Atlanta, GA: Centers for Disease Control and Prevention. Retrieved from www.surgeongeneral.gov/library/secondhandsmoke/report

U.S. Food and Drug Administration. (2016, August 8). *Extending authorities to all tobacco products, including e-cigarettes, cigars, and hookah.* Retrieved July 16, 2016, from www.fda.gov/TobaccoProducts/Labeling/RulesRegulationsGuidance/ucm388395.htm

van Dam, R. M., & Hu, F. B. (2005, July 6). Coffee consumption and risk of type 2 diabetes: A systematic review. *JAMA*, 294(1), 97–104. doi:10.1001/jama.294.1.97

van Dieren, S., Uiterwaal, C. S., & van der Schouw, Y. T. (2009). Coffee and tea consumption and risk of type 2 diabetes. *Diabetologia*, 52(12), 2561–2569. doi:10.1007/s00125-009-1516-3

van Dijk, A. E., Olthof, M. R., & Meeuse, J. C. (2009). Acute effects of decaffeinated coffee and the major coffee components chlorogenic acid and trigonelline on glucose tolerance. *Diabetes Care*, 32(6), 1023–1025. doi:10.2337/dc09-0207

van Duinen, H., Lorist, M. M., & Zijdewind, I. (2005). The effect of caffeine on cognitive task performance and motor fatigue. *Psychopharmacology (Berl)*, 180(3), 539–547.

Vetulani, J. (2001, May–June). Drug addiction: Part I. Psychoactive substances in the past and present. *Polish Journal of Pharmacology*, 53(3), 201–214.

Vu, A. T., Taylor, K. M., & Holman, M. R. (2015). Polycyclic aromatic hydrocarbons in the mainstream smoke of popular U.S. cigarettes. *Chemical Research in Toxicology*, 28(8), 1616–1626. doi:10.1021/acs.chemrestox.5b00190

Wakai, K., Inoue, M., & Mizoue, T. (2006). Tobacco smoking and lung cancer risk: An evaluation based on a systematic review of epidemiological evidence among the Japanese population. *Japanese Journal of Clinical Oncology*, 36(5), 309–324. doi:10.1093/jjco/hyl025

Wang, H., Li, X., & Guo, J. (2016, February 10). Distribution of toxic chemicals in particles of various sizes from mainstream cigarette smoke. *Inhalation Toxicology*, 1–6.

Warner, K. E., & Pollack, H. A. (2014, November 13). The nicotine fix. *The Atlantic*, pp. 1–28. Retrieved October 8, 2016, from www.theatlantic.com/national/archive/2014/11/the-nicotine-fix/382666/

Watson, J., Deary, I., & Kerr, D. (2002). Central and peripheral effects of sustained caffeine use: Tolerance is incomplete. *British Journal of Clinical Pharmacology*, 54(4), 400–406.

Watson, T. D., Sweeney, J. F., & Louis, H. (2014). Neurocognitive, psychological and behavioral correlates of binge drinking and use of alcohol with caffeinated beverages in college-aged adults. *The American Journal of Alcohol Abuse*, 40(1), 58–66. doi:10.3109/009952990.2013.843005

Whitten, L. (2009, November). Studies link family of genes to nicotine addiction. *NIDA Notes*, 22(6), 1, 10–14.

World Health Organization. (2009). *WHO Study Group on Tobacco Product Regulation: Report on the scientific basis of tobacco product regulation: Third report of a WHO study group.* Geneva, Switzerland: World Health Organization. Retrieved October 7, 2016, from www.worldcat.org/title/scientific-basis-of-tobacco-product-regulation-report-of-a-who-study-group/oclc/163571437

Wright, T. E., & Tam, E. (2010). Disparate rates of persistent smoking and drug use during pregnancy of women of Hawaiian ancestry. *Ethnicity & Disease*, 20(1 Supplement 1), S1–215–218.

Wu, W., Zhang, L., & Jain, R. B. (2005). Determination of carcinogenic tobacco-specific nitrosamines in mainstream smoke from U.S.-brand and non-U.S. brand cigarettes from 14 countries. *Nicotine & Tobacco Research*, 7(3), 443–451.

Yang, T. O., Crowe, B. J., & Cairns, B. J. (2015). Tea and coffee and risk of endometrial cancer: Cohort study and meta-analysis. *The American Journal of Clinical Nutrition*, 101(3), 570–578. doi:10.3945/ajcn.113.081836

Zevin, S., & Benowitz, N. L. (1999). Drug interactions with tobacco smoking. An update. *Clinical Pharmacokinetics*, 36(6), 425–438. doi:10.2165/00003088-199936060-00004

Zickler, P. (2003, March). Nicotine's multiple effects on the brain's reward system drive addiction. *NIDA Notes*, 17(6), 1–3. Retrieved October 7, 2016, from www.ehd.org/health_tobacco_19.php

Ziedonis, D., Hitsman, B., & Beckham, J. C. (2008). Tobacco use and cessation in psychiatric disorders: National Institute of Mental Health report. *Nicotine & Tobacco Research*, 10(12), 1691–1715. doi:10.1080/14622200802443569

5

WOMEN'S AMPHETAMINE AND COCAINE ABUSE

The *amphetamines* and *cocaine* are two major subclasses of the psychostimulants that are commonly used and abused by women in the U.S.[1] This chapter presents and discusses their pharmacology and medical and personal use and abuse by women during the new millennium. We begin with the amphetamines.

Amphetamines

The amphetamines (see Table 5.1) include the: (1) *prescription* amphetamines (e.g., mixed amphetamines, Adderall®) that are generally used to medically manage attention-deficit/hyperactivity disorder (A-D/HD);[2] and (2) *illicitly* produced and obtained amphetamines, particularly *methamphetamine* ("Crank," "Crystal Meth," "Glass," "Tweak"). At the beginning of the new millennium, the use of these amphetamines was about equal between women and men in the U.S. However, 2 decades later they are now most often used by women, particularly those who are 18 to 35 years-of-age. These women generally use the amphetamines to achieve such *desired* effects as:

- Euphoria
- Relief from hunger and fatigue
- Sexual arousal and pleasure
- Vigilance, or sustained concentration
- Wakefulness

[1] See Chapter 4, *Women's Caffeine and Nicotine Abuse*, for a discussion of the two other major subclasses of the psychostimulants that are commonly abused by women, *caffeine* and *nicotine*.

[2] Also, see the related discussion in the later section, "College/University Students."

TABLE 5.1 Amphetamines and Other Closely Related Psychostimulant

Generic Name	*Brand/Trade Names*	*Common Street Names*[a]
Amphetamines		
Amphetamine[b]		Ace; Amp; Co-Pilot
Dextroamphetamine	Dexedrine®	Co-Pilots; Dex; Hearts
Lisdexamfetamine	Vyvanase®	LDX
Mephentermine	Wyamine®	
Methamphetamine	Desoxyn®	Crank; Crystal Meth; Glass; Hillbilly Crack; Ice; Jib; Meth; Stove Top; Tina
Mixed Amphetamines[c]	Adderall®	Addies; Blueberries; Oranges; Tic-Tacs
Other Closely Related Psychostimulant		
Methylphenidate	Concerta®; Ritalin®	JIF; MPH; Rs; The Smart Drug

[a] Partial list. Examples of the most common street names are provided, when available. See Pagliaro and Pagliaro (2009) for a comprehensive listing of the drugs and substances of abuse and their common street names.

[b] Amphetamine, in its salt forms (i.e., amphetamine aspartate and amphetamine sulfate) is only legally available in the U.S. in the combination, mixed amphetamines product, *Adderall®*.

[c] This product contains the amphetamine salt forms, amphetamine aspartate and amphetamine sulfate. It also contains dextroamphetamine.

We begin with the basic pharmacology of the amphetamines—their *pharmacodynamics*, or proposed mechanisms of action; *pharmacokinetics*, or absorption, distribution, metabolism, and excretion; and common undesired, or harmful, effects and toxicities, including their potential for physical and psychological dependence.

Pharmacology

Chemically related to ephedrine, the active ingredient of the ancient herb, *Ephedra*, the amphetamines are *synthetic* drugs that produce dose-dependent actions on both the central and peripheral (i.e., sympathetic) nervous systems (Pagliaro & Pagliaro, 2004). Centrally, their actions involve the *endogenous* catecholamine excitatory neurotransmitters: *dopamine*; *epinephrine*; *norepinephrine*; and *serotonin* (see later section, "Pharmacodynamics: *Mechanisms of Action*"). Peripherally, they promote the actions of the sympathetic nervous system that, consequently, increase heart rate, constrict blood vessels, and elevate blood pressure. However, the amphetamines, being *more* potent than natural ephedrine, achieve *higher* levels of central and peripheral nervous system stimulation resulting in both greatly *heightened* alertness and psychomotor abilities along with significantly *diminished* feelings of drowsiness and fatigue. These actions have made the amphetamines attractive as "performance enhancers" to a variety of women, including aircraft pilots, athletes, college and university students, entertainers, long-haul truck drivers, soldiers, and surgeons.

Licit and Illicit Production

Both the amphetamines and methamphetamine are produced licitly and illicitly in the U.S. and in other countries. This production and distribution is discussed in the following sections in regard to women's access to, and use of these psychostimulants.

Amphetamines. The amphetamines that are commonly abused by women are chemically synthesized by chemists, either in *licit* pharmaceutical laboratories primarily as prescription products for medical use (e.g., mixed amphetamines, Adderall®) or in *illicit*, large scale, sophisticated, clandestine "super labs" (e.g., *methamphetamine*, "Crystal Meth"). Primarily controlled and directed by Mexican criminal organizations in Mexico and in Los Angeles, California, the super labs can produce ten or more pounds of methamphetamine per day. Other super labs are operated by major Asian and other criminal organizations, including outlaw motorcycle gangs (Pagliaro & Pagliaro, 2004; Shukla, Crump, & Chrisco, 2012).

Women, who abuse *prescription* amphetamines, obtain them by:

1. "Double doctoring" (see related discussion in Chapter 1, *Women's Opiate Analgesic Abuse*)
2. Stealing them from: family members, including children; friends; and work sites (e.g., hospitals and pharmacies)
3. Sex-for-drug exchanges
4. Purchase from "street dealers"

It is generally estimated that *licit* production accounts for a very small amount of the amphetamine that is abused by women and men in the U.S. (i.e., probably less than 10%). However, *illicit* production accounts for *most* of the amphetamine that is abused (approximately 90%).[3,4]

Methamphetamine. Women, who use methamphetamine, obtain it in similar ways as women who use other amphetamines, including: stealing; sex-for-drug exchanges;

---

[3] These are estimated percentages because there are *no* available records, or research data, that accurately account for either licit or illicit abuse among women in the U.S. during the new millennium.

[4] In addition, in parts of the U.S., illicit methamphetamine produced in Mexico (i.e., "Mexican Meth"), began to replace that domestically produced in illicit "home" laboratories (i.e., "home-cooked meth"). This change became established by 2007 and, since that time, the average purity of "Mexican Meth" has *increased* from approximately 37% to approximately 100% (Berkes, 2007; Buie & Tamburin, 2014) while the street price has significantly *decreased* (Pagliaro & Pagliaro, *Clinical Patient Data Files*). As noted by Shukla, Crump, and Chrisco (2012, p. 426):

> Transnational [criminal] organizations now control much of the methamphetamine supply in the U.S. and methamphetamine remains widely available.

or purchase from "street dealers." They also can *make* it. Methamphetamine is relatively easy to synthesize from inexpensive over-the-counter ingredients and commonly available supplies.[5] It is often illicitly synthesized in small, unsophisticated, clandestine labs across the U.S. that range from small basement laboratories (e.g., "mom and pop labs") to more sophisticated laboratories on college/university campuses. Methamphetamine also is synthesized in kitchens, bathrooms, and other places in the family home, including those where children often entertain themselves playing their favorite android and computer games or watching TV.

Methamphetamine is frequently synthesized from precursor drugs, such as amphetamine, phenylalanine, phenylpropanolamine, or pseudoephedrine[6] using the "anhydrous ammonia method" or the "red phosphorus method."[7,8] The anhydrous ammonia method is more often used in the production of *large* quantities of methamphetamine because of the ready and unregulated availability of nitrogen farm fertilizer (i.e., the source of anhydrous ammonia). To prevent, or at least significantly *diminish*, the widespread diversion of these precursor drugs for the illicit production of methamphetamine in the U.S., the *Comprehensive Methamphetamine Control Act* of 1996 was passed. In 2005, Congress passed a related law, the *Combat Methamphetamine Epidemic Act* (CMEA), that was followed by the *Methamphetamine Production Prevention Act of 2008*, which was implemented in 2011 (DEA, 2011).[9]

---

[5] These ingredients and supplies include: acetone; anhydrous ammonia; common cold and allergy tablets that contain pseudoephedrine; coffee filters; drain cleaner; isopropyl (rubbing) alcohol; lithium batteries; lye; Mason® jars; pillow cases; and toluene. (Also, see later list of supplies in text associated with the "shake and bake" method of production.)

[6] Alterations to the pharmaceutical formulation of pseudoephedrine have been used to impede the illicit production of methamphetamine from pseudoephedrine. For example, the Nexafed® pseudoephedrine tablet maintains bioequivalence with Sudafed® pseudoephedrine tablets, while utilizing the Impede® technology to limit the extraction of pseudoephedrine and its subsequent conversion to methamphetamine (Brzeczko, Leech, & Stark, 2013).

[7] Also, commonly referred to as either the "Birch Method" or the "Nazi Method" because this method of production was used during World War II to supply German soldiers with methamphetamine to increase alertness (Pagliaro & Pagliaro, 2004).

[8] N.B. Generally, amphetamine (i.e., dextroamphetamine) is only legally available by prescription while phenylalanine and pseudoephedrine, which are commonly found in common cold products, are generally legally available without a prescription (i.e., over-the-counter ["OTC"]).

[9] In this context, various state and federal regulations also have been enacted, including: (1) in pharmacies, keeping these and other related products (e.g., ephedrine; pseudoephedrine) "behind the counter" prior to sale; (2) limiting the amount of product sold; and (3) for Oregon and Mississippi, requiring a prescription for purchase. As identified by Messina, Marinelli-Casey, and West (2014):

> A review of state bills and regulations on over-the-counter purchases of these products reveals that as of 2005, 34 of the 50 states have passed bills to restrict access to and/or purchase of cold medications that include pseudoephedrine.
>
> *(p. 1874)*

However, the increasing adoption of the "shake and bake" method of methamphetamine production has *largely* nullified the past efforts aimed at controlling methamphetamine production (Hamilton, 2010). The "shake and bake" method only requires: a few packages of common "cold pills"; several corrosive, or flammable chemicals, readily purchased at most hardware or farm supply stores, Walmart-Stores, and similar stores; water; and an empty, 32- or 64-ounce plastic soda bottle to quickly and easily produce enough methamphetamine for a woman's personal use or for her to sell, on a very small scale (Carnevale Associates, 2011; Hall & Dunham, 2013; Office of National Drug Control Policy, 2010; Pagliaro & Pagliaro, 2009).

Various detailed lists of the typical supplies needed for the "shake and bake" method of illicit methamphetamine production can be found on the Internet. For example, the following list is from "Some Chick's Blog" (Shake and bake, n.d., p. 2):

- 2 32 oz. Gatorade® bottles
- 2 Mason® jars
- 3–4 ft. of aquarium tubing
- Aquarium air pump (optional)
- Fine coffee filters
- A funnel
- 75 g 100% lye
- 130 g 15-0-15 fertilizer (no weed killers)
- 2 96 ct. Pseudophedrine (crushed into fine powder)
- Coleman® lantern fuel
- 1.5g ice
- 2 AA lithium batteries
- Iodized salt
- Liquid Lightning® (drain cleaner)
- Pipe cutter
- Needle nose pliers
- Xacto® knife/scissors

Illicit methamphetamine producers generally identify *three* benefits of the "shake and bake" method, when compared to other methods of *illicit* methamphetamine production:

1. Ease of preparation (i.e., no need for skills or techniques related to chemistry)
2. Less expenditure (i.e., no need for costly, specialized chemical laboratory equipment)
3. Quick "cooking time" (i.e., using this method, a "batch" of methamphetamine can be easily produced in as little as 30 minutes)

The identification of illicit "meth labs" is crucial for law enforcement. Thus, various lists of related signs[10] of the presence of a possible "meth lab" have been compiled (e.g., Bartos, 2005). From these lists, we have provided three main areas for inspection outside, inside, and around meth labs and drug houses.

Signs inside "meth labs" include:

- Basic laboratory equipment (e.g., clear glass jugs; glassware; rubber tubing)
- Camp stoves, heat plates, or other heat sources
- Coffee filters with a white or red pasty or powdery substance
- Coolers or thermos bottles
- Cookware that contains powdery substances
- Empty cold/allergy medication packaging
- Strong odor of urine or unusual chemical odors such as acetone, ammonia, or ether
- Various chemicals or drugs in plain sight (e.g., cold/allergy medications, or ether)

Signs outside "meth labs" include:

- Empty containers of: acetone, antifreeze, drain cleaners, Freon®, Heet®, lye, starting fluids, or paint thinner
- Empty propane tanks

Signs of a "drug house" include:

- Heavily covered windows
- Little or no traffic during the day, but lots at night
- Never putting out the trash
- Reinforced doors
- Renters who pay landlords in cash
- Renters who are unfriendly, paranoid, or secretive
- Unemployed people who seem to have plenty of cash

Pharmacodynamics: Mechanisms of Action

The amphetamines are *indirect-acting* psychostimulants. As such, they *stimulate* the release of the biogenic amines (i.e., *dopamine*, *norepinephrine*, and *serotonin*) from the presynaptic nerve terminal storage vesicles that are primarily located in the midbrain. They also *inhibit* the reuptake of the biogenic amines, primarily by *blocking*

---

[10] The signs included in this listing are indicative of, but *not* definitive for, methamphetamine production activity.

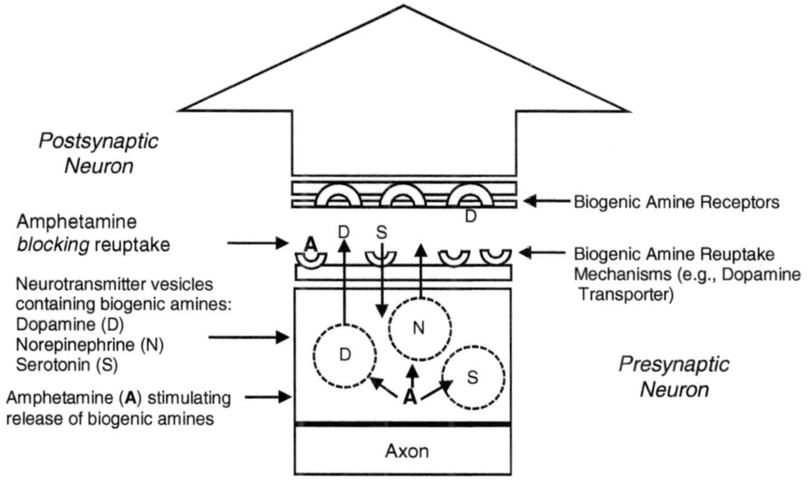

FIGURE 5.1 Amphetamines: Mechanism of Psychostimulant Action

the dopamine transporter and the monoamine transporter-2. Figure 5.1 provides a simplified, stylized representation of the principal sites and mechanisms of these psychostimulant actions.

In addition to their indirect effects on the CNS, the amphetamines also produce several physical effects on other body systems, such as: anorexia; bronchodilation; constriction of the sphincter of the urinary bladder; hypertension; mydriasis; and tachycardia. They also produce several other undesired, or harmful, effects and toxicities (see later section, *Undesired, or Harmful, Effects and Toxicities*).

Pharmacokinetics: Absorption, Distribution, Metabolism, and Excretion

The amphetamines are immediately and completely absorbed following intravenous injection. They also are readily absorbed following: oral ingestion; pulmonary inhalation (smoking, vaporizing); and nasal insufflation, or snorting. Following absorption, they are widely distributed in body tissues, and because they are lipid soluble, readily cross the blood-brain barrier. Urinary excretion is pH-dependent with acidic urine (pH *lower* than 7) *increasing* excretion and alkaline urine (pH *higher* than 7) *decreasing* excretion. These differences in urinary pH and excretion rates explain why women, who are regular, long-term amphetamine users, commonly consume antacids (e.g., calcium carbonate, Tums®) to *alkalinize* their urine. This action both *enhances* and *prolongs* the desired pharmacologic actions of the amphetamines. The half-life of elimination of the various amphetamines is approximately 10 hours, although it slightly differs from one specific amphetamine to another (e.g., from amphetamine sulfate to dextroamphetamine or methamphetamine) (Pagliaro & Pagliaro, 2009).

Popular Notion: That the half-life of elimination of a specific amphetamine (e.g., methamphetamine) depends on its method of use (i.e., route of administration).

NOT TRUE. While the method of use may affect the *rate* of absorption and, consequently, the *onset of action*, it does *not* affect the half-life of elimination.

Undesired, or Harmful, Effects and Toxicities

The amphetamines are associated with several undesired, or harmful, effects and toxicities that can be *acute* or *chronic*, *physical* or *mental*, *direct* or *indirect* and can affect virtually every body system (Pagliaro & Pagliaro, 2009). The *frequency* and *severity* of these effects are generally related to the:

1. Dosage used (e.g., 40 mg *versus* 1000 mg)
2. Method of use (e.g., oral ingestion *versus* intravenous injection—see later discussion)
3. Frequency of use (e.g., every hour over 1 or 2 days *versus* twice a week)
4. Pattern of use (e.g., occasional use *versus* regular, long-term use)
5. Mental health status at the time of use (e.g., a woman who has a contemporaneous diagnosis *versus* a woman who does *not*)
6. Physical health status at the time of use (e.g., a woman who has significant hypertension *versus* a woman who does *not*)
7. Specific personal characteristics (e.g., a woman who has a risk-taking personality trait *versus* a woman who does *not*)
8. Concurrent pharmacotherapy or use of other drugs and substances of abuse

Acute Toxicities. The acute toxicities associated with amphetamine use can be physical or mental and generally begin within 20 to 60 minutes after ingestion—or 30 to 60 seconds after intravenous injection or pulmonary inhalation.

ACUTE PHYSICAL TOXICITIES. Acute *physical* toxicities are *more* likely to occur among women who are novice or occasional users of amphetamine rather than women who are regular, long-term abusers, who, being *more* tolerant to the amphetamines, typically use *higher* dosages. The acute physical toxicities include: acute renal failure; bruxism; cardiac dysrhythmias; chest pain; coma; convulsions; cramps;

diaphoresis; dizziness; dysuria; headache; heart palpitations; hypertension; hyperthermia; metabolic acidosis; rhabdomyolysis; seizures; stroke; tachycardia; tachypnea; tremor; urinary retention; vomiting; and weight loss. Acute physical effects that are *indirectly* associated with use include local skin burns that occur with methamphetamine production.[11] However, the most *severe*, and *potentially fatal*, acute physical toxicities associated with amphetamine use are:

1. *Hypertensive crisis*, which is characterized by a drastic increase in blood pressure
2. *Hyperpyretic crisis*, which is characterized by a sustained elevated body temperature exceeding 106°F (41°C)

These two acute physical toxicities require emergency treatment, including medical support and monitoring of body systems.

ACUTE MENTAL TOXICITIES. Acute *mental* toxicities include: aggression; agitation; anxiety; compulsive behavior; confusion; delirium; euphoric grandiosity; hallucinations; hostility; hyperactivity; hypervigilance; impaired judgment; insomnia; irritability; loquacity (i.e., talkativeness) extending to pressured speech (i.e., loud and uncontrollable talking); mania; obsessive behavior; panic attacks; paranoia; and restlessness. Two, particularly serious mental toxicities, are *delirium* and *psychosis* (see later section, "Amphetamine Psychosis"), which can occur within 24 hours of amphetamine use.

ACUTE DIRECT AND INDIRECT TOXICITIES: INTRAVENOUS USE. Several acute toxicities have been related to two distinct phases of intravenous amphetamine use: (1) an *early phase*; and (2) a *late phase*. During the *early phase* of intravenous amphetamine use, women commonly inject 20 to 40 mg of amphetamine to achieve a desired *flash*, or *rush*. The *rush* is reportedly characterized by:

1. *Extreme* euphoria—a sense of *increased* physical energy, mental capacity, and self-confidence
2. *Heightened* sexual orgasm

During the *later phase*, women frequently inject increasingly *higher* dosages of amphetamine to achieve the desired actions that they experienced during the early phase. Unable to achieve their desired *rush*—primarily due to the development of tolerance—they continue to inject their amphetamine every 1 to 3 hours, around the clock, for several days. During this late phase, referred to as a *run*, they

[11] For related discussion, see the later section, *Women's Drug Trade Involvement*, "Production-Related Injuries."

generally remain awake and eat *very* little, if at all. After several days, the *run* typically ends for these women, when they:

1. Deplete their amphetamine supplies (e.g., the total available supply is used)
2. Are unable to obtain additional amphetamine because their funds are exhausted
3. Become so *mentally disorganized*, or *paranoid*, that they *cannot* continue their amphetamine use

Unable to continue their amphetamine use, they usually fall into a deep, but restless, sleep that lasts for 12 to 18 hours, or more. Upon awakening, they typically feel tired, weak, depressed, and hungry (Pagliaro & Pagliaro, *Clinical Patient Data Files*).

Chronic Toxicities. A range of chronic toxicities are associated with the regular, long-term *oral use* of 50 mg, or more, per day of the amphetamines. These toxicities include such *physical* toxicities as "meth mouth" and such *mental* toxicities as "diminished executive cognitive functioning/performance." Regular, long-term intravenous use also is associated with a range of chronic toxicities, as are higher dosages. These chronic toxicities, some of which may be permanent, or fatal, are discussed in the following sections.

"METH MOUTH." Methamphetamine-induced bruxism (also see later section, "Intravenous Use"), in conjunction with general prolonged neglect of oral hygiene, contributes to the loss of teeth and the associated distinctive appearance commonly referred to as "meth mouth" (Brown, Morisky, & Silverstein, 2013; Pagliaro & Pagliaro, *Clinical Patient Data Files*; Rommel, Rohleder, & Koerdt, 2016). This condition also is characterized by "rampant caries, periodontal diseases, and excessive tooth wear" (Rommel, Rohleder, & Wagenpfeil, 2016, p. 469).

In their study of 100 chronic methamphetamine abusers and 100 matched-pair controls, Rommel, Rohleder, and Wagenpfeil (2016) found that *total* saliva production among the methamphetamine users was significantly *lower* (i.e., more acidic) than that found for controls. These findings led Rommel and colleagues to posit that the noted differences in saliva production and pH also contribute to the increased risk for caries decay and dental erosions that are seen among regular, long-term methamphetamine users.

DIMINISHED EXECUTIVE FUNCTION. Higher order cognitive performance is affected by executive functions (i.e., mental processes associated with integration, synthesis, and problem solving) that are typically required for "task-oriented behaviors," including consciously planning, implementing, monitoring, and ceasing goal-directed behaviors. Minor and temporary deficits and fluctuations in executive function are largely situational. For example, occurring among most women at some time in their lives, they are more likely to be displayed when women are: extremely tired; experiencing reactive depression following a significant loss; or acutely intoxicated with alcohol (Pagliaro & Pagliaro, *Clinical Patient Data Files*).

Significant deficits in executive functioning also are associated with several mental disorders, including: attention-deficit/hyperactivity disorder (A-D/HD); autism; mental depression; obsessive-compulsive disorder (OCD); psychosis; and Tourette's syndrome. In addition, deficits in executive functioning typically occur with aging, both chronological and pathological (e.g., senile dementia). Among older women, a waning in memory processes is one of the major factors that contributes to declining executive functioning. Diminished executive functioning has been identified as both a *cause* and *result* of drug and substance abuse (e.g., Ersche, Clark, & London, 2006; Goldstein & Volkow, 2011).[12]

As found by Ersche, Clark, and London (2006), in their study of chronic amphetamine and opiate analgesic users:

> Chronic drug users display pronounced neurophysiological impairment in the domains of executive and memory function. Impairment persists after several years of drug abstinence and may reflect neuropathology in frontal and temporal cortices ... Compared to opiate users, amphetamine users showed more pronounced deficits on tasks of executive function...
>
> *(p. 1036)*

The researchers identified *no* gender differences. Thus, women, who used amphetamine, experienced as much impairment of executive functioning as did men, who used amphetamine (for related discussion, see later section, *Cocaine*). (Also, see related discussions in Chapter 1, *Women's Opiate Analgesic Abuse*; Chapter 2, *Women's Alcohol Abuse*; and Chapter 6, *Women's Psychodelic Abuse*.)

Methamphetamine-related diminished cognitive and executive functioning also includes: deficits in abstract thinking; learning; memory; and psychomotor speed. These deficits appear to be related to neurotoxicity involving the dopamine terminals. Neurotoxicity has long been associated with methamphetamine-induced damage to dopaminergic neurons in the basal ganglia and reduced dopamine transporter density in the caudate/putamen, nucleus accumbens, and prefrontal cortex. However, methamphetamine-induced neurotoxicity also may be due to down-regulation (i.e., temporary neuroadaptive changes). Consequently, it may be reversible with long-term abstinence from methamphetamine use.

---

12 Opposition to these findings include the critical review of Hart, Marvin, and Silver (2012, pp. 604–605), who found that:

> 1. Human laboratory data show that short-term, acute methamphetamine [use] *improves* cognitive performance of both methamphetamine abusers and nonusers in some domains...
> 2. The apparent methamphetamine abuse-cognitive impairment link, although widely publicized, has *not* been well-supported by research evidence.

Unfortunately, some of the neurotoxic effects, which have been associated with chronic amphetamine abuse, appear to be permanent—in which case, risk for parkinsonism, with advancing age, significantly increases (Ares-Santos, Granado, & Espadas, 2014; Matthew & Gedzior, 2015; Todd, Noyes, & Flavel, 2013). Research findings also indicate that the long-term use of higher dosages of methamphetamine selectively damages the striatal dopaminergic axons in the substantia nigra, resulting in permanent parkinsonian-like signs (e.g., pill-rolling tremor; shuffling gait) (Ares-Santos, Granados, & Espadas, 2014; Ares-Santos, Granado, & Moratalla, 2013).[13]

HIGHER DOSAGES. As the *dosage* of the amphetamine is *increased*, abdominal pain (severe); anorexia, with loss of body weight; blurred vision; chest pain; dizziness; emotional lability; headache; nausea; palpitations; tremor; and urinary retention may be experienced.

In addition, with the use of *higher* dosages of *methamphetamine*, cardiomyopathy and related medical complications (e.g., heart failure) may occur (e.g., Wijetunga, Seto, & Lindsay, 2003; Won, Hong, & Shohet, 2013; Yeo, Wijetunga, & Ito, 2007). For example, Turnipseed, Richards, and Kirk (2003), in their study of the acute coronary syndrome (ACS), noted that "ACS is common in patients hospitalized for chest pain after methamphetamine use" (p. 369). Diercks, Kirk, and Turnipseed (2007) similarly noted a significant incidence of coronary artery disease (CAD) among patients with positive urine screens for methamphetamine (or cocaine), who were admitted to their chest pain unit.[14]

The risk for cardiomyopathy appears to be significantly *higher* for women than men. As noted by Mau, Asao, and Efird (2009), it also appears to be *higher* for Native Hawaiian women, who have heart disease and other related risk factors (e.g., diabetes mellitus; hypertension; obesity). However, we believe, based on currently available data, that these risk factors probably apply to *all* women, particularly those who have the identified related risk factors.

Further increases in amphetamine dosage may be associated with other chronic toxicities, including automatic jerking movements and compulsive, stereotyped repetitive behaviors (i.e., *punding*) that may culminate in *toxic amphetamine psychosis* (see later discussion in the "Amphetamine Psychosis" section).

INTRAVENOUS USE. Chronic toxicities that are commonly associated with the *intravenous use* of amphetamines include: (1) grinding of the teeth (i.e., bruxism, associated with spasm of the jaw muscles, that usually occurs during sleep);[15]

---

[13] The affected area of the substantia nigra, which when visualized by transcranial sonography, assumes an abnormally enlarged and bright appearance. This change in appearance is referred to as *hyperechogenicity* (Todd, Noyes, & Flavel, 2013).

[14] Interestingly, only about 50% of methamphetamine or cocaine users, who present at an emergency department with symptoms of chest pain, accurately self-report their associated drug use (Lee, Vivier, & Diercks, 2009).

[15] Also, see related discussion in the earlier section, "Meth Mouth."

(2) touching and picking at the arms and face, usually related to the delusional sensation of something (e.g., bugs) crawling under the skin (i.e., *formication*);[16] (3) paranoia; (4) preoccupation with thinking processes and philosophical concerns about "meaning"; (5) compulsive, purposeless, stereotypic repetitive behavior, or *punding* (e.g., a need to take apart mechanical devices, such as a clock or motor, and put them back together again—or at least attempt to do so); and (6) amphetamine psychosis.

AMPHETAMINE PSYCHOSIS. Amphetamine psychosis, which has signs and symptoms that resemble paranoid schizophrenia in terms of observed behavior, is the major mental toxicity that is usually associated with the regular, long-term use of amphetamines over several weeks or months. However, amphetamine psychosis also may occur within two days following the ingestion of a single, large dose of amphetamine by a sensitive user. Once a woman has experienced an episode of amphetamine psychosis, she is at *increased* risk for its recurrence. This increased sensitivity to amphetamine psychosis is thought to be associated with a lowering of the threshold for this effect. In fact, amphetamine psychosis may recur in some women following the single ingestion of as little as 75 mg of amphetamine (Pagliaro & Pagliaro, *Clinical Patient Data Files*).

Efforts have been made to differentiate the clinical similarities and differences between amphetamine psychosis and schizophrenia. Although both conditions may display delusional thinking, depression, flattening of affect, and hallucinations, they differ in the etiology of the presenting thought disorder and its duration. In addition, aggressive and violent behavior is relatively *more* common during an amphetamine run when users, experiencing acute paranoia, can be found holding a loaded handgun or rifle, peering out a window for the "enemy," perhaps a "narc" (i.e., drug enforcement officer), from behind closed curtains. This behavior has been well-documented and has been recognized for some time now in medical, psychological, and legal contexts of practice (Pagliaro & Pagliaro, *Clinical Patient Data Files*).

Mild forms of psychotic-like behavior among women associated with their amphetamine use, generally can be treated by "talking them down" and by administering a sedative-hypnotic (i.e., diazepam, Valium®). *Acute* or *severe* forms of psychosis usually require medical treatment with a sedative-hypnotic (i.e., diazepam, Valium®) in combination with an antipsychotic (e.g., chlorpromazine, Thorazine®; haloperidol, Haldol®), which can promptly reverse many of the signs and symptoms of the psychosis (Buxton & Dove, 2008). Untreated, the psychosis generally resolves within 2 to 14 days.

---

[16] Over time, "picking" at the skin and consequent infections and scarring results in extensive disfiguration and associated characteristic facial appearance that resembles severe acne, with open sores, or lesions (Mullin, 2016; Pagliaro & Pagliaro, *Clinical Patient Data Files*).

FATALITIES. Although relatively uncommon, the use of amphetamines can be both *directly* and *indirectly* fatal. For example, amphetamine use has been *directly* related to the occurrence of: myocardial infarctions (Kaye, McKetin, & Duflou, 2007); cerebral vascular accidents; and overdosage deaths (see later section, "Overdosage"). However, these fatal toxicities *rarely* occur among amphetamine-tolerant, generally healthy women.

The use of amphetamines also has been *indirectly* related to: (1) fatal hepatitis and human immunodeficiency virus (HIV) infection, generally contracted by using contaminated needles and syringes; (2) fatalities related to the injection of an amphetamine dosage that was adulterated, or contaminated; and (3) fatal injuries occurring during *psychotic episodes* and *homicidal rages* (Pagliaro & Pagliaro, *Clinical Patient Data Files*). (Also, see following section.)

HIV INFECTION AND ACQUIRED IMMUNE DEFICIENCY SYNDROME (AIDS). In addition to significantly *increasing* women's risk for HIV infection by means of sharing contaminated needles and syringes (see previous discussion), amphetamine use also increases risky sexual behavior. Several studies and reviews (e.g., Pagliaro & Pagliaro, 2000) have described and documented this risk over the past 25 years. The use of amphetamines, particularly methamphetamine in *moderate* to *high* dosages, significantly *increases* sexual pleasure for many women by means of its associated action on neurotransmitters (see earlier section, *Pharmacodynamics: Mechanism of Action*). As found by Lorvick, Bourgois, and Wenger (2012, p. 385),[17] several women, in their study, shared that:

- "I love the way it makes me feel sexually"
- "It prolongs, um, my orgasms"
- "It makes me uninhibited"
- "It makes me feel sexy"

Consequently, women's methamphetamine use, commonly places them at *significant* risk for HIV infection and AIDS—directly because of engaging in high-risk sexual behavior, particularly unprotected sexual intercourse with multiple partners. As reported by Lorvick, Bourgois, and Wenger (2012), in their study of urban, mostly middle-aged impoverished women who abused methamphetamine: (1) "only 12% of women used condoms consistently during vaginal sex

---

[17] N.B. Lorvick, Bourgois, and Wenger (2012) appear to largely view the related interaction between methamphetamine use and sexual behavior as "supporting the pursuit of pleasure" and, perhaps consequently, being valued because it supports the "common-sense notion of agency as a measure of individual empowerment and efficacy" (pp. 385–386). We take a decidedly more jaundiced view of women's amphetamine abuse and sex. This is perhaps, at least in part, due to our memories of the harmful, disgusting, and degrading denigration of women that occurred during the 1990s in the context of women's attraction to *crack cocaine*, *crack houses*, and the associated lives of *crack whores*. (For related discussion, see Pagliaro and Pagliaro, 2000.)

with all types of partners"; and (2) "over three-quarters (79%)" of women "had multiple male sexual partners in the past six months" with "over a third" having "one or more female sexual partners" (p. 385).

Also of concern are the related tragic outcomes for women (e.g., neonatal infection; negative effects on mothering), emphasized by the finding that "African American women in 2010 comprised 64% of the estimated 9,500 *new* HIV infections in women" (Ivy, Miles, & Le, 2014, p. S266). Other women, who are at *high* risk for HIV infection are women of American Indian descent, who, to obtain methamphetamine for their personal use/abuse, engage in prostitution or sex-for-drug exchanges. These women often live in poverty either in inner-city neighborhoods or on reservations (Pagliaro & Pagliaro, *Clinical Patient Data Files*; Pagliaro, Pagliaro, & Thauberger, 1993). As shared by a woman from the Navajo Nation in Arizona:

> She indicated that she was constantly on the move and even kept two jobs: one for food and one to support her meth addiction. The addiction eventually led her to the street where she started prostituting to get meth.
>
> *(First Nations Centre, 2006, p. 19)*

PHYSICAL VIOLENCE. Regarding psychotic episodes and homicidal rages that required medical intervention, Glover-Kerkvliet (2009) identified that, per data provided by the *Federal Drug Abuse Warning Network* (DAWN):

> A greater than 50% increase in the number of ED visits related to methamphetamine abuse between 1995 and 2002, reaching about 73,000 ED visits or 4% of all drug-related visits in 2004.
>
> *(p. 5)*

Physical violence and associated injuries suffered by women who use *methamphetamine* accounts for most emergency department visits (Pagliaro & Pagliaro, *Clinical Patient Data Files*). Many perpetrators of this violence are the *intimate partners* of these women—who, commonly, also use methamphetamine.

As found by Cohen, Dickow, and Horner (2003, p. 377), from data obtained from a large multi-site study involving methamphetamine use, "80% of women reported abuse or violence from a partner." Going further, they noted that:

> Interpersonal violence is characteristic of the lifestyles of the majority of persons entering treatment for methamphetamine dependence.
>
> *(p. 381)*

In a study of 30 women currently in residential treatment for their methamphetamine abuse, Hamilton and Goeders (2010) identified that 67% of these women had violence perpetrated against them and 57% had perpetrated violence themselves. As they further explained, "the psychopharmacological effects of drugs contribute to increased arousal and irrational behavior, which contributes to aggression." They also noted that, "aggression is economically motivated (i.e., it occurs in relation to obtaining or selling drugs); [and] aggression is part of general deviance such that those who are involved in one type of deviance are involved in another" (p. 313). (Also, see discussion in the later section, "Women's Drug Trade Involvement.")

Physical and Psychological Dependence. The inability to discontinue their use of the amphetamines, particularly *methamphetamine*, has led to over a million people in the U.S., across the lifespan, to seek professional assistance from physicians, psychiatrists, psychologists, and other health and social care professionals—particularly in the western states of Arizona, California, Hawaii, New Mexico, and Texas—for the management of amphetamine dependence and related *tolerance* and *withdrawal.* A stark reflection of this situation is found in the outcomes of a national study analyzing trends in methamphetamine treatment among almost 250,000 pregnant women from 1994 to 2006:

> Methamphetamine has become the primary substance compelling treatment during pregnancy.
>
> *(Terplan, Smith, & Kozloski, 2009, p. 1285)*

TOLERANCE. Regular, long-term use of the amphetamines results in a *tolerance* to their desired psychostimulant actions and other related actions, particularly those that are centrally mediated, including cardiovascular effects and hyperthermia. Thus, women often increase their dosages to several grams per day in an effort to achieve desired psychostimulant actions and associated euphoria (Pagliaro & Pagliaro, *Clinical Patient Data Files*). However, tolerance to other chronic toxicities, such as amphetamine psychosis, does *not* generally occur. Thus, regular, long-term use of the amphetamines, particularly *high-dosage* use, will inevitably result in significantly *increasing* the risk for the development of amphetamine psychosis (see related discussion in earlier section, "Amphetamine Psychosis").

AMPHETAMINE WITHDRAWAL SYNDROME. A *true* amphetamine withdrawal syndrome, such as that which occurs following the abrupt discontinuation of the regular, long-term use of alcohol, opiate analgesics, or nicotine, and which can be *immediately* relieved with the resumed use of the drug or substance of abuse, has *not* been documented for any of the amphetamines, including methamphetamine. However, the abrupt discontinuation of regular, long-term patterns of *high* dosage *methamphetamine* use may result in signs and symptoms of *early-phase* withdrawal, which includes: anxiety; apathy; cognitive impairment; depressed mood (which may be severe); drug craving (often quite intense); fatigue; increased appetite; and sleep disturbances (e.g., excessive sleep).

Of note, it also is during *early-phase* withdrawal, which largely resolves within 1 week of the discontinuation of *amphetamine* or *methamphetamine* use, that most women, who abuse *methamphetamine*, perpetrate acts of violence against others, including their partners and children (Hamilton & Goeders, 2010). A *later-phase* withdrawal follows, characterized by similar, but significantly *less* severe signs and symptoms, that may last for an additional 2 weeks (McGregor, Srisurapanont, & Jittiwutikarn, 2005). There is *no* specific pharmacotherapy for the management of the signs and symptoms associated with amphetamine or methamphetamine withdrawal (Shoptaw, Kao, & Heinzerling, 2009). Medical management remains symptomatic (Pagliaro & Pagliaro, 2009).

Pregnancy, Lactation, and Mothering. As reported by the Committee on Health Care for Underserved Women (2011, p. 751):

> Among pregnant women, admissions for the treatment of methamphetamine abuse increased from 8% of federally funded treatment admissions in 1994 to 24% by 2006, with 73% of these admissions occurring in the western states.

Maternally ingested methamphetamine displays transplacental transfer to the fetus—as demonstrated by measurable levels in the neonate (Garcia-Bournissen, Rokach, & Karaskov, 2007). Fortunately, the use of *methamphetamine* by women during pregnancy has *not* been conclusively associated with any major physical birth defects, or *teratogenesis* (Pagliaro & Pagliaro, 2009, 2012). However, it has been associated with *expected* toxicities among women who are pregnant. In addition, there is *increased* risk for low birth weight and small-for-gestational-age births. Although not yet substantiated, it has been suggested that intrauterine exposure to *methamphetamine* and resultant effects on fetal growth and development may result in the expression of neurodevelopmental abnormalities during childhood (Eze, Smith, & LaGasse, 2016; Pagliaro & Pagliaro, 2012). Thus, as a precautionary measure, women who are pregnant should *not* use amphetamines, including methamphetamine. As well, women who use amphetamines should *discontinue* their use during pregnancy. In cases where use is necessary (e.g., medical management of A-D/HD), *extreme* caution is indicated.

The amphetamines are excreted in breast milk—often in concentrations that are 2 to 3 times *higher* than those found in maternal plasma. Breast-fed neonates and infants may experience expected pharmacologic effects including: agitation; crying; decreased body weight (generally associated with poor feeding behaviors and/or poor maternal-infant attachment); and irritability (Pagliaro & Pagliaro, 2009, 2012). Mothers who are breast-feeding should *not* use the amphetamines. Alternatively, mothers who are unable to discontinue their use of amphetamines, should *not* breast-feed.

In addition, methamphetamine abuse by women, who are mothers, particularly those who have neonates, infants, and young children in their custodial care, has been found, in several studies, to adversely affect both: (1) maternal-bonding; and (2) mothering (Pagliaro & Pagliaro, 2012). As identified by Derauf, LaGasse, and Smith (2007), "methamphetamine using women are more likely to have multiple, intertwined psychosocial risks that may result in maladaptive parenting and care-giving" (p. 281). Nair, Schuler, and Black (2003) also noted that "when drug use occurs in the context of multiple other risks, it may interfere with the mothers' ability to care for their children" (p. 993). Contributing factors, identified by the researchers, that could potentially *increase* "parenting problems and negative child outcomes" among drug abusing mothers included:

- Absence of a boyfriend, husband, or another intimate partner (e.g., being a "single parent")
- Domestic violence, including IPV, psychological abuse, and sexual abuse
- Family size (i.e., a high number of children)
- Homeless, or "living on the street"
- Incarceration, particularly with a longer sentence
- Major depressive disorder or other mental disorders
- Severity of drug and/or substance abuse

As identified in the analysis of data on the Navajo Nation from the Tuba City Health Facility, of the cases involving methamphetamine use, one-half of the cases involved women and, of these women, a significant number were pregnant young mothers. This situation has resulted in significant negative consequences for the Indian community. As shared by the director of the facility, it "creates a serious problem at home and in the community because children are neglected" (First Nations Centre, 2006, p. 20).

Tragically, for mothers who abuse methamphetamine—as well as for their families, including children—the abuse typically culminates in outcomes that are both unanticipated and undesired. For example, as reported by Schabner (2004):

> "I didn't have to deal with everyday life," the mother of two said. "I felt energetic. I felt like I could do everything." She said she realized how false that impression was when the local child protective services took her children away.
>
> *(p. 2)*

Or, as further illustrated:

> Kimbrough talked about her arrest following the death of her child, Timmy Jr. Born premature at 25 weeks on April 29, 2008, Timmy Jr. weighed 2 pounds 1 ounce, and lived only 19 minutes. When Kimbrough tested

> positive for methamphetamine, her two daughters were swiftly removed from her custody, and for 90 days, she was allowed only supervised visits. Social services mandated parenting classes and drug treatment.
>
> *(Calhoun, 2012, p. 1)*[18]

Mothering by women, who abuse amphetamines and other drugs and substances of abuse, can ultimately have the most extreme and horrific of consequences—as sadly reported in the following case:[19]

> Three people [with histories of drug and substance abuse, including the abuse of methamphetamine] have been charged in the brutal sexual assault, murder and dismemberment of a 10-year-old girl, including the girl's mother. The mother's boyfriend and his cousin were also charged … Police say Victoria [the child victim] was injected with methamphetamine, sexually assaulted, strangled, and stabbed before being dismembered [and her body burned].
>
> *(Contreras & Montoya Bryan, 2016, p. 1)*

Or, as tragically reported in a news story by NBC News/Reuters:

> A baby in Oklahoma died after her mother, high on methamphetamine and opioids, put the 10-day-old girl in a washing machine with a load of dirty laundry.
>
> *(Wilson & Shiffman, 2015, p. 3)*

Overdosage

Overdosages involving the amphetamines are common among women, particularly those who illicitly obtain their amphetamines "on the street" for intravenous injection (i.e., methamphetamine) or pulmonary inhalation (i.e., crystal meth) and, thus, *cannot* guarantee: (1) the purity of the "amphetamine" obtained, including if it is an amphetamine (e.g., crystal meth), or something else; and (2) its estimated dosage, or strength.

Psychostimulant-related deaths among women in the U.S. increased *threefold* during the first decade of the new millennium from 0.2 per 100,000 person-years in 2000, to 0.6 per 100,000 person-years in 2009 (Calcaterra & Binswanger, 2013, p. 11). The rates of psychostimulant deaths are *highest* among women: (1) of

---

18 Three months after being released on bond, Kimbrough was back in jail on charges of selling oxycodone to a confidential informant (Calhoun, 2012). (See related discussion in the later section, "Women's Drug Trade Involvement.")

19 See the *Comprehensive Subject Index* of this text for other specific locations in which mothering and parenting are discussed.

European continental descent; (2) of American Indian descent; and (3) who reside in the western states (Calcaterra & Binswanger, 2013; Kerley, Leban, & Copes, 2014).

Signs and symptoms of acute amphetamine overdosage include: agitation; constipation; hallucinations; overstimulation; panic; paranoia; restlessness; seizures; tachypnea; and tremor. Depression and fatigue usually follow the CNS stimulation (see earlier related discussion). Other signs and symptoms include: abdominal cramps; circulatory collapse; diarrhea; dysrhythmias; hypertension or hypotension; nausea; and vomiting. Hyperpyrexia and rhabdomyolysis (i.e., an acute, sometimes fatal reaction caused by the rapid destruction of skeletal muscle and release of proteins, such as myoglobin, that may cause damage to the kidneys resulting in failure) also can occur. Fatalities associated with amphetamine overdosage among women, particularly among those who are *novice* users, are usually preceded by hyperpyrexia, hypovolemic shock, and seizures.

The treatment of amphetamine overdosage involves supportive medical treatment to maintain vital body organ functions and pharmacotherapy to manage troublesome signs and symptoms. Both chlorpromazine (Thorazine®), a phenothiazine antipsychotic tranquilizer, and olanzapine (Zyprexa®), an atypical antipsychotic, effectively antagonize many of the toxic effects associated with the amphetamines. The benzodiazepine sedative-hypnotic/anticonvulsant, diazepam (Valium®) (see Chapter 3, *Women's Prescription Sedative-Hypnotic Abuse*), is generally effective for managing associated seizures. Ammonium chloride may be used to *acidify* the urine to increase the renal excretion of the amphetamines (see related discussion in the earlier section, *Pharmacology*, "Pharmacokinetics"). There is *no* known antidote.

Amphetamine poisoning can be *unintentional* (i.e., accidental)[20] or *intentional* (i.e., suicide attempt).[21] Most poisonings are associated with the ingestion of oral amphetamine formulations (i.e., capsules; tablets) and are generally treated with slurries of activated charcoal that, when appropriately administered, can prevent the further absorption of the ingested amphetamines from the stomach. Emetics should *not* be administered to induce vomiting because of the risk for precipitating seizures and the associated potential for the aspiration of vomitus.

---

[20] Farst, Duncan, and Moss (2007) first reported accidental poisoning of children associated with the illicit production of methamphetamine in home laboratories, identifying "cases of children harmed by ingesting caustic substances used in the production of methamphetamine in the home" (p. 341).

[21] Several studies of methamphetamine users in outpatient treatment (e.g., Glasner-Edwards, Mooney, & Marinelli-Casey, 2008; Zweben, Cohen, & Christian, 2004) have provided *strong* evidence to support a significant association with suicide attempts. As noted by Durrell, Kroutil, and Crits-Christoph (2008) in their related review and study of a "large sample of treatment-seeking methamphetamine users, 27% had reported a previous suicide attempt, and 43% had reported violent behavior problems" (p. 2). We, too, have noted this relationship in our own clinical practice (Pagliaro & Pagliaro, *Clinical Patient Data Files*). However, based on other available data, we would suggest that the relationship between methamphetamine use and suicide is *more* tangential—being related, for example, to an underlying intervening variable such as *major mental depression*. The mental depression also may be a *mediating* factor contributing to both IPV and suicide *ideation* or attempts.

Women's Medical and Personal Amphetamine Use and Abuse

Regarding young women, who abuse the amphetamines and other psychostimulant drugs, college/university students comprise a "special case" in terms of both type and frequency of amphetamine use, as well as reasons for use. In fact, college/university students are the *largest* group of women who report the illicit use of prescription amphetamines (i.e., drugs that are primarily prescribed for the management of A-D/HD, both for children and adults in the U.S.). This section presents and discusses this special case of women's drug and substance abuse. We begin with women's medical use and abuse.

Women's Medical Amphetamine Use/Abuse

Since the 1990s, women have been *increasingly* attracted to the use of the amphetamines, particularly *methamphetamine*, and closely related drugs that are primarily prescribed for the medical management of attention-deficit/hyperactivity disorder (A-D/HD).[22] These prescription drugs include:

1. *Mixed-amphetamines* (Adderall®; Addies; Tic Tacs), a combination drug that contains amphetamine and dextroamphetamine, as well as their salt forms
2. *Lisdexamfetamine* (Vyvanse®, LDX), a more recently developed amphetamine, a dextroamphetamine prodrug of the phenethylamine class and amphetamine class, that is beginning to be *more* widely used to treat A-D/HD (Blick & Keating, 2007; Popovic, Bhattacharya, & Sivaswamy, 2009)
3. *Methylphenidate* (Ritalin®, Rs, The Smart Drug), a psychostimulant of the phenethylamine and piperidine classes that is closely related to the amphetamines and, for decades, was extensively used to treat A-D/HD, and continues to be used for this indication
4. Racemic amphetamine sulfate (Evekeo®), approved by the FDA for the treatment of: A-D/HD for children 3 years-of-age and older, as well as adults; narcolepsy for children 6 years-of-age and older, as well as adults; and obesity (short-term treatment) for children 12 years-of-age and older, as well as adults (Abramowicz, 2015; Pagliaro & Pagliaro, 2009); and available as an extended-release, disintegrating tablet

While some women, who have A-D/HD, use their own prescription drugs to get *high*, most commonly, women, who do *not* have A-D/HD, buy or steal prescription drugs—to abuse (Wilens, Adler, & Adams, 2008). Other women may

[22] During the last half of the 20th century, the amphetamines (e.g., dextroamphetamine, Dexedrine®) were extensively prescribed in the U.S. to manage exogenous obesity—almost exclusively for women (Pagliaro & Pagliaro, 2004, 2009). Due to widespread abuse and poor, long-term efficacy, the medical use of amphetamines in this context, although still legal, has virtually disappeared from mainstream medical practice.

resort to "double doctoring," or "doctor shopping" (i.e., obtaining multiple prescriptions from multiple physicians, to obtain amphetamines from multiple pharmacies). They often pay in cash for their A-D/HD prescriptions and drugs, and, as noted by Cepeda, Fife, and Berwaerts (2015), travel a median of 92 miles in their "drug quests." (Also, see the later section, "Women's Personal Amphetamine Use/Abuse.")

College/university students reportedly comprise the *largest* group of women who acknowledge illicit use of *prescription* amphetamines and methylphenidate (Ritalin®) in the U.S. (e.g., Bogle & Smith, 2009; Clemow, 2015; Clemow & Walker, 2014; Pagliaro & Pagliaro, *Clinical Patient Data Files*; Varga, 2012). For example:

- 43% of 1,550 undergraduate students reported using prescription stimulants illicitly (Advokat, Guidry, & Martino, 2008)
- 31% of 115 undergraduate students from two universities, who were receiving prescriptions for A-D/HD, reported misuse during attendance at college (Rabiner, Anastopoulos, & Costello, 2009)

In addition, diversion of amphetamines and methylphenidate, which have been prescribed for the management of A-D/HD, is common among this group (e.g., Bogle & Smith, 2009; Clemow, 2015; Clemow & Walker, 2014; Pagliaro & Pagliaro, *Clinical Patient Data Files*; Wilens, Adler, & Adams, 2008). For example, from a random sample of 1,738 university students, Sepulveda, Thomas, and McCabe (2011), found that, among a cohort of 55 past-year "prescription stimulant users":

> Diversion of prescription stimulants was common (36%) and occurred more frequently among stimulant users (57%).
>
> *(p. 551)*

Rabiner, Anastopoulos, and Costello (2009) found that 26% of their sample of undergraduate students diverted their psychostimulant prescriptions to peers. While among those, who had never been prescribed a psychostimulant for the treatment of A-D/HD, diversion from family (e.g., younger siblings) and friends (e.g., college classmates) are the most common sources for the prescription psychostimulants (e.g., Cassidy, McNaughton & Varughese, 2015; Novak, Kroutil, & Williams, 2007).

The prescription formulation, mixed amphetamines (Adderall®), is generally *more* frequently used by college/university students than is the more closely related "chemical cousin," methylphenidate (Concerta®, Metadate®, Ritalin®). For example, in a web-based survey of a random sample of 4,580 college/university students, Teter, McCabe, and LaGrange (2006) found that, among the past-year illicit prescription psychostimulant users, approximately 75% reported use of mixed amphetamines (i.e., Adderall®) while only approximately 25%

reported use of methylphenidate (i.e., Concerta®; Metadate®; Ritalin®). In addition, among those who illicitly ingested prescription amphetamines, *immediate-release* formulations were significantly more likely to be used than the *extended-release* formulations (Cassidy, Varughese, & Russo, 2015; Upadhyaya, Kroutil, & Deas, 2010).[23]

Women, who are undergraduate, college/university students and who also abuse prescription amphetamines and other prescription psychostimulant drugs, can be generally distinguished by one or more of the following physical and behavioral characteristics:

- Belong to a sorority
- Engage in weekly partying that is significantly related to prescription amphetamine or other prescription psychostimulant use
- Frequently attend dance clubs
- Equally as likely to report past-year use of prescription amphetamines, or other prescription psychostimulants, as undergraduate men
- More likely to be of European continental descent than of African or Asian continental descent or Hispanic descent (Latina)
- More likely report *increased* rates of undesired, or harmful, effects and toxicities associated with the use of prescription amphetamines, or other prescription psychostimulant use, including insomnia and restlessness
- *Higher* incidence of concomitant, poly-drug and substance abuse

(Hartung, Canu, & Cleveland, 2013; Jardin, Looby, & Earleywine, 2011; Kelly, Wells, & Leclair, 2013; Teter, McCabe, & Boyd, 2003; Teter, McCabe, & LaGrange, 2006; Wilens, Adler, & Adams, 2008)

Several reasons have been identified by college/university women, in the U.S., for their use and abuse of the prescription amphetamines and other prescription psychostimulants, as well as the abuse of *illicit* amphetamines (e.g., methamphetamine). These reasons include, to:

- Achieve euphoria
- Initially experience the effects of using a specific psychostimulant
- Get "high"
- Intensify alertness

[23] Although illicit amphetamines are usually orally ingested, a significant number of college/university students report *intranasal* use (Pagliaro & Pagliaro, *Clinical Patient Data Files*). For example, Teter, McCabe, and LaGrange (2006), in their web-based survey of 4,580 college students, found that:

> Nearly every illicit user (95.3%) reported oral administration, and 38.1% reported snorting prescription stimulants.
>
> *(p. 1501)*

- Self-medicate in an attempt to relieve or manage a mental disorder (e.g., mental depression)
- Stay awake to "party" through the night or to go "clubbing."

(e.g., Teter, McCabe, & Cranford, 2005; Varga, 2012; Wilens, Adler, & Adams, 2008)

However, the *primary* reason provided by college/university women for their *illicit* use of the prescription amphetamines and other psychostimulants (i.e., methylphenidate) is to *improve* academic performance (e.g., Bogle & Smith, 2009; Pagliaro & Pagliaro, *Clinical Patient Data Files*; Rabiner, Anastopoulos, & Costello, 2009).

Women's Personal Amphetamine Use/Abuse[24]

During the 1980s, the use of the amphetamines among young women was largely replaced by the use of cocaine (see the following section, *Cocaine*). However, by the mid-1990s, there was a *renewed* interest in the use of the amphetamines, particularly *methamphetamine*, as an economic alternative to cocaine. This interest was fostered by the increased availability of both the *powdered* form of methamphetamine and the *crystalline* form ("Crystal Meth"). The use of the crystalline, or *smokable*, form had its origin in Hawaii from where it quickly spread to California (hence, the street name, "West Coast") and, subsequently, across the U.S. (Pagliaro & Pagliaro, 2009), where its use became ensconced across urban and rural areas in the Midwestern and southern states (hence, the street name, "Hillbilly Crack") (Gonzales, Mooney, & Rawson, 2010; Hauer, 2010; Sexton, Carlson, & Siegal, 2006).

A troubling trend that developed during the first decade of the new millennium was the *increased* use of methamphetamine, particularly by adolescent girls, 16 to 17 years-of-age (Wu, Schlenger, & Galvin, 2006). The use of methamphetamine, primarily the use of the *crystalline* form—"Crystal Meth," "Glass," or "Ice"—*soared*, from 2000 to 2010, because of its ready availability, relatively *low* cost, and ability to rapidly achieve *high* methamphetamine blood concentrations (and desired psychostimulant effects) without intravenous injection. Crystal Meth, smoked in much the same way as crack cocaine, also could produce a *longer* duration of desired psychostimulant effects than crack cocaine (i.e., 4 to 8 hours versus 15 to 60 minutes). As such, it quickly became the "poor woman's cocaine."

However, by 2010, the use of *methamphetamine* began to be slowly replaced with *cocaine*—the rich woman's drug (see later section in this chapter). It may seem ironic, or even surprising, to some readers that the same attributes that made

---

[24] When considering women and their amphetamine, particularly *methamphetamine*, use and abuse, it is important to keep in mind that an overwhelming majority (i.e., approximately 90%) are active poly-drug and substance users (Glover-Kerkvliet, 2009; NIDA, 2007; Pagliaro & Pagliaro, *Clinical Patient Data Files*).

methamphetamine so popular—its widespread availability, cheaper price, and longer duration of action in comparison to cocaine—are now contributing to its decline in popularity as it increasingly becomes known as the "poor woman's drug" (Pagliaro & Pagliaro, *Clinical Patient Data Files*). (See Table 5.2.)

TABLE 5.2 Comparison of *Cocaine* and *Methamphetamine*

Cocaine	*Methamphetamine*
Classification: Psychostimulant, natural	**Classification:** Psychostimulant (amphetamine), synthetic
Available Forms: Cocaine Base ("Crack") and Cocaine HCl ("Powder")	**Available form:** Powdered crystal
Desired Effects: Produces a *brief "high"* (*short* half-life of elimination)	**Desired Effects:** Produces *long-lasting* euphoria, sexual disinhibition, and other desired effects (*long* half-life of elimination)
Medical Use: Limited dental and medical use as a local anesthetic for short surgical and other procedures	**Medical Use:** Limited medical use for A-D/HD; exogenous obesity (maintenance or loss of body weight); narcolepsy
Personal Use: "Rich Woman's Drug" *primarily* used in the U.S. by women of African continental descent	**Personal Use:** "Poor Woman's Drug" *primarily* used in the U.S. by women of European continental descent
Methods of Use: Cocaine HCl powder is dissolved and intravenously injected; or nasally insufflated ("snorted"). Cocaine Base is heated, with a crack pipe or on the top of a discarded soda pop can or piece of tin foil, and the fumes inhaled.	**Methods of Use:** Methamphetamine is ingested; dissolved and intravenously injected; or nasally insufflated ("snorted"). It also is heated and inhaled from a glass pipe or from the top of a discarded soda pop can or piece of tin foil, and the fumes inhaled.
Mechanism of Action: Acts by *blocking* dopamine reuptake	**Mechanism of Action:** Acts by *increasing* dopamine release and *blocking* its reuptake
Metabolism/Elimination: 50% excreted in unchanged form in the urine over approximately 1 hour (pH dependent)	**Metabolism/Elimination:** 50% excreted in unchanged form in the urine over approximately 12 hours (pH dependent)
Abuse Potential: *High* abuse potential with extreme psychological craving. Cocaine does *not* display a true, or classical, withdrawal syndrome such as that which occurs with opiate analgesics and can be relieved with immediate resumed use.	**Abuse Potential:** *High* abuse potential. Methamphetamine does *not* display a true, or classical, withdrawal syndrome such as that which occurs with the opiate analgesics and can be relieved with immediate resumed use.
Street Names: *Blow; C; Coke; Nose Candy; Powder; Snow; Toot*	**Street Names:** *Crank; Crystal; Glass; Ice; Meth; Speed; Tina; Tweak*

Life-time prevalence of methamphetamine use among women in the U.S., 18 to 49 years-of-age, is approximately 7.3% (9% for men) (Durell, Kroutil, & Crits-Christoph, 2008). However, as noted, the use of *methamphetamine*, as with many other drugs and substances of abuse, waxes and wanes over time. As identified by Calcaterra and Binswanger (2013), "methamphetamine use *declined* significantly [in the U.S.] from 2002 to 2008, but *rose* again in 2009" (p. 2). Consequently, treatment statistics *vary* over the years—obviously, falling behind use statistics. Data available from the SAMHSA (2014), indicate that adolescent girls and women, from 15 years-of-age to 55 years-of-age, significantly outnumber (by percent) men in terms of methamphetamine being the *primary* drug responsible for treatment admissions. (Also, see Chapter 8, *Preventing and Treating Women's Drug and Substance Abuse*.)

As we identified from our analysis of data, which were collected from several sources (e.g., CDC, 2007; Durell, Kroutil, & Crits-Christoph, 2008; Maxwell & Rutkowski, 2008; and NIDA, 2007, 2013a), regarding adult methamphetamine abuse in the U.S., *ten* major trends in demographics and usage became well-established by the second decade of the new millennium:

1. Over 1 million adults, or 0.5% of the U.S. population, report using methamphetamine in the past year
2. Approximately 500,000 report using methamphetamine in the previous month
3. Approximately 5% report lifetime prevalence of use
4. Annually, over 100,000 ED visits are due to methamphetamine abuse
5. Methamphetamine abusers are approximately equally divided between women and men
6. On average, methamphetamine abusers commence use at 20 years-of-age
7. Most methamphetamine abusers are of European descent
8. The *highest* current rate of methamphetamine abuse is among adults, 18 to 25 years-of-age
9. Most methamphetamine abusers are in the West and Midwest[25]
10. The eastward spread of the methamphetamine epidemic slowed due to the *decreased* availability of the chemical precursor, pseudoephedrine[26]

During the methamphetamine epidemic that began in the U.S. during the 1990s, women comprised *less* than 50% of the users (Schabner, 2004). Well into the second decade of the new millennium, they now comprise *over* 50% of

[25] In addition, illicit psychostimulant (i.e., cocaine, methamphetamine) abuse, as well as "dealing," has been a significant and persistent problem among American Indians—particularly those residing on or near reservations in the Southwestern United States (First Nations Centre, 2006; Forcehimes, Venner, & Bogenschutz, 2011; Pagliaro & Pagliaro, *Clinical Patient Data Files*).

[26] The *decrease* in availability was directly due to the enactment of specific laws that purposely restricted the availability of ephedrine and pseudoephedrine to prevent, or reduce, their illicit conversion into methamphetamine (see earlier related discussion in the *Pharmacology*, "Methamphetamine" section).

methamphetamine users (Lyons, 2014).[27] When considering this trend, it is important to keep in mind that an overwhelming majority of women (i.e., approximately 90%), who abuse amphetamines, particularly *methamphetamine*, are poly-drug and substance users (Glover-Kerkvliet, 2009; NIDA, 2007; Pagliaro & Pagliaro, *Clinical Patient Data Files*). As adolescent girls and young women increasingly become involved with methamphetamine use, this trend is expected to continue.

Regarding this trend, it also is important to note that adolescent girls and women use amphetamines for some of the same, as well as for significantly different, reasons than do adolescent boys and men. Often introduced to the use of amphetamines by their boyfriends, *adolescent girls* primarily use amphetamines: (1) for their euphorigenic effects; (2) to decrease social inhibitions; (3) to enhance sexual pleasure; and (4) to gain acceptance, or to "fit in," with their peers. In comparison, *women* use the amphetamines: (1) for their euphorigenic effects; (2) to get *high*; (3) to feel *more* attractive and sexy; and (4) to *self-medicate*, often subconsciously, for their mental depression. They also use amphetamines: (5) as appetite suppressants to maintain, or lose, body weight; and (6) to *reduce* fatigue as they care for their homes and families as "super-moms," while they also attempt to deliver optimal job performances at work (Lyons, 2014; NIDA, 2007; Pagliaro & Pagliaro, *Clinical Patient Data Files*; Schabner, 2004; Schulzke, 2013). Consequently, a large, and still relatively well-hidden, group of women, who abuse *methamphetamine*, are rural or suburban women who, like other women, are *mothers*, *sex-for-drug exchangers*, *dealers*, and *producers*.

Women's Drug Trade Involvement. Other significant, methamphetamine-related trends include women's involvement in the drug trade and exchanging sex for methamphetamine. Regarding the former, up to 25% of women who abuse *methamphetamine* are actively involved in the drug trade, filling many diverse roles (Semple, Strathdee, & Zians, 2012). These roles include:

- "Look-out"
- Manufacturer
- "Mule"
- "Runner"
- Street-level dealer
- Wholesale/high-level dealer

> A woman attempted to smuggle methamphetamine into Texas from Mexico by hiding the drugs under her clothing and those of her infant child.
>
> *(Price, 2016, p. 1)*

Several reasons for becoming involved in the drug trade have been shared by women, who abuse methamphetamine, including: (1) monetary incentives; (2) to

---

27 For most other drugs and substance of abuse, *men* are the primary users with women comprising approximately one-third or less of the users (see relevant discussion in Chapters 1 to 4, and 6).

please a boyfriend or other significant partner; and (3) to achieve a feeling or sense of accomplishment and control (Boeri, 2013; Pagliaro & Pagliaro, *Clinical Patient Data Files*; Semple, Strathdee, & Zians, 2012).

Women's Sex-for-Drug Exchanges. Several researchers examining the phenomenon of women exchanging sex for methamphetamine (e.g., Corsi & Booth, 2008; Mimiaga, Fair, & Mayer, 2008; Watanabe-Galloway, Ryan, & Hansen, 2009) have identified that up to *one-third* of women who use *methamphetamine* exchange sex for the drug (e.g., Semple, Strathdee, & Zians, 2011).

Women's Methamphetamine Production: Effects on Mothers and Their Children. In a study of the impact of parent methamphetamine abuse on the development and well-being of school-aged children, Haight, Jacobsen, and Black (2005) found that:

> Children are brought by their methamphetamine abusing parents into a rural drug culture characterized by distinct antisocial beliefs and practices. Children's experience of this culture includes environmental danger, chaos, neglect, abuse, loss, and isolation … children develop antisocial beliefs and practices such as lying, stealing, drug use, and violence through direct teaching by their parents and indirectly, through observing [their] parents' own antisocial behavior.
>
> *(p. 949)*

As identified by Grant (2007):

> The illicit manufacturing and use of methamphetamine continues to be a significant and growing problem in the United States. Children are often found in homes where this activity is occurring and are affected by it on many levels.
>
> *(p. 31)*

For example, associated involvement with the criminal justice system, has resulted in *severe* negative effects on women and their children, including prolonged mother-child separation due to a mother's arrest and incarceration (Gold, 2016).[28] These effects have negatively impacted their roles as mothers resulting, quite commonly, in physical and psychological abuse and neglect of their children.

Regarding women's production of methamphetamine, "children are frequently found at the scene" of their mother's methamphetamine production "laboratory," which is often the kitchen or bathroom, in their apartment, home, or house trailer.

As a result, they are exposed to a countless number of toxic chemicals, including: (1) chemicals used in the production of methamphetamine;

[28] For additional related discussion, see the "Drug Courts" section in Chapter 8, *Preventing and Treating Women's Drug and Substance Abuse*.

(2) methamphetamine, itself; and (3) toxic wastes that are the "by-products" of the production process (Hohman, Oliver, & Wright, 2002, p. 373).[29] These women, and their children, also are susceptible to various injuries (e.g., burns) related to laboratory explosions and fires—injuries that may be severe and, sometimes, fatal (Pagliaro & Pagliaro, 2012; Winslow, Voorhees, & Pehl, 2007).

In addition, women, who produce, sell, and abuse methamphetamine in their homes, often have young children who reside with them, and who, consequently, may be inadvertently exposed to the toxic fumes associated with the production of methamphetamine. Common signs and symptoms of exposure to these toxic fumes include: abdominal pain; amber or dark-colored urine; blurred vision; chemical burns; chest pain; cognitive impairment; coughing; diarrhea; eye pain; fever; headaches; hallucinations; irritability; loss of body weight; skin irritation; sneezing; tachycardia; watery eyes, tearing, or other eye discharge; and vomiting (Horton, Berkowitz, & Kaye, 2003; Pagliaro & Pagliaro, 2012).[30]

Children, who live in households in which their mothers produce methamphetamine, also may suffer from maternal neglect identified by malnutrition and poor hygiene with associated infections (e.g., particularly involving the respiratory and urinary tracts) and infestations (e.g., body and head lice). They also may suffer forms of direct physical abuse often identified by patterns of bruising, broken bones, burns, and other physical injuries perpetrated by their mothers or others (e.g., mother's boyfriend) living in the home—often an abandoned residence, apartment, camper truck, hotel or motel room, house trailer, or remote, rural residence.

Children, whose mothers abuse and illicitly produce amphetamines, may also suffer various types of psychological abuse commonly identified by behavioral problems, learning difficulties, and mental depression. As identified by Lineberry and Bostwick (2006, p. 81):

> The on-call social worker had been summoned to evaluate the 6-year-old son [of a 23-year-old, single mother who has a history of methamphetamine

[29] Citing U.S. DEA data, Winslow, Voorhees, and Pehl (2007) noted that, for each pound of methamphetamine produced in "home laboratories," over 6 pounds of toxic waste are produced.

[30] For example, as noted by Burke, Lewis, and Latenser (2008), in their retrospective case-control study of adult burn patients, who were admitted for treatment, 10% who screened positive by urinalysis for methamphetamine use upon admission, were significantly *more* likely, than those who did *not*, to have: "*larger* burns in terms of affected body surface area (BSA); *higher* rates of inhalation injuries; and more nonthermal injuries" (p. 574). In a similar study comparing "meth patients with other burn patients," Blostein, Plaisier, and Maltz (2009, p. 1712), found that "meth patients": (1) suffer more frequent inhalation injuries; (2) need greater initial fluid resuscitation volume; (3) require endotracheal intubation more frequently; and (4) are more likely to have medical complications.

In a follow-up study, Davidson, Blostein, and Walsh (2013) found that "burn surgeries per patient were significantly increased in the current group" (p. 119). Others (e.g., Spann, McGwin, & Kerby, 2006) have reported similar findings, as well as, significantly increased rates of mortality among burn patients who suffered burns secondary to methamphetamine production laboratory explosion and fires.

> abuse]. She learns that the boy not only has had irregular school attendance but also has been experiencing academic difficulties and behavioral outbursts.

In this regard, the CDC (2007) cautioned that:

> Illegal methamphetamine production results in fires, explosions, spills, or air releases of hazardous chemicals (meth-chemical incidents), placing the meth producer and others nearby, including children, workers, and responders, at risk of injury or death and causing environmental contamination.
>
> *(p. 910)*

In 2015, the CDC noted that:

> During 2001–2012, a total of 1,325 meth-related incidents were reported in five states (Louisiana, Oregon, Utah, New York, and Wisconsin).
>
> *(Melnikova, Orr, & Wu, 2015, p. 909)*

Following is a list, from *high to low*, of the reported incidence of injuries associated with illicit methamphetamine production that was derived from the CDC 2015 surveillance report by Melnikova, Orr, and Wu (2015, p. 912):

- Respiratory irritation
- Burns
- Eye irritation
- Skin irritation
- Gastrointestinal distress
- Headache
- Dizziness
- Trauma

As noted by Connell-Carrick (2007), "Methamphetamine use and production is changing child welfare practice" (p. 125). To better deal with the significant risks posed to these children, several states (e.g., California) have created special "drug-endangered children's units" (Messina, Marinelli-Casey, & West, 2014). These units generally involve some degree of cooperation among various concerned agencies including, for example, child protective services (CPS), district attorney's offices, health and social care professionals, and police departments. (Also, see related discussion in the earlier section, "Women's Methamphetamine Production.")

In addition, several states have formally developed and adopted specific, related guidelines. For example, the state of Georgia, in a collaborative project with the Georgia Poison Center, developed a 15-page report entitled, *Guidelines for Managing Children Found at Clandestine Methamphetamine Laboratory Sites*). The explicit stated goals of these "Guidelines" are:

1. To assure the safety of the children found at meth laboratories
2. To assure the safety of law enforcement, health care providers, state agency personnel and the public interacting with and caring for children found at meth laboratories
3. To minimize the psychosocial trauma to the children while protecting their health and safety

(Geller, 2005, p. 5)

We now turn to *cocaine*.

Cocaine

Cocaine, in its powder form (i.e., *cocaine hydrochloride*), is intranasally insufflated or intravenously injected. In its base form (i.e., *crack* cocaine or *freebase* cocaine), it is vaporized and inhaled. Widely available across the U.S., it is commonly abused by women for such desired psychostimulant effects as intense euphoria and heightened sexual experiences. In this section of Chapter 5, we present and discuss the pharmacology of *cocaine*, including its: pharmacodynamics, or proposed mechanism of action; pharmacokinetics, or absorption, distribution, metabolism, and excretion; undesired, or harmful, effects and toxicities, including its potential for *psychological* dependence; and overdosage. We conclude the section with a presentation and discussion of women's medical and personal use and abuse of cocaine. We begin with the pharmacology of cocaine, which helps to explain why women, over the new millennium, both desire and abuse cocaine.

Pharmacology

Cocaine is an alkaloid primarily extracted from the leaves of two varieties of the coca plant (i.e., *Erythroxylon coca*), which is indigenous to the eastern slopes of the Andes Mountains of South America. The coca leaves from these plants contain typically, by weight, about 1% cocaine. The cocaine is generally produced for *illicit* distribution and sale in two forms, *cocaine hydrochloride* (HCl) and *crack cocaine*. Each of these forms has its own pharmacologic characteristics and patterns of use.

> Popular Notion: Crack cocaine is much *stronger* than cocaine powder and works at different brain centers.
>
> NOT TRUE. Once absorbed into the systemic circulation, both crack cocaine and cocaine powder work by the *same* mechanism of action and, at equivalent dosages, produce the same effects.

Cocaine Hydrochloride and Crack Cocaine

Cocaine Hydrochloride. Cocaine hydrochloride (cocaine HCl) is the salt form of cocaine that *readily* dissolves in water (i.e., 1 gram in 0.5 ml). A white powder that is generally intranasally insufflated, or "snorted," its *high* water solubility allows rapid absorption from the moist mucous membranes lining the nasal cavity. In addition, because of its *high* solubility in water, it is easily dissolved for intravenous injection.[31]

Crack Cocaine. Crack cocaine (i.e., cocaine base or freebase cocaine) is the natural form of cocaine that is directly extracted from the coca leaves. Only *slightly* soluble in water (i.e., 1 gram in 1,300 ml), it readily dissolves in ethanol (i.e., 1 gram in 7 ml), ether (i.e., 1 gram in 4 ml), and chloroform (i.e., 1 gram in 0.5 ml).[32] The melting point of crack cocaine is significantly *lower* than that for cocaine hydrochloride (i.e., 98° Celsius versus 195° Celsius). Thus, when heated, it vaporizes much more readily and is involved in less pyrolysis. Accordingly, pulmonary inhalation of the vaporized crack cocaine, or *smoking*, can achieve blood cocaine concentrations that are *equal* to those achieved by the intravenous injection of cocaine hydrochloride.

In addition, for pulmonary inhalation, because of the mechanisms inherent in pulmonary absorption, the onset of action is more rapid than with intravenous injection and it produces a subjectively *more* intense desired action. For these and other reasons (e.g., convenience; lower cost; avoidance of infections associated with intravenous injection, such as HIV infection), women, who use cocaine, often prefer the pulmonary inhalation of vaporized crack cocaine to any other method of cocaine use (e.g., intravenous injection; nasal insufflation).

Pharmacodynamics: Mechanism of Action

After absorption into the systemic circulation, cocaine is found in virtually *all* areas of the brain. However, it appears to preferentially accumulate in the caudate nucleus, the nucleus accumbens, and the ventral tegmental area. Cocaine *decreases* the dopamine transporter (DAT) clearance of dopamine from the synaptic cleft by blocking its reuptake into the presynaptic cells. It also appears to *block* the reuptake of other monoamines, including serotonin and norepinephrine. Consequently, cocaine increases the accumulation and activity of neurotransmitters in the synaptic cleft. A simplified representation of the proposed principal site and mechanism of cocaine's action is shown in Figure 5.2.

---

[31] Cocaine HCl, because of its high water solubility, also is used for selected medical and dental purposes, such as local anesthesia of the membranes of the oral, laryngeal, and nasal cavities.

[32] Thus, the requisite use of organic solvents (e.g., acetone, gasoline) in South American "jungle" laboratories to extract the cocaine from harvested cocaine leaves.

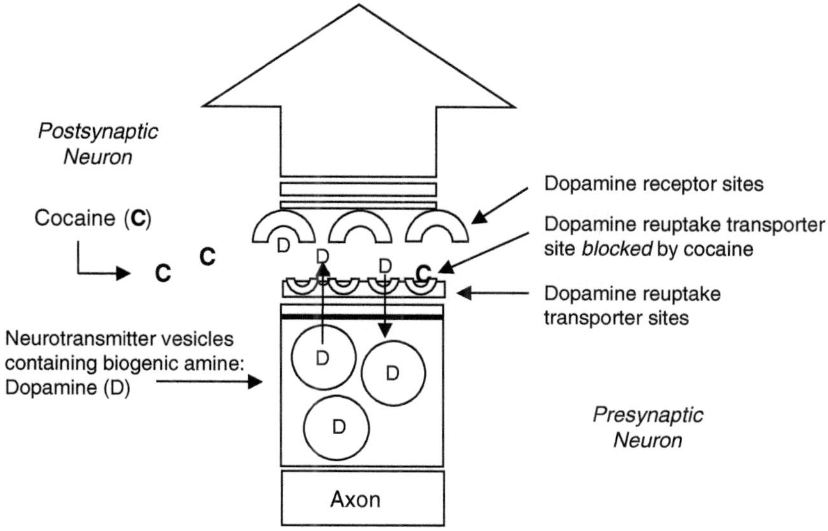

FIGURE 5.2 Cocaine: Mechanism of Psychostimulant Action

The ability of cocaine to *increase* neurotransmitter activity in the brain causes several *desired* effects that contribute to its continued use. These effects include: (1) an *intense* euphoria; (2) feelings of *increased* energy and competence; (3) *heightened* sociability and sexual desire; (4) *decreased* feelings of fatigue and hunger; and (5) *indifference* to pain and discomfort. Approximately 30 years ago, Dackis and Gold (1990) suggested that the action of cocaine could be divided into *three* phases: (1) the euphoric phase; (2) the excitation phase; and (3) the depression phase. This theory has remained a popular and useful one for explaining the observed actions and effects of cocaine.

During *Phase I*, cocaine stimulates the CNS, beginning with the cerebral cortex, by *decreasing* the reuptake of neurotransmitters (e.g., dopamine and serotonin). These actions generally result in euphoria and *mild* stimulation. As the amount of cocaine is *increased* by smoking, injecting, or snorting more lines, *Phase II*, the excitation phase, begins. During Phase II, more pronounced CNS stimulation occurs with various associated effects (e.g., anxiety; hypertension; mydriasis; rapid speaking; tachycardia; tremors; vomiting). However, as cocaine use continues, neurotransmitters in the CNS become depleted and *Phase III*, the depression phase, begins.

Phase III is characterized by a *depression* of the cortical areas of the CNS, which may progress to medullary depression and associated respiratory failure. This phase spontaneously resolves, but *not* until after the depleted endogenous neurotransmitters have had sufficient time to be *naturally* replenished. The associated mental depression experienced during this phase is commonly referred to as the "cocaine blues" (Pagliaro & Pagliaro, 2009).[33] (Also, see the later section, *Physical and Psychological Dependence*.)

Pharmacokinetics: Absorption, Distribution, Metabolism, and Excretion

The absorption, distribution, metabolism, and excretion of cocaine is affected by its: (1) formulation—cocaine hydrochloride or crack cocaine; (2) purity; and (3) method of use, or route of administration.

Absorption and Distribution. The mean *bioavailability* of cocaine is only approximately 33% after oral ingestion and, thus, women rarely use this method of administration. After intranasal insufflation, or "snorting," of cocaine hydrochloride, bioavailability is approximately 70%. However, the *rate* of intranasal absorption and the *total amount* absorbed may be significantly *reduced* by the *limited* surface area of the nasal mucosa and the local vasoconstriction that occurs in the nostrils as a direct pharmacological action of cocaine when "snorted." With intravenous injection, the bioavailability of cocaine is 100%. In comparison, when crack cocaine is vaporized or "smoked" with a glass "crack pipe" and inhaled into the lungs, pulmonary bioavailability is very *high* (i.e., over 90%), but incomplete, because a small portion of the dose is destroyed by pyrolysis[34] and a small, but relatively *larger* portion remains in the crack pipe.

Peak serum cocaine concentrations occur approximately 45 minutes after oral ingestion, 10 minutes after intranasal insufflation, and 1 minute after pulmonary inhalation (i.e., vaporization, or "smoking") or intravenous injection (i.e., "mainlining").

Metabolism. Cocaine is hydrolyzed and metabolized primarily in the liver to several metabolites, including: benzoylecgonine; ecgonine; ecgonine methyl ester; hydroxycocaine; hydroxybenzoylecgonine; and norcocaine. Esterases found in the plasma are predominately responsible for the formation of the major metabolite, benzoylecgonine. Esterases also are found in many other tissues, including hepatocytes.

---

[33] Mental depression, whether a result of the "cocaine blues," normal female hormone cycles from menarche through menopause, or situational variables (e.g., divorce; financial difficulties), is integrally related to women's cocaine use and abuse. For example, women often use cocaine as a means, consciously or, in in most cases, unconsciously, to self-medicate, or manage, their mental depression. As noted by Johnson, O'Leary, and Striley (2011, p. 1279), "current major depression appears to be associated with an increased risk for crack use among women."

[34] The major portion of the pyrolysis of crack cocaine is *methylecgonidine*. The amount of methylecgonidine that is produced, generally ranges from 1% to 5%, depending upon the temperature and rate of air flow in the crack pipe. The presence of methylecgonidine (i.e., anhydroecgonine methyl ester) has been used as a biological marker to differentiate (e.g., in forensic biological samples) crack cocaine smoking from other methods of cocaine use.

Concomitant use of alcohol and cocaine may result in up to 20% of the systemically available cocaine being converted to *cocaethylene*, a psychoactive ethyl homologue of cocaine. This interaction exclusively involves alcohol and cocaine. Women who use cocaine often comment that their concomitant use of alcohol appears to enhance, or prolong, the euphoria they experience with cocaine and mitigates the undesired effects associated with the use of alcohol (e.g., sedation). These effects may be explained, at least in part, by the formation of cocaethylene.

Excretion. The mean elimination half-life of cocaine is 1.25 hours. However, the elimination of cocaine appears to be influenced by urinary pH (as with the amphetamines). Consequently, cocaine elimination is increased in acidic urine (i.e., pH less than 7) and decreased in alkaline urine (i.e., pH greater than 7). In addition, the total body clearance of cocaine may be significantly *reduced* with the concurrent use of alcohol. (Also, see related discussion of *cocaethylene* in the previous section, *Metabolism*.)

Undesired, or Harmful, Effects and Toxicities

The use of cocaine has been commonly associated with several *acute* toxicities that are directly related to its specific pharmacologic actions on various body systems. The regular, long-term use of cocaine also has been implicated with the development of more *chronic* toxicities, including psychological dependence and, when used by adolescent girls and women during pregnancy, teratogenesis. Other toxicities have been specifically related to its adulteration and methods of use—intranasal insufflation, or snorting; pulmonary inhalation of the vaporized form, or smoking; and intravenous injection, or "mainlining" or "shooting up." These common toxicities are presented and discussed in the following sections.

Acute Toxicities. The use of cocaine has been associated with several acute toxicities, which are primarily related to its psychostimulant action, including: agitation; anxiety; apathy; cerebral vascular accident; difficulty concentrating; headache; hyperpyrexia; hypertension; insomnia; irritability; loss of sexual desire; memory impairment; mydriasis; myocardial infarction; panic attacks; seizures; suicide attempts; tachycardia; and tremors.

The acute toxicities of cocaine, which are directly related to its pharmacologic actions, depend upon the dose administered (i.e., the larger the dose, the greater the associated effect—in this context, toxicity). However, because cocaine is predominantly used in an *illicit* context and consequently, predominantly *illicitly* produced without stringent quality control standards, the dose administered depends upon the purity of the cocaine used. Studying the correlation between cocaine purity and trends in emergency department (ED) visits (i.e., as a measure of toxicity), Zhu, Wilson, and Stimpson (2014) found that:

> Cocaine purity is positively correlated with cocaine-related ED visits, and our findings suggest decreases in powder cocaine purity were associated with significant declines in ED visits.[35]
>
> *(p. 1015)*

Several other variables may play a role in the occurrence of these toxic effects and their severity. For example, the effect of HIV infection—as noted by Meyer, Little, and Fitzgerald (2014, p. 352), "crack cocaine use is associated with impaired memory in HIV-infected women more than uninfected women."

Chronic Toxicities. Regular, long-term use of cocaine has been associated with the development of additional toxicities, including: mental depression; paranoia; and psychological dependence (e.g., Pagliaro & Pagliaro, *Clinical Patient Data Files*; Pagliaro, Jaglalsingh, & Pagliaro, 1992). Increasing attention also is being given to data suggesting the association of regular, long-term use of cocaine with cognitive impairment, particularly deficits in executive cognitive functioning that involves decision making or problem solving (Bickel, Frank, & Moody, 2013; Moody, Franck, & Jarmolowicz, 2014). Cocaine psychosis and intimate partner violence are two other troubling undesired, or harmful, effects that are commonly associated with cocaine abuse. As found by Falck, Wang, and Carlson (2001), in their prospective study of women who abused crack cocaine, "since initiating crack use, 62% of the women reported suffering a physical attack" (p. 79).

COCAINE PSYCHOSIS. Cocaine psychosis is virtually indistinguishable from amphetamine psychosis, although it is usually of *shorter* duration (see earlier section in this chapter, *Amphetamines*). It also shares with amphetamine psychosis a similarity to paranoid schizophrenia. Both cocaine and amphetamine psychosis are often characterized by hypervigilance and paranoia and have been associated with an increased incidence of aggressive and violent behavior, including homicide (Pagliaro & Pagliaro, *Clinical Patient Data Files*).

INTIMATE PARTNER VIOLENCE. In a retrospective analysis of data from 96 related studies, Moore, Stuart, and Meehan (2008) found that, of *all* the drugs and substances of abuse, *cocaine* had the *strongest* relationship with *intimate partner violence* (IPV). (Also, see related discussion in the earlier *Amphetamines* section.) Although mental factors (e.g., personality traits; concurrent mental disorders; concomitant drug or substance use, including alcohol use) are very likely major contributing factors (Pagliaro & Pagliaro, *Clinical Patient Data Files*), IPV has been consistently found to be *strongly* associated with cocaine use (e.g., Ernst, Weiss, & Enright-Smith, 2008; Kraanen, Vedel, & Scholing, 2014; Siegal, Falck, & Wang, 2000; Smith,

---

[35] The finding was in the context of the related finding, which indicated that the average purity for cocaine powder in the greater Chicago area/market, fell from 65.2% in 2004 to 37% in 2010 (Zhu, Wilson, & Stimpson, 2014, p. 1013).

Homish, & Leonard, 2012; Winhusen & Lewis, 2013)—both in regard to women being *victims* and/or *perpetrators* of IPV.

For example, Gilbert, El-Bassel, and Chang (2012), in a longitudinal study of a representative sample of 241 low-income urban women receiving emergency care from an ED in the Bronx, New York, found that:

1. Crack or cocaine use was associated with an increased likelihood of injurious IPV and severe verbal abuse
2. Sexual IPV was significantly associated with subsequent use of crack or cocaine (p. 226)

Kalokhe, Paranjape, and Bell (2012) evaluated the incidence of IPV among HIV-infected crack cocaine users. Their sample was comprised of 343 participants, mostly of African continental descent and of low socioeconomic status. Results indicated that the overall "estimated IPV prevalence [in their sample] was 56%, highest in women (68%)" (p. 234).

Several studies (e.g., Illangasekare, Burke, & McDonnell, 2013) also have suggested that women who experienced *severe* IPV were several times *more* likely to be mentally depressed, than those who did *not* experience *severe* IPV. Cocaine, and/or amphetamine, use in this context may be explained, at least partially, as an attempt by these women to *self-medicate* their mental depression.

In addition to IPV, women, who use cocaine, have been noted in many studies to be subject to *increased* violence from multiple sources (e.g., drug dealers, "johns," pimps).[36] For example, Bungay, Johnson, and Varcoe (2010), in their critical ethnography of women's health and crack cocaine use in an inner-city neighborhood, identified that: "Everyday violence is perilously damaging for women who use crack" (p. 321).

Potentially Fatal Toxicities. Cocaine use has been related to fatal accidents, homicides, and suicides. However, there are *four* major, potentially fatal medical conditions associated with the abuse of cocaine that can occur regardless of a woman's age or her selected method of cocaine use:

1. Cardiotoxicity
2. CNS hemorrhage
3. Hyperpyrexia
4. Seizures

Other potentially fatal toxicities associated with cocaine abuse include: (1) toxicities that are associated with the inadvertent contamination, or deliberate

[36] Also, see later discussion in the sections, "Women's Sex-for-Drug Trading" and "Women's Drug Trade Involvement."

adulteration, of street supplies of cocaine *prior* to their distribution, sale, and use; and (2) toxicities that are related to the concomitant use of other drugs and substances of abuse, particularly alcohol and heroin (Bernstein, Bucciarelli, & Piper, 2007; Pagliaro & Pagliaro, 2009). Each of the four major potentially fatal medical conditions associated with cocaine use, as well as the significant threat posed by using adulterated cocaine, are discussed, in succession, in the following sections. (For related discussion, also see later section, "Overdosage.")

CARDIOTOXICITY. Cocaine's actions on the cardiovascular system have been associated with an increase in both heart rate and blood pressure. These actions, in turn, may lead to increased risk for dysrhythmias, end-stage renal disease, myocardial infarction, and stroke (Norris, Thornhill-Joynes, & Robinson, 2001; Phillips, Luk, & Soor, 2009; Pilgrim, Woodford, & Drummer, 2013). For example, Diercks, Kirk, and Turnipseed (2007) reported a significantly *high* rate of coronary artery disease among cocaine-using patients.

These severe, and possibly fatal, cardiotoxicities appear to occur, in part, because of the *decrease* in blood pH that is associated with cocaine use. The *acidemia* has been reported to cause scarring and disruption of the heart's electrical conduction system with prolongation of the QRS complex and QTc (i.e., corrected QT interval) duration on the electrocardiogram (ECG, EKG) (Wang, 1999). However, others have suggested molecular mechanisms of action for the cardiovascular effects associated with cocaine use, including: (1) interaction with cardiac calcium, potassium, and sodium (i.e., cation) channels (Turillazzi, Bello, & Neri, 2012); and (2) oxidative stress and resultant antioxidant cellular system injuries (Cerretani, Fineschi, & Bello, 2012).[37]

CENTRAL NERVOUS SYSTEM HEMORRHAGE. CNS hemorrhage (i.e., cerebrovascular accident, stroke) results from the combined effects of the vasoconstriction and increased cardiac output associated with cocaine use. CNS hemorrhage occurs more often among women who have cerebral aneurysms. Although it is estimated that approximately 1 in 20 people have a cerebral aneurysm, most women who use cocaine are unaware of this risk. This risk increases with age, irrespective of previous length of time of cocaine use.[38] In addition, a case-controlled study of stroke, in which participants were women (one-third) and men (two-thirds) of

---

[37] It should be noted that these different purported mechanisms of cocaine-induced cardiotoxicity are *not* mutually exclusive.

[38] Among hospitalized patients with aneurysmal subarachnoid hemorrhage, cocaine users are 3 times *more* likely to die than are nonusers (Chang, Kowalski, & Caserta, 2013). Similarly, in a large retrospective analysis of patients admitted to a stroke service from 2004 to 2007, Martin-Schild, Albright, and Hallevi (2010) found that:

> Patients with cocaine-associated intracerebral hemorrhage were nearly 3 times more likely to die during their acute hospitalization when compared to cocaine-negative patients.
>
> *(p. 680)*

African descent, who either abused crack cocaine or *did not* abuse crack cocaine, found that intracerebral hemorrhage occurred in twice as many participants who were crack cocaine abusers (i.e., 33.3% versus 17.2%) (Giraldo, Taqi, & Vaidean, 2012, p. 273).

HYPERPYREXIA. Cocaine-induced hyperpyrexia, a body temperature exceeding 104° Fahrenheit (41° Celsius), is usually caused by the combined effects of: (1) excessively stimulated body metabolism; and (2) vasoconstriction, which significantly impairs the ability of the body to cool itself. A body temperature of this magnitude can cause convulsions and coma, and may be fatal in up to 20% of cases. In non-fatal cases, irreversible brain damage may occur. Hyperpyrexia also is an associated sign that is observed in both cocaine-induced fatal excited delirium and cocaine-induced rhabdomyolysis.

SEIZURES. Seizures,[39] which may terminate in cardiovascular collapse, can be caused by several cocaine effects, including: (1) hyperactivity of the CNS; (2) increased body temperature; and (3) lack of sufficient oxygen in the CNS. On a molecular level, it has been proposed that the convulsions associated with cocaine use are mediated by means of interaction with $GABA_A$ receptors and NMDA receptors (Lason, 2001). Subsequently, Rolland, Karila, and Geoffroy (2011) extended this hypothesis by suggesting that the activation of the D1 receptor produces a kindling process involving the NMDA receptor phosphorylation state. Utilizing the case history of a 21-year-old woman, who chronically abused cocaine, they further postulated that the mechanism underlying cocaine-induced seizures could *overlap* with the mechanism underlying cocaine-induced psychosis.

ADULTERANTS. Adulterants (e.g., arsenic; benzocaine; corn starch; lactose, or milk sugar; quinine; sodium bicarbonate) are often used to *cut* various drugs and substances of abuse prior to selling them—most often to *increase* their bulk/volume and, consequently, to *increase* dealer profits. The adulterants that are used have been associated with several unique toxicities that can be *more* serious than those directly associated with the use of cocaine or other drugs and substances of abuse (see, for example, the related discussions in Chapter 1, *Women's Opiate Analgesic Abuse*). Unfortunately, the potential risk for unique and unexpected toxicities can occur whenever any illicitly manufactured drug or substance of abuse is prepared, sold, bought, and used.

For example, during 2008 to 2009, a specific adulterant, *levamisole*, was found in approximately two-thirds of all cocaine samples that were seized and analyzed by the U.S. government (Pagliaro & Pagliaro, 2009). Levamisole, a veterinary *deworming* agent (i.e., anthelminthic) also has been experimentally used in the treatment

[39] Among our patients and others, these seizures are commonly experienced/observed and are colloquially referred to by cocaine users as "doing the chicken" (Pagliaro & Pagliaro, *Clinical Patient Data Files*).

of some types of human cancers.[40] It has a stimulant action and may have been added to the illicit cocaine product to boost its effects. More likely, it was probably simply used to *cut* the cocaine to increase its weight and, consequently, the related profits of the distributor/seller.

The use of this adulterated cocaine was associated with several toxic effects, including: a flu-like syndrome; loss of the senses of smell and taste; leukopenia; and stomatitis. Levamisole also can cause agranulocytosis.[41] Over 30 cases of agranulocytosis, some *fatal*, were associated with using the adulterated cocaine in 2008 and 2009 (Czuchlewski, Brackney, & Ewers, 2010; Zhu, Legatt, & Turner, 2009). Subsequently, many cases of cutaneous vasculopathy associated with levamisole-adulterated cocaine use have been reported (e.g., Tran, Tan, & Marnejon, 2013; Ullrich, Koval, & Koval, 2011):

- "52-year-old woman who acutely developed an extensive bullous rash in the lower extremities after she snorted cocaine" (John, Manda, & Hamrock, 2011, p. 524)
- "A 48-year-old woman presented with a red, pruritic, and painful rash on her legs bilaterally after she snorted cocaine" (Shawwa, Alraiyes, & Eisa, 2013, p. 1)
- "44-year-old woman with a history of cocaine use … necrotic lesions of the nose led to its self-amputation … levamisole-induced vasculitis that required above-knee amputation" (Arora, Jain, & Bhanot, 2012, p. 19)

According to the *National Drug Abuse Warning Network* (DAWN), cocaine is involved in most of the admissions related to illegal drug and substance abuse reported by emergency departments (EDs) across the U.S. Approximately 0.5% of *all* emergency room admissions, on an annual basis, involve the use of cocaine (Office of National Drug Control Policy, 2010).

Toxicities Associated with Methods of Cocaine Use. Several toxicities have been commonly associated with the specific methods of cocaine use:

(1) Intranasal insufflation, or *snorting*
(2) Pulmonary inhalation, or *smoking*
(3) Intravenous injection, or *mainlining*

INTRANASAL INSUFFLATION, OR SNORTING. Intranasal insufflation of cocaine hydrochloride is associated with both *minor* irritation and *severe* injury to the nasal mucous membranes and the related underlying structures (e.g., nasal septum). Although *less* serious effects may occur, such as congestion (i.e., rhinitis) and

---

[40] It was withdrawn from American markets in 2005 because of concerns/reports of agranulocytosis (Buxton, Omura, & Kuo, 2015).

[41] The human leukocyte antigen (HLA)-B27 appears to confer a genetic predisposition to levamisole-induced agranulocytosis (Buxton, Omura, & Kuo, 2015).

eczema in and around the nostrils, more *serious* effects, such as nasal erosion and perforation of the nasal septum, also may occur, particularly with regular, long-term use (Vilela, Langford, & McCullagh, 2002).

The minor irritation and more serious injury are caused by: (1) the direct action of cocaine (i.e., vasoconstriction) on the surrounding skin and mucous membranes; and (2) the direct irritation of the hydrochloride salt form of cocaine, which, when it comes into contact with nasal secretions, forms a dilute, but irritating, solution of hydrochloric acid. The occurrence of these local effects, together with the relatively small surface area of the nasal mucosa, which restricts absorption rates to begin with, have helped to increase the popularity of the pulmonary inhalation, or smoking, of cocaine in its freebase, or crack, form—currently, the most popular method of cocaine use in the U.S. Unfortunately, this method of use (i.e., smoking) is associated with its own toxicities, particularly, pulmonary toxicities.

PULMONARY INHALATION, OR SMOKING. The toxicities associated with smoking cocaine result in both irritation and damage to the lungs, including pulmonary infiltrates and pneumonia. Acute exacerbation of asthma and bronchitis also may occur among users who already have these chronic medical conditions (i.e., COPDs) (Ali, Krugar, & Houghton, 2002; Gatof & Albert, 2002). In addition, the regular, long-term smoking of crack cocaine has been associated with alveolar and microvascular lung damage at the microscopic level—a condition that has been commonly referred to as "crack lung." For example:

> A 40-year-old woman with a history of recurrent "crack" cocaine use developed progressive shortness of breath over a period of years. Serial imaging revealed progressive interstitial fibrosis secondary to recurrent alveolar hemorrhage and inflammation from crack cocaine.
>
> *(Vidyasankar, Souza, & Lai, 2015, p. 77)*

INTRAVENOUS INJECTION, OR MAINLINING. The intravenous injection of cocaine has been related to several toxic effects. These effects include: the development of local infections and abscesses at the sites of injection; and the development of phlebitis when injected veins become irritated and inflamed as a response to being pierced with a needle and injected with an irritating solution of cocaine. Intravenous injection of cocaine also is associated with the development of thrombosis, which may be fatal.

These toxicities are *not* directly related to the action of cocaine, but rather to its chemistry (e.g., alkaline or basic pH; adulteration) and method of use—intravenous injection. Related to the method of use (i.e., piercing the protective skin barrier, causing injury to the epidermis, and dermis, as the needle is inserted through the skin to pierce the vein below), these effects may commonly occur with the intravenous use of *any* of the various drugs and substances of abuse. (Also, see Chapter 1, *Women's Opiate Analgesic Abuse*, Table 1.2.)

It is important to note that the intravenous injection of cocaine was a major contributing factor to the spread of the HIV infection during the late 1980s and 1990s (Pagliaro, Pagliaro, & Thauberger, 1993; Pagliaro & Pagliaro, 2000). "Coke burns," which are associated with the repeated inadvertent subcutaneous injection of cocaine by intravenous cocaine users, who miss the vein, are caused in much the same way as the intranasal irritation and damage that occurs with snorting cocaine (see previous discussion). These burns are related to the formation of dilute hydrochloric acid when the cocaine interacts with the subcutaneous body fluids.

Physical and Psychological Dependence. It has been estimated that of 100 women who try cocaine, 30 of the women will become *abusers*, and 10 will become *compulsive* users. Thus, for a significant number of women, who use cocaine, the cocaine *high* becomes the only—or, at least, primary—reason for living (i.e., cocaine use being preferred to personal likes, desires, or needs—including family, food, friends, recreation, sex, or career). This pattern of cocaine use often results in significant adverse social consequences for these women—and or their families and friends. (Also, see related discussion in the later section, *Women's Personal Cocaine Use/Abuse.*)

Over the last 2 decades, the consensus has been that there is *no* true physical dependence associated with the regular, long-term use of cocaine as defined by: (1) the development of tolerance with continued use; and (2) the occurrence of a withdrawal syndrome that is immediately relieved by the resumed use of the drug or substance of abuse—in this case, cocaine. Similar to the amphetamines, cocaine does *not* fit the classic definition of physical dependence because once the neurotransmitters are depleted, even if all the cocaine in the world was used, it would *not* relieve the undesired effects. Because cocaine indirectly stimulates the CNS, the endogenous neurotransmitters, which have been depleted in association with cocaine use, must be replenished before the use of cocaine can, again, achieve desired effects.

COCAINE WITHDRAWAL SYNDROME. The abrupt discontinuation of cocaine after regular, long-term use may result, however, in several undesired effects, including: anxiety; apathy; dysphoria; headaches; irritability; mental depression; mental fatigue (extreme); muscle cramps; psychomotor fatigue; sleep disturbances (e.g., insomnia); and vivid unpleasant dreams. These signs and symptoms may begin within a few hours of discontinuing cocaine use and generally resolve within 24 hours (Walsh, Stoops, & Moody, 2009). However, as previously noted, they *cannot* be relieved by resuming cocaine use.

Thus, the classic definitional criteria for a true cocaine withdrawal syndrome are *not* met (i.e., the development of tolerance and, upon abrupt discontinuation of use, signs and symptoms of withdrawal that can be relieved by the resumed use of the drug or substance of abuse). These signs and symptoms have been ascribed to the *severe* psychological dependence associated with the use of cocaine (i.e., craving). Interestingly, women are more likely than men to report craving for cocaine within 1 hour of discontinuing its use (Kennedy, Epstein, & Phillips, 2013).

The underlying cellular mechanism involved in cocaine withdrawal appears to be related to a decrease in mesolimbic dopamine activity (Hu, 2007; Kuhar & Pilotte, 1996). Dopamine modulates neuronal activity in the prefrontal cortex and is necessary for optimal cognitive functioning (Nogueira, Kalivas, & Lavin, 2006). The decrease in dopamine activity associated with cocaine withdrawal has been related to associated anhedonia and relapse (Kuhar & Pilotte, 1996; Walsh, Stoops, & Moody, 2009).

Pregnancy, Breast-Feeding, and Mothering. The use of cocaine by women during pregnancy, when breast-feeding, or when mothering neonates, infants, and young children can result in many harmful effects. These, sometimes deleterious effects are presented and discussed in the following sections.

COCAINE USE DURING PREGNANCY. Cocaine use by women who are pregnant is a significant problem in *most* major cities across the U.S. The three major factors associated with *high* rates of cocaine use during pregnancy are: (1) African continental descent; (2) deficient, or low, educational achievement; and (3) lower socioeconomic status. Numerous studies have documented the use of sex in exchange for crack cocaine (i.e., sex-for-drug exchanges), particularly among pregnant women of African descent.[42] For example, Sharpe (2001), in an ethnographic study of "34 poor Black women who exchanged sex for crack," found that "18 reported sex-for-crack pregnancies, and more than half of that number became pregnant this way more than once" (p. 612).

> Mother goes on crack cocaine binge in Florida motel giving birth in the bathtub and cutting the umbilical cord with her teeth ... newborn is in critical condition...
>
> *(Keneally, 2014, p. 1)*

(For additional related discussion, also see later section, "Women's Sex-for-Drug Trading.")

The use of cocaine by women during pregnancy is associated with intrauterine death, including spontaneous abortion; preterm delivery; and a variety of fetal physical abnormalities, including cerebral hemorrhages or infarctions, and intrauterine growth retardation (e.g., reduced head circumference).[43]

---

[42] See Pagliaro and Pagliaro (2000), for a comprehensive overview and discussion of related data *prior* to the new millennium.

[43] N.B. A causal relationship between cocaine use and the various observed fetal abnormalities has *not* been definitively established (i.e., there is *no* consensus in terms of common characteristics or features of the so-called "crack baby"—in stark contrast to the FAS/FASD (e.g., Pagliaro & Pagliaro, *Clinical Patient Data Files*; Schiller & Allen, 2005; Vidaeff, & Mastrobattista, 2003). This lack of a

In addition, cocaine use by pregnant women has been associated with low birth weight, seizures, and tachycardia among neonates and a significantly *higher* rate of developmental delays and learning disorders among preschoolers and school-age children (Pagliaro & Pagliaro, 2012). It also has been suggested by several researchers (e.g., Meyer & Zhang, 2009) that intrauterine cocaine exposure also may result in *increased* risk of heart disease as an adult. However, as identified by Viteri, Soto, and Bahado-Singh (2015):

> In summary, the literature available evaluating long-term effects on growth and neurodevelopment in children exposed to cocaine in utero is contradictory and likely subject to confounding bias as a result of the adverse social environment in which these children live.
>
> *(p. 408)*

Neonates, who are born to mothers who used *large* amounts of cocaine near term, also may experience CNS excitation (e.g., increased crying, irritability, and tremulousness). Thus, despite the lack of definitive confirmatory data, but with an abundance of caution, we strongly recommend that women, who are pregnant, should *not* use cocaine.

COCAINE AND BREAST-FEEDING. Women who are breast-feeding are cautioned *not* to use cocaine. Cocaine is excreted in women's breast milk. Thus, breast-fed neonates and infants may display characteristic CNS stimulation (e.g., irritability; seizures; tremulousness) and other expected effects (e.g., dilated pupils). Women who use cocaine, should *not* breast-feed their neonates or infants (Pagliaro & Pagliaro, 2002, 2009, 2012).

COCAINE AND MOTHERING. The disruption of maternal-infant and child attachment because of a mother's cocaine abuse may result in many harmful effects (Eiden, Schuetze, & Coles, 2011), including placing infants and children at extreme risk for neglect and abuse (Pagliaro & Pagliaro, *Clinical Patient Data Files*). In addition, as found by Mansoor, Morrow, and Accornero (2012) in their study of the relationship between prenatal maternal cocaine use and mother-child interactions:

> Prenatal and past-year maternal cocaine use seem to be associated with poorer quality in mother-child interaction during early childhood.
>
> *(p. 32)*

---

definitive relationship is due, in part, to the observation that women who use cocaine while pregnant are over 50 times more likely to also use other drugs and substances of abuse, including alcohol and nicotine—both of which have been recognized as human teratogens. (See Chapter 2, *Women's Alcohol Abuse*, and Chapter 4, *Women's Caffeine and Nicotine Abuse*.)

In addition, as described by Strathearn and Mayes (2010, p. 172) and Ryder and Brisgone (2013, p. 40), of increasing concern, particularly regarding alcohol and marijuana abuse—as well as cocaine abuse—is the apparent significant potential for "intergenerational transmission" of drug abuse and drug-related problems among *daughters*.

Overdosage

Cocaine overdosage may be fatal. Death is generally the result of cardiac dysrhythmias, hyperthermia, intracranial hemorrhage, respiratory arrest, or status epilepticus. *Acute* cocaine overdosage requires emergency medical support of body systems, with attention to *increasing* cocaine elimination. There is *no* known antidote (Pagliaro & Pagliaro, 2009, 2012).

Women's Medical and Personal Cocaine Use and Abuse

Women's Medical Cocaine Use/Abuse

The only currently approved medical use for cocaine in the U.S. is its use as a local anesthetic. A topical solution of cocaine (4% or 10%) is applied to accessible mucous membranes of the oral, laryngeal, or nasal cavities where it blocks the initiation and conduction of nerve impulses thereby eliciting a local anesthetic action. As noted in the position statement of the American Academy of Otolaryngology—Head and Neck Surgery, "No other single drug combines the anesthetic and vasoconstriction properties of cocaine" (2013, p. 1). The cocaine solution is *not* generally prescribed, nor is it particularly attractive to users who prefer the use and effects of cocaine hydrochloride and crack cocaine.[44]

Women's Personal Cocaine Use/Abuse

> With a crack hit, five minutes later you're running and chasing that feeling, that high.
>
> *(Ryder & Brisgone, 2013, p. 48)*

Various U.S. studies and reports estimate the annual use of cocaine among adults at approximately 2% (see Table 5.3). In comparison, the estimate for "past year use" of cocaine among university/college students is approximately 5% (University of

[44] An exception that we have noted in our clinical practices has included several dentists, who were abusing pharmaceutical grade cocaine topical solution administered through refilled, disposable nasal spray containers (e.g., empty Dristan® nasal spray containers)—kept readily available in their dental jacket pocket or hung from a chain or cord around their neck—reportedly, "to treat nasal congestion."

TABLE 5.3 New Millennial Annual Cocaine Use Estimates in the U.S.

Population Sample	*Reported Annual Cocaine Use Estimates*	*Reference Source*
12th-Grade Adolescents	**3.6%** (2.5% cocaine HCl and 1.1% crack cocaine)	NIDA (2013b)
12th-Grade Adolescents	**3.7%** (2.3% cocaine HCl and 1.4% crack cocaine)	NIDA (2016)
Adults, 18 to 25 years-of-age	**5.4%**	NIDA (2016)
Adults, 26 years-of-age and older	**1.7%** (1.4% cocaine HCl and 0.3% crack cocaine)	NIDA (2013b)
Hispanic Women	**1.4%**	U.S. Department of Health Resources and Human Services Administration (2011)
Non-Hispanic White Women	**1.7%**	U.S. Department of Health Resources and Human Services Administration (2011)
U.S. (general population)	**2.2%**	Kelley (2012)
U.S. (general population)	**2.3%**	*Which countries...* (2015)
Young Adults	**6.0%**	SAMHSA (2011)

Michigan, 2008).[45] In addition, it is estimated that approximately 40 million adolescent girls and women, 12 years-of-age and older (approximately 15% of the population), have used cocaine at least *once* in their lifetimes—a number that is generally maintained with approximately one million *new* users initiating cocaine use annually (Office of National Drug Control Policy, 2010). It also has been estimated that 5.3 million people in the U.S. (i.e., 1.6%), 12 years-of-age and older, including an estimated 2 million parents, have used cocaine in the previous year (NIDA, 2013b).

As the population of "baby boomers" continues to age during the first 2 decades of the new millennium, they continue many of their drug and substance use/abuse behaviors (Newmeyer, 2003; Pagliaro & Pagliaro, *Clinical Patient Data Files*; Schlaerth, Splawn, & Ong, 2004). For example, Rivers, Shirazi, and Aurora

[45] Using data obtained from a convenience sample of 4,580 undergraduate students from a major Midwestern research university, McCabe, Morales, and Cranford (2007) found that the *highest* reported use of cocaine (utilizing the data from the female students only) was among female students of European continental descent and Hispanic descent (i.e., 3.5%). The *lowest* reported use of cocaine was among female students of African and Asian continental descents (i.e., approximately 1%).

(2004) noted, in their sample derived from older patients presenting to an inner-city academic emergency department, that 2% tested positive for cocaine use.

Throughout the new millennium in the U.S., a *high* incidence of cocaine use among women was found to be related to several demographic factors, including: age; continental descent; history of alcoholism; homelessness; and socioeconomic status (e.g., Pagliaro & Pagliaro, *Clinical Patient Data Files*; Pope, Falck, & Carlson, 2011).[46] Other factors include involvement in sex-for-drug exchanges and drug dealing. Research findings, as related to each of these factors, are briefly highlighted in the following sections.

Demographic Factors. Demographic factors, particularly: age; continental descent; history of alcoholism; homelessness; and socioeconomic status are presented and discussed in the following sections.

AGE. Participants in a cohort study of *over* 200 "African American crack-using women," generally reported that their use of crack cocaine began in their mid-twenties (Wechsberg, Lam, & Zule, 2003, p. 669). A decade later, Whitehead, Trenz, and Keen (2014) found that cocaine use, "beginning at midlife," was significantly *higher* among *older* women. (Also, see earlier related comments concerning "baby boomers.")

However, club-going adolescent girls and young women (16 to 30 years-of-age)—who are usually poly-drug and substance of abuse users—reportedly have one of the *highest* rates of cocaine use (Grov, Kelly, & Parsons, 2009; Parsons, Grov, & Kelly, 2009; Ramo, Grov, & Delucchi, 2010).

HISTORY OF ALCOHOLISM. During the early part of the new millennium, a positive history of alcoholism in an immediate family member was associated with a risk for initiating cocaine use and subsequent dependence. However, the full nature of the genetic and/or sociocultural relationship has *not* yet been determined (Compton, Cottler, & Ridenour, 2002; Pagliaro & Pagliaro, *Clinical Patient Data Files*).[47]

---

46 An additional factor, "ovarian hormones," also appears to be a significant contributor to women's cocaine use. To date, most supporting data have come from animal studies. However, clinical studies of women tend to support the observations that: (1) progesterone, which is predominant during the luteal phase of the menstrual cycle, *attenuates*, or reduces, the reinforcing effects of cocaine (i.e., "drug liking"; euphoria; "high"); while (2) estrogen, which is predominant during the follicular phase, *enhances* the reinforcing effects of cocaine (e.g., Moran-Santa Maria, Flanagan, & Brady, 2014).

47 In a more recent study, Marks, Pike, and Stoops (2015) identified an interesting relationship between alcohol and cocaine use—although the mechanism has *not* yet been discerned. Recognizing that "alcohol consumption is a known antecedent to cocaine relapse," they conducted a double-blind, placebo-controlled, within-subjects study with 20 current cocaine users. The purpose of their study was to evaluate the effect of three different doses of alcohol on cocaine cue attentional bias. The result was that "alcohol administration increased craving for cocaine in a dose-dependent manner" (p. 1823).

CONTINENTAL DESCENT. A preference for cocaine or amphetamine (i.e., methamphetamine) appears to be generally divided in the U.S. by continental descent with women who abuse crack cocaine being predominantly of African continental descent, while women who abuse methamphetamine being predominantly of European continental descent (Esteban McCabe, Morales, & Cranford, 2007; Pagliaro & Pagliaro, 2009). For example, in a study of over 800 incarcerated women, the prevalence of cocaine dependence was significantly *higher* among incarcerated women of African descent, while the prevalence of methamphetamine dependence was significantly *higher* among those of European descent (Proctor, 2012, p. 278).

In another example, Palamar, Davies, and Ompad (2015), in their secondary analysis of data from the *National Survey on Drug Use and Health, 2009–2012*, determined that, in the U.S.:

1. Powder cocaine (i.e., cocaine HCl) was primarily used by women (and men) of European continental descent
2. Crack cocaine (i.e., cocaine base) was primarily used by women (and men) of African continental descent

Although available data appear to support arguments that preferences among women of different continental descents for cocaine or amphetamines may be primarily related to genetic differences, it is more likely that they reflect socioeconomic and sociocultural differences.

WOMEN'S HOMELESSNESS AND SOCIOECONOMIC STATUS. In their study of 260 *homeless* women in San Francisco, for whom "the median age was 47 and 70% were women of color" (p. 173), Riley, Shumway, and Knight (2015) found that almost *half* of their study participants used cocaine. In another study, Wenzel, Green, and Tucker (2009, p. 16) found, among their sample of *homeless* women, that those "with a greater proportion of drug users in their networks" had greater odds of using cocaine. Conducting a secondary analysis of the data from the *National Survey on Drug Use and Health, 2009–2012*, Palamar, Davies, and Ompad (2015) found that, among adults, "Crack users are at *higher* risk of arrest and tend to be of *lower* socioeconomic status compared to powder cocaine users" (p. 108).

Women's Sex-for-Drug Trading.[48] While drug and substance abuse has always had some association with sexual activity (e.g., use of date rape drugs—see, for example, Chapter 2, *Women's Alcohol Abuse* and Chapter 3, *Women's Prescription Sedative-Hypnotic Abuse*), it came to its zenith in the U.S. during the 1990s when it became inextricably ingrained in the crack cocaine subculture—particularly that affecting inner-city neighborhoods primarily comprised of families of African continental descent (Pagliaro & Pagliaro, 2000).

---

[48] Also, see related discussion in earlier section, *Cocaine Use During Pregnancy*.

Sadly, as noted by Ryder and Brisgone (2013):

> Neither the mothers nor the daughters of the Crack Era have fared well, and to ignore their stories is to watch the repetition of destructive patterns in future generations, regardless of the next "drug of choice."
>
> *(p. 58)*

Since that time, numerous studies and reports have documented the degradation and dehumanization of women (i.e., "crack whores")[49] by men within, and beyond, "crack houses." Unfortunately, this damaging degradation and dehumanization of women has continued into the new millennium (Pagliaro & Pagliaro, *Clinical Patient Data Files*). In the U.S., the victims of this exploitative and vile behavior have most often been women of African continental descent. As noted by Borders, Stewart, and Wright (2013):

> Crack cocaine use was positively associated with multiple sexual partners.
>
> *(p. 535)*

In addition:

> [Among] a racially diverse sample of cocaine users, both in treatment and community-dwelling, African American women reported rates of trading sex for drugs or money and number of sexual partners that were both higher than those reported by African American men and white or Hispanic women.
>
> *(p. 535)*

To better understand women's involvement in sex-for-drug trading, Edwards, Halpern, and Wechsberg (2006) examined "correlates of exchanging sex for drugs or money among women who use crack cocaine" (p. 420). Their study sample, 669 women of African continental descent, was part of the "Woman-Focused HIV Prevention with African American Crack Abusers Study." They found that *most* of the women in their study, who used crack cocaine (i.e., 66%), did *not* trade sex for cocaine. However, women who did trade sex for cocaine (i.e., 34%), had *high* risk factors for engaging in this behavior, including:

- Crack use for 15 or more days during the past month
- History of childhood physical and/or sexual abuse

---

[49] As identified by Simon (2016):

> Indeed, even street culture has always had its own dismissive names for a woman who has sex for drugs—"strawberry," "crackstatute," "toss up," "buffer," "bag bride"—placing her at the bottom of a hierarchy of already-marginalized people.
>
> *(p. 2)*

- Homelessness
- Most friends/associates also use drugs and substances of abuse

They also found two *protective* factors that were associated with a significantly *lower* percentage of involvement in sex-for-drug trading:

- Married or living with an intimate partner
- Full- or part-time employment

Unfortunately, women involved in trading/exchanging sex for drugs, particularly cocaine, are at a significant risk for HIV infection and, as documented by several researchers (e.g., Pagliaro, Pagliaro, & Thauberger, 1993), a corollary risk for spreading HIV to others. For example, Nilsson Schonnesson, Atkinson, and Williams (2008), in their study of "African-American crack cocaine smokers with HIV infection," found that, in direct relation to their cocaine use: (1) the numbers of sexual partners *increased*; and (2) the use of condoms became *more* inconsistent. In addition, Harzke, Williams, and Bowen (2009), in their study of African-American HIV-positive crack cocaine users, found that bingers were more likely to report: (1) lifetime trading of sex for drugs; (2) binges, on average, lasting for 3.7 days; (3) smoking, on average, 40 crack cocaine "rocks" during a binge; and, for 72% of bingers, (4) during their last binge, having sex, on average, with 3.1 *different* sexual partners (female and male).

> "I've … done party-and-play situations where the guy will share his blow with me in exchange for fucking," Alana relates. "The last time I did that, it was this guy I absolutely loathed and I explicitly told him I was there for the coke and not because I gave a shit about him."
>
> "He had a *gram* to share between us!" she exclaims. "I was pissed. On top of which, it was shitty blow and he didn't seem to care about conserving it—he cut it up on top of a CD case and was getting it everywhere. All I could think was, "We only have a fucking gram, you asshat, don't fucking waste it. I hate you so much right now."
>
> *(Simon, 2016, p. 3)*

In an earlier new millennial qualitative study of women who abused crack cocaine, Kail and Elberth (2002) identified that women's involvement in sex-for-drug trading also can significantly affect their entry into treatment, and is often overlooked. As shared by a participant in their study:

> Just the fact a woman has a way of making money and getting high she can always have something, can always get something and that makes it harder to come into treatment.
>
> *(p. 7)*

In the U.S., women's crack cocaine use, and the associated need for money to maintain its use, also led to their *increasing* direct involvement in the drug trade.

Women's Drug Trade Involvement. During the cocaine era of the 1990s, Federal Courts in the U.S. were hesitant to imprison women, particularly women who were pregnant and/or had young, dependent children in their care. This hesitance continued virtually unabated into the new millennium. However, it is beginning to change.[50]

> Males have made up at least 85% of the jail population since 2000. [However,] the female inmate population increased 18.1% between midyear 2010 and 2014, while the male population declined 3.2%.
>
> *(Minton & Zeng, 2015, p. 3)*

> Over the past three decades, the *increase* in the female prison population has continuously surpassed that of the male prison population in all 50 states, making women the fastest growing segment of the U.S. prison population.
>
> *(Allen, Flaherty, & Ely, 2010, p. 160)*

The *increasing* active involvement of women in the abuse of cocaine (e.g., Alleyne, 2006) and in the drug trade (e.g., Allen, Flaherty, & Ely, 2010)—albeit, usually at the lower end—have significantly contributed to these changes. Thus, in the U.S., it is generally estimated that 60% of women, who are incarcerated in federal prisons, are incarcerated due to drug trafficking offenses. In state prisons, approximately 25% of women, who are incarcerated, are incarcerated due to drug trafficking offenses (Bureau of Justice Statistics, 2013; Carson & Sabol, 2012).

> For a dozen years ... the unassuming woman owned five small wooden houses along the poor side street, filling them with her children, grand-children and other relatives who kept the lots tidy, watched out for trouble and pitched in with the family business ... an operation that monopolized crack cocaine sales in the area and employed her grown children and close acquaintances...
>
> *(Thompson, 2013, p. 1)*

---

50 These changes generally have not been viewed favorably by feminists and others. For example, the American Civil Liberties Union (2005), in relation to the *increasing* incarceration of women due to the U.S. "War on Drugs," stated:

> The war on drugs is having a specific, dramatic, and devastating impact on women that requires further study and attention when evaluating the success of drug policies that do far more harm than good in women's lives.
>
> *(p. 2)*

During the new millennium, women became *increasingly* involved in drug dealing and trafficking. Prototypical characteristics of these women include that they:

- Are single mothers
- Are socioeconomically disadvantaged
- Deal from their home or apartment
- "Front" for a boyfriend or their "baby daddy" (i.e., if arrested, courts tend to be *more* lenient with women than men, who also may have an extensive criminal record)
- Have a poor education
- Live in an ethnic ghetto
- Sell relatively small amounts of cocaine to support their own personal use, rather than using sex-for-drug trading or exchanging to do so
- Use cocaine
- Usually are receiving social assistance

> Two women were charged as cocaine and crack dealers near Seaford as one of them tried to flush a large bag of the drugs [less than 2 ounces] down a toilet, state police said on Tuesday.
>
> *(Brown, 2015, p. 1)*

However, most of the women, who are formally involved in drug dealing or trafficking, are paid for a specific activity and are *not* simply working to obtain a small amount of the drug for their own personal use. Many of these women work along the U.S./Mexico border, where the overwhelming majority of illicit drugs enter the U.S. (Pagliaro & Pagliaro, *Clinical Patient Data Files*).

> Listen, if you're looking for work I might be able to hook you up. I know of a good job, traveling … working as a mule … It's a cool job. You go, hand off the stuff, get your cash. And that's it. Like winning the lottery.
>
> *(Giacomello, 2014, p. 12)*

Unlike their "bosses," who live dangerous, but sometimes luxurious lives, more than 99% of these women, while also living dangerous, but *not* luxurious lives, work as "drug mules" smuggling drugs across the U.S.-Mexican border. Prior to crossing the border—on foot, by bus, by car, by train, or by commercial airline—these women generally either swallow "pepas," capsules of cocaine, or stuff packages of cocaine (i.e., "agaucates," avocados) as high as possible into their vaginas (Giacomello, 2014).

Whenever possible, to decrease suspicion and scrutiny by U.S. border guards, "bosses" use pregnant women and/or women with young children traveling on their own without a male companion. Once the cocaine is delivered into the U.S., the women are paid a stipulated wage/fee—generally, 500 pesos, or about

35 dollars U.S.—an amount significantly *more* than what they would receive for working at jobs otherwise available to them (e.g., cleaning; cooking; taking care of children or older people; washing clothes) (Giacomello, 2014; Pagliaro & Pagliaro, *Clinical Patient Data Files*; Wells, 2013).

As identified by Giacomello (2014), in her research study on women and drugs along the U.S./Mexico border:

> Most of them, either in the trade or as consumers, share the precarious existence common to many poor women throughout the Americas: social exclusion, gender-related violence, sexism, feminization of poverty, and single parenthood. [As explained by one of the women working as a drug mule,] "I have four children and I am a single mother. We don't do it because we're going to become millionaires, but because we're desperate."
>
> *(p. 2)*

References[51,52,53]

Abramowicz, M. (2015, September 28). Racemic amphetamine sulfate (Evekeo) for ADHD. *The Medical Letter on Drugs and Therapeutics*, 57(1478), 137–139.

Advokat, C. D., Guidry, D., & Martino, L. (2008). Licit and illicit use of medications for attention-deficit hyperactivity disorder in undergraduate college students. *Journal of College Health*, 56(6), 601–606. doi:10.3200/JACH.56.6.601-606

Ali, S. R., Krugar, M., & Houghton, J. (2002). Upper airway obstruction and acute lung injury associated with cocaine abuse. *International Journal of Clinical Practice*, 56(6), 484–485.

Allen, S., Flaherty, C., & Ely, G. (2010). Throwaway moms: Maternal incarceration and the criminalization of female poverty. *Affilia: Journal of Women and Social Work*, 25(2), 160–172. doi:10.1177/0886109910364345

Alleyne, V. (2006). Locked up means locked out: Women, addiction and incarceration. *Women and Therapy*, 29, 181–194.

American Academy of Otolaryngology—Head and Neck Surgery. (2013, May 6). *Position statement: Medical use of cocaine.* Retrieved March 11, 2016, from entnet.org, pp. 1–3: www.entnet.org/content/medical-use-cocaine

---

[51] As per publisher style, only the first three authors are listed for each reference.

[52] Several times the number of references listed were found, obtained, and analyzed by the authors during the preparation of this chapter. However, only the references that were cited at least once in the body of the text are included in the list. Major reasons for not citing other references, include that they: (1) did not provide any additional unique data; (2) were not well researched or written (i.e., were evaluated as not being valid or reliable); (3) were based predominantly, or exclusively, on animal studies; (4) provided usage statistics from outside the U.S.; and/or (5) were redundant with, or not as recent as, the already cited references.

[53] The reference citation, "Pagliaro & Pagliaro, *Clinical Patient Data Files*," refers to unpublished data collected, with permission, over the last 50 years by the authors, in the formal course of their professional academic roles as clinician scientists and professors—from their patients, research subjects, and students, from the 1970s to date.

American Civil Liberties Union. (2005). *Caught in the net: The impact of drug policies on women and families*. American Civil Liberties Union. Retrieved August 15, 2016, from www.aclu.org/images/asset_upload_file393_23513.pdf

Ares-Santos, S., Granado, N., & Espadas, I. (2014). Methamphetamine causes degeneration of dopamine cell bodies and terminals of the nigrostriatal pathway evidenced by silver staining. *Neuropsychopharmacology*, 39(5), 1066–1080. doi:10.1038/npp.2013.307

Ares-Santos, S., Granado, N., & Moratalla, R. (2013). The role of dopamine receptors in the neurotoxicity of methamphetamine. *Journal of Internal Medicine*, 273(5), 437–453. doi:10.1111/joim.12049

Arora, N. P., Jain, T., & Bhanot, R. (2012). Levamisole-induced leukocytoclastic vasculitis and neutropenia in a patient with cocaine use: An extensive case with necrosis of skin, soft tissue, and cartilage. *Addiction Science & Clinical Practice*, 7(19), 1–100. doi:10.1186/1940-0640-7-19

Bartos, L. (2005, July). Meth production is toxic to communities (methtoxic). *NEBLINE Newsletter*, pp. 1–4. Lincoln, NE: University of Nebraska-Lincoln. Retrieved November 2, 2016, from http://lancaster.uni.edu/family/methtoxic.shtml

Berkes, H. (2007, April 4). *Mexican "ice" replaces home-cooked meth in U.S.* Retrieved from National Public Radio (NPR), pp. 1–15: www.npr.org/templates/story/story.php?storyId=9193186

Bernstein, K. T., Bucciarelli, A., & Piper, T. M. (2007, March 9). Cocaine- and opiate-related fatal overdose in New York City, 1990–2000. *BMC Public Health*, 7, 31. doi:10.1186/1471-2458-7-31

Bickel, W. K., Franck, C. T., & Moody, L. (2013). Executive dysfunction among alcohol- and cocaine-dependent women: 2013. *APA 121st Annual Convention Proceedings* (p. NP). Honolulu, HI: American Psychological Association. doi:10.1037/e612522013-001

Blick, S. K., & Keating, G. M. (2007). Lisdexamfetamine. *Paediatric Drugs*, 9(2), 129–135.

Blostein, P. A., Plaisier, B. R., & Maltz, S. B. (2009). Methamphetamine production is hazardous to your health. *The Journal of Trauma*, 66(6), 1712–1717. doi:10.1097/TA.0b013e3181a0e589

Boeri, M. (2013). *Women on Ice: Methamphetamine use among suburban women*. New Brunswick, NJ: Rutgers University.

Bogle, K. E., & Smith, B. H. (2009). Illicit methylphenidate use: A review of prevalence, availability, pharmacology, and consequences. *Current Drug Abuse Reviews*, 2(2), 157–176.

Borders, T. F., Stewart, K. E., & Wright, P. B. (2013, November). Risky sex in rural America: Longitudinal changes in a community-based cohort of methamphetamine and cocaine users. *The American Journal on Addictions*, 22(6), 535–542. doi:10.1111/j.1521-0391.0391.12028.x

Brown, R. (2015, August 25). *Two women charged as cocaine, crack dealers.* Retrieved from The News Journal: rbrown@delawareonline.com

Brown, R. E., Morisky, D. E., & Silverstein, S. J. (2013). Meth mouth severity in response to drug-use patterns and dental access in methamphetamine users. *Journal of the California Dental Association*, 41(6), 421–428.

Brzeczko, A. W., Leech, R., & Stark, J. G. (2013, September). The advent of a new pseudoephedrine product to combat methamphetamine abuse. *American Journal of Drug and Alcohol Abuse*, 39(5), 284–290. doi:10.3109/00952990.2013.821476

Buie, J., & Tamburin, A. (2014, November 17). *Meth-lab busts down; dealers getting drug from Mexico.* Retrieved from The Tennessean: www.story/news/crime/2014/11/16/meth-labs-tn-dealers-turning-mexico/19141893/

Bungay, V., Johnson, J. L., & Varcoe, C. (2010). Women's health and use of crack cocaine in context: Structural and "everyday" violence. *The International Journal on Drug Policy*, 21(4), 321–329. doi:10.1016/j.drugpo.2009.12.008

Bureau of Justice Statistics. (2013, May 24). *Federal Criminal Case Processing Statistics Online Analysis Tool*. Federal Justice Statistics Resource Center. Retrieved June 24, 2016, from www.bjs.gov/fjsrc/index.cfm

Burke, B. A., Lewis, R. W., & Latenser, B. A. (2008). Methamphetamine-related burns in the cornbelt. *Journal of Burn Care & Research*, 29(4), 574–579. doi:10.1097/BCR.0b013e31817db832

Buxton, H. A., & Dove, N. A. (2008). The burden and management of crystal meth use. *CMAJ, Canadian Medical Association Journal*, 178(12), 1537–1539. doi:10.1503/cmaj.071234

Buxton, J. A., Omura, J., & Kuo, M. (2015, June 13). Genetic determinants of cocaine-associated agranulocytosis. *BMC Research Notes*, 8, 240. doi:10.1186/s13104-015-1219-4

Calcaterra, S., & Binswanger, I. A. (2013). Psychostimulant-related deaths as reported by a large national database. *Substance Abuse*, 34(2), 1–17. doi:10.1080/08897077.2012.726959

Calhoun, A. (2012, April 5). *The criminalization of bad mothers*. Retrieved July 12, 2016, from The New York Times: www.nytimes.com/2012/04/29/magazine/the-criminalization-of-bad-mothers.html?_r=0

Carnevale Associates. (2011, March). Update: The changing landscape of the methamphetamine epidemic. *Policy Brief*. Gaithersburg, MD: Carnevale Associates.

Carson, E. A., & Sabol, M. J. (2012, December). Prisoners in 2011 (NC1239808), Table 9. *State Prison Data*, 9. Washington, DC: U.S. Department of Justice Bureau of Justice Statistics. Retrieved June 24, 2016, from www.bjs.gov/content/pub/pdf/p11.pdf

Cassidy, T. A., McNaughton, E. C., & Varughese, S. (2015). Nonmedical use of prescription ADHD stimulant medications among adults in a substance abuse treatment population: Early findings from the NAVIPPRO surveillance system. *Journal of Attention Disorders*, 19(4), 275–283. doi:10.1177/1087054713493321

Cassidy, T. A., Varughese, S., & Russo, L. (2015). Nonmedical use and diversion of ADHD stimulants among U.S. adults ages 18–49: A national internet survey. *Journal of Attention Disorders*, 19(7), 630–640. doi:10.1177/1087054712468486

CDC, Centers for Disease Control and Prevention. (2007, January). *Methamphetamine use and risk for HIV/AIDS*. Retrieved from www.cdc.gov/hiv

Cepeda, M. S., Fife, D., & Berwaerts, J. (2015). Doctor shopping for medications used in the treatment of attention deficit hyperactivity disorder: Shoppers often pay in cash and cross state lines. *The American Journal of Drug and Alcohol Abuse*, 41(3), 226–229.

Cerretani, D., Fineschi, V., & Bello, S. (2012). Role of oxidative stress in cocaine-induced cardiotoxicity and cocaine-related death. *Current Medicinal Chemistry*, 19(33), 5619–5623.

Chang, T. R., Kowalski, R. G., & Caserta, F. (2013). Impact of acute cocaine use on aneurysmal subarachnoid hemorrhage. *Stroke*, 44(7), 1825–1829. doi:10.1161/STROKEAHA.111.000749

Clemow, D. B. (2015, December 23). Misuse of methylphenidate. *Current Topics in Behavioral Neurosciences*, [Epub ahead of print]. doi:10.1007/7854_2015_426

Clemow, D. B., & Walker, D. J. (2014). The potential for misuse and abuse of medications in ADHD: A review. *Postgraduate Medicine*, 126(5), 64–81. doi:10.3810/pgm.2014.09.2801

Cohen, J. B., Dickow, A., & Horner, K. (2003). Abuse and violence: History of men and women in treatment for methamphetamine dependence. *The American Journal on Addictions*, 12, 377–385. doi:10.1080/10550490390240701

Committee on Health Care for Underserved Women. (2011). Methamphetamine abuse in women of reproductive age (Committee Opinion No. 479). *Obstetrics & Gynecology*, 117, 751–755.

Compton, W. M., Cottler, L. B., & Ridenour, T. (2002). The specificity of family history of alcohol and drug abuse in cocaine abusers. *American Journal of Addiction*, 11(2), 85–94.

Connell-Carrick, K. (2007, May–June). Methamphetamine and the changing face of child welfare: Practice principles for child welfare workers. *Child Welfare*, 86(3), 125–144.

Contrearas, R., & Montoya Bryan, S. (2016, August 26). *Mother, 2 others arrested after horrific rape and murder of 10-year-old girl.* Retrieved August 26, 2016, from National | Globalnews.ca: http://globalnews.ca/news/2904176/mother-2-others-arrested-after-horrific-rape-and-murder-of-10-year-old-girl/

Corsi, K. F., & Booth, R. E. (2008). HIV sex risk behaviors among heterosexual methamphetamine users: Literature review from 2000 to present. *Current Drug Abuse Reviews*, 1(3), 292–296.

Czuchlewski, D. R., Brackney, M., & Ewers, C. (2010). Clinicopathologic features of agranulocytosis in the setting of levamisole-tainted cocaine. *American Journal of Clinical Pathology*, 133(3), 466–472. doi:10.1309/AJCPOPQNBP5THKP1

Dackis, C. A., & Gold, M. S. (1990). Addictiveness of central stimulants. *Advances in Alcohol & Substance Abuse*, 9(1–2), 9–26. doi:10.1300/J251v09n01_02

Davidson, S. B., Blostein, P. A., & Walsh, J. (2013, February). Resurgence of methamphetamine related burns and injuries: A follow-up study. *Burns*, 39(1), 119–125. doi:10.1016/j.burns.2012.03.003

DEA, Drug Enforcement Administration. (2011, December 1). Implementation of the Methamphetamine Production Prevention Act of 2008. Final rule. *Federal Register*, 76(231), 74696–74699.

Derauf, C., LaGasse, L. L., & Smith, L. M. (2007). Demographic and psychosocial characteristics of mothers using methamphetamine during pregnancy: Preliminary results of the Infant Development, Environment, and Lifestyle Study (IDEAL). *The Journal of Drug and Alcohol Abuse*, 33(2), 281–289. doi:10.1080/00952990601175029

Diercks, D. B., Kirk, J. D., & Turnipseed, S. D. (2007, December). Evaluation of patients with methamphetamine- and cocaine-related chest pain in a chest pain observation unit. *Critical Pathways in Cardiology*, 6(4), 161–164.

Durell, T. M., Kroutil, L. A., & Crits-Christoph, P. (2008). Prevalence of nonmedical methamphetamine use in the United States. *Substance Abuse Treatment, Prevention, and Policy*, 3, 1–10. doi:10.1186/1747-597X-3-19

Edwards, J. M., Halpern, C. T., & Wechsberg, W. M. (2006). Correlates of exchanging sex for drugs or money among women who use crack cocaine. *AIDS Education and Prevention*, 18(5), 420–429.

Eiden, R. D., Schuetze, P., & Coles, C. D. (2011). Maternal cocaine use and mother-infant interactions: Direct and moderated associations. *Neurotoxicology & Teratology*, 1, 120–128. doi:10.1016/j.ntt.2010.08.005

Ernst, A. A., Weiss, S. J., & Enright-Smith, S. (2008). Perpetrators of intimate partner violence use significantly more methamphetamine, cocaine, and alcohol than victims: A report by victims. *American Journal of Emergency Medicine*, 26(5), 592–596. doi:10.1016/j.ajem.2007.09.015

Ersche, K. D., Clark, L., & London, M. (2006). Profile of executive and memory function associated with amphetamine and opiate dependence. *Neuropsychopharmacology*, 31(5), 1036–1047. doi:10.1038/sj.npp.1300889

Esteban McCabe, S., Morales, M., & Cranford, J. A. (2007). Race/ethnicity and gender differences in drug use and abuse among college students. *Journal of Ethnicity in Substance Abuse*, 6(2), 75–95.

Eze, N., Smith, L. M., & LaGasse, L. L. (2016). School-aged outcomes following prenatal methamphetamine exposure: 7.5-year follow-up from the Infant Development, Environment, and Lifestyle Study. *Journal of Pediatrics*, 170, 34–38. doi:10.1016/j.peds.2015.11.070

Falck, R. S., Wang, J., & Carlson, R. G. (2001). The epidemiology of physical attack and rape among crack-using women. *Violence and Victims*, 16(1), 79–89.

Farst, K., Duncan, J. M., & Moss, M. (2007). Methamphetamine exposure presenting as caustic ingestions in children. *Annals of Emergency Medicine*, 49(3), 341–343. doi:10.1016/j.annemergmed.2006.05.020

First Nations Centre. (2006, May). *The emerging issue of crystal methamphetamine use in First Nations communities.* National Aboriginal Health Organization. Retrieved November 2, 2016

Forcehimes, A. A., Venner, K. L., & Bogenschutz, M. P. (2011). American Indian methamphetamine and other drug use in the Southwestern United States. *Cultural Diversity & Ethnic Minority Psychology*, 17(4), 366–376. doi:10.1037/a0025431

Garcia-Bournissen, F., Rokach, B., & Karaskov, T. (2007, September). Methamphetamine detection in maternal and neonatal hair: Implications for fetal safety. *Archives of Disease in Childhood. Fetal and Neonatal Edition*, 92(5), F351–F355. doi:10.1136/adc.2006.100156

Gatof, D., & Albert, R. K. (2002). Bilateral thumb burns leading to the diagnosis of crack lung. *Chest*, 121(1), 289–291.

Geller, R. (2005, July 19). *Guidelines for managing children found at clandestine methamphetamine laboratory sites*, 1–15. Atlanta, GA: Georgia Bureau of Investigation.

Giacomello, C. (2014). *How the drug trade criminalizes women disproportionately.* Retrieved June 24, 2016, from NACLA: https://nacla.org/news/2014/6/30/how-drug-trade-criminalizes-women-disproportionately

Gilbert, L., El-Bassel, N., & Chang, M. (2012). Substance use and partner violence among urban women seeking emergency care. *Psychology of Addictive Behaviors*, 26(2), 226–235. doi:10.1037/a0025869

Giraldo, E. A., Taqi, M. A., & Vaidean, G. D. (2012). A case-control study of stroke risk factors and outcomes in African American stroke patients with and without crack-cocaine abuse. *Neurocritical Care*, 16(2), 273–279. doi:10.1007/s12028-010-9410-x

Glasner-Edwards, S., Mooney, L. J., & Marinelli-Casey, P. (2008). Risk factors for suicide attempts in methamphetamine-dependent patients. *The American Journal on Addictions*, 17(1), 24–27. doi:10.1080/10550490701756070

Glover-Kerkvliet, J. (2009). The methamphetamine crisis in American Indian and Native Alaskan Communities: Toward a new research agenda. *Student Pulse*, 1(12), 1–11. Retrieved from Student Pulse: www.studentpulse.com/a?id=77

Gold, J. (2016, August 16). *California court helps kids by healing parents' addictions.* Retrieved from Shots—Health News: NPR: www.npr.org/sections/health-shots/2016/08/16/480960622/california-court-helps-kids-by-healing-parents-addiction

Goldstein, R. Z., & Volkow, N. D. (2011, November). Dysfunction of the prefrontal cortex in addiction: Neuroimaging findings and clinical implications. *Nature Reviews | Neuroscience*, 12, 652–669. Retrieved from www.nature.com/reviews/neuro

Gonzales, R., Mooney, L., & Rawson, R. A. (2010). The methamphetamine problem in the United States. *Annual Review of Public Health*, 31, 385–398. doi:10.1146/annurev.publhealth.012809.103600

Grant, P. (2007, February). Evaluation of children removed from a clandestine methamphetamine laboratory. *Journal of Emergency Nursing*, 33(1), 31–41. doi:10.1016/j.jen.2006.12.003

Grov, C., Kelly, B. C., & Parsons, J. T. (2009). Polydrug use among club-going young adults recruited through time-space sampling. *Substance Use & Misuse*, 44(6), 848–864. doi:10.1080/10826080802484702

Haight, W., Jacobsen, T., & Black, J. (2005). "In these bleak days": Parent methamphetamine abuse and child welfare in the rural Midwest. *Children and Youth Services Review*, 27(8), 949–971.

Hall, K., & Dunham, T. (2013, November 11). *The methiest states in the U.S. (Infographic).* Retrieved from HOFFPOST CRIME: www.huffingtonpost.com/2013/10/07/meth-states_n_4057372.html

Hamilton, A. B., & Goeders, N. E. (2010). Violence perpetrated by women who use methamphetamine. *Journal of Substance Use*, 15(5), 313–329. doi:10.3109/14659890903431611

Hamilton, K. (2010, May 19). *Methology 101: Old-school meth labs give way to "shake and bake."* Retrieved November 2, 2016, from St. Lewis News and Events | Riverfront Times: www.riverfronttimes.com/stlouis/methology-101-old-school-mth-labs-give-way-to-shake-and-bake/Cont?mode=print&old=2483461

Hart, C. L., Marvin, C. B., & Silver, R. (2012). Is cognitive functioning impaired in methamphetamine users? A critical review. *Neuropsychopharmacology*, 37, 586–608. Retrieved from www.neuropsychopharmacology.org

Hartung, C. M., Canu, W. H., & Cleveland, C. S. (2013). Stimulant medication use in college students: Comparison of appropriate users, misusers, and nonusers. *Psychology of Addictive Behaviors*, 27(3), 832–840. doi:10.1037/a0033822

Harzke, A. J., Williams, M. L., & Bowen, A. M. (2009, December). Binge use of crack cocaine and sexual risk behaviors among African-American, HIV-positive users. *AIDS and Behavior*, 13(6), 1106–1118. doi:10.1007/s10461-008-9450-9

Hauer, P. (2010). Systemic affects of methamphetamine use. *South Dakota Medicine*, 63(8), 285–287.

Hohman, M., Oliver, B. A., & Wright, W. (2002). Methamphetamine abuse and manufacture: The child welfare response. *Oxford Journals-Social Sciences-Social Work*, 49(3), 373–381.

Horton, D. K., Berkowitz, Z., & Kaye, W. E. (2003). The acute health consequences to children exposed to hazardous substances used in illicit methamphetamine production, 1996 to 2001. *Journal of Children's Health*, 1(1), 99–108.

Hu, X. T. (2007). Cocaine withdrawal and neuro-adaptations in ion channel function. *Molecular Neurobiology*, 35(1), 95–112.

Illangasekare, S. L., Burke, J. G., & McDonnell, K. A. (2013). The impact of intimate partner violence, substance use, and HIV on depressive symptoms among abused low-income urban women. *Journal of Interpersonal Violence*, 28(14), 2831–2848. doi:10.1177/0886260513488682

Ivy III, W., Miles, I., & Le, B. (2014). Correlates of HIV infection among African American women from 20 cities in the United States. *AIDS and Behavior*, 18(Supplement 3), S266–S275. doi:10.1007/s10461-013-0614-x

Jardin, B., Looby, A., & Earleywine, M. (2011). Characteristics of college students with attention-deficit hyperactivity disorder symptoms who misuse their medications. *Journal of American College Health*, 59(5), 373–377. doi:10.1080/07448481.2010.513073

John, S., Manda, S., & Hamrock, D. (2011). Cocaine-induced thrombotic vasculopathy. *The American Journal of Medical Sciences*, 342(6), 524–526. doi:10.1097/MAJ.0b013e31822979f1

Johnson, J. E., O'Leary, C. C., & Striley, C. W. (2011). Effects of major depression on crack use and arrests among women in drug court. *Addiction*, 106(7), 1279–1286. doi:10.1111/j.1360-0443.2011.03389.x

Kail, B. L., & Elberth, M. (2002). Moving the Latina substance abuser toward treatment: The role of gender and culture. *Journal of Ethnicity in Substance Abuse*, 1(3), 3–16.

Kalokhe, A. S., Paranjape, A., & Bell, C. E. (2012). Intimate partner violence among HIV-infected crack cocaine users. *AIDS Patient Care and STDS*, 26(4), 234–240. doi:10.1089/apc.2011.0275

Kaye, S., McKetin, R., & Duflou, J. (2007). Methamphetamine and cardiovascular pathology: A review of the evidence. *Addiction*, 102(8), 1204–1211. doi:10.1111/j.1360-0443.2007.01874.x

Kelley, M. B. (2012, June 29). *The top 11 cocaine-using countries in the world.* Retrieved March 10, 2016, from Business Insider, pp. 1–2: www.businessinsider.com/countries-most-cocaine-users-2012–6

Kelly, B. C., Wells, B. E., & Leclair, A. (2013). Prevalence and correlates of prescription drug misuse among socially active young adults. *International Journal of Drug Policy*, 24(4), 297–303. doi:1016/j.drugpo.2012.09.002

Keneally, M. (2014, April 16). *Mother goes on crack cocaine binge in Florida motel before giving birth in the bathtub and cutting the umbilical cord with her teeth.* Retrieved June 28, 2014, from MailOnline, pp. 1–10: www.dailymail.co.uk/news/article-2606148/Mother-goes-crack-cocaine-binge-Florida-motel-giving-birth-bathtub-cutting-umbilical-cord-teeth.html

Kennedy, A. P., Epstein, D. H., & Phillips, K. A. (2013). Sex differences in cocaine/heroin users: Drug-use triggers and craving in daily life. *Drug and Alcohol Dependence*, 132(1–2), 29–37. doi:10.1016/j.drugalcdep.2012.12.025

Kerley, K. R., Leban, L., & Copes, H. (2014). Methamphetamine using careers of White and Black women. *Deviant Behavior*, 35(6), 477–495. doi:10.1080/01639625.2013.859046

Kraanen, F. L., Vedel, E., & Scholing, A. (2014). Prediction of intimate partner violence by type of substance use disorder. *Journal of Substance Abuse Treatment*, 46(4), 532–539. doi:10.1016/j.jsat.2013.10.010

Kuhar, M. J., & Pilotte, N. S. (1996). Neurochemical changes in cocaine withdrawal. *Trends in Pharmacological Sciences*, 17(7), 260–264.

Lason, W. (2001). Neurochemical and pharmacological aspects of cocaine-induced seizures. *Polish Journal of Pharmacology*, 53(1), 57–60.

Lee, M. O., Vivier, P. M., & Diercks, D. B. (2009, August). Is the self-report of recent cocaine or methamphetamine use reliable in illicit stimulant drug users who present to the Emergency Department with chest pain? *The Journal of Emergency Medicine*, 37(2), 237–241. doi:10.1016/j.jemermed.2008.05.024

Lineberry, T. W., & Bostwick, J. M. (2006). Methamphetamine abuse: A perfect storm of complications. *Mayo Clinic Proceedings*, 81(1), 77–84.

Lorvick, J., Bourgois, P., & Wenger, L. D. (2012). Sexual pleasure and sexual risk among women who use methamphetamine: A mixed methods study. *International Journal of Drug Policy*, 23(5), 385–392. doi:10.1016/j.drugpo.2012.07.005

Lyons, K. (2014, February 27). *How young women desperate to be slim are using crystal meth to control their weight.* Retrieved July 4, 2014, from MailOnline: www.dailymail.co.uk/news/article-2568929/The-dangerous-weight-loss-drug-Young-women-taking-crystal-meth-helps-slim-down.html

Mansoor, E., Morrow, C. E., & Accornero, V. H. (2012). Longitudinal effects of prenatal cocaine use on mother-child interactions at ages 3 and 5 years. *Journal of Developmental and Behavioral Pediatrics*, 33(1), 32–41. doi:10.1097/DBP.0b013e31823968ab

Marks, K. R., Pike, E., & Stoops, W. W. (2015). Alcohol administration increases cocaine craving but not cocaine cue attentional bias. *Alcoholism, Clinical and Experimental Research*, 39(9), 1823–1831. doi:10.111/acer.12824

Martin-Schild, S., Albright, K. C., & Hallevi, H. (2010). Intracerebral hemorrhage in cocaine users. *Stroke*, 41(4), 680–684. doi:10.1161/STROKEAHA.109.573147

Matthew, B. J., & Gedzior, J. S. (2015). Drug-induced parkinsonism following chronic methamphetamine use by a patient on haloperidol decanoate. *The International Journal of Psychiatry in Medicine*, 50(4), 405–411. doi:10.1177/0091217415612736

Mau, M. K., Asao, K., & Efird, J. (2009). Risk factors associated with methamphetamine use and heart failure among native Hawaiians and other Pacific Island peoples. *Vascular Health and Risk Management*, 5(1), 45–52.

Maxwell, J. C., & Rutkowski, B. A. (2008). The prevalence of methamphetamine and amphetamine abuse in North America: A review of the indicators, 1992–2007. *Drug and Alcohol Review*, 27(3), 229–235. doi:10.1080/09595230801919460

McCabe, S. E., Morales, M., & Cranford, J. A. (2007). Race/ethnicity and gender differences in drug use and abuse among college students. *Journal of Ethnicity in Substance Abuse*, 6(2), 75–95.

McGregor, C., Srisurapanont, M., & Jittiwutikarn, J. (2005). The nature, time course, and severity of methamphetamine withdrawal. *Addiction*, 100(9), 1320–1329. doi:10.1111/j.1360-0443.2005.01160.x

Melnikova, N., Orr, M. F., & Wu, J. (2015, August 28). Injuries from methamphetamine-related chemical incidents—Five states, 2001–2002. *MMWR: Morbidity and Mortality Weekly Report*, 64(33), 909–912.

Messina, N., Marinelli-Casey, P., & West, K. (2014). Children exposed to methamphetamine use and manufacture. *Child Abuse & Neglect*, 38(11), 1872–1883. doi:10.1016/j.chiabu.2006.06.009

Meyer, K. D., & Zhang, L. (2009). Short- and long-term adverse effects of cocaine abuse during pregnancy on the heart development. *Therapeutic Advances in Cardiovascular Disease*, 3(1), 7–16. doi:10.1177/1753944708099877

Meyer, V. J., Little, D. M., & Fitzgerald, D. A. (2014). Crack cocaine use impairs anterior cingulate and prefrontal cortex function in women with HIV infection. *Journal of Neurovirology*, 20(4), 352–361. doi:10.1007/s13365-014-0250-x

Mimiaga, M. J., Fair, A. D., & Mayer, K. H. (2008). Experiences and sexual behaviors of HIV-infected MSM who acquired HIV in the context of crystal methamphetamine use. *AIDS Education & Prevention*, 20(1), 30–41.

Minton, T. D., & Zeng, Z. (2015, June). *Jail inmates at midyear 2014 (NCI248629)*. 3. Washington, DC: Bureau of Justice Statistics, Department of Justice. Retrieved June 24, 2016, from www.bjs.gov/content/pub/pdf/jim14.pdf

Moody, L., Franck, C., & Jarmolowicz, D. P. (2014). Executive functioning deficits in cocaine-dependent individuals. *Drug and Alcohol Dependence*, 140, e155.

Moore, T. M., Stuart, G. L., & Meehan, J. C. (2008). Drug abuse and aggression between intimate partners: A meta-analytic review. *Clinical Psychology Review*, 28(2), 247–274.

Moran-Santa Maria, M. M., Flanagan, J., & Brady, K. (2014). Ovarian hormones and drug abuse. *Current Psychiatry Reports*, 16(11), 511. doi:10.1007/s11920-014-0511-7

Mullin, G. (2016, January 28). *Faces of crystal meth: Shocking before and after pictures reveal damage of prolonged drug use.* Retrieved from World news.

Nair, P., Schuler, M. E., & Black, M. M. (2003). Cumulative environmental risk in substance abusing women: Early intervention, parenting stress, child abuse potential and child development. *Child Abuse & Neglect*, 27(9), 993–995.

Newmeyer, J. A. (2003, May). Patterns and trends of drug use in the San Francisco Bay Area. *Journal of Psychoactive Drugs*, 35(Supplement 1), 127–132. doi:10.1080/02791072.2003.10400507

NIDA, National Institute on Drug Abuse. (2007, June 27). *Crystal methamphetamine use in young adults may be higher than previously reported.* Retrieved from ScienceDaily: www.sciencedaily.com/releases/2007/06/070627095343:

NIDA, National Institute on Drug Abuse. (2013a, September). *What is the scope of methamphetamine abuse in the United States?* Retrieved April 11, 2016, from National Institute on Drug Abuse (NIDA): www.drugabuse.gov/pubications/research-reports/methamphetamine/what-scope-methamphetamine-abuse-in-united-states

NIDA, National Institute on Drug Abuse. (2013b, December). *Cocaine.* Retrieved from Cocaine | National Institute on Drug Abuse (NDA), pp. 1–6: www.drugabuse.gov/drugs-abuse/cocaine

NIDA, National Institute on Drug Abuse. (2016). *Cocaine.* National Institute on Drug Abuse. Retrieved from www.drugabuse.gov/drugs-abuse/cocaine

Nilsson Schonnesson, L., Atkinson, J., & Williams, M. L. (2008, September). A cluster analysis of drug use and sexual HIV risks and their correlates in a sample of African-American crack cocaine smokers with HIV infection. *Drug and Alcohol Dependence*, 97(1–2), 44–53. doi:10.1016/j.drugalcdep.2008.03.023

Nogueira, L., Kalivas, P. W., & Lavin, A. (2006). Long-term neuroadaptations produced by withdrawal from repeated cocaine treatment: Role of dopaminergic receptors in modulating cortical excitability. *The Journal of Neuroscience*, 26(47), 12308–12313. doi:10.1523/JNEUROSCI.3206-06.2006

Norris, K. C., Thornhill-Joynes, M., & Robinson, C. (2001). Cocaine use, hypertension, and end-stage renal disease. *American Journal of Kidney Diseases*, 38(3), 523–528. doi:10.1053/ajkd.2001.26845

Novak, S. P., Kroutil, L. A., & Williams, R. L. (2007, October 31). The nonmedical use of prescription ADHD medications: Results from a national internet panel. *Substance Abuse Treatment, Prevention, and Policy*, 2, 32. doi:10.1186/1747-597X-2-32

Office of National Drug Control Policy (ONDCP). (2010, July). *Fact Sheet: Methamphetamine trends in the United States.* Retrieved April 5, 2016, from www.WhiteHouseDrugPolicy.gov

Pagliaro, A. M., & Pagliaro, L. A. (2000). *Substance use among women: A reference and resource guide.* Philadelphia, PA: Brunner/Mazel.

Pagliaro, A. M., Pagliaro, L. A., & Thauberger, P. C. (1993). Knowledge, behaviours, and risk perception of intravenous drug users in relation to HIV infection and AIDS: The PIARG projects. *Advances in Medical Psychotherapy*, 6, 1–28.

Pagliaro, L. A., & Pagliaro, A. M. (Eds.). (2002). *Problems in pediatric drug therapy* (4th ed.). Washington, DC: American Pharmaceutical Association.

Pagliaro, L. A., & Pagliaro, A. M. (2004). *Pagliaros' comprehensive guide to drugs and substances of abuse* (1st ed.). Washington, DC: American Pharmacists Association.

Pagliaro, L. A., & Pagliaro, A. M. (2009). *Pagliaros' comprehensive guide to drugs and substances of abuse* (2nd ed.). Washington, DC: American Pharmacists Association.

Pagliaro, L. A., & Pagliaro, A. M. (2012). *Handbook of child and adolescent drug and substance abuse.* Hoboken, NJ: Wiley & Sons.

Pagliaro, L. A., Jaglalsingh, L. H., & Pagliaro, A. M. (1992). Cocaine use and depression. *Canadian Medical Association Journal*, 147, 1636–1637.

Palamar, J. J., Davies, S., & Ompad, D. C. (2015). Powder cocaine and crack use in the United States: An examination of risk for arrest and socioeconomic disparities in use. *Drug and Alcohol Dependence*, 149, 108–116. doi:10.1016/j.drugalcdep.2015.01.029

Parsons, J. T., Grov, C., & Kelly, B. C. (2009). Club drug use and dependence among young adults recruited through time-space sampling. *Public Health Reports*, 124(2), 246–254.

Phillips, K., Luk, A., & Soor, G. S. (2009). Cocaine cardiotoxicity: A review of the pathophysiology, pathology, and treatment options. *American Journal of Cardiovascular Drugs*, 9(3), 177–196. doi:10.2165/00129784-200909030-00005

Pilgrim, J. L., Woodford, N., & Drummer, O. H. (2013). Cocaine in sudden and unexpected death: A review of 49 post-mortem cases. *Forensic Science International*, 227(1–3), 52–59. doi:10.1016/j.forsciint.2012.08.037

Pope, S. K., Falck, R. S., & Carlson, R. G. (2011). Characteristics of rural crack and powder cocaine users: Gender and other correlates. *The American Journal of Drug and Alcohol Abuse*, 37(6), 491–496. doi:10.3109/00952990.2011.600380

Popovic, B., Bhattacharya, P., & Sivaswamy, L. (2009). Lisdexamfetamine: A prodrug for the treatment of attention-deficit/hyperactivity disorder. *American Journal of Health-System Pharmacy*, 66(22), 2005–2012. doi:10.2146/ajhp080353

Price, B. (2016, August 10). *Texas woman uses infant child to smuggle meth from Mexico.* Retrieved August 16, 2016, from Breitbart.com: www.breitbart.com/texas/2016/08/10/texas-woman-uses-infant-child-smuggle-meth-mexico/

Proctor, S. L. (2012). Substance use disorder prevalence among female state prison inmates. *American Journal of Drug and Alcohol Abuse*, 38(4), 278–285. doi:10.3109/00952990.2012.668596

Rabiner, D. L., Anastopoulos, A. D., & Costello, E. J. (2009). The misuse and diversion of prescribed ADHD medications by college students. *Journal of Attention Disorders*, 13(2), 144–153. doi:10.1177/1087054708320414

Ramo, D. E., Grov, C., & Delucchi, K. (2010). Typology of club drug use among young adults recruited using time-space sampling. *Drug and Alcohol Dependence*, 107(2–3), 119–127. doi:10.1016/j.drugalcdep.2009.09.014

Riley, E. D., Shumway, M., & Knight, K. R. (2015). Risk factors for stimulant use among homeless and unstably housed adult women. *Drug and Alcohol Dependence*, 153, 173–179. doi:10.1016/j.drugalcdep.2015.05.023

Rivers, E., Shirazi, E., & Aurora, T. (2004). Cocaine use in elder patients presenting to an inner-city emergency department. *Academic Emergency Medicine*, 11(8), 874–877.

Rolland, B., Karila, L., & Geoffroy, P. A. (2011). Shared vulnerability between seizures and psychosis in cocaine addiction? *Epilepsy & Behavior*, 22(3), 596–598. doi:10.1016/j.yebeh.2011.08.004

Rommel, N., Rohleder, N. H., & Koerdt, S. (2016, May 26). Sympathomimetic effects of chronic methamphetamine abuse on oral health: A cross-sectional study. *BMC Oral Health*, 16(1), 59. doi:10.1186/s12903-016-0218-8

Rommel, N., Rohleder, N. H., & Wagenpfeil, S. (2016, April). The impact of the new scene drug "crystal meth" on oral health: A case-control study. *Clinical Oral Investigations*, 20(3), 469–475. doi:10.1007/s00784-015-1527-z

Ryder, J. A., & Brisgone, R. E. (2013). Cracked perspectives: Reflections of women and girls in the aftermath of the crack cocaine era. *Feminist Criminology*, 8(1), 40–62. doi:10.1177/1557085112444899

SAMHSA, Substance Abuse and Mental Health Services Administration. (2011). *Results from the 2010 National Survey on Drug Use and Health (NSDUH): Summary of National Findings, NSDUH Series H-41, HHS Publication No. (SMA) 11–4658)*. Rockville, MD: Substance Abuse and Mental Health Services Administration.

SAMHSA, Substance Abuse and Mental Health Services Administration. (2014, April 3). *The TEDS Report: Gender differences in primary substance of abuse across age groups.* U.S. Department of Health and Human Services, Center for Behavioral Health Statistics and Quality, Rockville, MD.

Schabner, D. (2004, October 25). *Meth use by women on the rise.* Retrieved July 4, 2014, from ABC News: http://abcnews.go.com/US/print?id=185310

Schiller, C., & Allen, P. J. (2005). Follow-up of infants prenatally exposed to cocaine. *Pediatric Nursing*, 31(5), 427–436.

Schlaerth, K. R., Splawn, R. G., & Ong, J. (2004). Change in the pattern of illegal drug use in an inner city population over 50: An observational study. *Journal of Addictive Diseases*, 23(2), 95–107. doi:10.1300/J069v23n02_07

Schulzke, E. (2013, May 24). *Mothers on meth: New book highlights family struggles in the suburbs.* Retrieved July 4, 2014, from Deseret News: www.deseretnews.com/article/print/865580620/Mothers-on-meth-New-book-highlights-family-struggles-in-the-suburbs.html

Semple, S. J., Strathdee, S. A., & Zians, J. (2011). Correlates of trading sex for methamphetamine in a sample of HIV-negative heterosexual methamphetamine users. *Journal of Psychoactive Drugs*, 43(2), 79–88.

Semple, S. J., Strathdee, S. A., & Zians, J. (2012). Correlates of drug dealing in female methamphetamine users. *Journal of Urban Health: Bulletin of the New York Academy of Medicine*, 90(3), 529–541. doi:10.1007/s11524-012-9748-9

Sepulveda, D. R., Thomas, L. M., & McCabe, S. E. (2011). Misuse of prescribed stimulant medication for ADHD and associated patterns of substance use: Preliminary analysis among college students. *Journal of Pharmacy Practice*, 24(6), 551–560. doi:10.1177/0897190011426558

Sexton, R. L., Carlson, R. G., & Siegal, H. (2006). The role of African-American clergy in providing informal services to drug users in the rural South: Preliminary ethnographic findings. *Journal of Ethnicity in Substance Abuse*, 5(1), 1–21. doi:10.1300/J233v05n01_01

Shake and bake or one pot meth making. (n.d.). Retrieved November 2, 2016, from Some Chick's Blog All About Meth, pp. 1–11: http://somechicksblog.com/make-meth/shake-and-bake-or-one-pot-meth-making

Sharpe, T. T. (2001). Sex-for-crack-cocaine exchange, poor black women, and pregnancy. *Qualitative Health Research*, 11(5), 612–630.

Shawwa, K., Alraiyes, A. H., & Eisa, N. (2013, August 30). Cocaine-induced leg ulceration. *BMJ Case Reports*, 1–2.

Shoptaw, S. J., Kao, U., & Heinzerling, K. (2009, April 15). Treatment for amphetamine withdrawal. *Cochrane Database of Systematic Reviews*, 2009(2), CD003021. doi:10.1002/14651858.CD003021.pub2

Shukla, R. K., Crump, J. L., & Chrisco, E. S. (2012, November). An evolving problem: Methamphetamine production and trafficking in the United States. *The International Journal on Drug Policy*, 23(6), 426–435. doi:10.1016/_drugpo.2012.07.004

Siegal, H. A., Falck, R. S., & Wang, J. (2000). Crack-cocaine users as victims of physical attack. *Journal of the National Medical Association*, 92(2), 76–82.

Simon, C. (2016, July 12). *You know that cliché of trading sex for drugs? Here's the real thing*. TheInfluence, pp. 1–8. Retrieved from http://theinfluence.org/you-know-that-cliche-of-trading-sex-for-drugs-heres-the-real-thing/

Smith, P. H., Homish, G. G., & Leonard, K. E. (2012). Intimate partner violence and specific substance use disorders: Findings from the National Epidemiologic Survey on Alcohol and Related Conditions. *Psychology of Addictive Behaviors*, 26(2), 236–245. doi:10.1037/a0024855

Spann, M. D., McGwin, G., & Kerby, J. D. (2006, July–August). Characteristics of burn patients injured in methamphetamine laboratory explosions. *Journal of Burn Care & Research*, 27(4), 496–501. doi:10.1097/01.BCR.0000226056.81279.C9

Strathearn, L., & Mayes, L. C. (2010). Cocaine addiction in mothers: Potential effects on maternal care and infant development. *Annals of the New York Academy of Sciences*, 1187, 172–183. doi:10.1111/j.1749-6632.2009.05142.x

Terplan, M., Smith, E. J., & Kozloski, M. J. (2009). Methamphetamine use among pregnant women. *Obstetrics & Gynecology*, 113(6), 1285–1291. doi:10.1097/AOG.0b013e3181a5ec6f

Teter, C. J., McCabe, S. E., & Boyd, C. J. (2003). Illicit methylphenidate use in an undergraduate student sample: Prevalence and risk factors. *Pharmacotherapy: The Journal of Human Pharmacology and Drug Therapy*, 23(5), 609–617.

Teter, C. J., McCabe, S. E., & Cranford, J. A. (2005). Prevalence and motives for illicit use of prescription stimulants in an undergraduate student sample. *Journal of American College Health*, 53(6), 253–262. doi:10.3200/JACH.53.6.253-262

Teter, C. J., McCabe, S. E., & LaGrange, K. (2006). Illicit use of specific prescription stimulants among college students: Prevalence, motives, and routes of administration. *Pharmacotherapy: The Journal of Human Pharmacology and Drug Therapy*, 1501–1510. doi:10.1592/phco.26.10.1501

Thompson, C. (2013, October 6). *NY woman who ran family drug ring faces prison.* Retrieved June 28, 2014, from The Big Story, pp. 1–6: http://bigstory.ap.org/article/ny-woman-who-ran-drug-ring-faces-prison

Todd, G., Noyes, C., & Flavel, S. C. (2013). Illicit stimulant use is associated with abnormal substantia nigra morphology in humans. *PLoS One*, 8(2), e56438. doi:10.1371/journal.pone.0056438

Tran, H., Tan, D., & Marnejon, T. P. (2013). Cutaneous vasculopathy associated with levamisole-adulterated cocaine. *Clinical Medicine & Research*, 11(1), 26–30. doi:10.3121/cmr.2012.1085

Turillazzi, E., Bello, S., & Neri, M. (2012). Cardiovascular effects of cocaine: Cellular, ionic and molecular mechanisms. *Current Medicinal Chemistry*, 19(33), 5664–5676.

Turnipseed, S. D., Richards, J. R., & Kirk, J. D. (2003). Frequency of acute coronary syndrome in patients presenting to the emergency department with chest pain after methamphetamine use. *The Journal of Emergency Medicine*, 24(4), 369–373.

U.S. Department of Health Resources and Services Administration. (2011). *Illicit drug use.* Retrieved from Maternal and Child Health Bureau: www.mchb.hrsa.gov/whusa11/hstat/hshb/pages/205idu.html?printfriendly

Ullrich, K., Koval, R., & Koval, E. (2011). Five consecutive cases of a cutaneous vasculopathy in users of levamisole-adulterated cocaine. *Journal of Clinical Rheumatology*, 17(4), 193–196. doi:10.1097/RHU.0b013e31820e6822

University of Michigan. (2008, October). *Monitoring the future: National Survey Results on Drug Use, 1975–2007: Volume II: college students and adults ages 19–45, 2007.* Ann Arbor, MI: University of Michigan.

Upadhyaya, H. P., Kroutil, L. A., & Deas, D. (2010). Stimulant formulation and motivation for nonmedical use of prescription attention-deficit/hyperactivity disorder medications in a college-aged population. *The American Journal of Addictions*, 19(6), 569–577. doi:10.1111/j.1521-0391.2010.00078.x

Varga, M. D. (2012). Adderall abuse on college campuses: A comprehensive literature review. *Journal of Evidence-Based Social Work*, 9(3), 293–313. doi:10.1080/15433714.2010.525402

Vidaeff, A. C., & Mastrobattista, J. M. (2003). In utero cocaine exposure: A thorny mix of science and mythology. *American Journal of Perinatology*, 20(4), 165–172.

Vidyasankar, G., Souza, C., & Lai, C. (2015). A severe complication of crack cocaine use. *Canadian Respiratory Journal*, 22(2), 77–79.

Vilela, R. J., Langford, C., & McCullagh, L. (2002). Cocaine-induced oronasal fistulas with external nasal erosion but without palate involvement. *Ear, Nose, & Throat Journal*, 81(8), 562–563.

Viteri, O. A., Soto, E. E., & Bahado-Singh, R. A. (2015). Fetal anomalies and long-term effects associated with substance abuse in pregnancy: A literature review. *American Journal of Perinatology*, 32(5), 405–416. doi:10.1055/s-0034-1393932

Walsh, S. L., Stoops, W. W., & Moody, D. E. (2009). Repeated dosing with oral cocaine in humans: Assessment of direct effects, withdrawal, and pharmacokinetics. *Experimental and Clinical Psychopharmacology*, 17(4), 205–216. doi:10.1037/a0016469

Wang, R. Y. (1999). pH-dependent cocaine-induced cardiotoxicity. *The American Journal of Emergency Medicine*, 17(4), 364–369.

Watanabe-Galloway, S., Ryan, S., & Hansen, K. (2009). Effects of methamphetamine abuse beyond individual users. *Journal of Psychoactive Drugs*, 41(3), 241–248.

Wechsberg, W. M., Lam, W. K., & Zule, W. (2003). Violence, homelessness, and HIV risk among crack-using African-American women. *Substance Use & Misuse*, 38(3–6), 669–700.

Wells, M. (2013, March 31). *Rise in women trafficking drugs on Mexico-US border.* Retrieved June 24, 2016, from InSight Crime: www.insightcrime.org/news-briefs/rise-women-drug-traffickers-mexico-us-border

Wenzel, S. L., Green JR, H. D., & Tucker, J. S. (2009). The social context of homeless women's alcohol and drug use. *Drug and Alcohol Dependence*, 105(1–2), 16–23. doi:10.1016.j.drugalcdep.2009.05.026

Which countries consume the most cocaine and how does it get there? (2015). Retrieved March 10, 2016, from The LAD Bible, pp. 1–15: www.theladbible.com/articles/which-countries-consume-the-most-cocaine-and-how-does-it-get-there

Whitehead, N. E., Trenz, R. C., & Keen 2nd, L. (2014). Younger versus older African Americans: Patterns and prevalence of recent illicit drug use. *Journal of Ethnicity in Substance Abuse*, 13(2), 126–138. doi:10.1080/15332640.2014.883581

Wijetunga, M., Seto, T., & Lindsay, J. (2003). Crystal methamphetamine-associated cardiomyopathy: Tip of the iceberg? *Journal of Toxicology: Clinical Toxicology*, 41(7), 981–986.

Wilens, T. E., Adler, L. A., & Adams, J. (2008). Misuse and diversion of stimulants prescribed for ADHD: A systematic review of the literature. *Journal of the American Academy of Child & Adolescent Psychiatry*, 47(1), 21–31. doi:10.1097/chi.0b013e31815a56f1

Wilson, D., & Shiffman, J. (2015, December 7). *Newborns die after going home with moms fighting drug addiction.* Retrieved October 11, 2016, from NBC News: www.nbcnews.com/news/us-news/newborns-die-after-going-home-moms-fighting-drug-addiction-n475531

Winhusen, T., & Lewis, D. (2013). Sex differences in disinhibition and its relationship to physical abuse in a sample of stimulant-dependent patients. *Drug and Alcohol Dependence*, 129(1–2), 158–162. doi:10.1016/j.drugalcdep.2012.09.014

Winslow, B. T., Voorhees, K. I., & Pehl, K. A. (2007). Methamphetamine abuse. *American Family Physician*, 76(8), 1169–1174.

Won, S., Hong, R. A., & Shohet, R. V. (2013). Methamphetamine-associated cardiomyopathy. *Clinical Cardiology*, 36(12), 737–742. doi:10.1002/clc.22195

Wu, L. T., Schlenger, W. E., & Galvin, D. M. (2006). Concurrent use of methamphetamine, MDMA, LSD, ketamine, GHB, and flunitrazepam among American youths. *Drug and Alcohol Dependence*, 84(1), 102–113.

Yeo, K. K., Wijetunga, M., & Ito, H. (2007). The association of methamphetamine use and cardiomyopathy in young patients. *The American Journal of Medicine*, 120(2), 165–171. doi:10.1016/j.amjmed.2006.01.024

Zhu, H., Wilson, F. A., & Stimpson, J. P. (2014). Correlation between cocaine prices and purity with trends in emergency department visits in a major metropolitan area. *Journal of Urban Health: Bulletin of the New York Academy of Medicine*, 91(5), 1009–1018. doi:10.1007/s11524-014-9899-y

Zhu, N. Y., Legatt, D. F., & Turner, A. R. (2009). Agranulocytosis after consumption of cocaine adulterated with levamisole. *Annals of Internal Medicine*, 150(4), 287–289.

Zweben, J. E., Cohen, J. B., & Christian, D. (2004). Psychiatric symptoms in methamphetamine users. *The American Journal on Addictions*, 13(2), 181–190.

6

WOMEN'S PSYCHODELIC ABUSE

The psych**o**delics[1] comprise a group of drugs and substances of abuse that were originally named, *psych**e**delics*, by Osmond (1957) to differentiate them from *hallucinogens*. As explained by Cohen (1967), the term, *hallucinogen*, was generally used to denote drugs and substances of abuse that produced a *temporary madness*, whereas the term, *psych**e**delics*, was used to denote drugs and substances of abuse that induced *valuable states of self-transcendence and mystical unity* (p. 301).

Various other names, such as *phantasticants* and *illusinogens*, were used to reflect the vivid sensory experiences and common visual illusions and misperceptions associated with the psychodelics. In addition, various terms associated with the specific professional stance of the person proposing the term (e.g., mystic; physician; psychologist), also were used, such as: *psychotogens* (i.e., inducers of psychosis); *psychotomimetics* (i.e., mimickers of psychosis); *schizophrenomimetics* (i.e., mimickers of schizophrenia); *mysticomimetics* (i.e., mimickers of mystic states); and *psychotomystics* (i.e., mimickers of psychosis and mystic states).

The synthesis of 3,4-methylenedioxymethamphetamine (MDMA, "Ecstasy") and other related drugs, led to the common use of such terms as, *empathogens* (i.e., drugs that produce feelings of *empathy* toward others) and *entactogens* (i.e., *touch*, or *hug drugs* that produce feelings of *closeness*, *belonging*, and *love*). For clarity, and in keeping with the terms used to denote the other two major groups of psychotropics discussed in this text (i.e., *psych**o**depressants* and *psych**o**stimulants*), we have selected to use the term, *psych**o**delics*.[2]

---

1 To avoid confusion, a boldface "**o**" and "**e**" are used in this brief chapter introduction to emphasize the slight difference between the *older* term, "psych**e**delic," and the more recent term used in this chapter and text, "psych**o**delic."

2 We began using this term following the development of our classification system, which was constructed to clarify the confusion we encountered in published journal articles and textbooks and

The psychodelics consist of three subclasses: (1) *amphetamine-like* psychodelics; (2) *d-lysergic-acid diethylamide* (LSD) and *LSD-like* psychodelics; and (3) *miscellaneous* psychodelics (see Table 6.1).[3] This chapter focuses on the psychodelics from each of these subclasses that are *most* commonly used by women in the U.S. during the new millennium. We begin with the synthetic, amphetamine-like psychodelic, *methylenedioxymethamphetamine* (MDMA). We then present and discuss *lysergic acid diethylamide* (LSD)—the prototype for the LSD-like psychodelics. We conclude with the miscellaneous psychodelics, *cannabis*—particularly, in the form of marijuana—and *phencyclidine* (PCP).

Popular Notion: The use of psychodelics peaked during the 1960s and has been on the decline ever since.

NOT TRUE. See the following sections of this chapter.

Several factors are largely responsible for the *high* rates of psychodelic use observed among women during the new millennium—rates that are *higher* for women than at any other time in the history of the U.S., including the "hippie subculture era" of the 1960s. These factors include:

1. Adoption of *more* accepting attitudes toward women's use of psychodelics
2. Decriminalization/legalization of cannabis in most states
3. Relatively new and convenient sources of availability

---

among health and social care professionals, including both undergraduate and graduate students, and patients in regard to the identification of *abusable* and *nonabusable* psychotropic drugs. The system also simplified the categorization and organization of *all* of the *abusable* psychotropics—natural, synthetic, and semisynthetic—into *three* major classes along with their associated subclasses. Over the new millennium, we found this system consistent with our intent and designated the three major classes of the drugs and substances of abuse *simply* as: *psychodepressants*, *psychostimulants*, and *psychodelics*. (See, for example, Pagliaro & Pagliaro, 2000, 2004, 2009, 2012.)

3 Published statistics regarding psychodelic abuse among new millennial women in the U.S., as a population group, are generally unavailable. Consequently, reported statistics are often extrapolated from data reported for: (1) subpopulations of women (e.g., those of a certain continental or other descent; those who are a certain age; those who are homeless or incarcerated); or (2) mixed population groups that use drugs and substances of abuse. For example, the Substance Abuse and Mental Health Services Administration (SAMHSA, 2014) reported that annual rates of drug and substance use by young adults are approximately: 2%, for LSD; 4%, for MDMA; and 33%, for marijuana. Although the reported statistics vary, it also is consistently reported (e.g., Boyd, McCabe, & d'Arcy, 2003) that, among samples of young adults (e.g., undergraduate college/university students, including co-eds), marijuana is the most frequently used illicit drug followed by MDMA.

TABLE 6.1 Psychodelics

Sub-Classification Generic Name[a] CHEMICAL SUBCLASS	Common Street Names[b]
Amphetamine-Like Psychodelics—Phenethylamines	
4-Bromo-2,5-dimethoxyphenethylamine	Bromo; 2-CB; Nexus
2,5-Dimethoxy-4-methylamphetamine	DOM; STP
Mescaline	Buttons; Cactus; *Peyote*
3,4-Methylenedioxyamphetamine	Adam, Love Drug; MDA
3,4-Methylenedioxyethylamphetamine	Eve; MDE; MDEA
3,4-Methylenedioxymethamphetamine	Dancing Shoes; Ecstasy; MDMA; XTC
N-Methyl-1-(3,4-methylenedioxyphenyl)-2-butanamine	Eden; Fido-Dido; MBDB
4-Methylthioamphetamine	4-MTA; Flat Liners; Golden Eagle
Nutmeg	Magic; Noz Moscada; Muskatbaum
Paramethoxyamphetamine	Death; Mitsubishi; PMA
3,4,5-Trimethoxyamphetamine	Mescalamphetamine; TMA
LSD & LSD-Like Psychodelics—Indoles, Tryptamines, and Indoles/Tryptamines	
INDOLES	
Amanita muscaria	Flesh of the gods; Fly Agaric; Soma
Harmala alkaloids	Yage; Yaje
Lysergic acid amide	Blue Stars; LSA; Morning Glory
Lysergic acid diethylamide	Acid; LSD; Twenty-Five
TRYPTAMINES[c,d]	
Alpha-ethyltryptamine	Alpha-ET; ET; Love Pearls
N,N-Diethyltryptamine	DET
N,N-Dipropyltryptamine	DIPT
5-Hydroxy-N,N-dimethyltryptamine[e]	Bufo; 5-OH-DMT; Toad
5-Methoxy-N,N-dimethyltryptamine	5-MeO-DMT
INDOLES/TRYPTAMINES	
Alpha-methyltryptamine	3-IT; AMT; Spirals
N,N-Dimethyltryptamine	45 Minute Trip; Businessman's Lunch; DMT
5-Methoxy-N,N-diisopropyltryptamine	Foxy; Foxy Methoxy; 5-MeO-DIPT
Psilocin	Magic Mushrooms; Pizza Toppings; Shrooms
Psilocybin	Fungus; Sacred Mushrooms; Smurf Hats
Miscellaneous Psychodelics	
Cannabis	Ganja; Grass; Weed
Ibogaine[f]	Bocca; Iboga; *Lebuga*
Ketamine	Cat; K; Special K; Vitamin K
Phencyclidine	Angel Dust; PCP; Peace Pill
Piperazine derivatives	A2; Fly; Nemesis
Salvia divinorum	Big Sal; Diviner's Mint; *Ska Maria Pastora*

TABLE 6.1 *(cont.)*

[a] There are *no* brand/trade names for the psychodelics, other than those for the therapeutically approved and available cannabinoids—dronabinol (Marinol®) in the U.S, and nabilone (Cesamet®) in Canada.

[b] *Partial* list. Examples of the most common street names are provided, when available. See Pagliaro and Pagliaro (2009) for a comprehensive listing of the drugs and substances of abuse and their common street names.

[c] Virtually all the tryptamines are classified as *LSD-like psychodelics* because of their observed psychotropic actions. However, they also are classified as tryptamines in this taxonomy because each has the amino acid, *tryptamine*, as its core chemical structure.

[d] Psilocybin (i.e., O-phosphoryl-4-hydroxy-N,N-ethyltryptamine) and psilocin (i.e., 4-hydroxy-N,N-dimethyltryptamine) also can be added to this taxonomy.

[e] Also, known as *bufotenine*. There is some question as to its psychodelic action, but the lack of psychodelic activity in human subjects may be simply due to its poor ability to cross the blood-brain barrier.

[f] At *lower* dosages, ibogaine acts as a *psychostimulant*, primarily affecting the NMDA receptors. At *higher* dosages, it acts as a *psychodelic*, primarily involving the serotonin receptors.

During the first 2 decades of the new millennium, the availability of *all* the various psychodelics *increased* significantly in the U.S. (and elsewhere) as a result of the *Dark Web* and the online, illicit drug marketplace, *Silk Road 3* (Barratt, Ferris, & Winstock, 2014; Van Hout & Bingham, 2013). While most of the psychodelics and other drugs and substances of abuse sold on the Silk Road, are purchased by men, fully a quarter are purchased by women. In addition, many of the men, who purchase psychodelics and other drugs and substances of abuse from this marketplace, share their purchases with either their wives and girlfriends or sell them to other women who desire them.

Methylenedioxymethamphetamine (MDMA)

Commonly known on-the-street as "Ecstasy," "E," "Molly,"[4] and other common names, MDMA is primarily used to achieve such *desired* empathogenic/entatogenic actions as feelings of elation, sensory pleasure, and emotional closeness. As identified by Hysek, Schmid, and Simmler (2014), MDMA increases and intensifies, "explicit and implicit emotional empathy," particularly among women (p. 1645). The use of MDMA also is associated with *mild* hallucinations that can last for 4 to 8 hours without the anxiety, dissociation, perceptual distortion, or other *undesired* effects commonly associated with the use of other psychodelics (e.g., LSD). Desired *psychostimulant* effects associated with MDMA use include: alleviation of fatigue; heightened perceptions; increased energy; stress relief; and wakefulness. These desired pharmacological effects, particularly the feelings of euphoria, understanding, and closeness to others (i.e., "pro-social effects"), have made MDMA especially

[4] The popular street name, "Molly," is derived from the word "molecule," and is commonly used by new millennial women.

appealing to young women (Kirkpatrick & de Wit, 2015; Pagliaro & Pagliaro, 2009; Piper, 2007; Wardle, Kirkpatrick, & de Wit, 2014; Wu, Grady, & Rosales, 2011).

Pharmacology

MDMA is a *synthetic* psychodelic related to the amphetamines, which explains its *psychostimulant* actions. The attachment of a *methylenedioxy* group to the aromatic ring makes MDMA also structurally similar to the *natural* psychodelic, *mescaline*. MDMA was originally synthesized as an appetite suppressant in 1914 by the German pharmaceutical company, *Merck*. However, there was little interest in MDMA for the next 60 years, at which time it was rediscovered and popularized by the *hippies* during the *counter-culture movement*.

Pharmacodynamics: Mechanism of Action

The feelings of elation, emotional closeness, and sensory pleasure that are associated with the use of MDMA are thought to be caused by the: (1) release of neurotransmitters, primarily serotonin (i.e., 5-hydroxytryptamine, 5-HT); and (2) prevention of their reuptake (i.e., MDMA acts as an *indirect* biogenic amine agonist). This mechanism of action involves the interaction of MDMA with 5-HT transporters (SERTs) as substrates. In addition, several researchers (e.g., Meyer, 2013; Parrott, Lock, & Conner, 2008) suggest that the MDMA-associated neuro-hormonal release—particularly, the release of cortisol and oxytocin—may be a key underlying factor in producing the observed effects typically associated with MDMA use.

Parrott, Lock, and Conner (2008) noted that cortisol release is *increased* by such stimulatory factors as physical activity, thermal stress, and psychostimulant drugs. Parrott (2009), citing data from a previous study that found that cortisol levels *increased* significantly (i.e., by 800%) among participants when "dance clubbing" on MDMA, concluded that:

> In MDMA-using dance clubbers, the cortisol levels are … possibly due to the combined factors of stimulant drug, physical exertion and psychosocial stimulation.
>
> *(p. 148)*

As identified by Hysek, Schmid, and Simmler (2014), in their "placebo-controlled, double-blind, random-order, cross-over design" study of "32 healthy volunteers"—including 16 women:

> MDMA increased plasma levels of cortisol and prolactin, which are markers of serotonergic and noradrenergic activity, and of oxytocin, which has been associated with prosocial behavior.
>
> *(p. 1645)*

The identified situational, or contextual, factors, as well as the MDMA dosage ingested, probably explain, or at least account for, *most* of the observed variance in individual response to MDMA use.

In addition, McGregor, Callaghan, and Hunt (2008) advanced the theory that the neuropeptide, oxytocin, may play an integral and significant role in the action of MDMA.[5] As noted by the researchers, oxytocin often has been referred to as the *social neuropeptide* because of its *pro-social* and *pro-sexual* effects (i.e., as has been associated with MDMA use). This action appears to be mediated by way of oxytocin-dopamine interactions that occur in the mesolimbic region of the brain. However, the mechanism of action for MDMA, as for many other drugs and substances of abuse, putatively involve several different mechanisms. In addition, these mechanisms can, themselves, vary in extent and magnitude of contribution to the action of MDMA based upon several underlying variables (e.g., age, gender, and genetics).

Pharmacokinetics: Absorption, Distribution, Metabolism, and Excretion

MDMA is readily absorbed from the GI tract following oral ingestion and has an onset of action generally occurring within 30 minutes. Peak serum concentrations are achieved within 1 to 3 hours. The half-life of elimination is approximately 7 hours with the effects of MDMA generally lasting for *only* 3 to 6 hours (DrugFacts, 2016).

MDMA is metabolized in the liver, primarily by the hepatic microsomal enzyme cytochrome P450-2D6,[6] to an *active* metabolite, *methylenedioxyamphetamine* (MDA, "Adam"). The half-life of MDA (i.e., 12 to 36 hours) is *longer* than that of its active parent drug, MDMA, and is associated with *more* neurotoxicity (Pagliaro & Pagliaro, 2009).

Undesired, or Harmful, Effects and Toxicities

The use of MDMA is associated with both *acute* and *chronic* toxicities. These and other *undesired*, or harmful, effects and toxicities are presented in the following sections. Interestingly, several researchers (e.g., Ogeil, Rajaratnam, & Broadbear, 2013; Wu, Grady, & Rosales, 2011) have reported that, when compared to men, women, who use MDMA, have a *higher* incidence of toxicity, and/or a *greater* severity of toxicity. For example, as reported by Rosenson, Smollin, and Sporer (2007):

---

[5] Although oxytocin is probably best known for its physiological effects, such as *increasing* contractions during parturition and *increasing* milk ejection during lactation and breast-feeding, it also is known for several significant psychological effects. For example, oxytocin has been specifically associated with: (1) an *increased* ability to cope with stress, elevated mood, increased sociability, and trust; and (2) *decreased* feelings of anxiety, aggression, and irritability.

[6] Consequently, enzyme *inducers* and *inhibitors* of cytochrome P450-2D6 can significantly *increase* or *decrease*, respectively, the half-life of elimination of MDMA.

> Female sex was associated with increased odds of hyponatremia and increased odds of hyponatremia-associated coma among persons with ecstasy intoxication.[7]
>
> *(p. 164)*

Acute and Chronic Toxicities. The use of MDMA is associated with several *acute toxicities*, including: agitation; anxiety; blurred vision; bruxism; cardiac dysrhythmias; diaphoresis; dissociated signs and symptoms;[8] hallucinations (mild); headache; hepatitis (drug-induced); hyperkinesia; hypertension; hyponatremia;[9] impulsive behavior; increased body temperature;[10] mental confusion; mydriasis; nausea; seizures; tachycardia; and urinary retention (Pagliaro & Pagliaro, 2009; Smith, Larive, & Romanelli, 2002). Regarding *chronic toxicities*, the regular, long-term use of MDMA is associated with: insomnia; neurogenic bladder; soreness of the jaw muscles related to jaw clenching (i.e., trismus) or teeth grinding (i.e., bruxism); and weight loss.

The regular, long-term use of MDMA also is directly associated with the *loss* of serotonergic axons in the corpus striatum and other areas associated with higher levels of brain functioning, including the frontal cortex (Quednow, Jessen, & Kuhn, 2006). Young women may be at risk for these MDMA-related neurotoxicities (Montoya, Sorrentino, & Lukas, 2002). Of increasing concern, are findings that some neurotoxic effects do *not* appear to abate, even several years after the discontinuation of MDMA use. Consequently, these neurotoxic effects may be permanent (Gouzoulis-Mayfrank & Daumann, 2006, 2009; Pagliaro & Pagliaro, 2009).

Several researchers support this contention in regard to more serious neurotoxic effects affecting attention and memory, particularly, verbal memory[11] (Parrott, 2006; Piper, 2007). For example, as identified by Parrott (2006):

---

7 Also, see related discussion in the later section, "Overdosage."

8 Dissociated signs and symptoms are *not* usually reported, particularly when MDMA has been used alone (i.e., apart from the typical pattern of multidrug abuse by women who abuse MDMA). However, these signs and symptoms have been induced in controlled laboratory studies (e.g., van Heugten-Van der Kloet, Giesbrecht, & van Wel, 2015) following typical single doses to volunteer subjects. These MDMA-associated signs and symptoms generally exceed those observed among patients with schizophrenia.

9 Generally mild, except in cases of overdosage (see related discussion in later section, "Overdosage.") In a related study, van Dijken, Blom, and Hene (2013) noted that "most cases (significantly more cases) of hyponatremia occurred in females" (p. 2277). Also, see earlier related observations by Rosenson, Smollin, and Sporer (2007).

10 The increase in body temperature is usually minimal (i.e., 0.5° to 1.0°C) with *low* to *moderate* dosages (Parrott, 2012). However, increases in body temperature can be significant with *higher* dosages and can result in hyperthermia (see related discussion in the later section, "Overdosage").

11 Memory and other neurological impairments associated with regular, long-term use of MDMA are *not* always experienced by all users (Gouzoulis-Mayfrank & Daumann, 2006; Gouzoulis-Mayfrank, Fischermann, & Rezk, 2005). The reason for this apparent variation in response to MDMA is unknown. However, it is most likely associated with the: (1) concomitant use of other neurotoxic

> Most heavy (ecstasy/MDMA) users report memory or other psychobiological problems … confirmed by objective deficits in working memory, attention, frontal-executive memory tasks, and episodic memory tasks.
>
> *(p. 147)*

As found by Quednow, Jessen, and Kuhn (2006):

> Abstinent MDMA users have memory deficits … users revealed impairments in learning, consolidation, recall and recognition.
>
> *(p. 373)*

In another example, as reported by Roberts, Nestor, and Garavan (2009):

> Ecstasy users performed significantly worse in learning and memory compared to controls and cannabis users.
>
> *(p. 71)*

In addition, *mental depression* (i.e., "mid-week blues") has been reported by both occasional and regular, long-term MDMA users. Usually occurring 2 to 5 days following the last use of MDMA, it is unclear as to whether the depressive symptomatology is related to: (1) the specific pharmacological mechanisms associated with MDMA; or (2) a negative placebo effect, such as a young woman wishing that she was back in the MDMA-clubbing scene again. In any event, *severe* MDMA-midweek blues is *more* often reported by women than men, who similarly use MDMA (Falck, Wang, & Carlson, 2006; Meyer, 2013). (Also, see related discussion in following section, *Physical and Psychological Dependence*, "Withdrawal Syndrome.")

Physical and Psychological Dependence. Whereas, the regular, long-term use of most psychodelics (e.g., LSD; PCP) has *not* been associated with physical and psychological dependence, the regular, long-term use of MDMA has been *increasingly* associated with *both* physical and psychological dependence (Leung & Cottler, 2008; Wu, Ringwalt, & Weiss, 2009)—albeit, reportedly significantly *less* severe in nature than that associated with alcohol, methamphetamines, opiate analgesics, or smoking tobacco/nicotine (Meyer, 2013).

TOLERANCE. *Acute* tolerance to MDMA has been identified. Repeated MDMA use over a *short* period (i.e., repeated doses over 2 to 4 hours) may result in acute tolerance. This short-term reduction or absence of desired MDMA effects (e.g.,

---

drugs and substances of abuse (e.g., alcohol; methamphetamine)—for example, over 90% of MDMA users also report use of cannabis (Parrott, 2006); (2) dosage of MDMA used; and (3) genetic predisposition. In addition, several researchers (e.g., Parrott, 2006, p. 147) have suggested that the venues in which MDMA is typically used (i.e., "hot and crowded dances/raves") may significantly raise the body temperature of users and, consequently, contribute to the observed neuropsychobiological effects (including noted deficits in learning and memory).

euphoria)—as well as other effects (e.g., increased heart rate)—is believed to be due to the *inhibition* of serotonin synthesis and/or *depletion* of serotonin stores (Farre, Tomillero, & Perez-Mana, 2015; Gallagher, Hadjiefthyvoulou, & Fisk, 2014; Hysek, Simmler, & Schillinger, 2014; Peiro, Farre, & Roset, 2013).

WITHDRAWAL SYNDROME. An MDMA withdrawal syndrome also has been identified (Pagliaro & Pagliaro, 2009). The withdrawal syndrome generally occurs 3 to 5 days following the abrupt discontinuation of regular long-term MDMA use and is characterized by feelings of *dysphoria*. The relationship of the MDMA withdrawal syndrome to "mid-week blues," is possible, but has *not* been formally established.

Overdosage

During the first decade of the new millennium, over 300 overdosage fatalities were associated with MDMA in the U.S. (CDC, 2010; Pagliaro & Pagliaro, 2009).[12] In many of these cases, uncharacteristic behavior and vomiting were initially observed, followed by seizures, disorientation or coma, and death. Death was usually associated with: acute renal failure; cardiac dysrhythmia; cerebrovascular accident; disseminated intravascular coagulation; hyperkalemia; hyperthermia; hyponatremic encephalopathy; renal toxicity; and rhabdomyolysis (Pagliaro & Pagliaro, 2009; Patel, Belson, & Longwater, 2005).

MDMA-induced *hyperthermia* commonly occurs among women who have experienced a significant acute overdosage, and significantly contributes to associated morbidity and mortality. The major factors that appear to contribute to the severity of MDMA-induced hyperthermia, particularly among young women, include the: (1) dose of MDMA ingested; (2) temperature of the immediate surroundings (e.g., dance club; rave); and (3) amount of physical exertion—usually related to continuous dancing throughout the night (Armenian, Mamantov, & Tsutaoka, 2013; Pagliaro & Pagliaro, 2009).

MDMA-induced *renal toxicity* is most often related to: (1) acute renal injury (e.g., non-traumatic rhabdomyolysis); or (2) severe hyponatremia (Campbell & Rosner, 2008; Ghatol & Kazory, 2012). As identified by Campbell and Rosner (2008), the factors contributing to MDMA-associated hyponatremia include:

- MDMA-induced secretion of arginine vasopressin (AVP), or antidiuretic hormone (ADH)
- MDMA-induced thirst
- Ready availability of fluids
- Encouragement to drink a lot of fluids at dance clubs or rave dance parties
- Absorption of hypotonic solutions from the GI tract

---

[12] Most of these deaths have been accidental and related to dehydration and hyperthermia. Suicide involving MDMA use, such as that verified in a 15-year-old adolescent girl—are relatively rare events (Fernando, Gilbert, & Carroll, 2012).

The severe MDMA-induced hyponatremia is most often observed among young women (Rosenson, Smollin, & Sporer, 2007; van Dijken, Blom, & Hene, 2013). It is commonly medically managed with infusions of hypertonic saline solution (Pagliaro & Pagliaro, 2009). Malignant hypotension also may significantly contribute to the acute renal injury (Campbell & Rosner, 2008).

A clear picture as to the cause and sequelae of MDMA overdosage is difficult to obtain because the overwhelming majority of MDMA users (i.e., 80% to 90%) are known poly-drug and substance abusers, who commonly report the concomitant use of alcohol, LSD, and other drugs and substances of abuse, including cannabis (e.g., Ho, Karimi-Tabesh, & Koren, 2001; Pagliaro & Pagliaro, 2009). It also should be noted that street samples of MDMA are commonly misrepresented, adulterated, and/or deliberately "cut" with other drugs—drugs that can contribute to, or exacerbate, the signs and symptoms of MDMA overdosage (CDC, 2010). As noted by the NIDA (DrugFacts, 2016):

> Much of the Molly seized by the police contains additives such as cocaine, ketamine, methamphetamine, over-the-counter cough medicine, or synthetic cathinones (i.e., "bath salts").
>
> *(p. 3)*

As further noted by the NHTSA, National Highway Traffic Safety Administration (2016):

> Potency of street samples is highly variable, and tablets sold as "ecstasy" may in fact contain little or no MDMA, but may contain caffeine, ephedrine, phenylpropanolamine, paramethoxyamphetamine (PMA), methylenedioxyamphetamine (MDA), dextromethorphan, amphetamine, methamphetamine, and ketamine.
>
> *(p. 1)*

It also has been suggested that, what is often identified as MDMA overdosage, may, in many cases, be the *serotonin syndrome*. The serotonin syndrome may occur because of the interaction of MDMA with a selective serotonin reuptake inhibitor (SSRI), such as the antidepressant, fluoxetine (Prozac®), or other interacting drugs (Pilgrim, Gerostamoulos, & Drummer, 2011; Schifano, 2004). In addition, many of the signs and symptoms of fatal MDMA overdosage (e.g., hyponatremic encephalopathy) can be related to several other risk factors, including the concurrent oral ingestion of an excessive amount of beer or water.[13] In any case, the serious and

[13] MDMA use, even in healthy volunteers, has resulted in an increase in vasopressin secretion with consequent reduced sodium concentrations and polydipsia because of its effects on the serotonergic system. When excess fluids (e.g., beer, water) have been ingested, resultant hyponatremia and/or hypervolemia may occur (Campbell & Rosner, 2008; Traub, Hoffman, & Nelson, 2002). (Also, see earlier, related discussion.)

potentially fatal consequences of MDMA overdosage require emergency medical evaluation and support of body systems. There is *no* known antidote.

Women's Medical and Personal MDMA Use and Abuse

Whereas medical abuse has been extremely limited, the *personal* use of MDMA among women, during the new millennium, has a short, but interesting history.

Women's Medical MDMA Use/Abuse

MDMA was *not* actively promoted/marketed following its synthesis and introduction as an appetite suppressant in 1914. MDMA was briefly used as a possible adjunct to psychotherapy for the treatment of posttraumatic stress disorder (PTSD) (Jerome, Schuster, & Yazar-Klosinski, 2013; Meyer, 2013). However, it currently has *no* FDA-approved therapeutic medical indication for use in the U.S.

Women's Personal MDMA Use/Abuse

Women's personal use and abuse of MDMA has an interesting history. After a relatively slow start, its use virtually exploded worldwide, particularly in response to two trends that began in the 1980s: (1) *raving*; and (2) *clubbing*. As described by the CDC (2010):

> A rave is an all-night dance party with electronic music. When raves first emerged in the late 1980s, they were underground parties usually held at abandoned warehouses and outdoor sites. Since then, raves have become organized commercial events staged by promoters at established venues, often with high ticket prices and elaborate laser light effects.
>
> *(p. 1)*

The new millennium witnessed continued widespread use of MDMA in the U.S., particularly among middle-class, young women of European continental descent (Parsons, Grov, & Kelly, 2009). These women have little difficulty obtaining MDMA from supplies that are primarily produced in Western Europe—particularly Belgium, Luxembourg, and the Netherlands—and imported for distribution and sale across the U.S.—often through Canada or Mexico (Shukla, Crump, & Chrisco, 2012). Women usually ingest *illicitly* produced MDMA capsules and tablets. However, other women intranasally insufflate, or "snort," their MDMA after emptying the powdered drug from a capsule, or crushing a tablet into a fine powder. Rarely, some women dissolve the powder and intravenously inject their MDMA (Pagliaro & Pagliaro, *Clinical Patient Data Files*).

Wu, Schlenger, and Galvin (2006), in their review of data from the *National Survey on Drug Use and Health* (NSDUH), found, in their sample of non-institutionalized household members, 16 years-of-age to 23 years-of-age, that 13.6% of participants reported "lifetime prevalence of MDMA use" and 6% of participants reported "past year use."

Several factors *highly* correlate with MDMA use among new millennial women. These factors include:

- High sensation-seeking personality
- History of childhood physical abuse
- Initiation of drug and substance abuse during childhood
- Low academic achievement
- Multiple ethnicity or continental descent
- Parental drug and substance use
- Peer drug and substance use
- Poly-drug and substance use

(e.g., Pagliaro & Pagliaro, Clinical Patient Data Files; *Wu, Schlenger, & Galvin, 2006)*[14]

In addition, several researchers (e.g., Boyd, McCabe, & d'Arcy, 2003; Parsons, Kelly, & Wells, 2006; Ramo, Grov, & Delucchi, 2010; Santos, Rapues, & Wilson, 2014) have identified that the use of MDMA is *highest* among young women who are:

1. Bisexual, lesbian, or transgendered
2. Homeless or *living-on-the-streets*
3. Regular attendees of dance club parties and rave events
4. Enrolled in a treatment program aimed at discontinuing their drug and substance use

Interestingly, Wu, Grady, and Rosales (2011) found that, after controlling for demographics, "young, low-income women who use ecstasy experience higher levels of stress than nonusers" (p. 404) and, subsequently, are at *higher* risk for participating in risky sexual behavior (e.g., *higher* number of lifetime sexual partners).

A *major* factor associated with millennial women's MDMA use in the U.S. is their access to a relatively *new* source from which to obtain their MDMA, as well as virtually any other drug or substance of abuse they desire. This source is the *Dark Net* (darknet). Winstock (2016), reviewing related data from the 2015 *Global Drug Survey* of 23 different countries, found that the purchase of drugs from the darknet was significant—ranging from a high of 18% of respondents from Sweden to a low of 0.4% of respondents from Greece. The *average* percent of purchases, by country, was reported at 4.5%. The U.S. reported 8% (p. 21).

---

[14] Women commonly use MDMA concurrently with alcohol and/or marijuana (NIDA, 2016). In addition, a significant number of women use MDMA with cocaine, methamphetamine, and opiate analgesics (Meyer, 2013).

Winstock (2016, p. 20), based upon responses obtained from study participants regarding the benefits and issues related to a *darknet* drug purchase versus a *conventional* drug purchase, discovered several "clear benefits" associated with darknet purchases:

- Reduced rates of exposure to violence
- Less adulterated drugs
- More confidence in product quality
- Removal from street dealing

Typically, women, who want to purchase a drug or substance of abuse, sign into a service (e.g., TOR) that masks the purchaser's identity, and then proceed to a digital black market site (e.g., *Silk Road 3*), and complete the purchase using "bitcoins." The drug or substance of abuse is then sent *directly* to the purchaser by postal service or courier delivery.

Lysergic Acid Diethylamide (LSD)

Lysergic acid diethylamide (LSD), commonly known as "acid," "blotter," "dots," "kool-aid," "trips," and a myriad of other names, produces *profound* psychodelic actions. These actions include:

- *Micropsia*, seeing things much *smaller* than they are
- *Macropsia*, seeing things much *larger* than they are
- *Synesthesias*, blending, or mixing, of sensory input such as *hearing* colors and *seeing* sounds
- *Temporal disintegration*, perceiving time as passing *extremely* slowly—such as, watching "grass grow" or "paint dry"
- *Visual illusions* and *hallucinations*
- *Vivid thoughts and memories*, including "flashbacks"

These psychodelic actions have been particularly attractive to adolescent girls and young women, as well as to their male counterparts, for over 7 decades. The pharmacology of LSD and women's medical and personal abuse of LSD are presented and discussed in the following sections.

Pharmacology

LSD is a semi-synthetic derivative of an ergot alkaloid and is considered to be the *most* widely used indole psychodelic in the U.S. (see Table 6.1). It was first synthesized in 1938 by Albert Hoffman from lysergic acid that occurs naturally in ergot fungi, which grows on wheat and rye. LSD was the 25th in a series of ergot derivatives. Hence, once identified, the substance was initially named "LSD-25." Preliminary animal studies did *not* yield significant results and interest in the compound rapidly diminished. In fact, little was done until April 16, 1943, when Hoffman prepared a fresh supply of the compound. Inadvertently absorbing a small amount on his fingertips (due to poor laboratory techniques), he quickly and pleasantly became overcome by both an intense stimulation of the imagination and altered state of awareness of the world (i.e., resultant illusions and hallucinations). Three days later, he deliberately ingested 250 mcg of the compound (under controlled, experimental conditions), to confirm his first "accidental"experience with LSD (Hoffman, 1970, 1980; Pagliaro & Pagliaro, 2004). The rest of the story, as they say, is history.

Pharmacodynamics: Mechanism of Action

Although *vast* amounts of data have now accumulated regarding LSD's general pharmacology, its *exact* mechanism of action remains largely unknown (Passie, Halpern, & Stichtenoth, 2008). It has been suggested that LSD interacts as a partial agonist with the serotonin 5-HT(2A) receptors (Gonzalez-Maeso & Sealfon, 2009), particularly those expressed on neocortical pyramidal cells (Nichols, 2004). More recent data suggest that:

> LSD reduces connectivity within brain networks and reduces the extent to which separate networks remain distinct in their patterns of firing.
>
> *(American College of Neuropsychopharmacology, 2015, p. 1)*

The resultant "more chaotic" brain state suggested by this proposed mechanism of LSD action, is consistent with both the: (1) prodromal phase of psychosis/schizophrenia; and (2) characterization/nomenclature that refers to the psychodelics as "psychotogens" or "schizophrenomimetics" (as described in the chapter introduction).

Pharmacokinetics: Absorption, Distribution, Metabolism, and Excretion

Following oral ingestion, the onset of action of LSD is generally within 30 to 60 minutes. The *intensity* of psychodelic effects, such as the experience of perceptual changes, is dose-related and, thus, depends on the *amount* of LSD used. It also depends on the personality, predisposition, or tendencies of the user to react in a particular way, and the context of use (i.e., *drug, set, and setting*). The effects produced by LSD generally peak within 1 to 6 hours and usually dissipate within 8 to 12 hours. The terminal half-life of elimination reportedly ranges from 3 to 15 hours (Dolder, Schmid, & Haschke, 2015). Additional pharmacokinetic data are *not* available (Pagliaro & Pagliaro, 2009).

Undesired, or Harmful, Effects and Toxicities

LSD use has been associated with several physical and mental toxicities that also are generally related to "drug, set, and setting" and can be troubling. Its use also has been associated with other long recognized, and generally *more* serious, mental toxicities.

Physical and Mental Toxicities. The *physical toxicities* associated with LSD use include: anorexia; blurred vision; diaphoresis; dry mouth; heart palpitations; hypertension; incoordination; insomnia; mydriasis; and tachycardia. *Mental toxicities* include: anxiety; difficulty locating the source of a sound; distortions of body image; fear of fragmentation, or disintegration of self; mood swings from happiness to sadness; and prolonged visual afterimages. While troublesome, these mental toxicities are generally short-lived. However, they can be extremely frightening when experienced in the context of a "bad trip" or "flashback" (see following section, "More Serious Toxicities").

More Serious Toxicities. The relatively common, and *more* serious, mental toxicities associated with LSD use are well recognized, and include: mental depression; *severe* panic reactions (i.e., "bad trips"); paranoia; and prolonged psychosis, particularly among women who use LSD and have a predisposition for these toxicities (i.e., are pre-schizophrenic and/or have a positive family history of schizophrenia) (Pagliaro & Pagliaro, *Clinical Patient Data Files*). These common, and more serious, toxicities have been classified into *four substance-induced* disorders according to the American Psychiatric Association's DSM taxonomy:

1. *Anxiety disorder*, characterized by nervous behavior or panic, which can occur during, or following, LSD intoxication
2. *Hallucinogen persisting perception disorder*, the transient recurrence of perceptual disturbances associated with previous LSD intoxication (i.e., "flashbacks"), which can occur days, months, or even years after the last use of LSD and, particularly because of their unplanned, or unexpected occurrence, commonly result in clinically or socially significant stress or impairment
3. *Mood disorder*, characterized by depression and risk for suicide attempts, or completions, which can occur during, or following, LSD intoxication and persist for more than 24 hours
4. *Psychotic disorder*, characterized by disordered thinking, extreme alterations in emotions, and hallucinations, which can occur during LSD intoxication and resolve within hours, or progress to a *long-term schizophreniform disorder*

These *more* serious LSD-induced disorders are managed in various ways. (Also, see Chapter 7, *Identifying Women's Contemporaneous Diagnoses*.) For example: sedative-hypnotic pharmacotherapy (e.g., diazepam, Valium®) may be required to relieve the signs and symptoms associated with anxiety disorder; or antipsychotic pharmacotherapy (e.g., haloperidol, Haldol®) may be required to relieve the signs and symptoms associated with psychosis.

Hallucinogen-persisting perception disorder, or *flashbacks*, typically involve *visual* hallucinations, but also may involve olfactory, tactile, or other sensory hallucinations that can last for minutes to hours. Flashbacks may be triggered by any type of environmental stimuli, but are commonly associated with the frequent use of LSD and the people, places, and things related to the initial use of LSD.[15] Flashbacks also have been related to physical or mental stress (Pagliaro & Pagliaro, *Clinical Patient Data Files*). Flashbacks should be treated in the same way as LSD psychosis (see following brief discussion in this section). Virtually all flashbacks have the potential to be unpleasant because they are unplanned and unexpected. Although they are encountered more commonly when LSD has been used several times, flashbacks also can occur following an initial use of LSD.[16]

LSD-induced psychosis, which is similar to *amphetamine-induced psychosis*, is more likely to occur with the repeated use of LSD. The psychosis generally resolves on its own with the discontinuation of LSD use or, if necessary, responds well to appropriate antipsychotic pharmacotherapy. However, the psychosis may last for several days or several months, even with treatment. Less severe "bad trips" are usually temporary and last for approximately 24 hours. They generally can be successfully managed in a familiar environment by providing reassurance and other psychological support. Antipsychotic pharmacotherapy (e.g., chlorpromazine, Thorazine®), which antagonizes most of the pharmacologic actions of LSD, usually is *not* required (Pagliaro & Pagliaro, 2009).

A common identified observation regarding women's chronic, lifetime use of LSD and an associated major mental disorder (MMD) is that the MMD generally occurs when a woman has:

1. A predisposing, or genetic, tendency for the MMD
2. Other significant risk factors (e.g., environmental risk factor; concomitant, predisposing drug or substance abuse)

In the absence of these factors, lifetime LSD use has *not* been significantly associated with an *increased* likelihood of: suicide attempt, or completion; serious psychological distress; or mental health treatment (Hendricks, Thorne, & Clark, 2015; Johansen & Krebs, 2015; Krebs & Johansen, 2013). Thus, it appears that women, who use LSD and develop signs and symptoms of psychosis/schizophrenia, generally have a pre-existing positive family history of schizophrenia.

---

[15] We have suggested, for example, that flashbacks, like the déjà vu experience, may be related, at least in some cases, to olfactory memory (Pagliaro, 1991).

[16] More recently, particularly with the generally lower dosages of LSD that are being used during the new millennium (i.e., approximately half the dosage that was commonly used during the 1960s and 1970s), the incidence of flashbacks has been significantly *reduced*—to the point that they are becoming a relatively uncommon event (Pagliaro & Pagliaro, *Clinical Patient Data Files*).

Physical and Psychological Dependence. Although LSD use has been associated with tolerance, its use has *not* been associated with a specific LSD withdrawal syndrome when regular, long-term use is abruptly discontinued.

TOLERANCE. Women's abuse of LSD is associated with *tolerance* to both physical and psychological effects. It also has been associated with *cross tolerance*, and *reverse tolerance*. Regarding specific physical effects, *lower tolerance* develops to the cardiovascular effects of LSD (i.e., these effects are more resistant to tolerance). The extent of tolerance to LSD can be significant—in the same order of magnitude as that observed with alcohol, or other sedative-hypnotics, and phencyclidine (PCP). Following 3 to 4 days of nonuse, developed tolerance dissipates (i.e., sensitivity to the *desired* effects of LSD rapidly return) (Scholey, Parrott, & Buchanan, 2004).

CROSS-TOLERANCE AND REVERSE TOLERANCE. Cross-tolerance has been reported to occur among LSD, MDMA, mescaline, and psilocybin—suggesting a common molecular mechanism of action. *Reverse* tolerance, or increased sensitivity to the actions of LSD, rarely has been reported (Pagliaro & Pagliaro, *Clinical Patient Data Files*).

LSD WITHDRAWAL SYNDROME. There is *no* available evidence, anecdotal or otherwise, that supports the existence/occurrence of an LSD withdrawal syndrome when regular, long-term use is abruptly discontinued. Thus, physical dependence (as traditionally defined) is *not* associated with the personal use of LSD.

Pregnancy and Lactation. No data have been published that demonstrate a clear link between maternal use of LSD and teratogenesis (i.e., congenital malformation, including chromosomal damage among offspring). Excretion into breast milk also has *not* yet been demonstrated (Pagliaro & Pagliaro, 2002, 2012).

Overdosage

LSD has a *high* LD_{50} and, thus, is relatively safe to use. Although LSD has *not* been *directly* associated with overdosage fatalities, it has been *indirectly* associated with several accidental deaths and completed suicides. These fatalities occurred among women when they were under the influence of its psychodelic actions (e.g., a woman, believing she can "fly like a bird," may fatally jump off the roof of a building to her death; a woman, believing she is being chased by an illusionary figure, may run across the street in terror and be fatally struck by a passing motor vehicle).

Women's Medical and Personal LSD Use and Abuse

Women's Medical LSD Use/Abuse

LSD *never* received FDA approval for medical use, although it was briefly used as an adjunct to psychotherapy and for military experiments (Pagliaro & Pagliaro,

2004; Pagliaro & Pagliaro, *Clinical Patient Data Files*). It is *not* currently approved in the U.S. for *any* medical indication.

Women's Personal LSD Use/Abuse

Embodied by the *hippies* as a *Turn on, Tune-in, Drop Out* antiestablishment drug that was musically eternalized by The Beatles, The Rolling Stones, and Bob Dylan, women's LSD use flourished during the 1960s only to significantly *decline* during the 1970s and 1980s. During the 1990s, LSD *and other* psychodelic drugs (at significantly *lower* dosages than those typically used during the 1960s) underwent *renewed popularity* when their use *exploded* as they became a major part of women's attendance at dance clubs and raves. Thus, during the new millennium, women in the U.S. have used LSD extensively and by *every* method of administration possible.

Most women ingest a tiny LSD microdot tablet or place it under the tongue. Some women ingest a sugar cube, gelatin square (or other shaped "window pane"), or small piece of blotter paper, upon which a drop of LSD solution was instilled. Regardless of method of use, one of the few available national drug surveys of psychodelic use found that, in 2014, approximately 11% of U.S. adults, 26 years-of-age and older, reported lifetime use of LSD (NIDA, 2016). While the use of LSD by women during the new millennium is relatively common, the dosage and frequency of use are generally much *lower* than that observed during the 1960s (Pagliaro & Pagliaro, *Clinical Patient Data Base*).

Cannabis

> *Cannabis is the most commonly used illicit drug worldwide.*
>
> *(Power, Verweij, & Zuhair, 2014, p. 1201)*

Thus, it should *not* be surprising that for adolescent girls and young women, cannabis, in the form of *marijuana*, is the *most* widely known and used psychodelic in the U.S. (Pagliaro & Pagliaro, 2009, 2012).[17]

As identified by Radhakrishnan, Wilkinson, and D'Souza (2014):

> Cannabis is the most commonly used illicit drug by adults, with 18.1 million current users in the U.S. and approximately 5 million daily cannabis users.
>
> *(p. 1)*

[17] Perhaps surprising, given its widespread availability and patterns of medical and personal use across the U.S., published current statistics regarding the use of marijuana, particularly among women, are relatively scarce. For example, there are *no* available national surveys of rates of marijuana use for specific population groups and patterns of use (e.g., percent THC, amount used, and frequency of use). In addition, valid and reliable data are unavailable for subpopulation groups in terms of those who have engaged in "past month," "past year," or "lifetime" marijuana use. However, the consensus

As similarly identified by Azofeifa, Mattson, and Schauer (2016):

> In the United States, marijuana is the most commonly used illicit drug. In 2013, 7.5% (19.8 million) of the U.S. population … 12 years of age or older … reported using marijuana during the preceding month.
>
> *(p. 1)*

In addition, with the legalization of medicinal marijuana and the increased availability of high-percentage THC varieties in newly opened dispensaries, and various methods of use (e.g., colorful, electronic marijuana smoking devices; fancy vaporizers and bongs; exotic hookahs; and candies and other treats), it is extremely likely that rates of marijuana use are increasing (for further related discussion, see later section, "Women's Medical Cannabis Use/Abuse.")

Pharmacology

Whereas *pharmacology* is the study of origin, nature, chemistry, effects, and uses of drugs, a related science, *pharmacognacy*,[18] focuses more specifically on the medicinal use of plants and other natural substances. For this reason, and because of the high rates of cannabis use by women in the U.S., we begin with an additional section on its pharmacognacy. We then continue with the pharmacology of cannabis, a member of the miscellaneous subclass of psychodelics. Categorized as one of three products of cannabis (i.e., marijuana, hashish, and hashish oil), marijuana—commonly referred to as: "bud"; "dope"; "grass"; "Mary Jane"; "pot"; and "weed"—remains the most popular. We conclude the section with *Women's Medical and Personal Cannabis Use/Abuse*.

Pharmacognacy and Botany of Cannabis

Several species of *cannabis* exist, including *Cannabis lativa* and *Cannabis sativa* (Indian hemp). *Cannabis sativa* is the principal variety from which marijuana, hashish, and hashish oil are prepared. Within the species of *Cannabis sativa*, there are several varieties including *Cannabis sativa indica*, *Cannabis sativa ruderalis*, and *Cannabis sativa sativa*. These varieties significantly differ in regard to their concentration of delta-9-tetrahydrocannabinol (THC), the major active psychodelic ingredient found in *cannabis*,[19] with the *indica* varieties having the *highest* concentrations.[20]

---

appears to be that marijuana is one of the *most* commonly used substances of abuse among women in the U.S.

[18] *Pharmacognacy* is the study of the recognition, preparation, and use of bioactive natural products, particularly medicinal drugs that are extracted or otherwise obtained from plants and other natural sources.

[19] Other major cannabinoids found in cannabis include, for example, *cannabidiol* and *cannabinol*.

[20] N.B. Some botanical taxonomies classify *indica*, *ruderalis*, and *sativa* as belonging to different species of cannabis.

The *highest* concentration of THC is found in the *bracts*, or small leaves, at the base of the *cannabis* flowers, and their resin. The next highest concentration is found in the flowering tops, and then, in *decreasing* order, the upper leaves, large stems, and seeds, with the roots having the *lowest* concentration. The female plants tend to have a much *higher* THC concentration than the male plants. Thus, the reason for advertisements and sales of tools (e.g., ultraviolet lights) in drug-paraphernalia stores (i.e., headshops, hemp stores) and drug culture magazines (e.g., *High Times*) to detect plant sex.

The desire for higher THC concentrations also accounts for the popularity of *sinsemilla*—unfertilized female cannabis plants that are cultivated specifically for their higher THC concentration. The cultivation of *sinsemilla* is generally accomplished by planting only female seeds, or by destroying the male plants before pollen is produced and the female plants are fertilized. These procedures allow the unfertilized female plants to *flower* more abundantly and, consequently, to produce more THC-containing resin.

Cannabis is produced worldwide as illustrated by the names given to the many varieties that are distributed and sold across the U.S. These names include, for example: *Acapulco Gold*; *BC Bud*; *Cambodian Red*; *Hawaiian Buds*; *Indian Hash*; *Jamaican Ganja*; *Lebanese Hash*; *Moroccan Kif*; *New Mexico Sinse*; *Panama Gold*; *Thai Sticks*; and *Ukrainian Ditch Weed*. In addition to worldwide distribution and sale, several states (i.e., Alabama, California, Florida, Hawaii, Kentucky, North Carolina, Oregon, Tennessee, Washington, West Virginia, Wisconsin) produce cannabis to the extent that it is the state's most significant cash crop (albeit, predominantly illicit) with the combined annual revenues reaching the tens of billions of dollars (Pagliaro & Pagliaro, 2009).[21]

> The domestic marijuana crop is: larger than cotton in Alabama; larger than grapes, vegetables, and hay combined in California; larger than peanuts

---

[21] As individual states (e.g., California, Colorado, Washington) begin to *re-legalize* marijuana (i.e., marijuana was legal and unregulated in the U.S. prior to the early 20th century [Pagliaro & Pagliaro, 2004]), both for medicinal and personal (i.e., *recreational*) use, tens of millions of dollars in tax revenue are being added to state tax coffers. For example, Colorado collected approximately $40 million in additional tax dollars in 2014 (La Corte, 2014; Phillips Erb, 2014). As reported by the Colorado Department of Revenue, for 2016:

> Total marijuana tax revenue includes the 2.9% retail and medical marijuana sales tax, 10% retail marijuana special sales tax, 15% marijuana excise tax, and retail/medical marijuana application and license fees.
>
> (*p. 1*)

In the state of Washington, legal marijuana sales yielded over $70 million in tax revenue during the 2014/2015 fiscal year (Williams, 2015). It has been estimated that if marijuana sales were legalized in all 50 states, the associated tax revenue generated could exceed 3 billion dollars annually (Ferner, 2014). (Also, see related discussion later in this chapter.)

> in Georgia; and larger than tobacco in both South Carolina and North Carolina.
>
> *(Gettman, 2006, p. 1)*

However, despite its worldwide production and commerce, approximately 50% of the cannabis that is used in the U.S. is smuggled in from *one* specific country, Mexico.[22]

As noted earlier in the introduction to this section:

> Marijuana is the most frequently used illicit substance in the U.S.
>
> *(Cerda, Wall, & Keyes, 2012, p. 22)*

Marijuana (i.e., *grass, pot, weed*) is the dried, shredded plant form (generally *flowers* and *leaves*) of cannabis.[23] Marijuana is generally grayish-green or greenish-brown in color and, when compared to hashish or hashish oil, contains significantly *lower* concentrations of THC. Marijuana is prepared for pulmonary inhalation (i.e., smoking, or *toking*) using methods that are similar to those used for preparing tobacco leaves for smoking. However, marijuana generally requires less time and involvement regarding curing and drying.

Hashish is prepared from the dried resin and compressed flowers of the cannabis plant and is generally light brown to black in color. Prepared and distributed for use in compressed blocks or cubes, it has a relatively *high* concentration of THC. *Hashish oil* is prepared from hashish by the means of extraction with an organic solvent, often isopropyl alcohol (i.e., "rubbing alcohol"). It is then filtered and concentrated. Hashish oil contains the *highest* concentration of THC ranging in color from clear to almost black. Food coloring often is added for color enhancement.

The concentration of THC in marijuana, hashish, and hashish oil can generally range from:

- 1% to 10% for marijuana cigarettes (i.e., *doobies; joints; reefers*)[24]
- 15% to 25% for hashish
- Up to 60% for hashish oil

---

22 Over the first decade of the new millennium, increasing amounts of high potency marijuana (i.e., 15% to 25% THC) also began to enter the U.S. from Canada, produced predominantly from indoor growing operations (i.e., *grow ops*) in the Province of British Columbia (i.e., *BC Bud*).

23 *Kif* (kaif, keef, kief), an Arabic word meaning *well-being* or *pleasure*, was originally the name given to a powder that was made from the dried flowers of the female *cannabis* plant. Indigenous to the Rif mountain area of northern Morocco, it was usually mixed with tobacco (1 part to 2 parts) prior to smoking (Nahas, Zeidenberg, & Lefebure, 1975). Although the use of kif in the U.S. has been reported over the years, its use is relatively uncommon (Pagliaro & Pagliaro, *Clinical Patient Data Files*). The term is now more commonly used to denote marijuana or hashish that is from Morocco.

24 Also, the same for *blunts* (i.e., marijuana that is rolled in tobacco leaves or a cigar wrap).

While these concentrations vary depending on the specific part of the plant (e.g., buds, leaves, or stems) from which they were prepared, it also depends on the: (1) quality and source of the *cannabis*—the state, province, or country of origin (e.g., British Columbia, Canada; Hawaii, U.S.; Mexico); and (2) cultivation techniques (e.g., hydroponic cultivation). It is extremely important to recognize that, since the beginning of the new millennium, THC concentrations have significantly *increased*, on average, from 25% to 300% across the U.S. primarily depending upon: (1) pre-millennial comparison year; (2) form of cannabis; (3) type/variety of cannabis; and (4) location.

During the new millennium, the average, *high* potency, marijuana joint contained approximately *150 mg* of THC. By comparison, an average, *high* potency, marijuana joint during the 1960s and 1970s, contained approximately *10 mg* of THC. In this regard, it is important to keep in mind that the amount of THC that reaches the lungs and is absorbed into the blood stream is variable and depends on: (1) the amount of THC in the cannabis that is smoked; (2) the smoking technique used, including the rate, depth, and length of inhalation before exhaling (i.e., the *drag* or *hit*); and (3) the amount of THC that is destroyed by pyrolysis.[25]

Pharmacodynamics: Mechanism of Action

Over 400 different chemicals have been identified in cannabis smoke, including ammonia, benzo(a)pyrene, carbon monoxide, cresols, hydrogen cyanide, nitric oxide, phenols, and tars.[26] These chemicals include approximately 60 different *cannabinoids* (i.e., chemicals that are only naturally found in *cannabis* plants). Of these, the principal active cannabinoid, in terms of psychodelic actions, is delta-9-tetrahydrocannabinol, *THC*.

A variety of clearly defined dose-related effects, from euphoria to toxic psychosis, have been associated with the psychotropic actions of THC. *Lower* dosages may produce: decreased intraocular pressure; drowsiness; euphoria; hypertension; increased appetite; memory impairment; reddened eyes; relaxation; tachycardia; and temporal disintegration. *Moderate* dosages may produce: anxiety; decreased muscle strength and motor performance; decreased visual acuity; and paranoia. *Higher* dosages may produce: confused thinking; delusions; hallucinations; synesthesia; and toxic psychosis.

---

[25] N.B. Given the interest in vaporization as a use of nicotine delivery (see related discussion of e-cigarettes in Chapter 4, *Women's Caffeine and Nicotine Abuse*) it is important to note that, despite some well-documented degradation of THC by pyrolysis, several researchers (e.g., Eisenberg, Ogintz, & Almog, 2014; Hartman, Brown, & Milavetz, 2015) have demonstrated that vaporization is an effective means for THC delivery.

[26] Several of these chemicals are *known* human carcinogens (e.g., benzo(a)pyrene, a highly carcinogenic hydrocarbon found in coal tar; cresols; phenols; and tars). (Also, see later section, *Undesired, or Harmful, Effects and Toxicities.*)

> The interchanging of the senses ... the hashish eater knows what it is ... to smell colors, to see sounds, and, much more frequently, to see feelings.
>
> *(Ludlow, 1857, p. 72)*

The mechanism by which THC exerts its psychodelic and other effects is *not* yet fully understood. However, important strides have been made since the beginning of the new millennium in this regard. Undoubtedly, the greatest advancement has been the identification of the endocannabinoid system—the *endogenous* system of cannabinoid receptors and agonists, or ligands (Breivogel & Childers, 1998).[27] Overall, the endocannabinoid system appears to primarily act as a neuromodulator of the CNS by affecting the release of several identified neurotransmitters, including: acetylcholine; dopamine; endorphins; gamma-aminobutyric acid (GABA); glutamate; noradrenaline; and serotonin (Lopez-Moreno, Gonzalez-Cuevas, & Moreno, 2008; Moreira & Lutz, 2008). Two major cannabinoid G-protein coupled receptor subtypes appear to exist, Subtype 1 (i.e., CB1 receptors) and Subtype 2 (i.e., CB2 receptors) (Pertwee, 2000).

CB1 receptors are primarily present on central and peripheral neurons, predominantly within the CNS (Pertwee, 2000). These receptors appear to mediate the: (1) inhibition of adenylate cyclase and various calcium channels; (2) stimulation of potassium channels; and (3) activation of mitogen-activated protein kinase (Ameri, 1999). The endocannabinoid activity of these receptors suggests a role in the modulation of neurotransmitter release and action (e.g., increasing dopaminergic neuronal activity in the ventral tegmental area-mesolimbic pathway) (Di Marzo, Melck, & Bisogno, 1998).

CB2 receptors are primarily present on immune cells, predominantly outside of the CNS (Klein, Lane, & Newton, 2000). These receptors appear to mediate the activation of mitogen-activated protein kinase and the inhibition of adenylate cyclase (Ameri, 1999). The endocannabinoid activity of these receptors (e.g., enhanced physiological response to cytokines) suggests a role in immunosuppression and anti-inflammatory action (Nocerino, Amato, & Izzo, 2000). In addition, although *not* yet confirmed, these mechanisms may play an active role in the treatment of other medical disorders such as chronic neuropathic pain that is often refractory of standard pharmacotherapeutic interventions (Eisenburg, Orgintz & Almog, 2014; Wilsey, Marcotte, & Deutsch, 2013).

Pharmacokinetics: Absorption, Distribution, Metabolism, and Excretion

Following oral ingestion, THC bioavailability is *low* (i.e., approximately 10%) because of *extensive* first-pass hepatic metabolism. Following pulmonary inhalation,

[27] Anandamide (N-archidonoyl ethanolamine) and arachidonoylglycerol have been identified as the major endogenous agonists, or ligands, of the endocannabinoid receptors. These endogenous

THC bioavailability is much *higher* having a mean of 27% (range, 17% to 37%) due to its *rapid* absorption from the lungs and avoidance of first-pass hepatic metabolism. Once in the blood stream, oxidative metabolism, primarily in the liver, produces both its *active* metabolite, 11-hydroxy-delta-9-tetrahydrocannabinol (11-OH-THC), and its *inactive* metabolite, 11-nor-hydroxy-delta-9-tetrahydrocannabinol (THCCOOH). Interestingly, blood THC concentrations peak *prior* to the end of pulmonary inhalation of cannabis; 11-OH-THC blood concentrations peak just *after* the end of pulmonary inhalation of cannabis; and THCCOOH blood concentrations peak 1.5 to 2 hours *after* the pulmonary inhalation of cannabis.

THC is approximately 97% protein bound, while its active metabolite 11-OH-THC is *more* highly protein bound (i.e., 99%). The apparent volume of distribution of THC is approximately 10 liters per kg, primarily because of its *high* lipid solubility. Some researchers report a THC mean initial alpha distribution half-life of elimination of approximately 30 hours. However, the later beta phase elimination half-life is about 3.5 days because of its preferential concentration and storage in the spleen and body fat (range, 1 to 7 days). In addition, it has long been recognized that cannabis smoke has the potential, like tobacco smoke, to induce hepatic microsomal isoenzymes. In this regard, regular, long-term cannabis users generally eliminate THC *more* rapidly (half-life of elimination, approximately 28 hours) than nonusers (half-life of elimination, approximately 57 hours).

Total body clearance of THC generally ranges from 750 to 1,200 ml/minute. The elimination half-life of its *inactive* metabolite, THCCOOH, is 2 to 6 days. *Both* metabolites are excreted in the urine and are also secreted back into the gut, by means of enterohepatic recirculation, where they are *reabsorbed* or excreted in the feces.

THC and its two major metabolites, 11-OH-THC and THCCOOH, are present in the urine as glucuronide conjugates. *Low* concentrations of both THC metabolites can often be detected in the feces and urine for *more* than 5 weeks after cannabis was last used. Although, urinary concentrations of THC that exceed 1.5 ng/ml are suggestive of cannabis use during the previous 8 hours, because of pharmacokinetic variance and extreme inter-individual variability, a presumptive blood concentration of THC, *cannot* be reliably related to a specific measurable level of cognitive or behavioral impairment. The *blood to plasma concentration ratio* for THC is 0.55.

The urine tests currently used for detecting cannabis use can detect concentrations of THC and its major *inactive* metabolite, THCCOOH as low as 1 ng/ml of urine with good validity and reliability. However, the validity of urine tests is *not* always accurate because false positive results can occur due to the: (1) interference of certain other drugs that might have been concurrently used (e.g., ibuprofen,

chemicals elicit several of the pharmacologic actions associated with the use of THC (Maccarrone & Finazzi-Agro, 2002; Martin, Mechoulam, & Razdan, 1999).

Motrin®); and (2) inability of a test to differentiate between cannabis that was deliberately and directly inhaled and cannabis that was passively and indirectly inhaled (i.e., as sidestream, or secondhand, fumes—*smoke* or *vapor*).

In addition, the ingestion of large quantities of products that contain hemp seed oil may produce *false positive* results if the cutoff values designated by the laboratory for the urine test are too low. Urine tests also can give *false negative* results. These false negative results are much more likely to occur when the urine test sample is deliberately adulterated with an in vitro adulterant (e.g., pyridinium chlorochromate, which is found in "Urine Luck®," a product specifically developed to invalidate urine tests).

Undesired, or Harmful, Effects and Toxicities

Popular Notion: Cannabis is a relatively non-toxic, natural psychodelic that does *little* harm.

NOT TRUE. Cannabis use can do *much* harm.

There are several characteristic signs and symptoms associated with women's *acute* cannabis use, primarily the: (1) pungent odor of the cannabis smoke on clothing and in closed areas where it was smoked (e.g., automobile; bathroom; bedroom; office); and (2) reddened, or *blood shot*, eyes. Common toxicities that are associated with the use of cannabis can be readily divided into those associated with *short-term use* (i.e., generally, *acute* effects) and those associated with *regular, long-term* use (i.e., generally, *chronic* effects).[28,29]

---

28 The intensity and clinical significance of these toxicities depend, to a significant degree, upon the amount of THC absorbed, the environmental setting or circumstances of use, and physical, mental, and social characteristics of the user. For example, among adults in the 50+ age group, *increasing* marijuana use has been associated with *increasing* injuries. In this regard, Choi, Marti, and DiNitto (2017), in their sample of 14,715 adults, over the age of 50 (including 8,336 women), found that:

> Past year injury rates were 18.9% for nonusers and 28.8% for users (3.9% of the 50+ age group), and past-year ED visit rates were 23.5% for nonusers and 30.9% for users ($p < .001$) (p. 1).

29 A better understanding of cannabis pharmacology (see earlier section, *Pharmacodynamics: Mechanism of Action*) provides possible mechanistic explanations for many of these observed undesired, or harmful, effects and toxicities. For example, the undesired effects involving human immune response are likely mediated by interactions involving THC, or other cannabinoids, with the CB2 receptor. The mental depression and psychosis are likely mediated by the effects of the endocannabinoid system on the neurotransmitters, dopamine and serotonin. In addition, a genetic expression of various harmful effects may also contribute to associated mental disorders (e.g., the development of schizophrenia, as noted by Power, Verweij, and Zuhair, 2014). (Also, see related discussion in Chapter 7, *Identifying Women's Contemporaneous Diagnoses.*)

Short-Term Use. Short-term cannabis use is generally associated with the following toxicities:

- Academic or work achievement, *decreased*
- Anxiety
- Appetite, *increased*
- Blood pressure, *increased*
- Burn injuries (Jehle, Nazir, & Bhavsar, 2015)
- Cognitive impairment (i.e., impaired executive functioning)
- Confusion
- Delusions
- Depersonalization
- Drowsiness
- Hallucinations
- Memory impairment, particularly short-term memory
- Panic reaction
- Paranoia
- Psychomotor impairment (with related motor vehicle crashes)
- Psychotic disorders (also see later section, "Psychosis," for further discussion)
- Pulmonary irritation (e.g., coughs; colds)
- Reddened eyes
- Synesthesia
- Tachycardia
- Temporal disintegration
- Toxic delirium
- Visual acuity, *decreased*

Regular, Long-Term Use. Over the 1970s, 1980s, and 1990s, the potency of cannabis *increased* fivefold, from an average THC content of 2% to a THC content of 10% (Harrison, Backenheimer, & Inciardi, 1996).[30] The *increase* in potency reflected a preferential change among users from *Cannabis (sativa) sativa* to *Cannabis (sativa) indica* and the increased selective cultivation of *sinsemilla* varieties (see earlier discussion). Consequently, several toxicities have *now* been associated with the *regular, long-term use of cannabis*.[31] These toxicities include:

---

[30] As briefly discussed earlier, these "standard" THC concentrations continued to rise during the new millennium.

[31] It may seem logical to conclude, based upon these observations, that potential cannabis users, being aware of the significant increases in the THC concentrations of current cannabis products, would take appropriate precautions (e.g., avoidance of cannabis use or reduction of dosage, or amount consumed or inhaled). However, new millennial concerns with medicalization, decriminalization, and legalization of marijuana use in many cities and states across the U.S., have significantly affected people's attitudes (Cerda, Wall, & Keyes, 2012; Samuels, 2015). For example, *decreased* perception

- Academic or work achievement, decreased
- Cannabinoid hyperemesis syndrome (CHS) (Beech, Sterrett, & Babiuk, 2015)[32]
- Cannabis withdrawal syndrome, relatively mild
- *Cognitive impairment*[33]
- Disruption of normal ovulation
- Immunosuppression[34]
- Interference with prenatal development, potential for (see later section, *Pregnancy and Lactation*)[35]
- Lethargy
- Lung cancer[36]

---

of significant risk associated with the current use of marijuana has been positively associated with: (1) younger age; (2) high school graduation; (3) family income greater than $75k annually; and (4) current marijuana use (Pacek, Mauro, & Martins, 2015). In addition, Certa, Wall, and Keyes (2012) noted two related and potentially problematic, but expected trends: (1) that residents of states with *marijuana laws* (e.g., regarding decriminalization) had *higher* odds of marijuana use; and (2) that states, which *legalized* marijuana use, had *higher* rates of marijuana use.

32 *Cannabinoid hyperemesis syndrome* (CHS) is a rare condition that was first officially recognized early in the new millennium (Allen, de Moore, & Heddle, 2004). It is typically characterized by: (1) abdominal pain; (2) intractable nausea and vomiting that occurs in a cyclic pattern; and (3) relief, albeit temporary, by compulsive bathing/showering in *hot* water (Alaniz, Liss, & Metz, 2015; Simonetto, Oxentenko, & Herman, 2012). Episodes generally last for 2 to 4 days.

Although the exact mechanism underlying the syndrome remains unknown, it is only observed in chronic cannabis users (i.e., generally regular, long-term daily or weekly users) (Allen, de Moore, & Heddle, 2004; Simonetto, Oxentenko, & Herman, 2012). In addition, although the significance is unclear, hypophosphatemia has been observed in some patients presenting with CHS (Cadman, 2017). It should be noted that CHS shares several clinical similarities with the Cyclic Vomiting Syndrome, for which it is often confused—particularly when appropriate attention is *not* given to a history of cannabis use (Galli, Sawaya, & Friedenberg, 2011).

Various therapeutic interventions for CHS, including standard pharmacotherapy for vomiting with 5-HT3 or D2-receptor antagonists, have been attempted with *little* or *no* success. As noted by Hermes-Laufer, Del Puppo, and Inan (2012), and widely supported by many others (e.g., Sorensen, De Santo, & Borgelt, 2016):

> The only long-term satisfying treatment option [for CHS] is the complete abstinence from cannabis consumption.
>
> *(p. 1)*

However, this treatment option may be difficult to successfully implement with women who are dependent on cannabis.

33 The neuropsychological dysfunction (e.g., cognitive impairment; memory impairment), which is associated with the acute use of cannabis, is *not* associated with regular, long-term use following a period of abstinence (van Holst & Schilt, 2011).

34 The immunosuppression appears to be modulated by interaction with the CB2 receptor (see earlier section, *Pharmacodynamics: Mechanism of Action*).

35 Also, for men: decreased sperm count and motility; and gynecomastia.

36 Although there is a paucity of available reliable published data, lung cancer would be an expected chronic toxicity associated with regular, long-term cannabis smoking. This toxic effect would be expected because of: (1) the presence of known human carcinogens in cannabis smoke in concentrations significantly higher than those found in tobacco cigarette smoke (Ashton, 2001; Pagliaro, 1983); and (2) the method of smoking cannabis (i.e., inhaling the cannabis smoke deeply into the lungs and holding it in the lungs as long as possible). This smoking technique is

- Mental depression
- Physical dependence
- Psychosis (see additional related discussion in later section, "Psychosis")
- Pulmonary irritation (e.g., cough and colds, with the eventual development of related COPD [i.e., asthma; bronchitis])

Although these and other toxicities associated with regular, long-term use have been documented in the published literature, relatively *few* serious toxicities have been *directly* associated with cannabis use. The available evidence, from controlled clinical studies and common sense, point to *four* additional major toxicities that are *directly* linked to the regular, long-term use of cannabis: (1) *amotivational syndrome*; (2) *motor vehicle and other crashes*, including airplane, train, and truck crashes; (3) *psychosis*; and (4) *pulmonary toxicity*. (Also, see later sections, *Physical and Psychological Dependence* and *Pregnancy and Lactation*.)

AMOTIVATIONAL SYNDROME. Amotivational syndrome, or *burn out*, is identified among women who are regular, long-term cannabis users.[37] Generally, after several months to years of using cannabis to *mellow out* or to forget their problems, these women tend to lose interest in their homes, work and social environments, and the daily "challenges" of life. They typically content themselves, alone, each day, doing little else than looking through favorite magazines, listening to music, watching their favorite television programs, and playing android or iPhone games on their cell phones while they smoke cannabis. As noted by Castle (2013):

> An "amotivational syndrome" has been described in chronic, heavy cannabis users. The syndrome resembles the negative symptoms of schizophrenia and is characterized by apathy, amotivation, social withdrawal, narrowing of interests, lethargy, impaired memory, impaired concentration, disturbed judgment, and impaired occupational achievement.
>
> *(p. 2)*

Whether the use of cannabis causes the syndrome, or whether it merely brings out a woman's latent personality characteristics, has *not* yet been clearly determined.

---

thought to maximize the contact of the smoke with the alveoli and, hence, increase the amount of THC absorbed by the capillaries for distribution through the circulatory system). Reportedly, vaporization of the marijuana significantly *decreases* or *eliminates* this risk. (See later related discussion.)

37 This syndrome, generally recognized since the 1970s, is supported by evidence that is largely anecdotal and is derived from uncontrolled studies. Several researchers question the validity of this syndrome and suggest that, what is observed, is simply the expected behavior associated with chronic, long-term intoxication among cannabis users (e.g., Johns, 2001).

MOTOR VEHICLE AND OTHER CRASHES.

Popular Notion: It is relatively safe to smoke marijuana while driving a car. NOT TRUE. See following discussion.

Several large meta-analyses have found that acute cannabis intoxication results in a significant *increase* in the odds ratios of being involved in a motor vehicle crash. For example, Li, Brady, and DiMaggio (2012) reported that:

> The results of this meta-analysis suggest that marijuana use by drivers is associated with a significantly increased risk of being involved in motor vehicle crashes.
>
> *(p. 65)*

As found by Asbridge, Hayden, and Cartwright (2012):

> Acute cannabis consumption is associated with an increased risk of a motor vehicle crash, especially for fatal collisions.
>
> *(p. 1)*

Women, who are regular, long-term cannabis users, are at *greatest* risk for motor vehicle and other crashes, particularly if they: (1) use *high* potency cannabis; (2) are 65 years-of-age or older; or (3) are drivers who concomitantly abuse both cannabis and alcohol, which can result in deleterious, synergistic effects—associated with different mechanisms of action—on driving ability (Hartman & Huestis, 2013; Pagliaro & Pagliaro, 2009; Stein, Caviness, & Anderson, 2014).[38]

While many cannabis researchers generally agree that there is a *direct* relationship between cannabis intoxication and *decreased* driving performance, others (e.g., Sewell, Poling, & Sofuoglu, 2009) continue to argue the contrary, positing the following assumptions as a basis for their position:

1. That alcohol, which is legal and, generally, socially acceptable, impairs driving performance to a significantly greater extent than does cannabis
2. That cannabis users are *less* likely to smoke and drive than to drink and drive

[38] N.B. It is particularly important to recognize that the incidence of related MVAs is increasing (e.g., Christophersen, Morland, & Stewart, 2016) and we fully expect it to continue to do so over the next decade or so as increasing numbers of states legalize marijuana use or decriminalize its possession and use. For example, Couper and Peterson (2014), in their comprehensive study of drug use and MVAs—pre- and post-legalization in Washington state—found that, while other drug use remained constant, marijuana use significantly *increased* (i.e., from 25% to *over* 50%).

3. That cannabis users, because cognition is significantly *less* compromised than with alcohol use, are consciously aware of the "impairment" associated with their cannabis use, and, therefore, take conscious precautions (e.g., driving more slowly) to compensate and prevent associated motor vehicle crashes[39]

We believe, however, that it is socially irresponsible to disregard the significance of cannabis use in relation to motor vehicle crashes by simply stating that the statistics are *not* as bad as those associated with alcohol use. The fact is that drivers, who are under the influence of cannabis, cannot drive as well as they can when they are *no*t under the influence of cannabis. The driving impairment—which is *directly* related to the acute toxicities associated with cannabis use—becomes *increasingly* severe in direct relation to *increasingly* high cannabis dosages (i.e., using *larger* amounts of cannabis or using cannabis that is *more* potent in terms of relative THC concentration) (e.g., Ramaekers, Berghaus, & van Laar, 2004; Sewell, Poling, & Sofuoglu, 2009).

In addition, as previously noted, when cannabis is used in combination with alcohol—a common practice, particularly among young women—the research is abundantly clear that the degree of driving impairment is significantly *greater* than that caused using either cannabis or alcohol, alone (e.g., Crowley & Courtney, 2003; Ramaekers, Berghaus, & van Laar, 2004; Sewell, Poling, & Sofuoglu, 2009).

> The sister-in-law of the woman who killed herself and seven others when she hit another car head-on while driving the wrong way on the Tacomic State Parkway in July, told investigators that the woman smoked marijuana regularly and was a heavy drinker, according to a lawyer for the family of two of the victims...
>
> A toxicology report indicated that [the woman] had a blood-alcohol level of 0.19, more than twice the legal limit, and a significant level of tetrahydrocannabinol, the active ingredient in marijuana.
>
> *(O'Connor & Schweber, 2009, p. 1)*

Although this case may have involved an *autocide*, the seriousness of impaired driving associated with cannabis use *cannot* be overemphasized. Women, as well as other drivers, who smoke cannabis, should not "smoke and drive."[40]

---

[39] Sewell, Poling, and Sofuoglu (2009) *do* point out that their third assumption is negated when both cannabis and alcohol are used concomitantly.

[40] Despite this admonition, and its support in the professional and scientific literature, the effects of cannabis use on driving performance has *not* as yet been ingrained into the public psyche in the U.S. To illustrate the lack of awareness that is commonly observed among members of the public regarding the deleterious effects of cannabis use on motor vehicle driving performance, we share the following two anecdotal cases that we have personally observed. In the first case,

PSYCHOSIS—*SCHIZOPHRENIA*. Currently, it is widely accepted and acknowledged that the use of cannabis is associated with a wide variety of schizophrenia-like effects, including positive, negative, and cognitive symptoms.[41]

Positive symptoms include:

- Abnormalities in time perception
- Conceptual disorganization
- Delusions, usually grandiose
- Depersonalization
- Derealization
- Feelings of unreality
- Fragmented thinking
- Hallucinations (i.e., perceptual alterations)
- Paranoid thoughts/extreme suspiciousness
- Thought alienation

Negative symptoms include:

- Affective flattening
- Alogia
- Amotivation
- Anhedonia
- Apathetic withdrawal
- Asocial behavior
- Avolition
- Diminished thought content
- Lack of spontaneity

---

a middle-aged woman, whose driver's license had been revoked because of an impaired driving conviction, requested that her adolescent daughter—a daily user of marijuana—be her designated driver. In another case, an elderly woman was in the waiting room of her ophthalmologist's office with her daughter, who was her designated driver, which she needed because her eyes were being dilated as part of her examination. After a while, the woman's daughter told her mother that she needed to "go out for a smoke" and to "stretch a bit" to relieve her back pain. As the daughter left the waiting room, another elderly patient shared that he had recently lost his son to lung cancer and that, perhaps the woman's daughter should stop smoking. The mother quickly clarified that it was okay. Her daughter was *not* going out to smoke a tobacco cigarette, but was going out to smoke her medical marijuana, which she used to manage her chronic back pain (Pagliaro & Pagliaro, *Clinical Patient Data Files*.)

41 This has *not* always been the case, particularly in the United States and in the related published western clinical and scientific literature. For example, we were among the first to formally identify this relationship in presentations and publications during the 1970s and 1980s (e.g., Pagliaro, 1983, 1988) based upon both our clinical experience (i.e., Pagliaro & Pagliaro, *Clinical Patient Data Files*) and review of related East Indian literature. However, we commonly received "push back" that either this observation was: (1) inaccurate; or (2) accurate for use in India, but *not* in the United States.

- Lack of spontaneous speech
- Paucity of thought
- Psychomotor retardation
- Reduced rapport
- Short, unembellished conversation

Cognitive symptoms include:

- Decreased attention
- Impaired executive functioning
- Reduced ability for abstract thought
- Reduced problem-solving ability
- Short-term memory deficits
- Working memory deficits

Depending upon a woman's personal characteristics (e.g., age; genetics, including gender and race) and the characteristics and pattern of cannabis use (e.g., THC concentration; amount used; frequency of use), these symptoms can range in both severity (i.e., from mild to severe) and duration (i.e., from transient to "permanent"). Thus, noted effects among women, who use cannabis, are *not* uniform and monolithic. The etiological relationship between women's cannabis use and psychosis (i.e., schizophrenia) symptomatology is also believed to be largely mediated by a shared mechanism involving the endogenous "cannabinoid" receptor, specifically the CB1 receptor (Cohen, Solowij, & Carr, 2008; D'Souza, 2007; Leweke & Koethe, 2008). (Also, see earlier section, *Pharmacodynamics: Mechanism of Action.*)

It is important to recognize that women who are diagnosed with schizophrenia, often use cannabis to self-medicate their symptomatology in an effort to control or manage undesired signs and symptoms (Castle, 2013). For other women, whose schizophrenia is directly cannabis-induced, symptoms can be either: (1) transient, in which case they may be considered to be an undesired, or harmful, effect or an adverse drug reaction/experience associated with cannabis use; or (2) long-term or "permanent," in which case the use of cannabis likely elicited or exacerbated the onset, or display, of schizophrenia—particularly in susceptible women (Castle, 2013; Radhakrishnan, Wilkinson, & D'Souza, 2014).[42] It also should be noted that women, who have been diagnosed with schizophrenia, but who are in remission, may have a relapse accompanied by full-blown symptomatology triggered by resumed cannabis use (Pagliaro & Pagliaro, *Clinical Patient Data Files*). (Also,

[42] Women who have "polymorphisms of COMT and AKT1 genes may be at increased risk for psychotic disorders in association with cannabinoids" (Radhakrishnan, Wilkinson, & D'Souza, 2014, p. 1).

see related detailed discussion in Chapter 7, *Identifying Women's Contemporaneous Diagnoses*, "WCDs: Psychotic Disorders—Schizophrenia," Cannabis Use Disorder [CUD]) & Schizophrenia, section.)

PULMONARY TOXICITIES. Cannabis smoking, among women who smoke tobacco cigarettes or have chronic obstructive pulmonary disease (COPD), is associated with significant pulmonary disease due to *increased* irritation and damage to lung tissue and results in the further compromise of lung function (Hancox, Poulton, & Ely, 2010; Lee & Hancox, 2011; Pagliaro & Pagliaro, 2009; Taylor, Fergusson, & Milne, 2002).

Pulmonary toxicity has been observed among *heavy* cannabis users and is, primarily, related to the components (e.g., ammonia, hydrogen cyanide, and nitric oxide) in cannabis smoke other than THC (Marijuana smoke, 2007; Pagliaro, 1983, 1988). Therefore, the severity of these effects depends more on the amount of cannabis smoked, the smoking techniques employed by the user, and the combustion properties of the smoking material used to smoke the cannabis rather than on its actual THC content (Impact on lungs, 2007; Marijuana smokers, 2008; Pagliaro & Pagliaro, 2009).[43]

For example, regarding effects on airway obstruction, Aldington, Williams, and Nowitz (2007)—utilizing high-resolution computed tomography (HRCT) scanning, pulmonary function tests, and a smoking questionnaire—found that "one cannabis joint had a similar effect to 2.5–5 tobacco cigarettes" (p. 1058). Although replication studies and confirmatory data are currently lacking, we have long warned of the risk of cannabis smoking as a carcinogen or co-carcinogen contributing to lung cancer in genetically susceptible women. Joshi, Joshi, and Bartter (2014), in their review of the effects of marijuana smoke on the respiratory system, noted that:

> The immuno-histopathologic and epidemiologic evidence in marijuana users suggest biological plausibility of marijuana smoking as a risk for the development of lung cancer.
>
> *(p. 173)*

---

[43] Over 400 chemicals—primarily a result of pyrolysis—can be found in marijuana smoke, including many of the same chemicals that are found in tobacco smoke. When marijuana is smoked, it yields *more* tar than tobacco. In addition, the tar from marijuana smoke has *higher* concentrations of certain carcinogens (e.g., benzo(a)pyrene) than are found in the tar from tobacco smoke. Thus, it is probable that marijuana smoking will produce *more* lung cancer when compared to tobacco smoking, which currently is the leading cause of lung cancer. Based upon the chemical constituents found in the pyrolysis products of marijuana smoke versus the pyrolysis products of tobacco smoke, and comparative differences in smoking techniques for marijuana versus tobacco (i.e., smoking the entire joint and inhaling the marijuana smoke *more* deeply into the lungs where it is held in the lower respiratory tract for a longer period of time), we have, for several decades (e.g., Pagliaro, 1983; Pagliaro & Pagliaro, 1996 2004, 2009) estimated that smoking one joint of marijuana exposes smokers to as much irritation and associated damage to the respiratory system, along with subsequent risk for lung cancer, as smoking one package (i.e., 20) filter-tipped tobacco cigarettes.

Tashkin (2013), as well as other researchers, suggested that the association between cannabis smoking and lung cancer is only evident with "heavy, long term use," not with light or moderate use (p. 239).

In addition, the respiratory toxicity associated with smoking cannabis can, on occasion, be due to a contaminant, or additive, to the cannabis. For example, Gilbert, Baram, and Cavarocchi (2013) reported two cases of "respiratory failure soon after they had smoked 'wet' marijuana cigarettes" (p. 64). "Wet" marijuana cigarettes, or joints, are typically dipped, prior to smoking, in either *formaldehyde*, known on the street as "embalming fluid," or *phencyclidine* (PCP). (Also, see later discussion in this chapter, *Phencyclidine (PCP)*.)

Physical and Psychological Dependence. The question as to whether the regular, long-term use of cannabis results in physical dependence has been extensively argued over the last century. The new millennial consensus is that it does.[44] The regular, long-term, *high* dosage use of cannabis is clearly recognized as being associated with the development of physical dependence (Khalsa, Genser, & Francis, 2002; Maldonado & Rodriguez de Fonseca, 2002). In the U.S., the increase in the average potency of cannabis since the 1960s (as noted in earlier sections), has been tremendous (i.e., a five to tenfold increase in THC concentration) and appears to have significantly *increased* the probability for developing physical dependence, reflected in the *cannabis use disorder*, or, more likely, the recognition of the clinical significance of the *cannabis withdrawal syndrome*.

CANNABIS USE DISORDER. Women, who develop cannabis use disorder, generally are women who have experienced *higher* rates of anxiety disorders, including panic attacks, than other women and *significantly* higher rates than men, who develop *cannabis use disorder* (Buckner, Heimberg, & Schneier, 2012; Pagliaro & Pagliaro, *Clinical Patient Data Files*). In addition, for women of African continental descent and those of Puerto Rican descent, initiating marijuana use at an early age and long-term use of marijuana were associated with anger, depression, and other mental disturbances (Pahl, Brook, & Koppel, 2011).

For women, the length of time from *initiation* of cannabis use to the development of physical or psychological dependence (i.e., tolerance, craving, and withdrawal syndrome), or CUD—as well as time to entrance into treatment—is generally significantly *shorter* than that for men (Ehlers, Gizer, & Vieten, 2010; Hernandez-Avila, Rounsaville, & Kranzler, 2004; Khan, Secades-Villa, & Okuda,

[44] For example, since its 4th edition in 1994, the *Diagnostic and Statistical Manual of Mental Disorders* (DSM) (American Psychiatric Association, 2000) has listed cannabis dependence in its taxonomy based largely upon noted tolerance and a well-recognized withdrawal syndrome. However, until the last decade of the 20th century, it was generally thought that only psychological dependence, *not* physical dependence, was likely to develop with the regular, long-term use of cannabis. Currently, the DSM-5 subsumes these related conditions under the rubric of *cannabis use disorder (CUD)*—the continued use of cannabis regardless of significant impairment that can range from mild to severe.

2013). This phenomenon is referred to as *telescoping*. Women of African continental descent, particularly those whose marijuana use *preceded* their alcohol use, are significantly more likely to experience *telescoping* than are women of European continental descent (Sartor, Agrawal, & Lynskey, 2013).[45]

CANNABIS WITHDRAWAL SYNDROME. Following the abrupt discontinuation of regular, long-term cannabis use, women commonly experience the cannabis withdrawal syndrome. The occurrence of the cannabis withdrawal syndrome is supported by *two* major pieces of evidence: (1) pharmacological characterization of the endocannabinoid system (see earlier discussion in the *Mechanism of Action* section); and (2) acute demonstration of characteristic signs and symptoms when the CB1 cannabinoid receptor *antagonist* is administered to an active cannabis user as part of a controlled research study (e.g., Budney & Hughes, 2006; Cooper & Haney, 2009).

These signs and symptoms, which are dependent on dose and duration of use, include: aggression; anger, *increased*; anorexia; anxiety; cramping; craving for cannabis; increased dreaming, often strange or *wild*; insomnia; irritability; mental depression; nausea; nervousness; nightmares; restlessness; rebound increase in rapid eye movement (REM) sleep; shakiness; sweating; violent outbursts; and weight loss (Cornelius, Chung, & Martin, 2008). Chills, hypersomnia, hyperthermia, tremor, and weakness also may occur. The onset of withdrawal is generally within 2 to 4 days of ceasing cannabis use. The signs and symptoms generally peak within 1 week and can persist for up to 30 days (Pagliaro & Pagliaro, 2009; Preuss, Watzke, & Zimmermann, 2010).

The overwhelming majority of women who experience cannabis withdrawal report the characteristic signs and symptoms of this syndrome, but also report a *wide* variance in the *severity* of these signs and symptoms. Both the risk for CUD and this variance appear to be associated with several factors, including: (1) amount and potency of the cannabis used; (2) duration of regular, long-term use; (3) genetic predisposition; (4) history of childhood physical or sexual abuse (Sartor, Agrawal, & Grant, 2015; Sartor, Waldron, & Duncan, 2013; Simpson & Miller, 2002); (5) concurrent use of other drugs and substances of abuse; and (6) major depressive or psychotic disorder—the factor that appears to account for *most* of the observed variance (e.g., Arendt, Rosenburg, & Foldager, 2007; Khan, Secades-Villa, & Okuda, 2013; Preuss, Watzke, & Zimmermann, 2010).

Interestingly, Herrmann, Weerts, and Vandrey (2015), in their study of treatment-seeking cannabis users, who were primarily of African descent, found that:

> Women had higher overall scores than men [on the Marijuana Withdrawal Checklist] and women had higher scores than men on 6 individual symptoms

[45] Telescoping also has been noted among women regarding the use of other drugs and substances of abuse, such as alcohol. (For further discussion, see "telescoping" in the *Index* for a comprehensive list of page citations.)

in 2 domains, mood symptoms (i.e., irritability, restlessness, increased anger, violent outbursts), and gastrointestinal symptoms (i.e., nausea, stomach pain). (p. 415).

Pregnancy, Lactation, and Mothering. Although THC crosses the placenta, studies of *infrequent* or *moderate* use during pregnancy have *not* been significantly associated with teratogenic effects. However, some studies and reports (e.g., Bryant, 2015; Fried & Smith, 2001; Richardson, Ryan, & Willford, 2002) suggest that *higher* order cognitive functioning among children, such as attentional processes and analysis/hypothesis testing, is *negatively* correlated with in utero exposure to cannabis. We also note concerns regarding possible long-term negative effects of in utero exposure upon subsequent memory processes (e.g., encoding and retrieval mechanisms) (Pagliaro & Pagliaro, 2009). Also, THC is excreted into breast milk and expected effects (e.g., drowsiness) can be observed among breast-fed neonates and infants.

In addition, because the endocannabinoid system appears to be involved in brain development—cell proliferation and differentiation—several authors (e.g., Cannabis damages, 2009; Crane, Schuster, & Gonzalez, 2013; Long-term cannabis, 2008; Schneider, 2008; Trezza, Cuomo, & Vanderschuren, 2008) have expressed concerns that there is a significant risk for cannabis toxicity during periods of high neuronal plasticity (e.g., prenatal period, late adolescence, and early adulthood) and, consequently, associated toxicities on executive functioning, including problem solving and other higher cognitive functions. We, too, share this concern.

Thus, it is a further cause for concern that *cannabis* use has become the primary reason for seeking inpatient treatment for SUDs among pregnant adolescent girls and young women. In 2007, 45.9% of the admissions of pregnant adolescent girls and young women for inpatient treatment across the U.S., were primarily related to cannabis use (SAMHSA, 2014). This statistic reflects a significant change from the statistics reported in 1992 when admission for pregnant adolescents and young women for treatment of SUDs were primarily related to alcohol abuse—with marijuana use accounting for only 19.3% of other admissions at that time.

Another noted change among millennial pregnant women in the U.S. is the finding that they are more likely to usually use two or more drugs simultaneously when pregnant. Buchi, Suarez, and Varner (2013), in their analysis of data obtained from women in labor and delivery units across Utah, found that the most frequent detected psychotropic drugs were:

- Alcohol
- Cocaine
- Marijuana

- Methamphetamine
- Opiate analgesics

These findings appear to be generally consistent among pregnant women across the U.S. However, regional differences—primarily due to age, drug availability, and sociocultural/ethnic factors, as well as, continental descent—affect the drugs and substances used by pregnant women.

In response to the *increasing* use of cannabis by women during pregnancy, particularly at a time of growing social acceptance of its use, Gunn, Rosales, and Center (2016) sought to assess maternal and fetal outcomes regarding the effects of cannabis use during pregnancy. Retrospective meta-analysis of 24 studies from 7 electronic databases was conducted. Major findings included significantly increased odds ratio of: (1) anemia among women who used cannabis during pregnancy; (2) decreased birth weight among neonates exposed to cannabis in utero; and (3) increased need for placement of neonates, who were born to mothers who used cannabis during pregnancy, in neonatal intensive care units (NICUs).

The increased use of cannabis by women in the U.S., who are pregnant, also has brought attention to undesired, or harmful, effects and toxicities that were generally considered rare in this population group. For example, Alaniz, Liss, and Metz (2015) identified the cannabinoid hyperemesis syndrome in this clinical context (also see earlier related discussion):

> We report a case of a pregnant 28-year-old woman with multiple admissions for episodic nausea and vomiting resulting in Malory-Weiss esophageal tears, dehydration, and abdominal pain who was noted to be showering compulsively during her hospitalizations. After an extensive workup for the etiology of her intractable nausea and pain, she was diagnosed with cannabinoid hyperemesis syndrome.
>
> *(p. 1484)*

Adolescent girls and young women should *not* smoke or otherwise use cannabis because of the potential risks to their offspring (Pagliaro, 1995; Pagliaro & Pagliaro, 2002). In addition to the concerns already stipulated, the National Institutes of Health (NIH) reported that the risk for stillbirth increases up to 2.3-fold in association with maternal marijuana use (Hill & Reed, 2013; Metz & Stickrath, 2015).

Cannabis use by young mothers of infants and young children may also negatively affect their parenting (Pagliaro & Pagliaro, *Clinical Patient Data Files*). It also has been associated with a *higher* incidence of marijuana use by offspring later in their life. For these reasons, several professional organizations (e.g., The American Congress of Obstetricians and Gynecologists [ACOG]) have made formal recommendations that the use of marijuana be totally avoided among all pregnant and breast-feeding women (ACOG, 2015a, 2015b).

Overdosage

Surprisingly, given the 10,000-plus years of cannabis use among the earliest human populations (Pagliaro & Pagliaro, 2004, 2009), the toxicities associated with its use have not yet been fully evaluated (Pope Jr., Gruber, & Hudson, 2001). However, it appears that fatal overdosages are relatively rare. In fact, during the last two centuries, the general medical consensus has been that the occasional use of cannabis is *not* particularly harmful and that the intermittent use of *low potency* cannabis is *not* generally associated with obvious signs and symptoms of toxicity (ARF/WHO, 1981).

In support of the relative "safety" of cannabis use is the observation that its use among middle-aged *men* was associated with a *reduction* in suicides—in comparison to states in which cannabis use was not legalized (Anderson, Rees, & Sabia, 2014).[46]

Women's Medical and Personal Cannabis Use and Abuse

During the new millennium, there have been several changes in both the medical and personal use and abuse of cannabis among women in the U.S.

Women's Medical Cannabis Use/Abuse

Cannabis, in the form of its chemical surrogate, THC, or dronabinol (Marinol®), is approved by the FDA for the medical management of:

1. Anorexia with weight loss in patients with AIDS
2. Mild to moderate nausea and vomiting associated with cancer chemotherapy

In addition, most states have individually legalized (contrary to U.S. federal law) the medicinal use of cannabis in a variety of formulations for the treatment of a wide variety of physical and mental conditions. For example, these conditions, as approved by the state of California,[47] include:

---

[46] It has been postulated that middle-aged men now have an additional method (i.e., marijuana use) to cope with "life's pains, disappointments, and impossible tasks" (Andersson, Rees, & Sabia, 2014). However, a later comprehensive review of over 600,000 suicide deaths documented in the *National Vital Statistics System Multiple Cause of Death* files, found "no statistically significant association between medical marijuana policy and suicide risk" (Grucza, Hur, & Agrawal, 2015, p. 68).

[47] Lists of eligible conditions can vary from state to state depending upon the specific wording of the related legislation.

- Acquired immune deficiency syndrome (AIDS)
- Anorexia
- Arthritis
- Cachexia
- Cancer pain
- Chronic pain
- Glaucoma
- Migraine headaches
- Nausea (severe)
- Persistent muscle spasms (e.g., as related to multiple sclerosis)
- Seizures (e.g., epilepsy)
- Any other chronic or persistent medical sign or symptom that either: (1) limits the ability to conduct a major life activity as defined in the *Americans With Disabilities Act* of 1990, Public Law 101–3336; or (2) if *not* alleviated, "may cause serious harm to the patient's safety or physical or mental health" (e.g., medical marijuana has been prescribed for children and adolescents for the treatment of attention-deficit/hyperactivity disorder (A-D/HD).

In states that have formally approved the medical use of marijuana—through the enactment of related legislation—women who have a medical prescription, as well as men, can legally purchase, possess, and use varying prescribed amounts of marijuana. Marijuana also can be "home-grown" for personal use.[48] However, it is more commonly purchased from specialized marijuana dispensaries.

Women's Personal Cannabis Use/Abuse

During the new millennium, women's personal use and abuse of marijuana is increasingly guided by related changing trends in public attitudes toward marijuana use. For example, as noted by Motel (2015, pp. 1–3), these trends include:

- Support for marijuana legalization—which is rapidly and significantly outpacing opposition[49]
- 68% of women say marijuana should be legalized in the U.S.
- 70% of Americans say alcohol is *more* harmful to a person's health than marijuana

---

[48] In addition, several states (i.e., Alaska, California, Colorado, Massachusetts, Nevada, Oregon, and Washington) have *legalized* the non-medical recreational/social use of marijuana (Levin, 2016; Miller, 2016).

[49] For example, most adults in the U.S. (i.e., 53%) *favor* marijuana legalization—with 44% opposed. In addition, it has been noted that most adults of African or European continental descent support the legalization of marijuana use in the U.S. (Motel, 2015).

- 57% of Americans would *not* be bothered if a store or business selling legal marijuana opened up in their neighborhood
- Half of Americans say they have tried marijuana
- Several states, and the District of Columbia, have *legalized* recreational/social marijuana use

In addition, as noted by Azofeifa, Mattson, and Schauer (2016)—and previously discussed earlier in this chapter:

> A decrease in the perception of great risk from smoking marijuana combined with increases in the perception of availability (i.e., fairly easy or very easy to obtain marijuana) and fewer punitive legal penalties (e.g., no penalty) for the possession of marijuana for personal use might play a role in increased use among adults.
>
> *(p. 1)*

In the U.S., fewer women than men (i.e., 4 million versus 5 million, respectively) report past-year use of marijuana (NIDA, 2016; SAMHSA, 2014). However, the numbers for both appear to be significantly and rapidly increasing. For example, according to a 2016 Gallup poll of over 1,000 adults in all 50 states and the District of Columbia:

> The percentage of American adults who say they currently smoke marijuana has nearly doubled since 2013. Thirteen percent of adults in the U.S. now say they currently smoke pot—up from 7 percent in 2013.
>
> *(Miller, 2016, p. 3)*

As noted earlier in this chapter, valid and reliable national statistics for marijuana use among women are unavailable. However, some interesting associated findings have been reported. For example, De Genna, Cornelius, and Goldschmidt (2015) examined the generally held tenet that becoming a mother is a point of developmental transition that is generally associated with "desistance from substance use." Specifically, regarding cannabis use, they conducted a prospective study of 456 pregnant adolescent girls and women, 13 to 42 years-of-age, who were recruited from a prenatal clinic and interviewed about their cannabis use 1 year prior to their pregnancy; during each trimester of pregnancy; and at 6, 10, 14, and 16 years following their pregnancy. The researchers found that the mothers in their study, who became pregnant at a younger age, were significantly *more* likely to: (1) endorse cannabis use; (2) use cannabis while pregnant; and (3) continue to regularly use cannabis over the subsequent 17 years' post-partum.

Women who use marijuana, generally employ two common methods of use: (1) oral ingestion; and (2) pulmonary inhalation (i.e., smoking; vaporizing). The more recent legalization of medicinal marijuana in many states has resulted in the development of a wide variety of edible marijuana products (e.g., brownies;

butters; cakes; caramels; chocolates; granola bars; and lollipops).[50] These edible products can be purchased at marijuana dispensaries as an alternative to smoking or vaporizing the extensive varieties of marijuana buds and leaves that also are legally sold in these dispensaries.

However, because the bioavailability of ingested marijuana products is approximately 10%, the dosage of marijuana required must be approximately *5* times *higher* than the dosage that is inhaled in order to achieve equivalent actions.[51] This difference in dosage is required because pulmonary absorption from the lungs is much greater than that from the GI tract. Thus, smoking, or *toking*, is the *most* common method of use for all three forms of cannabis. In addition to rolling the cannabis into a cigarette paper to form a *reefer*, or *joint*, to smoke (i.e., *toke*), cannabis users also may use a traditional conical pipe, small-bowled pipe, or water pipe—also referred to as a *bong*, *chillum*, *galyan*, *goza*, *hookah*, *narghile*, or *shisha*—to inhale the cannabis smoke with minimal generation and exhalation of sidestream smoke (Chaouachi, 2009).[52]

Hookahs. Hookahs have become increasingly popular among new millennial women, especially young women. (Also, see Chapter 4, *Women's Caffeine and Nicotine Abuse*, for related discussion.) Favorable attitudes regarding hookah use have been reported in up to 90% of research participants (Krauss, Sowles, & Moreno, 2015). Approximately 15% to 20% of high school senior girls in the U.S. and 20% to 40% of U.S. college/university students have reported hookah use during the past year (CDC, 2015a). The reported rates of hookah use among young women and men are approximately equal. Factors that tend to support *high* levels of hookah use include: (1) social acceptability; (2) having friends and family members who smoke; and (3) believing that hookah smoking is *less* harmful than cigarette smoking (Morris, Fiala, & Pawlak, 2012).

---

50 During the 19th century, cannabis also was orally ingested as candy bonbons or baked into foods, such as cookies and brownies, and eaten. The oral method of use continued through the 1950s, 1960s, and 1970s by women who often used a classic hashish fudge recipe which was offered by Alice B. Toklas (1954).

51 Although hashish oil may be injected, this method of use is relatively rare because of the associated severe pain and inflammation that occurs at the injection site secondarily to the injection of an oil. This pain and inflammation also are the reasons why, whenever possible, most injectable drugs are prepared as aqueous solutions or suspensions. Therefore, like other types of cannabis, it is more often ingested or inhaled by smoking or vaporizing.

52 A more recent method used by new millennial women, particularly younger women, is referred to as "dabbing." Dabbing involves passing butane gas over dried marijuana to make a gummy resin of THC and its related cannabinoids (often referred to as *butane hash oil*, or *BHO*, because of the method of production). The "dabs," which also are referred to as "budder" or "earwax," can typically have a THC concentration as *high* as 60% to 80%. The "dabs" are then pressed through a filter and used in bongs, water pipes, or vaporizers (including e-cigarettes and e-hookahs). The major concerns with this method of use—in addition to the much *higher* concentrations of THC than are generally achieved with other methods of use—is the danger of explosions and fires associated with "dabbing" (Pagliaro & Pagliaro, *Clinical Patient Data Files*).

Women are increasingly recognizing that, when they inhale cannabis smoke deeply into their lungs to enhance THC absorption and resultant *high* blood THC concentrations, along with the THC, they also are inhaling other chemicals and constituents—including carcinogens (see following section).

However, hookah smoking also is associated with several other undesired effects and toxicities. For example, in addition to potential for physical and psychological dependence associated with the drugs and substances that may be smoked (e.g., cannabis; tobacco), the charcoal used to heat the cannabis or tobacco can produce, when heated, *high* levels of carbon monoxide, heavy metals, and cancer-causing chemicals. In addition, when women share the same mouthpiece with others as they pass the mouthpiece from one to another during smoking sessions, they can spread communicable diseases: including: bronchitis; oral herpes, syphilis, or gonorrhea; and tuberculosis (American Lung Association, 2016, p. 1; CDC, 2015a, 2015b; Pagliaro & Pagliaro, *Clinical Patient Data Files*). Thus, young women are increasingly turning to the use of an electronic hookah, or *e-hookah*, a relatively new product available for vaporizing cannabis that is similar to the e-cigarette (see related discussion in Chapter 4, *Women's Caffeine and Nicotine Abuse*).

E-hookahs. Vaporizing cannabis involves using a commercial vaporizer (e.g., Syge® inhaler device; Volcano® forced-air vaporizer) to heat the cannabis and evaporate the THC into a gas that, when inhaled, delivers up to 95% of the evaporated THC with significantly less carbon monoxide and other toxins (e.g., tars found in cannabis smoke). In addition, the required temperature is significantly *lower* than that needed for smoking and, thus, the cannabis is *not* burned, diminishing the production of associated carcinogens and, consequently, related cancer risk.

Thus, the noted benefits of e-hookah use, according to many women, include:

- Being smaller in size than the traditional hookah, the e-hookah can be more conveniently carried from place to place
- Using a battery as a heat source rather than burning charcoal, the e-hookah produces cleaner and less toxic smoke than the traditional hookah
- Restricted by fewer laws and regulations, the e-hookah can be *more* widely used, both publicly and privately

Phencyclidine (PCP)

Phencyclidine (PCP),[53] known as *Angel Dust*, *Fry*, *Hog*, *PeaCe Pill*, *Rocket Fuel*, and many other street names, was originally synthesized in 1958 for use as a surgical dissociative anesthetic (i.e., Sernyl®). Since that time, *lower* doses of PCP have been abused by women to: (1) achieve a *buzz*, or an alcohol-like disinhibitory euphoria

[53] The common abbreviation for phencyclidine, "PCP," is derived from its chemical name: 1-(1-**p**henyl**c**yclohexyl) **p**iperidine.

and elevated mood; (2) promote relaxation; (3) relieve pain; and (4) reduce sexual inhibitions. Women also abuse PCP to achieve such *psychodelic* effects as:

- Feelings of unreality
- Distortions in the perception of time, space, and body image (i.e., hallucinations and illusions)

Pharmacology

This section provides a brief overview of the proposed mechanism of action of PCP and its absorption, distribution, metabolism, and excretion. It also presents and discusses the undesired, or harmful, effects and relatively *serious* toxicities associated with the use of PCP, including: (1) aggressive and violent behavior, or *bad trips*; (2) PCP psychosis; and (3) the *less* commonly occurring delusional and mood disorders. The signs and symptoms of physical and psychological dependence, PCP overdosage, and the *indirect* causes of associated PCP fatalities also are presented.[54]

Pharmacodynamics: Mechanism of Action

The exact mechanism by which PCP exerts its psychodelic actions has *not* been determined. However, *noncompetitive* antagonism of the N-Methyl-D-aspartate (NMDA) receptor channel complexes, located in the cortex and limbic regions of the brain, has been postulated as a primary contributory mechanism. The antagonism is thought to block the action of the excitatory amino acids, aspartate and glutamate (Morris, Cochran, & Pratt, 2005). PCP also inhibits GABA and increases dopamine concentrations by both: (1) increasing the synthesis of dopamine; and (2) inhibiting its presynaptic reuptake. In addition, PCP possesses significant anticholinergic activity. The acute effects of PCP begin within 5 minutes after pulmonary inhalation, or within 1 hour after oral ingestion, and can last for up to 24 hours.

Pharmacokinetics: Absorption, Distribution, Metabolism, and Excretion

PCP is well-absorbed from all routes of administration. However, 50% of the PCP, which is smoked, such as that used to "dip" tobacco cigarettes or marijuana joints for an extra "buzz," is degraded, or lost, because of the heat and pyrolysis associated with smoking. When smoked, the onset of action is generally within 5 minutes.

[54] As a result of the difficulties with the "street synthesis" of PCP (i.e., ranging from lack of availability of needed precursor chemicals to lack of needed laboratory facilities and "cooks," who are familiar with associated recipes and production techniques), street samples are often contaminated with precursors and byproducts—each of which *increases* the toxicity of the PCP product in unique and often unexpected and harmful ways (e.g., unintentional production of *PCC*, a PCP precursor that releases cyanide).

However, the onset of action when ingested or intranasally insufflated (i.e., *sniffed*; *snorted*) can be *delayed* for up to 30 minutes. PCP is extensively metabolized to inactive metabolites in the liver primarily by the hepatic microsomal isoenzyme P450-3A. Approximately 5% to 20% of PCP is excreted in unchanged form in the urine. The half-life of elimination is approximately 17 hours (West, Helman, & McKeown, 2015).

PCP is commonly included in urine drug screening tests. For example, those requested when a woman is admitted to an emergency department (ED) in an unconscious, or unresponsive state. These tests generally involve an immunoassay (e.g., Siemens Syva EMIT II Immunoassay®) that are subject to false-positive results. False-positive results for PCP can result from the use of tramadol (Ultram®) or dextromethorphan (Benylin DM®) a synthetic opiate derivative antitussive (Ly, Thornton, & Buono, 2012; Rengarajan & Mullins, 2013).

Undesired, or Harmful, Effects and Toxicities

Almost 3 decades ago, Carroll (1990) summarized published retrospective studies that examined the effects of PCP and identified two different categories of *dose-related* effects: (1) *subjective effects* that appear to vary dramatically in relation to personality type, or predisposition, of the user; and (2) *secondary effects* that appear to vary dramatically during *different* episodes of PCP use by the *same* user. The use of *lower* dosages of PCP, was associated with cognitive impairment in most cases in addition to desired effects. The use of *higher* dosages was associated with a *wasted psychological state*, characterized by: anxiety; confusion; disordered thinking; disorientation; fear of death; incoordination; illusions; irritability; obsession with trivial matters; panic; paranoia; and restlessness.

Surveys of PCP users have generally found that the desired effects of PCP are experienced only about half of the time, while undesired, or harmful, effects are experienced during the other half of the time.[55] As described by Domino[56] and Luby (2012):

> It was astounding to us that phencyclidine became a major street drug of abuse … Few of our volunteer subjects were ever willing to take the drug a second time. One former resident still recalls her PCP experience as intensely psychologically painful.
>
> *(p. 916)*

---

[55] This response may be, at least in part, due to drug interactions. As noted by West, Helman, and McKeown (2015):

> Of PCP-related ED visits in 2011, 72% involved PCP combined with other drugs.
>
> *(p. 1)*

[56] One of the original PCP human-study researchers.

As reported by many regular, long-term PCP users, in addition to their *desired* effects, it is this *unpredictable* action of PCP that also makes it—seemingly *contrary* to common sense—*attractive* to use (Pagliaro & Pagliaro, *Clinical Patient Data Files*). It also has been suggested that women, as well as men, who experience a *positive* subjective experience are more likely to develop a pattern of regular, long-term use than those who initially experience *dysphoria*, or other undesired effects.

Several common toxicities associated with PCP use also appear to be dose-related. *Lower* dosages of PCP are generally associated with: amnesia; ataxia; decreased sensitivity to pain; dry mouth; edema; impaired judgment; muscle rigidity; polydipsia with polyuria; rapid mood swings; and speech disturbances. *Higher* dosages are generally associated with: abnormal breathing; a facial expression characterized by a *blank stare*; bradycardia; coma; compulsive and repetitive movements; convulsions; hallucinations; hypotension; incoherent speech; and vomiting. Both *lower* and *higher* dosages of PCP have been associated with: aggressive and violent behavior; agitation; amnesia; belligerence; flashbacks; nystagmus, both vertical and horizontal; paranoia; and PCP psychosis (Peters, Kelder, & Meshack, 2005; Pagliaro & Pagliaro, 2009). Several of these undesired effects and toxicities are presented and briefly discussed in the following sections, specifically *amnesia*, *aggressive and violent behavior*, *bad trips*, *delusional and mood disorders*, and *PCP psychosis*—all of which can be quite serious.

Amnesia. Once PCP is ingested or smoked, amnesia can begin and last until effects begin to wear off.[57] During this time, users may behave uncharacteristically in ways that, while not generally harmful, may be later identified as being bizarre (e.g., removing their clothing and running around naked). At the other extreme, they may perform brutal and violent acts that may be fatal. Usually, the user *blacks out* and, later, has *no* conscious memory of the event that occurred during the violent episode (Pagliaro & Pagliaro, 2009). Although embarrassing acts or even injurious fatal attacks may occur while *high* on PCP, its amnestic effects probably contribute to continued use (i.e., the potentially aversive behaviors are *not* remembered by the user and, thus, do not serve as a deterrent to future use). In addition, the PCP-induced memory impairment has resulted in the use of the amnesia defense in some criminal trials to establish diminished capacity (e.g., Berman & Coccaro, 1998; Pagliaro & Pagliaro, *Clinical Patient Data Files*). (Also, see following section, "Aggressive and Violent Behavior.")

Aggressive and Violent Behavior. One of the most troublesome toxicities associated with the regular, long-term use of PCP is its tendency to precipitate, or aggravate, aggressive and violent behavior—behavior that is often bizarre, sudden, and unexpected. Three contexts of aggressive and violent behavior have been

[57] This anterograde amnesia is similar to that associated with the use of alcohol or the benzodiazepine group of sedative-hypnotics (see related discussion in Chapter 3, *Women's Prescription Sedative-Hypnotic Abuse*).

observed: (1) toxic organic brain disorders (i.e., psychosis); (2) primitive sadistic criminal behaviors (e.g., brutal murders; extreme self-mutilation); and (3) *bad trips* (see following section). The use of PCP also has been associated with Intimate Partner Violence (IPV) (e.g., Crane, Easton, & Devine, 2013). (Also, see *Intimate Partner Violence* section in Chapter 5, *Women's Amphetamine and Cocaine Abuse*.)[58]

While the disinhibition caused by PCP may explain uncharacteristic behavior, the *aggressive* and *violent* behavior associated with PCP use is most likely related to underlying, or latent, psychological characteristics of the user (e.g., anger; depression; fear; hostility). The *superhuman* strength that has been observed among PCP users during these episodes is probably due to the analgesic and dissociative *anesthetic* effects of PCP. By decreasing or eliminating the pain, users can perform aggressive and violent acts with, what appears to be *superhuman* strength that they would otherwise *not* be able to perform because of the associated injuries to body tissues and resultant pain. As such, PCP users do *not* become superhuman, they only *think* or *feel* that they are.[59]

Bad Trips. The bad trips associated with PCP use occur suddenly and unexpectedly among users and are characterized by sudden and severe acts of violence against themselves and others. Generally, users who experience a bad trip have previously used PCP with the achievement of expected desirable effects (e.g., alcohol-like euphoria). For these reasons, it has been suggested that the bad trips may be due to the contamination of street supplies of PCP with formaldehyde or other impurities that could cause these effects (Marceaux, Dilks, & Hixson, 2008).

Delusional and Mood Disorders. PCP-induced delusional disorder may emerge up to a week following a PCP overdosage and is characterized by: (1) mild cognitive impairment; (2) ritualistic stereotypic behavior; (3) dysphoria; (4) rambling, garbled, and incoherent speech; and (5) a disheveled or an eccentric appearance. The mood disorder may present within 1 or 2 weeks following PCP use and is characterized by a prominent and persistently depressed, elevated, or expansive mood

---

58 Although data are limited, they suggest that PCP use might be a risk factor for IPV. For example, in their related study, Crane, Easton, and Devine (2013) found that:

> The association between PCP use and violence may extend into IPV as partner violence was *more* common among PCP users than cannabis or combined cannabis and problematic alcohol users in the current sample.
>
> *(p. 8)*

59 The unpredictable toxicities associated with PCP have contributed to its street folk lore and to its *increased* popularity of use among certain groups of users. For example, adolescent boys and young men of Hispanic descent, particularly those who are involved in criminal youth gangs (Pagliaro & Pagliaro, *Clinical Patient Data Files*), are attracted to PCP and other drugs and substances of abuse that have unpredictable, and possibly horrific, consequences associated with their use (i.e., their willingness to use such a dangerous drug is evidence that they are "macho").

with feelings of anxiety, irritability, somatization, panic attacks, hallucinations, and delusions. Although these two mental disorders are relatively uncommon, they may be long-lasting and have been associated with suicide attempts.

PCP Psychosis. Although available data do *not* provide strong evidence implicating the regular, long-term use of PCP with major body organ (e.g., cardiac; hepatic; renal) or cellular damage, they do provide evidence for the occurrence of several toxicities, including a PCP psychosis—a psychosis that is similar in many regards to amphetamine-induced psychosis (Murray, 2002). PCP psychosis can occur after a single use of PCP—whether not the user has a prior positive history of mental illness. However, it is more likely to occur among users who have previously used PCP or who have a genetic predisposition, or family history, of schizophrenia. The psychosis may last for several days or months, even with appropriate medical management (e.g., antipsychotic pharmacotherapy, such as haloperidol, Haldol®). It also may spontaneously recur with subsequent PCP use, even when lower dosages of PCP are used.

PCP is pharmacologically recognized as a *psychotomimetic.* In this regard, it has been used to study psychosis, particularly that associated with catatonic or negative features (Pagliaro & Pagliaro, 2009). Common signs and symptoms that occur to a moderate to high degree among *both* PCP users and patients with schizophrenia, include: affect disorder; ambivalence; attention disorder; autistic dreamy states; concreteness; depersonalization; loosening of associations; and over-inclusive thoughts (Domino & Luby, 2012, p. 917).

Physical and Psychological Dependence. In response to the epidemic use of PCP reported during the late 1960s and 1970s, a considerable amount of research was undertaken in an effort to identify its abuse potential and addiction liability. The general results of this research were that: (1) PCP is *not* associated with the development of physical dependence; (2) PCP use is *not* associated with a *definite* physical withdrawal syndrome in relation to the abrupt discontinuation of regular, long-term use, although tolerance, the need to increase the amount of PCP used in order to achieve *initial* desired pharmacologic actions, appears to occur; (3) the development of cross-tolerance between PCP and other drugs and substances of abuse has *not* been reported; and (4) PCP is associated with various degrees of psychological dependence, the development of which is characterized by varying degrees of mental depression, lack of energy, and physical distress upon abrupt discontinuation of PCP use.

Pregnancy and Lactation. The maternal use of PCP during pregnancy has been implicated with birth defects, including neonatal dysmorphogenesis, characterized by distorted facial features, low birth weight, and small head circumference. However, this reported teratogenic effect is *poorly* documented and has been deemed to be generally clinically *insignificant* (i.e., if it does occur, then it is *extremely* rare). The long-term effects of prenatal PCP exposure on the later development of infants and children, including effects on learning, have been raised, but remain inconclusive (Pagliaro & Pagliaro, 1996, 2009, 2012).

Overdosage

The signs and symptoms of PCP overdosage, which may be fatal, include: agitation; ataxia; coma; hyperthermia; nystagmus; psychosis; rhabdomyolysis; and seizures. Similar to LSD overdosage, the associated fatalities are often *indirectly* caused and are related to accidental injuries, drownings, and physical trauma. Overdosage fatalities also may involve homicides and suicides. Most PCP overdosage victims, who present to the emergency department, only require medical observation and supportive care (D'Onofrio, McCausland, & Tarabar, 2006). There is no known antidote. If necessary, benzodiazepine (e.g., diazepam, Valium®) pharmacotherapy may be used to manage associated anxiety and fear. An antipsychotic *without* high anticholinergic actions (e.g., haloperidol, Haldol®, or risperidone, Risperdal®) may be of benefit for the management of the behavioral toxicities associated with PCP overdosage (MacNeal, Cone, & Sinha, 2012; Pagliaro & Pagliaro, 2009).

As noted by Bey and Patel (2007):

> Non-traumatic causes of death [among PCP users] include cardiopulmonary arrest, intracranial hemorrhage, hypertension, and hyperkalemia secondary to rhabdomyolysis. [However,] most deaths among PCP-intoxicated patients are the result of *self-inflicted* violent behavior (e.g., jumping from buildings; walking into traffic) associated with PCP use.
>
> *(p. 11)*

Women's Medical and Personal PCP Use and Abuse

Women's Medical PCP Use/Abuse

PCP was developed for use in veterinary medicine as an animal tranquilizer. It also was used, subsequently, as an anesthetic for people who were undergoing various surgical procedures. When a *low to moderate* dose of PCP (Sernylan®) was intravenously administered according to recommended dosing schedules, it was physically well-tolerated during surgery and produced few undesired physical effects (e.g., excessive changes in blood pressure; depth and rate of respirations; or heart rate) during surgery. However, during the immediate recovery period following surgery, several troublesome psychological effects were observed among patients, including agitation, hallucinations, and violent behavior. Thus, PCP was withdrawn from medical use and was replaced with a derivative—the dissociative anesthetic, *ketamine*.[60]

---

[60] Ketamine (Ketalar®) is similar to PCP. It is a dissociative anesthetic that minimally suppresses breathing. It has a relatively rapid onset of action (i.e., less than 5 minutes by IM or IV injection and

Women's Personal PCP Use/Abuse

PCP had already gained popularity among many groups of users (e.g., members of organized motorcycle gangs, or *OMGs*) and, when no longer able to obtain legal pharmaceutical grade PCP for their use, these groups of users soon found that PCP could be illegally produced and sold on the street in various forms for intravenous injection, intranasal insufflation, oral ingestion, or pulmonary inhalation (e.g., smoking a *Sherman*).[61]

The Hell's Angels OMG was extremely successful in producing tremendous profits in relation to the production, distribution, and sale of PCP across the U.S. during the early 1970s. It was during this time, and because of their "marketing campaign," that PCP received its most popular street names (i.e., *Angel Dust* and *Hog*), which continue to be commonly used today.

It is generally estimated that approximately 1 in 20 young adults, 18 to 25 years-of-age, has used PCP during the previous year (Pagliaro & Pagliaro, *Clinical Patient Data Files*). However, this estimate may be *low* because accurate data regarding the actual use of PCP by young adults is relatively difficult to obtain for several reasons, including: (1) young adults who use PCP cannot be reached in common surveys of college/university students, respectively, because they may *not*, for various reasons, attend college/university (e.g., choose to be a "stay-at-home" parent; "drop out" of college/university, join the military, or obtain other part- or full-time jobs prior to graduation); (2) PCP use does *not* often result in emergency department visits for which data would usually be available; and (3) PCP, primarily for economic reasons, is *not* always screened for and, consequently detected in blood or urine screening tests.

However, one of the few available national drug surveys of psychodelic use found that, in 2014, approximately 3% of adults in the U.S. (26 years-of-age and older) reported lifetime use of PCP (NIDA, 2016).

Contributing to PCP's ability to "fly under the radar" is its changing pattern of use over the last decade, including its use: (1) in combination with other drugs

---

less than 30 minutes when administered orally). Ketamine is metabolized by the hepatic microsomal enzyme system (CYP3A4) with greater than 90% excreted, both in its unchanged form and as its major metabolite, norketamine, in the urine. The duration of action is approximately 1 hour and the half-life of elimination is approximately 3 hours. The primary mechanism of action of ketamine is as a non-competitive antagonist of the NMDA receptor (Pagliaro & Pagliaro, 2009).

The acute undesired, or harmful, effects associated with ketamine include amnesia and cognitive impairment, particularly of executive functioning. Ketamine, commonly known on the street as "Cat," "K," "Kit-Kat," or "Special K," is abused for its psychodelic effects. With *high* dosages or regular, long-term use, some users describe the experience of going into the "K-hole"—a state of *extreme* dissociation with both auditory and visual hallucinations (Li, Vicknasingam, & Cheung, 2011; Pagliaro & Pagliaro, *Clinical Patient Data Files*).

[61] *Shermans* are small, cigarette-like cigars, or cigarillos, that, along with tobacco cigarettes and marijuana "joints," are often "dipped" in a solution of PCP and embalming fluid (i.e., formaldehyde) and then dried before smoking. The laced embalming fluid and PCP product is commonly referred to as "fry," "illy," or "wet" (Modesto-Lowe & Petry, 2001; Pagliaro & Pagliaro, *Clinical Patient Data Files*; Peters, Kelder, & Meshack, 2005).

and substances of abuse, particularly marijuana; (2) in *lower* dosages; and (3) by increasingly diverse sociocultural groups. For example, in their study of U.S. adults of African continental descent,18 to 40 years-of-age, and current crack cocaine and PCP ("fry") users, Peters, Williams, and Ross (2008) found that their sample of cocaine and PCP users was *significantly* more likely, than a sample of matched non-PCP users, to:

1. Use marijuana
2. Use codeine cough syrup
3. Use methamphetamine
4. Engage in sex-for-drug exchanges
5. Be diagnosed with gonorrhea

References[62,63,64]

ACOG, The American Congress of Obstetricians and Gynecologists. (2015a, July). *Marijuana use during pregnancy and lactation (Committee Opinion, No. 637).* Retrieved from ACOG.org, pp. 1–5: www.acog.org/Resources-And-Publications/Committee-Opinions/Committee-on-Obstetric-Practice/Marijuana-Use-During-Pregnancy-and-Lactation

ACOG, The American Congress of Obstetricians and Gynecologists. (2015b, June 22). *Ob-gyns warn against marijuana use for pregnant women.* Retrieved from ACOG.org, pp. 1–2: www.acog.org/About-ACOG/News-Room/News-Releases/2015/Ob-gyns-Warn-Against-Marijuana-Use-for-Pregnant-Women

Alaniz, V. I., Liss, J., & Metz, T. D. (2015). Cannabinoid hyperemesis syndrome: A cause of refractory nausea and vomiting in pregnancy. *Obstetrics & Gynecology*, 125(6), 1484–1486. doi:10.1097/AOG.0000000000000595

Aldington, S., Williams, M., & Nowitz, M. (2007). Effects of cannabis on pulmonary structure, function and symptoms. *Thorax*, 62(12), 1058–1063.

Allen, J. H., de Moore, G. M., & Heddle, R. (2004). Cannabinoid hyperemesis: Cyclical hyperemesis in association with chronic cannabis abuse. *Gut*, 53(11), 1566–1570. doi:10.1136/gut.2003.036350

Ameri, A. (1999). The effects of cannabinoids on the brain. *Progress in Neurobiology*, 58(4), 315–348.

[62] As per publisher style, only the first three authors are listed for each reference.

[63] Several times the number of references listed were found, obtained, and analyzed by the authors during the preparation of this chapter. However, only the references that were cited at least once in the body of the text are included in the list. Major reasons for not citing other references, include that they: (1) did not provide any additional unique data; (2) were not well researched or written (i.e., were evaluated as not being valid or reliable); (3) were based predominantly, or exclusively, on animal studies; (4) provided usage statistics from outside the U.S.; and/or (5) were redundant with, or not as recent as, the already cited references.

[64] The reference citation, "Pagliaro & Pagliaro, *Clinical Patient Data Files*," refers to unpublished data collected, with permission, over the last 50 years by the authors, in the formal course of their professional academic roles as clinician scientists and professors—from their patients, research subjects, and students, from the 1970s to date.

American College of Neuropsychopharmacology. (2015, December 10). *LSD changes consciousness by reorganizing human brain networks.* Retrieved February 1, 2016, from ScienceDaily, pp. 1–6: www.sciencedaily.com/releases/2015/12/151210144910.htm

American Lung Association. (2016). *Hookah smoking: A growing threat to public health.* Washington, DC: American Lung Association. Retrieved June 6, 2016.

American Psychiatric Association. (2000). *Diagnostic and statistical manual of mental disorders* (4th ed.). Washington, DC: American Psychiatric Association.

Anderson, D. M., Rees, D. I., & Sabia, J. J. (2014). Medical marijuana laws and suicides by gender and age. *American Journal of Public Health*, 104(12), 2369–2376. doi:10.2105/AJPH.2013.301612

Arendt, M., Rosenberg, R., & Foldager, L. (2007). Withdrawal symptoms do not predict relapse among subjects treated for cannabis dependence. *American Journal on Addictions*, 16(6), 461–467.

ARF/WHO, Addiction Research Foundation/World Health Organization. (1981). *Report of an ARF/WHO Scientific (6) Meeting on the Adverse Health and Behavioral Consequences of Cannabis Use.* Toronto: Addiction Research Foundation.

Armenian, P., Mamantov, T. M., & Tsutaoka, B. T. (2013). Multiple MDMA (Ecstasy) overdoses at a rave event: A case series. *Journal of Intensive Care Medicine*, 28(4), 252–258. doi:10.1177/0885066612445982

Asbridge, M., Hayden, J. A., & Cartwright, J. L. (2012, February 9). Acute cannabis consumption and motor vehicle collision risk: Systematic review of observational studies and meta-analysis. *BMJ*, 344. doi:10.1136/bmj.e536

Ashton, C. B. (2001). Pharmacology and effects of cannabis: A brief review. *The British Journal of Psychiatry*, 178(2), 101–106. doi:10.1192/bjp.178.2.101

Azofeifa, A., Mattson, M. E., & Schauer, G. (2016, September 2). National estimates of marijuana use and related indicators—National survey on drug use and health, United States, 2002–2014. *MMWR, Morbidity and Mortality Weekly Report*, 65(11), pp. 1–25.

Barratt, M. J., Ferris, J. A., & Winstock, A. R. (2014). Use of Silk Road, the online drug marketplace, in the United Kingdom, Australia and the United States. *Addiction*, 109(5), 774–783. doi:10.1111/add.12470

Beech, R. A., Sterrett, D. R., & Babiuk, J. (2015). Cannabinoid hyperemesis syndrome: A case report and literature review. *Journal of Oral and Maxillofacial Surgery*, 73(10), 1907–1910. doi:10.1016/joms.2015.03.059

Berman, M. E., & Coccaro, E. F. (1998). Neurobiologic correlates of violence: Relevance to criminal responsibility. *Behavioral Sciences and the Law*, 16(3), 303–318. doi:10.1002/(SICI)1099-0798(199822)16:3<285::AID-BSL308>3.0.C0;2–4

Bey, T., & Patel, A. (2007, February). Phencyclidine intoxication and adverse effects: A clinical and pharmacological review of an illicit drug. *The California Journal of Emergency Medicine*, VIII(1), 9–14.

Boyd, C. J., McCabe, S. E., & d'Arcy, H. (2003). Ecstasy use among college undergraduates: Gender, race and sexual identity. *Journal of Substance Abuse Treatment*, 24(3), 209–215.

Breivogel, C. S., & Childers, S. R. (1998). The functional neuroanatomy of brain cannabinoid receptors. *Neurobiology of Disease*, 5(6 Part B), 417–431. doi:10.1006/nbdi.1998.0229

Bryant, A. (2015, June 22). Marijuana: ACOG encourages abstinence while pregnant or breast-feeding. *Obstetrics & Gynecology*, ACOG Committee on Obstetric Practice. (Committee opinion no. 637). Retrieved April 18, 2016, from NEJM Journal Watch, p. 1: http://dx.doi.org/10.1097/AOG.0000000000000993

Buchi, K. F., Suarez, C., & Varner, M. W. (2013). The prevalence of prenatal opioid and other drug use in Utah. *American Journal of Perinatology*, 30(3), 241–244. doi:10.1055/s-0032-1323586

Buckner, J. D., Heimberg, R. G., & Schneier, F. R. (2012). The relationship between cannabis use disorders and social anxiety disorder in the National Epidemiological Study of Alcohol and Related Conditions (NESARC). *Drug and Alcohol Dependence*, 124(1–2), 128–134.

Budney, A. J., & Hughes, J. R. (2006). The cannabis withdrawal syndrome. *Current Opinion in Psychiatry*, 19(3), 233–238.

Cadman, P. E. (2017). Hypophosphatemia in users of cannabis. *American Journal of Kidney Diseases*, 69(1), 152–155. doi:10.1053/j.ajkd.2016.06.028

Campbell, G. A., & Rosner, M. H. (2008). The agony of ecstasy: MDMA (3,4-methylenedioxymethamphetamine) and the kidney. *Clinical Journal of the American Society of Nephrology*, 3(6), 1852–1860. doi:10.2215/CJN.02080508

Cannabis damages young brains more than originally thought, study finds. (2009, December 20). Retrieved from ScienceDaily, pp. 1–2: www.sciencedaily.com/releases/2009/12/091217115834.htm

Carroll, M. E. (1990). PCP and hallucinogens. In C. K. Erickson, M. A. Javors, & W. W. Morgan (Eds.), *Addiction potential of abused drugs and drug classes* (pp. 167–190). New York, NY: John Wiley & Sons.

Castle, D. J. (2013). Cannabis and psychosis: What causes what? *Faculty of 1000 Medicine Reports*, 5(1), 1–4. doi:10.3410/M5-1

CDC, Centers for Disease Control and Prevention. (2010). Ecstasy overdoses at a New Year's Eve rave—Los Angeles, California, 2010. *MMWR, Morbidity and Mortality Weekly Report*, 59(22), pp. 677–681.

CDC, Centers for Disease Control and Prevention. (2015a, September 14). *Hookahs.* Retrieved June 25, 2016, from Office on Smoking and Health: www.cdc.gov/chronicdisease/

CDC, Centers for Disease Control and Prevention. (2015b, November 9). *Dangers of hookah smoking*. Retrieved June 25, 2016, from www.cdc.gov/chronicdisease/

Cerda, M., Wall, M., & Keyes, K. M. (2012). Medical marijuana laws in 50 states: Investigating the relationship between state legalization of medical marijuana and marijuana use, abuse and dependence. *Drug and Alcohol Dependence*, 120(1–3), 22–27. doi:10.1016/j.drugalcdep.2011.06.011

Chaouachi, K. (2009). Hookah (shisha, narghile) smoking and environmental tobacco smoke (ETS). A critical review of the relevant literature and the public health consequences. *International Journal of Environmental Research and Public Health*, 6(2), 798–843. doi:10.3390/ijerph6020798

Choi, N. G., Marti, C. N., & DiNitto, D. M. (2017, May 8). Older adults' marijuana use, injuries, and emergency department visits. *American Journal of Drug and Alcohol Abuse*, [Epub ahead of print], 1–9. doi: 10.1080/00952990.2017.1318891

Christophersen, A. S., Morland, J., & Stewart, K. (2016). International trends in alcohol and drug use among vehicle drivers. *Forensic Science Review*, 28(1), 37–66.

Cohen, M., Solowij, N., & Carr, V. (2008). Cannabis, cannabinoids and schizophrenia: Integration of the evidence. *Australian & New Zealand Journal of Psychiatry*, 42(5), 357–368. doi:10.1080/00048670801961156

Cohen, S. (1967). Psychotomimetic agents. *Annual Review of Pharmacology*, 7, 301–318. doi:10.1146/annurev.pa.07.040167.001505

Colorado Department of Revenue. (2016). *Colorado marijuana tax data.* Retrieved April 13, 2016, from Department of Revenue, pp. 1–2: www.colorado.gov/pacific/revenue/colorado-marijuana-tax-data

Cooper, Z. D., & Haney, M. (2009). Actions of delta-9-tetrahydrocannabinol in cannabis: Relation to use, abuse, dependence. *International Review of Psychiatry*, 21(2), 104–112.

Cornelius, J. R., Chung, T., & Martin, C. (2008). Cannabis withdrawal is common among treatment-seeking adolescents with cannabis dependence and major depression, and is associated with rapid relapse to dependence. *Addictive Behaviors*, 33(11), 1500–1505.

Couper, F. J., & Peterson, B. L. (2014). The prevalence of marijuana in suspected impaired driving cases in Washington state. *Journal of Analytical Toxicology*, 38(8), 569–574. doi:10.1093/jat/bku090

Crane, C. A., Easton, C. J., & Devine, S. (2013). The association between phencyclidine use and partner violence: An initial examination. *Journal of Addictive Diseases*, 32(2), 150–157. doi:10.1080/10550887.2013.797279

Crane, N. A., Schuster, R. M., & Gonzalez, R. (2013). Preliminary evidence for a sex-specific relationship between amount of cannabis use and neurocognitive performance in young adult cannabis users. *Journal of International Psychology and Sociology*, 19(9), 1009–1015. doi:10.1017/S135561771300088X

Crowley, J., & Courtney, R. (2003). *The relationship between drug use, impaired driving and traffic accidents.* Retrieved from Illicit Drugs in Road Traffic Symposium: www.pomidou.coe.int/English/route/route en_187.html

De Genna, N. M., Cornelius, M. D., & Goldschmidt, L. (2015, November 1). Maternal age and trajectories of cannabis use. *Drug and Alcohol Dependence*, 156, 199–206. doi:10.1016/j.drugalcdep.2015.09.014

Di Marzo, V., Melck, D., & Bisogno, T. (1998). Endocannabinoids: Endogenous cannabinoid receptor ligands with neuromodulatory action. *Trends in Neurosciences*, 21(12), 521–528.

Dolder, P. C., Schmid, Y., & Haschke, M. (2015, June 22). Pharmacokinetics and concentration-effect relationship of oral LSD in humans. *International Journal of Neuropsychopharmacology*, 1–7. doi:10.1093/ijnp/pyv072

Domino, E. F., & Luby, E. D. (2012). Phencyclidine/schizophrenia: One view toward the past, the other to the future. *Schizophrenia Bulletin*, 38(5), 914–919. doi:10.1093/schbul/sbs011

D'Onofrio, G., McCausland, J. B., & Tarabar, A. F. (2006). Illy: Clinical and public health implications of a street drug. *Substance Abuse*, 27(4), 45–51.

DrugFacts: MDMA (Ecstasy/Molly). (2016, February). Retrieved April 10, 2016, from National Institute on Drug Abuse (NIDA), pp. 1–5: www.drugabuse.gov/publications/drugfacts/mdma-ecstasymolly

D'Souza, D. C. (2007). Cannabinoids and psychosis. *International Review of Neurobiology*, 78, 289–326. doi:10.1016/S0074-7742(06)78010-2

Ehlers, C. L., Gizer, I. R., & Vieten, C. (2010). Cannabis dependence in the San Francisco Family Study: Age of onset of use, DSM-IV symptoms, withdrawal, and heritability. *Addictive Behaviors*, 35(2), 102–110. doi:10.1016/j.addbeh.2009.09.009

Eisenberg, E., Ogintz, M., & Almog, S. (2014). The pharmacokinetics, efficacy, safety, and ease of use of a novel portable metered-dose cannabis inhaler in patients with chronic neuropathic pain: A phase 1a study. *Journal of Pain and Palliative Care Pharmacotherapy*, 28(3), 216–225. doi:10.3109/15360288.2014.941130

Falck, R. S., Wang, J., & Carlson, R. G. (2006). Prevalence and correlates of current depressive symptomatology among a community sample of MDMA users in Ohio. *Addictive Behaviors*, 31(1), 90–101. doi:10.1016/j.addbeh.2005.04.017

Farre, M., Tomillero, A., & Perez-Mana, C. (2015). Human pharmacology of 3,4-methylenedioxymethamphetamine (MDMA, ecstasy) after repeated doses taken 4 h apart. *European Neuropsychopharmacology*, 25(10), 1637–1649. doi:10.1016/j.euroneuro.2015.05.007

Fernando, T., Gilbert, J. D., & Carroll, C. M. (2012). Ecstasy and suicide. *Journal of Forensic Sciences*, 57(4), 1137–1139. doi:10.1111/j.1556-4029.2012.02107.x

Ferner, M. (2014, September 22). *Marijuana tax revenue may top $3 billion a year with legalization*. Retrieved April 13, 2016, from HOFFPOST POLITICS: www.huffingtonpost.com/2014/09/22/legal-marijuana-taxes_n_5863860.html

Fried, P. A., & Smith, A. M. (2001). A literature review of the consequences of prenatal marihuana exposure. An emerging theme of a deficiency in aspects of executive function. *Neurotoxicology and Teratology*, 23(1), 1–11.

Gallagher, D. T., Hadjiefthyvoulou, F., & Fisk, J. E. (2014). Prospective memory deficits in illicit polydrug users are associated with the average long-term typical dose of ecstasy typically consumed in a single session. *Neuropsychology*, 28(1), 43–54. doi:10.1037/neu0000004

Galli, J. A., Sawaya, R. A., & Friedenberg, F. K. (2011, December). Cannabinoid hyperemesis syndrome. *Current Drug Abuse Reviews*, 4(4), 241–249.

Gettman, J. (2006, December). *Marijuana production in the United States (2006)*. Retrieved August 1, 2015, from The Bulletin of Cannabis Reform, pp. 1–28: www.drugscience.org/bcr/index.html

Ghatol, A., & Kazory, A. (2012). Ecstasy-associated acute severe hypnonatremia and cerebral edema: A role for osmotic diuresis? *The Journal of Emergency Medicine*, 42(6), e137–e140. doi:10.1016/j.jemermed.2009.05.001

Gilbert, C. R., Baram, M., & Cavarocchi, N. C. (2013). "Smoking wet": Respiratory failure related to smoking tainted marijuana cigarettes. *Texas Heart Institute Journal*, 40(1), 64–67.

Gonzalez-Maeso, J., & Sealfon, S. C. (2009). Psychedelics and schizophrenia. *Trends in Neurosciences*, 32(4), 225–232. doi:10.1016/j.tins.2008.12.005

Gouzoulis-Mayfrank, E., & Daumann, J. (2006). Neurotoxicity of methylenedioxymethamphetamines (MDMA; ecstasy) in humans: How strong is the evidence for persistent brain damage? *Addiction*, 101(3), 348–361. doi:10.1111/j.1360-0443.2006.01314.x

Gouzoulis-Mayfrank, E., & Daumann, J. (2009). Neurotoxicity of drugs of abuse—The case of methylenedioxymethamphetamines (MDMA, ecstasy), and amphetamines. *Dialogues in Clinical Neuroscience*, 11(3), 305–317.

Gouzoulis-Mayfrank, E., Fischermann, T., & Rezk, M. (2005). Memory performance in polyvalent MDMA (ecstasy) users who continue or discontinue MDMA use. *Drug and Alcohol Dependence*, 78(3), 317–323. doi:10.1016/j.drugalcdep.2004.12.002

Grucza, R. A., Hur, M., & Agrawal, A. (2015, July 1). A reexamination of medical marijuana policies in relation to suicide risk. *Drug and Alcohol Dependence*, 152, 68–72. doi:10.1016/j.drugalcdep.2015.04.014

Gunn, J. K., Rosales, C. B., & Center, K. E. (2016). Prenatal exposure to cannabis and maternal and child health outcomes: A systematic review and meta-analysis. *BMJ Open*, 6, 1–7. doi:10.1136/bmjopen-2015–009986

Hancox, R. J., Poulton, R., & Ely, M. (2010). Effects of cannabis on lung function: A population-based cohort study. *European Respiratory Journal*, 35(1), 42–47. doi:10.1183/09031936.00065009

Harrison, L. D., Backenheimer, M., & Inciardi, J. A. (1996). Cannabis use in the United States: Implications for policy. In P. Cohen, & A. Sas, *Cannabisbeleid in Duitsland, Frankrijk en de Verenigde Staten* (pp. 179–276). Amsterdam: Centrum voor Drugsonderzoek.

Hartman, R. L., Brown, T. L., & Milavetz, G. (2015). Controlled cannabis vaporizer administration: Blood and plasma cannabinoids with and without alcohol. *Clinical Chemistry*, 61(6), 850–869. doi:10.1373/clinchem.2015.238287

Hartman, R. L., & Huestis, M. A. (2013). Cannabis effects on driving skills. *Clinical Chemistry*, 59(3), 478–492. doi:10.1373/clinchem.2012.194381

Hendricks, P. S., Thorne, C. B., & Clark, C. B. (2015). Classic psychedelic use is associated with reduced psychological distress and suicidality in the United States adult population. *Journal of Psychopharmacology*, 29(3), 280–288. doi:10.1177/0269881114565653

Hermes-Laufer, J., Del Puppo, L., & Inan, I. (2016). Cannabinoid hyperemesis syndrome: A case report of cyclic severe hyperemesis and abdominal pain with long-term cannabis use. *Case Reports in Gastrointestinal Medicine*. doi:10.1155/2016/2815901

Hernandez-Avila, C. A., Rounsaville, B. J., & Kranzler, H. R. (2004). Opioid-, cannabis- and alcohol-dependent women show more rapid progression to substance abuse treatment. *Drug and Alcohol Dependence*, 74(3), 265–272.

Herrmann, E. S., Weerts, E. M., & Vandrey, R. (2015). Sex differences in cannabis withdrawal symptoms among treatment-seeking cannabis users. *Experimental and Clinical Psychopharmacology*, 23(6), 415–421. doi: 10.1037/pha0000053

Hill, M., & Reed, K. (2013). Pregnancy, breast-feeding, and marijuana: A review article. *Obstetrical & Gynecological Survey*, 68(10), 710–718. doi:10.1097/01.ogx.0000435371.51584.d1

Ho, E., Karimi-Tabesh, L., & Koren, G. (2001). Characteristics of pregnant women who use ecstasy (3, 4-methylenedioxymethamphetamine). *Neurotoxicology and Teratology*, 23(6), 561–567.

Hoffman, A. (1970). Notes and documents concerning the discovery of LSD. *Agents and Actions*, 1(3), 148–150.

Hoffman, A. (1980). How LSD originated. *Journal of Psychedelic Drugs*, 11(1–2), 53–60.

Hysek, C. M., Schmid, Y., & Simmler, L. D. (2014). MDMA enhances emotional empathy and prosocial behavior. *Social Cognitive & Affective Neuroscience*, 9(11), 1645–1652. doi:10.1093/scan/nst161

Hysek, C. M., Simmler, L. D., & Schillinger, N. (2014). Pharmacokinetic and pharmacodynamic effects of methylphenidate and MDMA administered alone or in combination. *International Journal of Neuropsychopharmacology*, 17(3), 371–381. doi:10,1017/S1461145713001132

Impact on lungs of one cannabis joint equal to up to five cigarettes. (2007, August 2). Retrieved from ScienceDaily, pp. 1–2: www.sciencedaily.com/releases/2007/07/070731085550.htm

Jehle Jr, C. C., Nazir, N., & Bhavsar, D. (2015). The rapidly increasing trend of cannabis use in burn injury. *Journal of Burn Care & Research*, 36(1), e12–e17. doi:10.1097/BCR.0000000000000192

Jerome, L., Schuster, S., & Yazar-Klosinski, B. B. (2013). Can MDMA play a role in the treatment of substance abuse? *Current Drug Abuse Reviews*, 6(1), 54–62.

Johansen, P. O., & Krebs, T. S. (2015). Psychedelics not linked to mental health problems or suicidal behavior: A population study. *Journal of Psychopharmacology*, 29(3), 270–279. doi:10.1177/0269881114568039

Johns, A. (2001). Psychiatric effects of cannabis. *The British Journal of Psychiatry*, 178, 116–122.

Joshi, M., Joshi, A., & Bartter, T. (2014). Marijuana and lung diseases. *Current Opinion in Pulmonary Medicine*, 20(2), 173–179. doi:10.1097/MCP.0000000000000026

Khalsa, J. H., Genser, S., & Francis, H. (2002). Clinical consequences of marijuana. *Journal of Clinical Pharmacology*, 42(Supplement 11), 7S–10S.

Khan, S. S., Secades-Villa, R., & Okuda, M. (2013). Gender differences in cannabis use disorders: Results from the National Epidemiologic Survey of Alcohol and Related Conditions. *Drug and Alcohol Dependence*, 130(1–3), 101–108. doi:10.1016/j.drugalcdep.2012.10.015

Kirkpatrick, M. G., & de Wit, H. (2015). MDMA: A social drug in a social context. *Psychopharmacology (Berlin)*, 232(6), 1155–1163. doi:10.1007/s00213-014-3752-6

Klein, T. W., Lane, B., & Newton, C. A. (2000). The cannabinoid system and cytokine network. *Proceedings of the Society for Experimental Biology and Medicine*, 225(1), 1–8.

Krauss, M. J., Sowles, S. J., & Moreno, M. (2015, July 30). Hookah-related twitter chatter: A content analysis. *Preventing Chronic Disease*, 12(e121), 1–9. doi:10.5888/pcd12.150140

Krebs, T. S., & Johansen, P. O. (2013, August 19). Psychedelics and mental health: A population study. *PLoS One*, 8(8), e63972. doi:10/1371/journal.pone.0063972

La Corte, R. (2014, November 20). *Washington marijuana tax revenue more than predicted*. Retrieved from King 5.com: www.king5.com/story/news/local/2014/11/20/washington-state-marijuana-tax-revenue/19325309/

Lee, M. H., & Hancox, R. J. (2011). Effects of smoking cannabis on lung function. *Expert Review of Respiratory Medicine*, 5(4), 537–546. doi:10.1586/ers.11.40

Leung, K. S., & Cottler, L. B. (2008). Ecstasy and other club drugs: A review of recent epidemiologic studies. *Current Opinion in Psychiatry*, 21(3), 234–241. doi:10.1097/YCO.0b013e3282f9b1f1

Levin, S. (2016, November 9). California, Nevada and Massachusetts vote to legalize recreational marijuana. *The Guardian*, pp. 1–5. San Francisco. Retrieved November 9, 2016, from www.theguardian.com/us-news/2016/nov/08/state-ballot-initiative-election-results-live-marijuana-death-penalty-healthcare

Leweke, F. M., & Koethe, D. (2008). Cannabis and psychiatric disorders: It is not only addiction. *Addiction Biology*, 13(2), 264–275. doi:10.1111/j.1369-1600.2008.00106.x

Li, J., Vicknasingam, B., & Cheung, Y. (2011). To use or not to use: An update on licit and illicit ketamine use. *Substance Abuse and Rehabilitation*, 2, 11–20. doi:10.2147/SAR.S15458

Li, M. C., Brady, J. E., & DiMaggio, C. J. (2012). Marijuana use and motor vehicle crashes. *Epidemiologic Reviews*, 34, 65–72. doi:10.1093/epirev/mxr017

Long-term cannabis users may have structural brain abnormalities. (2008, June 3). Retrieved from ScienceDaily.com, p. 1: www.sciencedaily.com/releases/2008/06/080602160845.htm

Lopez-Moreno, J. A., Gonzalez-Cuevas, G., & Moreno, G. (2008). The pharmacology of the endocannabinoid system: Functional and structural interactions with other neurotransmitter systems and their repercussions in behavioral addiction. *Addiction Biology*, 13(2), 160–187. doi:10.1111/j.1369-1600.2008.00105.x

Ludlow, F. H. (1857). *The hashish eater: Being passages from the life of a Pythagorean*. New York, NY: S. G. Rains.

Ly, B. T., Thornton, S. L., & Buono, C. (2012). False-positive urine phencyclidine immunoassay screen caused by interference by tramadol and its metabolites. *Annals of Emergency Medicine*, 59(6), 545–547. doi:10.1016/j.annemergmed.2011.08.013

Maccarrone, M., & Finazzi-Agro, A. (2002). Endocannabinoids and their actions. *Vitamins and Hormones*, 65, 225–255.

MacNeal, J. J., Cone, D. C., & Sinha, V. (2012). Use of haloperidol in PCP-intoxicated individuals. *Clinical Toxicology (Philadelphia, PA)*, 59(9), 851–853. doi:10.3109/15563650.2012.722222

Maldonado, R., & Rodriguez de Fonseca, F. (2002). Cannabinoid addiction: Behavioral models and neural correlates. *Journal of Neuroscience*, 22(9), 3326–3331.

Marceaux, J. C., Dilks, L. S., & Hixson, S. (2008). Neuropsychological effects of formaldehyde use. *Journal of Psychoactive Drugs*, 40(2), 207–210. doi:10.1080/02791072.2008.10400632

Marijuana smoke contains higher levels of certain toxins than tobacco smoke. (2007, December 18). Retrieved from ScienceDaily.com, p. 1: www.sciencedaily.com/releases/2007/12/071217110328.htm

Marijuana smokers face rapid lung destruction—As much as 20 years ahead of tobacco smokers. (2008, January 27). Retrieved from ScienceDaily.com, pp. 1–2: www.sciencedaily.com/releases/2008/01/0801231040017.htm

Martin, B. R., Mechoulam, R., & Razdan, R. K. (1999). Discovery and characterization of endogenous cannabinoids. *Life Sciences*, 65(6–7), 573–595.

McGregor, I. S., Callaghan, P. D., & Hunt, G. E. (2008). From ultrasocial to antisocial: A role for oxytocin in the acute reinforcing effects and long-term adverse consequences of drug use? *British Journal of Pharmacology*, 154, 358–368. doi:10.1038/bjp.2008.132

Metz, T. D., & Stickrath, E. H. (2015). Marijuana use in pregnancy and lactation: A review of the evidence. *American Journal of Obstetrics & Gynecology*, 213(6), 761–778. doi:10.1016/j.ajog.2015.05.025

Meyer, J. S. (2013, November 21). 3,4-methylenedioxymethamphetamine (MDMA): Current perspectives. *Substance Abuse and Rehabilitation*, 4, 83–99. doi:10.2147/SAR.S37258

Miller, S. G. (2016, August 8). High numbers? 1 in 8 US adults smokes pot. *Live Science*, 1–10.

Modesto-Lowe, V., & Petry, N. M. (2001). Recognizing and managing "illy" intoxication. *Psychiatric Services*, 52, 1660.

Montoya, A. G., Sorrentino, R., & Lukas, S. E. (2002). Long-term neuropsychiatric consequences of "ecstasy" (MDMA): A review. *Harvard Review of Psychiatry*, 10(4), 212–220.

Moreira, F. A., & Lutz, B. (2008). The endocannabinoid system: Emotion, learning and addiction. *Addictive Behaviors*, 13(2), 196–212. doi:10.1111/j.1369-1600.2008.00104.x

Morris, B. J., Cochran, S. M., & Pratt, J. A. (2005). PCP: From pharmacology to modeling schizophrenia. *Current Opinion in Pharmacology*, 5(1), 101–106.

Morris, D. S., Fiala, S. C., & Pawlak, R. (2012, November 15). Opportunities for policy interventions to reduce youth hookah smoking in the United States. *Preventing Chronic Disease*, 9, 1–4. doi:org.org/10.5888/pcd9.120082

Motel, S. (2015, April 14). *6 facts about marijuana.* Retrieved April 14, 2016, from PewResearchCenter: www.pewresearch.org/author/smotel/

Murray, J. B. (2002). Phencyclidine (PCP): A dangerous drug, but useful in schizophrenia research. *The Journal of Psychology*, 136(3), 319–327.

Nahas, G. G., Zeidenberg, P., & Lefebure, C. (1975). Kif in Morocco. *International Journal of the Addictions*, 10(6), 977–993. doi:10.3109/10826087509028355

NHTSA, National Highway Traffic Safety Administration. (2016). *Drugs and human performance fact sheets.* Retrieved April 10, 2016, from Methylenedioxymethamphetamine (MDMA, Ecstasy), pp. 1–5: www.nhtsa.gov/people/injury/research/job185drugs/methylenedioxymethamphetamine.htm

Nichols, D. E. (2004). Hallucinogens. *Pharmacology & Therapeutics*, 101(2), 131–181. doi:10.1016/j.pharmthera.2003.11.002

NIDA, National Institute on Drug Abuse. (2016, January). *Substance use in women and men.* Retrieved January 12, 2016, from Substance use in women and men, pp. 1–4: www.drugabuse.gov/related-topics/trends-statistics/infographics/substance-use-in-women-men

Nocerino, E., Amato, M., & Izzo, A. A. (2000). Cannabis and cannabinoid receptors. *Fitoterapia,* 71(Supplement 1), S6–S12.

O'Connor, A., & Schweber, N. (2009, November 6). *Driver said to have used marijuana regularly.* Retrieved September 29, 2016, from The New York Times, pp. 1–2: www.nytimes.com/2009/11/07/nyregion/07taconic.html?_r=0

Ogeil, R. P., Rajaratnam, S. M., & Broadbear, J. H. (2013). Male and female ecstasy users: Differences in patterns of use, sleep quality and mental health outcomes. *Drug and Alcohol Dependence,* 132(1–2), 223–230. doi:10.1016/j.drugalcdep.2013.02.002

Osmond, H. (1957). A review of the clinical effects of psychotomimetic agents. *Annals of the New York Academy of Sciences,* 66(3), 418–434.

Pacek, L. R., Mauro, P. M., & Martins, S. S. (2015). Perceived risk of regular cannabis use in the United States from 2002 to 2012: Differences by sex, age, and race/ethnicity. *Drug and Alcohol Dependence,* 149, 232–244. doi:10.1016/j.drugalcdep.2015.02.009

Pagliaro, A. M., & Pagliaro, L. A. (1996). *Substance use among children and adolescents: Its nature, extent, and effects from conception to adulthood.* New York, NY: John Wiley & Sons.

Pagliaro, A. M., & Pagliaro, L. A. (2000). *Substance use among women: A reference and research guide.* Philadelphia, PA: Brunner/Mazel.

Pagliaro, L. A. (1983). Up in smoke? A brief overview of marijuana toxicity. *Kerygma, Issue* 41, 1–4.

Pagliaro, L. A. (1988, June). Marijuana and hashish: What are the risks? *Let's Talk,* 13, 12–14.

Pagliaro, L. A. (1991). The deja vu phenomena (letter). *American Journal of Psychiatry,* 148, 1418.

Pagliaro, L. A. (1995). Pharmacopsychology updates: Marijuana reconsidered. *Psymposium,* 5(2), 12–13.

Pagliaro, L. A., & Pagliaro, A. M. (Eds.). (2002). *Problems in pediatric drug therapy* (4th ed.). Washington, DC: American Pharmaceutical Association.

Pagliaro, L. A., & Pagliaro, A. M. (2004). *Pagliaros' comprehensive guide to drugs and substances of abuse.* Washington, DC: American Pharmacists Association.

Pagliaro, L. A., & Pagliaro, A. M. (2009). *Pagliaros' comprehensive guide to drugs and substances of abuse* (2nd ed.). Washington, DC: American Pharmacists Association.

Pagliaro, L. A., & Pagliaro, A. M. (2012). *Handbook of child and adolescent drug and substance abuse.* Hoboken, NJ: Wiley & Sons.

Pahl, K., Brook, J. S., & Koppel, J. (2011). Trajectories of marijuana use and psychological adjustment among urban African American and Puerto Rican women. *Psychological Medicine,* 41(8), 1775–1783. doi:10.1017/S0033291710002345

Parrott, A. C. (2006). MDMA in humans: Factors which affect the neuropsychobiological profiles of recreational ecstasy users, the integrative role of bioenergetic stress. *Journal of Psychopharmacology,* 20(2), 147–163.

Parrott, A. C. (2009). Cortisol and 3,4-methylenedioxymethamphetamine: Neurohormonal aspects of bioenergetic stress in ecstasy users. *Neuropsychobiology,* 60(3–4), 148–158. doi:10.1159/000253551

Parrott, A. C. (2012). MDMA and temperature: A review of the thermal effects of "Ecstasy" in humans. *Drug and Alcohol Dependence,* 121(1–2), 1–9. doi:10.1016/j.drugalcdep.2011.08.012

Parrott, A. C., Lock, J., & Conner, A. C. (2008). Dance clubbing on MDMA and during abstinence from Ecstasy/MDMA: Prospective neuroendocrine and psychobiological changes. *Neuropsychobiology*, 57(4), 165–180. doi:10.1159/000147470

Parsons, J. T., Grov, C., & Kelly, B. C. (2009). Club drug use and dependence among young adults recruited through time-space sampling. *Public Health Reports*, 124(2), 246–254.

Parsons, J. T., Kelly, B. C., & Wells, B. E. (2006). Differences in club drug use between heterosexual and lesbian/bisexual females. *Addictive Behaviors*, 31(12), 2344–2349.

Passie, T., Halpern, J. H., & Stichtenoth, D. O. (2008). The pharmacology of lysergic acid diethylamide: A review. *CNS Neuroscience and Therapeutics*, 14(4), 295–314.

Patel, M. M., Belson, M. G., & Longwater, A. B. (2005). Methylenedioxymethamphetamine (ecstasy)-related hyperthermia. *The Journal of Emergency Medicine*, 29(4), 451–454.

Peiro, A. M., Farre, M., & Roset, P. N. (2013). Human pharmacology of 3,4-methylenedioxymethamphetamine (MDMA, ecstasy) after repeated doses taken 2 h apart. *Psychopharmacology (Berlin)*, 225(4), 883–893. doi:10.1007/s00213-012-2894-7

Pertwee, R. G. (2000). Cannabinoid receptor ligands: Clinical and neuropharmacological considerations, relevant to future drug discovery and development. *Expert Opinion on Investigative Drugs*, 9(7), 1553–1571.

Peters Jr., R. J., Kelder, H., & Meshack, A. (2005). Beliefs and social norms about cigarettes or marijuana sticks laced with embalming fluid and phencyclidine (PCP): Why youth use "fry." *Substance Use and Misuse*, 40(1), 125–135.

Peters Jr., R. J., Williams, M., & Ross, M. W. (2008). The use of fry (embalming fluid and PCP-laced cigarettes or marijuana sticks) among crack cocaine smokers. *Journal of Drug Education*, 38(3), 285–295.

Phillips Erb, K. (2014, March 11). *It's no toke: Colorado pulls in millions in marijuana tax revenue—Forbes.* Retrieved April 13, 2016, from Forbes: www.forbes.com/sites/kellyphillipserb/2014/03/11/its-no-toke-colorado-pulls-in-millions-in-marijuana-tax-revenue/#65d443f44d4a

Pilgrim, J. L., Gerostamoulos, D., & Drummer, O. H. (2011). Deaths involving MDMA and the concomitant use of pharmaceutical drugs. *Journal of Analytical Toxicology*, 35(4), 219–226.

Piper, B. J. (2007). A developmental comparison of the neurobehavioral effects of ecstasy (MDMA). *Neurotoxicology and Teratology*, 29(2), 288–300. doi:10.1016/j.ntt.2006.10.002

Pope Jr, H. G., Gruber, A. J., & Hudson, J. I. (2001). Neuropsychological performance in long-term cannabis users. *Archives of General Psychiatry*, 58(10), 909–915.

Power, R. A., Verweij, K. J., & Zuhair, M. (2014). Genetic predisposition to schizophrenia associated with increased use of cannabis. *Molecular Psychiatry*, 19(11), 1201–1204. doi:10.1038/mp.2014.51

Preuss, U. W., Watzke, A. B., & Zimmermann, J. (2010). Cannabis withdrawal severity and short-term course among cannabis-dependent adolescent and young adult inpatients. *Drug and Alcohol Dependence*, 106(2–3), 133–141.

Quednow, B. B., Jessen, F., & Kuhn, K. U. (2006, May). *Memory deficits in abstinent MDMA (ecstasy) users: Neuropsychological evidence of frontal dysfunction.* Retrieved March 30, 2016, from PubMed—NCBI, pp. 373–384: www.ncbi.nim.gov/pubmed/16574711

Radhakrishnan, R., Wilkinson, S. T., & D'Souza, D. C. (2014). Gone to pot—A review of the association between cannabis and psychosis. *Frontiers in Psychiatry*, 5(Article 54), 1–24. doi:10.3389/psyt.2014.00054

Ramaekers, J. G., Berghaus, G., & van Laar, M. (2004). Dose related risk of motor vehicle crashes after cannabis use. *Drug and Alcohol Dependence*, 73(2), 109–119.

Ramo, D. E., Grov, C., & Delucchi, K. (2010). Typology of club drug use among young adults recruited using time-space sampling. *Drug and Alcohol Dependence*, 107(2–3), 119–127.

Rengarajan, A., & Mullins, M. E. (2013). How often do false-positive phencyclidine urine screens occur with use of common medications? *Clinical Toxicology (Philadelphia, PA)*, 51(6), 493–496. doi:10.3109/15563650.2013.801982

Richardson, G. A., Ryan, C., & Willford, J. (2002). Prenatal alcohol and marijuana exposure: Effects on neuropsychological outcomes at 10 years. *Neurotoxicology and Teratology*, 24(3), 309–320.

Roberts, G. M., Nestor, L., & Garavan, H. (2009, October 6). Learning and memory deficits in ecstasy users and their neural correlates during a face-learning task. *Brain Research*, 71–81. doi:10.1016/j.brainres.2009.07.040

Rosenson, J., Smollin, C., & Sporer, K. A. (2007). Patterns of ecstasy-associated hyponatremia in California. *Annals of Emergency Medicine*, 49(2), 164–171. doi:10.1016/j.annemergmed.2006.09.018

SAMHSA, Substance Abuse and Mental Health Services Administration. (2014). *Results from the 2013 National Survey on Drug Use and Health: Summary of National Findings (No. SMA 14–4863, NSDUH Series H-48)*. Rockville, MD: Substance Abuse and Mental Health Services Administration.

Samuels, A. (2015, July 16). Study: Marijuana disapproval rate down among millennials. *USA Today College News*. Retrieved from USA Today College News.

Santos, G. M., Rapues, J., & Wilson, E. C. (2014). Alcohol and substance use among transgender women in San Francisco: Prevalence and association with human immunodeficiency virus infection. *Drug and Alcohol Review*, 33(3), 287–295. doi:10.1111/dar.12116

Sartor, C. E., Agrawal, A., & Grant, J. D. (2015). Differences between African-American and European-American women in the association of childhood sexual abuse with initiation of marijuana use and progression to problem use. *Journal of Studies on Alcohol and Drugs*, 76(4), 569–577.

Sartor, C. E., Agrawal, A., & Lynskey, M. T. (2013). Cannabis or alcohol first? Differences by ethnicity and in risk for rapid progression to cannabis-related problems among women. *Psychological Medicine*, 43(4), 813–823. doi:10.1017/S0033291712001493

Sartor, C. E., Waldron, M., & Duncan, A. E. (2013). Childhood sexual abuse and early substance use in adolescent girls: The role of familial influences. *Addiction*, 108(5), 993–1000. doi:10.1111/add.12115

Schifano, F. (2004). A bitter pill. Overview of ecstasy (MDMA, MDA) related fatalities. *Psychopharmacology (Berlin)*, 173(3–4), 242–248. doi:10.1007/s00213-003-1730-5

Schneider, M. (2008). Puberty as a highly vulnerable developmental period for the consequences of cannabis exposure. *Addiction Biology*, 13(2), 253–263.

Scholey, A. B., Parrott, A. C., & Buchanan, T. (2004). Increased intensity of ecstasy and polydrug usage in the more experienced recreational ecstasy/MDMA users: A WWW study. *Addictive Behaviors*, 29(4), 743–752. doi:10.1016/j.addbeh.2004.02.022

Sewell, R. A., Poling, J., & Sofuoglu, M. (2009). The effect of cannabis compared with alcohol on driving. *The American Journal on Addictions*, 18(3), 185–193. doi:10.1080/10550490902786934

Shukla, R. K., Crump, J. L., & Chrisco, E. S. (2012). An evolving problem: Methamphetamine production and trafficking in the United States. *International Journal of Drug Policy*, 23(6), 426–435. doi:10.1016/j.drugpo.2012.07.004

Simonetto, D. A., Oxentenko, A. S., & Herman, M. L. (2012). Cannabinoid hyperemesis: A case series of 98 patients. *Mayo Clinic Proceedings*, 87(2), 114–119. doi:10.1016/j.mayocp.2011.10.005

Simpson, T. L., & Miller, W. R. (2002). Concomitance between childhood sexual and physical abuse and substance use problems. A review. *Clinical Psychology Review*, 22(1), 27–77. doi:10.1016/S0272-7358(00)00088-X

Smith, K. M., Larive, L. L., & Romanelli, F. (2002). Club drugs: Methylenedioxymethamphetamine, flunitrazepam, ketamine hydrochloride, and gamma-hydroxybutyrate. *American Journal of Health-System Pharmacy: AJHP*, 59(11), 1067–1076.

Sorensen, C. J., DeSanto, K., & Borgelt, L. (2016, December 20). Cannabinoid hyperemesis syndrome: Diagnosis, pathophysiology, and treatment—A systematic review. *Journal of Medical Toxicology*, 13(1), 71–87. doi: 10.1007/s13181-016-0595-z

Stein, M. D., Caviness, C. M., & Anderson, B. J. (2014). Alcohol use potentiates marijuana problem severity in young adult women. *Women's Health Issues*, 24(1), e77–e82. doi:10.1016/j.whi.2013.10.005

Tashkin, D. P. (2013). Effects of marijuana smoking on the lung. *Annals of the American Thoracic Society*, 10(3), 239–247. doi:10.1513/AnnalsATS.201212-127FR

Taylor, D. R., Fergusson, D. M., & Milne, B. J. (2002). A longitudinal study of the effects of tobacco and cannabis exposure on lung function in young adults. *Addiction*, 97(8), 1055–1061.

Toklas, A. B. (1954). *The Alice B. Toklas cookbook*. New York, NY: Harper Collins.

Traub, S. J., Hoffman, R. S., & Nelson, L. S. (2002). The "ecstasy" hangover: Hyponatremia due to 3,4-methylenedioxymethamphetamine. *Journal of Urban Health*, 79(4), 549–555.

Trezza, V., Cuomo, V., & Vanderschuren, L. J. (2008). Cannabis and the developing brain: Insights from behavior. *European Journal of Pharmacology* , 585(2–3), 441–452.

van Dijken, G. D., Blom, R. E., & Hene, R. J. (2013). High incidence of mild hyponatremia in females using ecstasy at a rave party. *Nephrology Dialysis Transplantation*, 28(9), 2277–2283. doi:10.1093/ndt/gft023

van Heugten-Van der Kloet, D., Giesbrecht, T., & van Wel, J. (2015). MDMA, cannabis, and cocaine produce acute dissociative symptoms. *Psychiatry Research*, 228(3), 907–912. doi:10.1016/j.psychres.2015.04.028

van Holst, R. J., & Schilt, T. (2011). Drug-related decrease in neuropsychological functions of abstinent drug users. *Current Drug Abuse Reviews*, 4(1), 42–56.

Van Hout, M. C., & Bingham, T. (2013). "Surfing the Silk Road": A study of users' experiences. *International Journal of Drug Policy*, 24(6), 524–529. doi:10.1016/j.drugpo.2013.08.011

Wardle, M. C., Kirkpatrick, M. G., & de Wit, H. (2014). "Ecstasy" as a social drug: MDMA preferentially affects responses to emotional stimuli with social content. *Social Cognitive & Affective Neuroscience*, 9(8), 1076–1081. doi:10.1093/scan/nsu035

West, P. L., Helman, R. S., & McKeown, N. J. (2015, April 20). *Phencyclidine toxicity*. Retrieved from Medscape, pp. 1–3: http://emedicine.medscape.com/article/816348-overview

Williams, S. (2015, July 12). *Washington's marijuana tax revenue tops estimates, but big problems still exist*. Retrieved April 13, 2016, from The Motley Fool, pp. 1–8: www.fool.com/investing/general/2015/07/12/washingtons-marijuana-tax-revenue-tops-estimates-b.aspx

Wilsey, B., Marcotte, T., & Deutsch, R. (2013). Low-dose vaporized cannabis significantly improves neuropathic pain. *The Journal of Pain*, 14(2), 136–148. doi:10.1016/j.pain.2012.10.009

Winstock, A. (2016). *What did we learn from GDS2015? An overview of our key findings.* Retrieved January 12, 2016, from The Global Drug Survey 2015 findings, pp. 1–27: www.globaldrugsurvey.com/the-global-drug-survey-2015-findings/

Wu, L. T., Ringwalt, C. L., & Weiss, R. D. (2009). Hallucinogen-related disorders in a national sample of adolescents: The influence of ecstasy/MDMA use. *Drug and Alcohol Dependence*, 104(1–2), 156–166.

Wu, L. T., Schlenger, W. E., & Galvin, D. M. (2006). Concurrent use of methamphetamine, MDMA, LSD, ketamine, GHB, and flunitrazepam among American youths. *Drug and Alcohol Dependence*, 84(1), 102–113.

Wu, Z. H., Grady, J. J., & Rosales, S. (2011). Ecstasy use and its correlates among young, low-income women. *Substance Use & Misuse*, 46(4), 404–410. doi:10.3109/10826084.2010.501680

7

IDENTIFYING WOMEN'S CONTEMPORANEOUS DIAGNOSES

Contemporaneous diagnosis is a term that we use in this chapter to denote the identification of one, or more, *active* alcohol use disorders (AUDs), and/or one, or more, *active* substance use disorders (SUDs), and/or one, or more, *active* other mental disorders (OMDs) that, occur among women, during the same period of time.[1] Over the years, several closely related terms have been commonly used to denote this complex and varied combination of women's mental disorders, such as:

- *Dual addiction—concomitant alcoholism and drug abuse* (Kreek & Stimmel, 1984)
- *Dual disorder—concurrent diagnosis of alcoholism plus a psychiatric diagnosis* (Daley, Moss, & Campbell, 1987, p. 3)
- *Dual diagnosis—coexistence of a substance use disorder and a separate psychiatric disorder … ranging from a single episode of alcohol abuse to severe daily intravenous opiate dependence* (Stowell, 1991, p. 98)
- *Comorbidity—substance abuse with psychiatric illness … cases of two diagnosable entities in the realm of substance abuse and mental illness* (Belfer, 1993, p. 70)
- *Dual diagnosis—co-occurrence of another disorder (psychiatric or medical) … independent of an addictive disorder* (Miller, Leukefeld, & Jefferson, 1994, p. 169; Pagliaro, 1990, p. 23)

The diversity of these terms and definitions, which has continued into the new millennium, contributes to much semantic confusion in both the published literature and in clinical settings. For example, Drake, Essock, and Sharner (2001, p. 469) defined *dual diagnosis*, as the co-occurrence of *substance abuse* and *severe*

---

[1] This definition can be reflected in a parsimonious manner by the following equation: *(AUD[s] +/- SUD[s]) + (OMD[s]) = contemporaneous diagnosis.*

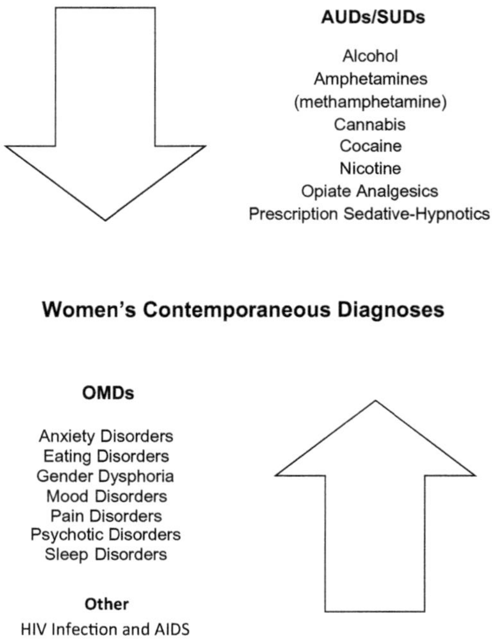

FIGURE 7.1 Mental Disorders Commonly Involved in Women's Contemporaneous Diagnoses

mental illness (i.e., *long-term* psychiatric disorder). In another example, Slesnick and Prestopnik (2005, p. 179) used *multiple diagnosis—two or more mental health diagnoses in addition to a substance use diagnosis.*

To actively address and to try to clarify, or at least minimize, this semantic confusion, we offer the term, *women's contemporaneous diagnosis* (WCD), which we use throughout this text. We define WCD as the diagnosis of one, or more, AUDs, SUDs, *and/or* OMDs[2] among young, middle-aged, or older women, that may, or may *not*, be *directly* related, but are present at the same time (see Figure 7.1).

As originally recognized by Keller, Lavori, and Beardslee (1992), the presence of one or more AUDs and/or SUDs[3] and/or OMDs, is more common than once thought. In fact, among the women in their study, who had been diagnosed with a SUD, almost three-quarters (74%) had *2* to *4* OMDs. More recently, Nauert (2014), using data obtained from the 2012 *National Survey on Drug Use and Health*, found that approximately 8.4 million adults in the U.S. had *both* a SUD and an OMD.

[2] In addition, for the sake of parsimony, and to further reduce semantic confusion, we define the term, *other mental disorder*, as including *all* emotional disorders, mental illnesses, psychiatric disorders, and psychological disorders typically *diagnosed* and *treated* by psychiatrists and psychologists.

[3] Adding to the semantic confusion, many, but not all authors *include* "AUDs" within the label of "SUDs."

In cases in which AUDs, SUDs, and/or OMDs are *directly* related, the AUDs and/or SUDs are *most* commonly either an *antecedent* to, or a *consequence* of, the OMD.[4] An example of the former, is a 19-year-old girl, who, over a few weeks of heavy, *high*-grade marijuana use, develops paranoid psychosis. An example of the latter, is a young woman, who began to regularly use cocaine to *self-medicate* her undiagnosed depression. In many cases, women with OMDs often consciously or unconsciously use drugs and substances of abuse in an attempt to "self-medicate" their OMD(s) (see Table 7.1).

Figure 7.2 illustrates the many possible relationships that can contemporaneously occur among and between AUDs, SUDs, and OMDs.[5]

TABLE 7.1 Drugs and Substances of Abuse Often Used by Women to *Self-Medicate* Other Mental Disorders[a]

Other Mental Disorders	*Drugs or Substances of Abuse Used for Self-Medication*	*Comments*	*References (Examples)*
Anxiety Disorder *(also see, Panic Disorder; Posttraumatic Stress Disorder)*	Alcohol Cannabis	Used to reduce *high* anxiety or "to cope." Both alcohol and cannabis are used to self-medicate anxiety and are associated with a significantly *increased* risk of suicide attempts.	Alegria, Hasin, and Nunes, 2010; Armeli, Todd, & Conner, 2008; Bolton, Cox, & Clara, 2006; Robinson, Sareen, & Cox, 2009.
Bipolar Disorder (BD)	Alcohol	Used to ameliorate manic signs and symptoms (e.g., distractions; flight of ideas; irritability).	Bolton, Robinson, & Sareen, 2009.
Eating Disorders	Amphetamines Caffeine Cocaine Nicotine	Used to control hunger and to help to promote loss/maintenance of body weight.	Greenfield, Back, & Lawson, 2010.

[4] Usually, the distinction as to whether, or not, a mental disorder (e.g., major depressive disorder [MDD]) is an *antecedent to* or a *consequence of* an AUD and/or SUD, is *not* particularly relevant in many clinical contexts. However, in cases where it is an *antecedent*, intervention aimed at its amelioration will also help to ameliorate the related AUD and/or SUD.

[5] These relationships can often be further complicated when young women are considered because they may be actively developing a SUD, and have one or more diagnostic signs and symptoms, but may *not* yet have developed *sufficient* signs and symptoms to meet established diagnostic criteria (i.e., DSM, ICD, or other diagnostic criteria) to satisfy a formal diagnosis of a SUD.

TABLE 7.1 *(cont.)*

Other Mental Disorders	*Drugs or Substances of Abuse Used for Self-Medication*	*Comments*	*References (Examples)*
Major Depressive Disorder (MDD)	Alcohol Cannabis Cocaine Nicotine	Alcohol, a psychodepressant, and cannabis, a psychodelic, are used in an attempt to "forget about" depressing thoughts. Cocaine and nicotine, both of which are psychostimulants, are used to *relieve* the signs and symptoms of depression by *elevating* mood, at least temporarily.	Pagliaro, Jaglalsingh, & Pagliaro, 1992.
Panic Disorder/ Individual Panic Attacks	Alcohol Benzodiazepines Cannabis Opiate Analgesics	Used to manage symptoms of PD or individual panic attacks (e.g., "freaking out").	Valentiner, Mounts, & Deacon, 2004.
Psychotic Disorder (Schizophrenia)	Caffeine Cannabis Nicotine	Used *primarily* to manage negative symptoms (e.g., affect regulation and socialization).	Dekker, Linszen, & De Haan, 2009; Krystal, D'Souza, & Gallinat, 2006; Williams & Gandhi, 2008.
Posttraumatic Stress Disorder (PTSD)	Alcohol Cannabis Opiate Analgesics	Used to *diminish* associated anxieties and fears and to help "stop thinking" about the precipitating PTSD-*eliciting* event.	Leeies, Pagura, & Sareen, 2010; Ouimette, Read, & Wade, 2010.
Sleep Disorders (Insomnia)	Alcohol Benzodiazepines Cannabis Z-Drugs	Used to try to *fall,* or *stay, asleep.*	Pagliaro & Pagliaro, *Clinical Patient Data Files.*

[a] All psychodepressants and psychostimulants have been associated with their own characteristic withdrawal syndromes. Women may continue to use respective drugs and substances of abuse as a means of *self-medication* to prevent, or self-manage, the associated signs and symptoms of their withdrawal syndromes (see Chapters 1–5). An interesting and important note is that the *psychodelics* are *not* used as a means of self-medication to ameliorate the signs and symptoms of withdrawal because their use is *not* generally associated with a formal withdrawal syndrome (see Chapter 6, *Women's Psychodelic Abuse*).

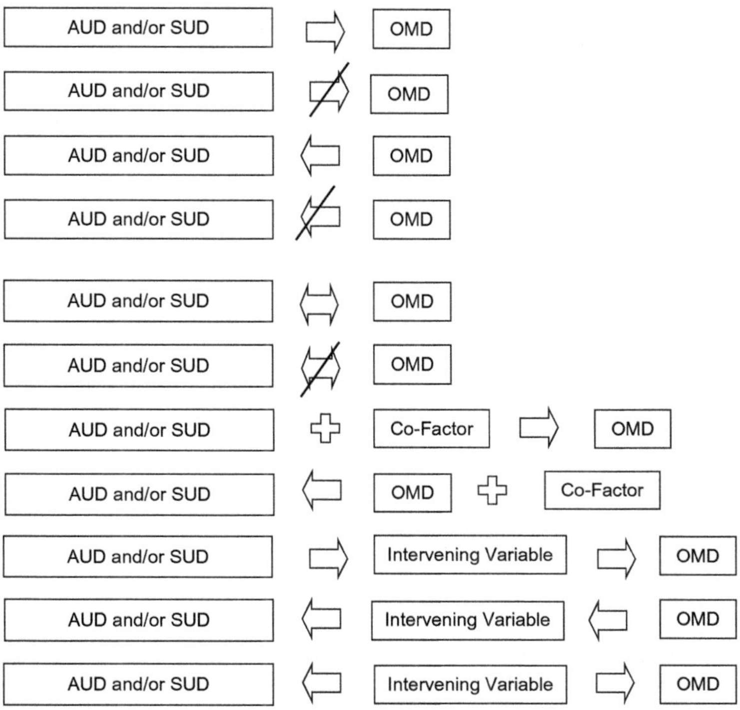

FIGURE 7.2 Possible Relationships Among Mental Disorders in the Context of Women's Contemporaneous Diagnoses

As previously noted, a significant percentage of women, who present with a *primary* diagnosis of an AUD and/or a SUD, can be expected to have a contemporaneous diagnosis.[6] Although several studies and reports have suggested that a contemporaneous diagnosis can be generally expected in approximately 10% to 20% of patients who have an AUD and/or a SUD, the published literature (e.g., Drake, Essock, & Sharner, 2001; Miller, Belkin, & Gibbons, 1994), and the authors' clinical experiences, suggest that the incidence of contemporaneous diagnosis is significantly *higher* (i.e., over 50% and often closer to 100%) among patients whose primary disorder is a significant AUD and/or SUD (e.g., increasingly harmful drug or substance abuse; poly-drug and substance abuse) (Pagliaro & Pagliaro,

[6] In our clinical practice, which specializes in the treatment of contemporaneous diagnoses, we have noted that most of our patients were generally unaware that they had a contemporaneous diagnosis. Generally, the contemporaneous diagnosis had *not* been previously diagnosed and the patients were only consciously aware that they were *depressed* or that they had a *drinking problem* (i.e., the reason for their referral). They were *not* aware that they had two, and generally more, mental disorders and that these *active* disorders were generally highly interrelated (Pagliaro & Pagliaro, *Clinical Patient Data Files*).

Clinical Patient Data Files). Our clinical experience in this regard, which spans over 40 years, supports the claim that the incidence of contemporaneous diagnoses generally is directly proportional to the *severity* of the AUD and/or SUD.

Women with contemporaneous diagnoses often present with other major and significant related health and social care needs or requirements (Pagliaro & Pagliaro, *Clinical Patient Data Files*). These additional needs and requirements include *increased* rates of:

- Academic difficulties (e.g., absenteeism; *dropping out* of, or not completing, high school or college/university; low academic performance)
- Arrest and incarceration[7]
- Difficulty making friends (i.e., poor interpersonal relationships)
- Difficulty maintaining major interpersonal relationships (e.g., with their children, parents, and significant others)
- Job loss and unemployment
- High-risk pregnancy
- Homelessness and reliance on social assistance
- Hospitalization or institutionalization
- Medical disorders (e.g., AIDS; hepatitis; tuberculosis)
- Mothering practices that are abusive or negligent (i.e., mothers with AUDs, and/or SUDs, and OMDs have significantly *higher* rates of committing acts of child abuse and neglect than mothers who do not)[8]
- Non-compliance with prescribed pharmacotherapy and other treatment interventions (e.g., family therapy; group therapy; individual psychotherapy)
- *Poor* responses, or no response, to treatment interventions
- Recidivism, or relapse, in response to treatment intervention
- Suicide, attempted or completed[9]

---

[7] For example, Zlotnick, Clarke, and Friedmann (2008), in their study of offenders newly admitted to a prison substance abuse program, noted that:

> Women were significantly more likely than men to report a lifetime disorder and a lifetime severe disorder. Furthermore, gender differences emerged in the pattern of lifetime psychiatric comorbidity. Women reported greater lifetime major depression, PTSD, eating disorder, and borderline personality disorder.
>
> *(p. 403)*

[8] In addition, mothers with contemporaneous diagnoses, who have neonates or young infants, often have *increased* difficulties regarding healthy maternal-infant bonding, including greater risk for anaclitic depression among infants (Pagliaro & Pagliaro, *Clinical Patient Data Files*; Rasmussen, Borelli, & Decoste, 2016; Ryder & Brisgone, 2013; Suchman, Decoste, & Rosenberger, 2012).

[9] Many researchers (e.g., Pagliaro & Pagliaro 2000; Pagliaro & Pagliaro, *Clinical Patient Data Files*) found a significant relationship between continental descent and AUDs, or SUDs, and suicide among women in the U.S. Hahm, Tzu-Han Chang, and Tong (2014), in their comprehensive review of the published literature concerning suicide among women, also found that suicidal and self-harming behaviors among women of Asian continental descent are significantly mediated by their drug and substance abuse.

Also, these women often display increasingly high-risk behaviors for HIV infection (e.g., unprotected sex with multiple partners; sharing contaminated needles and syringes) (Pagliaro, Pagliaro, & Thauberger, 1993). In this regard, the need for the designation of an identified contemporaneous diagnosis with the addition of a diagnosis of HIV infection (Pagliaro & Pagliaro, 1992) has become increasingly recognized. (See the later section in this chapter, *WCD and Human Immunodeficiency Virus Infection*.)

Women who have a contemporaneous diagnosis may present with any number of possible AUDs, SUDs, and OMDs, often making identification difficult or seemingly impossible. In fact, there seems to be an unending number of combinations and permutations of these co-occurring disorders as illustrated in Figure 7.2. As noted by Stowell (1991), over 25 years ago: "dual diagnosis patients are [generally] heterogeneous as to their psychiatric diagnoses, as well as the various substances they abuse" (p. 98). However, a review of the published literature suggests that, regarding the identification of women's contemporaneous diagnoses (WCDs), the following *seven* drugs and substances of abuse are the most commonly and frequently involved:[10]

- Alcohol
- Amphetamines (methamphetamine)
- Cannabis
- Cocaine
- Nicotine
- Opiate analgesics
- Prescription sedative-hypnotics

In addition, most OMDs involve one or more of the following *seven* categories of mental disorders, which are presented and discussed in the following sections:

1. Anxiety Disorders, including panic disorder (PD), posttraumatic stress disorder (PTSD),[11] and social anxiety disorder (SAD)[12]

---

10 Also, see respective Chapters, 1 through 6, for additional related discussion of each of the seven listed major drugs and substances of abuse that are discussed, specifically in regard to WCDs, in the following sections.

11 Other related terms that are commonly used, but which are *not* included in the DSM, include: *Complex posttraumatic stress disorder* (C-PTSD); *complex trauma* (CT); and *developmental trauma disorder* (DTD), which are associated with interpersonal and social stress that has been endured for a long period (e.g., being cruelly treated by parents or other caregivers; being held hostage by terrorists; being ruthlessly kidnapped or imprisoned).

12 N.B. The abbreviation, "SAD," also is commonly used to denote another mental disorder, "seasonal affective disorder." As such, it serves as a further example of the problems inherent in using abbreviations in a clinical context. Health and social care professionals are urged to minimize the use of abbreviations and, when use is necessary, ensure that the intended meaning is made explicit.

2. Eating Disorders, including anorexia nervosa (AN), bulimia nervosa (BN), and compulsive dieting
3. Gender Dysphoria, as well as, racial dysphoria and ethnic identity disorder
4. Mood Disorders, including bipolar disorder (BD) and major depressive disorder (MDD)
5. Pain Disorders
6. Psychotic Disorders (e.g., schizophrenia)
7. Sleep Disorders (e.g., insomnia)

WCDs: Anxiety Disorders

Contemporaneous diagnoses involving an AUD and/or a SUD with an anxiety disorder (i.e., PD; PTSD) are particularly common among women in the U.S. (Conway, Compton, & Stinson, 2006; Falck, Carlson, & Wang, 2006; Grant, Stinson, & Dawson, 2004; Lai, Cleary, & Sitharthan, 2015; Morris, Stewart, & Ham, 2005). In fact, several researchers (e.g., Stromwall & Larson, 2004) have reported that women are significantly more likely than men to experience anxiety disorders. These anxiety disorders are often associated with a "history of repetitive childhood physical and/or sexual assault" that tends to be chronic, or long-term. The chronic traumatic nature of this pattern of physical and sexual abuse gives rise to several types of anxiety disorders among women, including PD and PTSD (Greenfield, Back, & Lawson, 2010; Pagliaro & Pagliaro, *Clinical Patient Data Files*).

Health and social care professionals are reminded about the importance of sensitivity—compassion, empathy, kindness, understanding, and warmth—when planning, selecting, initiating, and successfully completing therapeutic interventions for women, particularly those who have contemporaneous diagnoses involving histories of mental/physical/sexual abuse. In this context, the provision of gender-specific treatment options may, in many cases, significantly *decrease* a woman's anxiety, and, thus, facilitate her group involvement and participation in the therapeutic process of recovery. (Also, see the later section in this chapter, *WCDs: Gender Dysphoria*, for further related discussion.) In addition, adequate and appropriate attention must be given to the increased risk for suicide among these women (for related discussion, see the later section in this chapter, *WCDs: Mood Disorders*).

Panic Disorder (PD) and Individual Panic Attacks

In the formulation of a WCD that includes PD and/or individual panic attacks, one or more different drugs and substances of abuse can be involved (e.g., Goodwin, Lieb, & Hoefler, 2004).[13] These drugs and substances of abuse most frequently include:

---

[13] Additionally, it is common for women to use *more* than one drug or substance of abuse from the following list to "self-medicate," or "cope," with their anxiety (Pagliaro & Pagliaro, *Clinical Patient Data Files*). For example, McHugh, Votaw, and Bogunovic (2017), in their study of adults undergoing

- Alcohol
- Benzodiazepines
- Cannabis
- Cocaine
- MDMA
- Nicotine
- Opiate analgesics
- Prescription sedative-hypnotics

Although the relationship between a drug or substance of abuse and PD, or individual panic attacks, can be variable (see Figure 7.2), *three* major contextual relationships have been identified:

1. *Women* may use a drug or substance of abuse, such as *cannabis*, *cocaine*, or *MDMA* (ecstasy) that induces PD, or individual panic attacks, as a *direct* result of its pharmacological actions[14]
2. *Women* may abruptly discontinue the regular, long-term use of a drug or substance of abuse, such as *alcohol* or *nicotine*, that *induces* PD or individual panic attacks
3. *Women* may personally use a drug or substance of abuse, particularly: *alcohol*; *benzodiazepines*; *opiate* analgesics; and *prescription sedative-hypnotics* to "self-medicate" their PD, or individual panic attacks, in an attempt to ameliorate related symptoms

In addition, an AUD and/or a SUD and a PD may be *independently* related to each other—as well as to another factor or co-factor, such as a medical condition or procedure, including induced abortion (see Figure 7.2).

Posttraumatic Stress Disorder (PTSD)

As found by Stromwall and Larson (2004), in their study of 754 women and men, who were receiving community mental health services:

> Women were almost seven times more likely than men in this sample to have a diagnosis of posttraumatic stress disorder in conjunction with substance abuse.
>
> *(p. 81)*

---

treatment for "opioid use disorders," found that women, but *not* men, used benzodiazepines to cope with anxiety.

14 N.B. Recognizing the significance of WCDs and women's needs for optimal professional health and social care attention and services, we do *not* agree with, nor follow, the DSM diagnostic criterion that a panic disorder must *not* be due to the direct pharmacologic effect of a drug or substance of abuse.

The most common cause of PTSD among women is trauma that, generally, is directly related to acute, or relatively brief, but extremely terrifying, experiences— or to prolonged torture or years of extreme physical, psychological, and/or sexual abuse (e.g., Najavits, Weiss, & Shaw, 1997). (For additional related discussion, see later section in this chapter, *WCDs: Gender Dysphoria.*) Another common cause of PTSD among women, which also may have begun during childhood or adolescence, is *bullying* by other children and adolescents (Pagliaro & Pagliaro, *Clinical Patient Data Files*).

Women, who have PTSD, reportedly are 3 to 5 times *more* likely to develop an AUD and/or a SUD[15] than women who do *not* (Ouimette & Brown, 2003; Reed, Anthony, & Breslau, 2007). As found by Sullivan, Weiss, and Flanagan (2016), in their study of PTSD and daily co-occurrence of drug and alcohol use among women experiencing intimate partner violence (IPV):

> Women with PTSD, compared to those without, were nearly 15 times more likely to have days of co-occurrence of drug and alcohol use and nearly 7 times more likely to have days of drug use alone.
>
> *(p. 36)*

In this context, WCDs, AUDs and/or SUDs, particularly those involving other psychodepressants, are frequently implicated (Eggleston, Calhoun, & Svikis, 2009; Johnson, Cottier, & Callahan O'Leary, 2010).[16] As noted by Najavits, Weiss, and Shaw (1997), 20 years ago, the rates of PTSD ranged from 30% to 60% among women, who abused drugs and substances of abuse. The *highest* occurrence of WCDs involving an AUD and/or SUD and PTSD has been reported for women incarcerated in urban and rural jails (Lynch, Dehart, & Belknap, 2014).[17] Findings from this report may be partially accounted for by the observation by Cohen,

---

[15] Although a variety of SUDs, including those involving cocaine or opiate analgesics, have been related to PTSD among women, AUDs are *most* commonly encountered. Interestingly, research suggests that the intensity or severity of the involved AUD can be better predicted by the woman's positive *alcohol expectancies* (i.e., her perceptions of the relief provided by alcohol use) than by the *severity* of the PTSD (Pederson, Myers, & Browne, 2014; Schaumberg, Vinci, & Raiker, 2015).

[16] In addition, eating disorders also have been reported to occur with a *high* incidence in this context. As noted by Killeen, Brewerton, and Campbell, in their study of women with PTSD and comorbid SUDs (2015):

> Eating disorders occur more frequently in SUD populations than in the general population, with the highest reported rates of co-occurrence in individuals with bulimia nervosa and AUDs.
>
> *(p. 547)*

See related discussion in the following section, *WCDs: Eating Disorders.*

[17] N.B. Another group of women, for which a significant incidence of PTSD and concurrent SUD(s) has been documented by several researchers (e.g., Bowe & Rosenheck, 2015), is women veterans. This number is *increasing* primarily in response to the growing numbers of women in the U.S. military, particularly those in active combat roles.

Field, and Campbell (2013), that, when a SUD and PTSD are left untreated, IPV is exacerbated, as are related poor outcomes for women in terms of successful intervention/treatment of the AUD and/or SUD and PTSD.[18]

As noted by Franco (2007):

> American women are more at risk for PTSD than men as a result of the high frequency of sexual and domestic physical abuse that women experience.
>
> *(p. 103)*

For example:

> U.S. pop star Lady Gaga says she has been suffering from posttraumatic stress disorder (PTSD) since being raped at the age of 19.
>
> *(BBC, 2016, p. 1)*[19]

Numerous researchers have found that the incidence of physical or sexual abuse among women, who abuse drugs and substances of abuse, and who also have PTSD, commonly exceed 50% (Greenfield, Back, & Lawson, 2010). In addition, as noted by Tuchman (2010):

> Prevalence rates of intimate partner violence among women in drug treatment have been found to range between 25% and 57%. These rates of intimate partner violence are substantially higher than the range of 1.5% to 16% prevalence rates found in epidemiological surveys of community-based samples of non-drug using women.
>
> *(p. 131)*

Many agree that the associated use of drugs and substances of abuse often begins as an attempt to assuage the fear, negative emotions, nightmares, and pain—including feelings of shame and helplessness related to bullying, IPV, imprisonment, or sexual abuse—that commonly are associated with PTSD among women (Ouimette & Brown, 2003; Reed, Anthony, & Breslau, 2007; Schaumberg, Vinci, & Raiker, 2015).[20] Although, as noted by Brady, Killeen, and Brewerton (2000), this situation lends itself to becoming a vicious cycle because the acute

---

[18] Correspondingly, Myers, Browne, and Norman (2015), in their study of female survivors of IPV, who were enrolled in treatment for both related PTSD and AUD, found that women who were *most* likely to actively engage in treatment: (1) were older; (2) had fewer dependents; (3) had more *severe* PTSD symptoms; and (4) had a *longer* history of heavy drinking.

[19] Rape, including "drug- or alcohol-facilitated/incapacitated rape," is often associated with PTSD and suicide ideation (Gilmore, Walsh, & Badour, 2017, p. 1).

[20] N.B. Interestingly, women, who are exposed to PTSD-level traumas, and do *not* succumb, or otherwise develop criteria for a diagnosis of PTSD, are *not* at increased risk for the subsequent development of an AUD or a SUD (Breslau, 2002; Breslau, Davis, & Schultz, 2003). Perhaps, reflective of existential philosophy, these *survivors become stronger at the broken places* (Hemingway, 1929).

withdrawal associated with the abrupt discontinuation of drugs and substances of abuse, tends to aggravate, heighten, intensify, or worsen, the signs and symptoms that their use was meant to ameliorate.

Another "caution" regarding the treatment of PTSD, which involves the drugs and substances of abuse, is specifically related to concerns involving marijuana use. In the past, and for some time, marijuana has been frequently used to self-medicate the signs and symptoms of anxiety disorders, including PTSD (Pagliaro & Pagliaro, *Clinical Patient Data Files*).[21] More recently, several states have legalized the use of medicinal marijuana for the treatment of PTSD. (See related discussion in Chapter 6, *Women's Psychodelic Abuse*, "Cannabis" section.) However, this specific use of marijuana is *not* devoid of significant risks. For example, in an observational study of 2,276 veterans with PTSD, who were admitted to specialized Veterans Association (VA) treatment programs, Wilkinson, Stefanovics, and Rosenheck (2015) found that:

> Marijuana use was significantly associated with worse outcomes in PTSD symptom severity, violent behavior, and measures of alcohol and drug use when compared with stoppers and never-users … initiating marijuana use after treatment was associated with worse PTSD symptoms, more violent behavior, and alcohol use. Marijuana may actually worsen PTSD symptoms or nullify the benefits of specialized, intensive treatment. Cessation or prevention of use may be an important goal of treatment.
>
> *(p. 1174)*

WCDs: Eating Disorders

> In general, overconcern about body weight puts women at risk for problematic drinking, as evidenced by the high comorbidity between eating disorders and AUDs. This is not only true for women with restrictive and purging eating disorders, but also women who are overweight or obese.
>
> *(Glanton Holzhauer, Zenner, & Wulfert, 2016, p. 122)*

Eating disorders, which commonly occur primarily among women,[22] have been widely recognized and clinically addressed in the U.S. since the middle of the

---

21 For example, several women, including both patients and colleagues, have shared with us over the years that they "deal with" their "fear of flying" by smoking a marijuana joint, or reefer, prior to going to the airport. Upon arrival at the airport, they have a drink or two at the airport bar, or swallow an "Ativan®" (i.e., lorazepam, a benzodiazepine), prior to boarding their flight (Pagliaro & Pagliaro, *Clinical Patient Data Files*).

22 Several authors (e.g., Greenfield, Back, & Lawson, 2010) have reported that, in the U.S., when compared to men, over 90% of eating disorders occur among women.

last century. However, they have *not* been generally recognized as a formal integral component of WCDs until the new millennium (e.g., Cohen, Greenfield, & Gordon, 2010; Dansky, Brewerton, & Kilpatrick, 2000; Killeen, Brewerton, & Campbell, 2015). The three eating disorders most commonly identified among women during the new millennium in the U.S. are:

1. *Anorexia nervosa* (AN), national incidence 4%
2. *Bulimia nervosa* (BN), national incidence 2%
3. *Binge eating disorder* (BED), national incidence, 2%

(Smink, van Hoeken, & Hoek, 2013)

The incidence of comorbid eating disorders among women appears to vary by continental and other descent. For example, in their study that included approximately 650 women, who had participated in the *Collaboration Study on the Genetics of Alcoholism*, Hesselbrock, Hesselbrock, and Segal (2003) found that: (1) *AN* occurred primarily among women of European descent; (2) *BN* occurred primarily among women of European descent, closely followed in lifetime incidence by women of African descent; and (3) women of Hispanic descent did *not* report either of the eating disorders (i.e., *overall*, eating disorders, and related WDCs, occur predominantly among women in the U.S. who are of European descent).

Eating disorders also are commonly encountered among older women, particularly "baby boomers," who were born between the post-World War II years, 1946–1964. For example, in their review of related published literature, Mangweth-Matzek, Hoek, and Pope (2014) found that:

> Pathological eating behaviors and frank eating disorders are surprisingly common in older women, as are associated body-image disturbances.
>
> *(p. 431)*

Finally, although still frequently overlooked, eating disorders also commonly occur among women who are seeking treatment for AUDs and SUDs (Bulik, Klump, & Thornton, 2004; Franko, Dorer, & Keel, 2008; Warren, Lindsay, & White, 2013; Wu, Gersing, & Swartz, 2013). For example, in a study of women residing at Oxford Houses—low-cost, self-governed homes for long-term drug and substance abuse treatment across the U.S.—Czarlinski, Aase, and Jason (2012) found that 75% of woman residents, who had eating disorders, also reported drug and substance abuse. As noted by the researchers:

> Present findings suggest that young adult and middle-aged women in recovery from an SUD appear to be at a high risk for binge eating disorder.
>
> *(p. 190)*

In another study of women in treatment for substance abuse, Warren, Lindsay, and White (2013) found that:

> The majority of participants were concerned about gaining weight during treatment and/or that weight gain could trigger drug relapse.
>
> *(p. 494)*

In this context, Cohen, Greenfield, and Gordon (2010) noted that, in their sample of "substance abusing women with co-occurring PTSD," women, who reported at least one episode of binge eating during the previous month, were significantly *less* likely to respond favorably to SUD/PTSD group therapy. Also, in a related context, Elmquist, Shorey, and Anderson (2015), in their study of 122 women enrolled in residential treatment for SUDs, found that:

> Eating disorder symptoms were significantly associated with decisions to leave treatment against medical advice after controlling for age, years of education, depressive symptoms, alcohol problems, and drug problems.
>
> *(p. 233)*

Several researchers (e.g., Becker & Grilo, 2015) also have identified that anxiety and mood disorders (see related sections in this chapter) are commonly encountered among women who have both a SUD and an eating disorder.[23] In this regard, it has been suggested by several researchers (e.g., Greenfield, Back, & Lawson, 2010; Schoemaker, Smit, & Bijl, 2002) that contemporaneous disorders among women involving an: (1) AUD and/or SUD; (2) eating disorder; and (3) mood disorder may be related by various underlying, common etiological mechanisms, including:[24]

- Personality, or personality factors—such as avoidant-insecure subtypes or behaviorally dysregulated personality that facilitate the development of both eating disorders and SUDs (e.g., Thompson-Brenner, Eddy, & Franko, 2008)
- "Self-medication" (i.e., "emotional" eating; substance abuse) to alleviate negative affect, specifically regarding the anxiety disorder(s) and mood disorder(s) (e.g., Spence & Courbasson, 2012)

---

23 Eating disorders, specifically AN and BN, also have been noted to occur among adults with A-D/HD (Cumyn, French, & Hechtman, 2009).

24 In addition, several researchers note that these intervening relationships may be contextual and *not* fixed. For example, Dunn, Neighbors, and Fossos, 2009) identified that:

> Associations between disordered eating behaviors and negative consequences resulting from alcohol and drug use among collegiate women suggest that temporal precedence depends on the particular symptoms and substances assessed.
>
> *(p. 114)*

- History of physical and/or sexual abuse, which predisposes women to contemporaneous diagnoses (e.g., Greenfield, Back, & Lawson, 2010; Schoemaker, Smit, & Bijl, 2002)

It has become common knowledge that women frequently use the psychostimulants for their anorexiant effects (e.g., to lose or maintain body weight). (Also, see Chapter 4, *Women's Caffeine and Nicotine Abuse*, and Chapter 5, *Women's Amphetamine and Cocaine Abuse*.) As identified by others, women who have contemporaneous diagnoses involving eating disorders are particularly prone to have *higher* rates of caffeine (e.g., Burgalassi, Ramacciotti, & Bianchi, 2009) and nicotine use (e.g., White and Grilo (2006). (See Chapter 4, *Women's Caffeine and Nicotine Abuse*.) In addition, because of the well-recognized *increased* appetite, or feeling of hunger (i.e., "munchies"), associated with cannabis use (see Chapter 6, *Women's Psychodelic Abuse*), it is *not* surprising that several researchers (e.g., Herzog, Franko, & Dorer, 2006) have reported a *high* incidence of cannabis use among women, who have eating disorders.

WCDs: Gender Dysphoria

AUDs, particularly, and/or SUDs (e.g., cannabis use disorder, cocaine use disorder) are often involved with gender dysphoria[25] in the formulation of WCDs. Gender dysphoria is diagnosed among young, middle-aged, and older women, including bisexual, lesbian, and trans women (i.e., male-to-female, or "MTF"). AUDs and/or SUDs can be directly related to gender dysphoria, as well as OMDs including IPV and MDD, within the context of a woman's lifestyle and experiences that are often associated with mental, physical, or sexual abuse (e.g., Dunlap, Golub, & Johnson, 2003; Kendler, Bulik, & Silberg, 2000). The abuse is often perpetrated by a *trusted adult*, including a parent or other family member, teacher, or athletic coach. An adolescent girl also may have been victimized by a boyfriend or girlfriend of similar age or by an adult sexual predator. They also may become involved in sex-for-drug exchanges and sex slavery.

As noted by Bulik, Prescott, and Kendler (2001), child sexual abuse "tends to function more as a non-specific risk factor that is associated with increased later risk for a range of psychiatric and substance use syndromes" (p. 448). The victims of childhood sexual abuse are often first diagnosed with MDD or PTSD, which is then followed by a diagnosis of a SUD (Cohen, Mannarino, & Zhitova, 2003; Hussey, Chang, & Kotch, 2006; Simpson & Miller, 2002). Perhaps, *not* surprisingly, given the nature and extent of associated childhood suffering, related

---

[25] *Gender dysphoria*, previously identified as gender identity disorder by DSM, can be defined as a state of unease, or dissatisfaction, with the life that a person experiences because of the sex (i.e., female or male genitalia, or DNA) and gender (i.e., social and cultural differences assigned to males or females) that they were assigned at birth.

AUDs and/or SUDs among adolescents (and adults) tend to be severe and to have a more morbid course, including a poor long-term prognosis (Pagliaro & Pagliaro, *Clinical Patient Data Files*; Westermeyer, Wahmanholm, & Thuras, 2001). (For further related discussion, also see previous sections, *WCDs: Anxiety Disorders*, "PTSD," and the following section, *WCDs: Mood Disorders*, "MDD.")

Adolescent girls and young women, who have gender dysphoria, also are at significant risk for AUDs and/or SUDs (e.g., Keuroghlian, Reisner, & White, 2015; Nelson, Heath, & Lynskey, 2006). In addition, girls and young women, who are lesbian, are at *increased* risk of AUDs, particularly, and/or SUDs (Hughes, 2005; Rosario, 2008; Rosario, Schrimshaw, & Hunter, 2004, 2008). They also are at risk for HIV infection (see later section, *WCDs: Human Immunodeficiency Virus Infection*). Histories of childhood sexual abuse, bullying, depression, and family rejection are significant among these adolescent girls and young women and appear to play a major role regarding the development of AUDs and/or SUDs (Cochran, Mays, & Alegria, 2007; Hughes, 2003; Padilla, Crisp, & Rew, 2010; Ryan, Huebner, & Diaz, 2009). For related discussion, also see previous section, *WCDs: Anxiety Disorders*, "PTSD" and the following section, *WCDs: Mood Disorders*.

WCDs: Mood Disorders

Similar to the anxiety disorders, *mood disorders* are frequently involved in contemporaneous diagnoses (Falck, Carlson, & Wang, 2006; Grant, Stinson, & Dawson, 2004; Lai, Cleary, & Sitharthan, 2015; Stromwall & Larson, 2004), particularly among women. Bolton, Robinson, and Sareen (2009), in their analysis of the data from 43,000 community-dwelling adults with diagnoses of mental illness and who participated in the *National Epidemiologic Survey on Alcohol and Related Conditions* (NESARC), found that:

> Almost one-quarter of individuals with mood disorders (24.1%) used alcohol or drugs to relieve symptoms.
>
> *(p. 367)*

As explained by Conway, Compton, and Stinson (2006):

> Greater comorbidity between mood and anxiety and drug use disorders among women may reflect greater deviance and psychopathology among drug-using women than men.
>
> *(p. 247)*

It has been noted (e.g., Bolton, Robinson, & Sareen, 2009) that "self-medication" with the drugs and substances of abuse is common among adults with mood disorders, particularly bipolar disorder. This section considers AUDs and/or SUDs that are commonly involved in the formulation of WCDs that involve *two* particular mood disorders: (1) *bipolar disorder* (BD); and (2) *major depressive disorder* (MDD).

Bipolar Disorder (BD)

Bipolar disorder commonly occurs with AUDs and/or SUDs in the formulation of WCDs (Hunt, Malhi, & Cleary, 2016; Sonne & Brady, 2002; Strakowski, DelBello, & Fleck, 2000). The occurrence of this WCD is variable (Krishnan, 2005).[26] It is estimated that about half of the adults, who have bipolar disorder, also "have an alcohol abuse problem at some point of their lifetime" (Azorin, Bowden, & Garay, 2010, p. 37). Further, as noted by Hunt, Malhi, and Cleary (2016), in their retrospective meta-analysis of nine household surveys involving over 218,000 subjects:

> The meta-analysis revealed that people with an alcohol use disorder were 4.1 times of greater risk of having a BD compared to those without an AUD. The risks were even higher for illicit drug users where they were 5.0 times of greater risk of having BD compared to non-users.
>
> *(p. 1)*

In addition, it has often been noted (e.g., Heffner, Strawn, & DelBello, 2011) that nicotine dependence, as denoted by cigarette smoking, is significantly *more* prevalent among adults with bipolar disorder than those without the disorder.

In some case reports and studies, the BD *precedes* the AUD and/or SUD and, in others, it *follows* (see Figure 7.2). However, for the clear majority of cases, BD appears to *precede* the development of an AUD and/or SUD (Goldstein & Bukstein, 2010). This observation is consistent with the finding of Bolton, Robinson, and Sareen (2009) that the: (1) *highest* incidence of self-medication among community-dwelling adults with mental illness was among those with a diagnosis of BD; and (2) observed incidence was 41%. For example, Carrie Fisher, a well-known actress and author, was quite open about her life-long battle with BD and her related abuse of alcohol, nicotine, opiate analgesics, and other drugs and substances of abuse—in response to, or to "deal with" her mental disorder (Howard, 2016). In an interview, which appeared in *Psychology Today*, she shared that:

> Her drug use was a way to "dial down" the manic in her. And in some respects, it was a form of self-medication … At her worst, she took 30 Percodan® a day.[27]
>
> *(Ma, 2001, p. 3)*

---

[26] An often-overlooked group, in regard to this particular WCD, is elderly women (Lala & Sajatovic, 2012).

[27] Percodan® is a combination analgesic that contains the opiate analgesic, oxycodone (see Chapter 1, *Women's Opiate Analgesic Abuse*).

Among those with an AUD and/or SUD and BD, risk for suicide attempts, and completion, is significantly increased (Carra, Bartoli, & Crocamo, 2014; Finseth, Morken, & Andreassen, 2012; Sublette, Carballo, & Moreno, 2009; Yoon, Chen, & Yi, 2011). In this regard, it should be noted that BD among women is characterized by a predominance of depression (Azorin, Belzeaux, & Kaladjian, 2013; Nivoli, Pacchiarotti, & Rosa, 2011) and this factor very likely contributes in a significant manner to the observed *high* rates of suicide attempts and completions. (Also, see related discussion on suicide in the following section, *Major Depressive Disorder.*)

Major Depressive Disorder (MDD)

In their review of the co-occurrence of MDD and SUDs, Davis, Uezato, and Newell (2008) found that:

> Nearly one-third of patients with major depressive disorder also have substance use disorders.
>
> *(p. 14)*

In comparison, among veterans identified by the Veterans Health Administration (VHA) during 2012 as having MDD, approximately 20% had a concurrent AUD (Yoon, Petrakis, & Rosenheck, 2015).[28]

Contemporaneous diagnoses that involve AUD(s) and/or SUD(s) and MDD are *more* often identified among women than men (Caton, Xie, & Drake, 2014; Falck, Carlson, & Wang, 2006; Gamble, Talbot, & Cashman-Brown, 2013). They also are occurring at an *increasing* rate among *older* women in the U.S.

Alcohol Use Disorder (AUD) and MDD

Genetic factors have been cited as a major contributing factor to the comorbidity of alcoholism and MDD. As noted by Nurnberger, Foroud, and Flury (2002), "This combination of alcoholism and depression tends to run in families" (p. 233). In addition, Austin and Irwin (2010), in their analysis of data from the *Lesbian Social Life Study* that involved responses from 1,141 "self-identified Southern lesbians," found that alcohol abuse was *most* commonly associated with depression.

Reporting on data obtained from the *National Epidemiologic Survey on Alcoholism and Related Conditions*, which sampled over 43,000 respondents in the U.S., 18 years-of-age or older, Hasin, Goodwin, and Stinson (2005) found *lifetime* estimates of MDD to be approximately 13%, and *12-month* estimates of MDD to be approximately 5%. Of some concern is the observation that the reported incidence of

[28] The study did *not* include SUDs.

MDD has significantly *increased* from 1980 to 2010. For some time, a major contributor to this increase has been the related *increase* in the contemporaneous diagnoses involving AUD and MDD among *older* women (Satre, Sterling, & Mackin, 2011).

Depression is often integrally related to situational life factors among women of all ages and all socioeconomic levels. However, for women between menarche and menopause, depression also is directly related to hormone secretions during the luteal phase of the menstrual cycle and this contributes directly to the premenstrual dysphoric disorder (PMDD) (Miller, Girgis, & Gupta, 2009; Zukov, Ptacek, & Raboch, 2010). (For related discussion concerning the effects of the menstrual cycle, also see Chapter 8, *Preventing and Treating Women's Drug and Substance Abuse*.)

The diagnosis of depression, in all its various forms, also is potentially *more* varied and *more* complex among women. For example, Holbrook and Kaltenbach (2012), in a study of pregnant women enrolled in a drug and substance abuse treatment program, found that 30.4% had *moderate to severe* prenatal depression and 43.7% had postnatal depression—in addition to an AUD.[29] The significance of this contemporaneous diagnosis among pregnant and post-partum women, has *not* been fully recognized although several specific intervention programs have been developed and implemented, including CARES (Worley, Conners, & Crone, 2005).

However, as noted by Seay and Kohl (2015), the contemporaneous occurrence of depression and SUDs is "highly prevalent among mothers involved with the child welfare system" and, these mothers "had the poorest self-reported parenting and child behavior problems over time" (i.e., were the poorest historians in terms of the accurate self-identification and reporting of significant parenting and child behavior problems) (p. 899).

As with OMDs, MDD can occur as an *antecedent* or *consequence* of an AUD and/or a SUD, particularly when *psychodepressants* are involved[30,31] (Wu & Blazer, 2014). As noted by Greenbaum, Prange, and Friedman (1991):

> Among the dually diagnosed, controversy exists as to whether substance abuse is a symptom of an underlying mental health problem or conversely, whether the mental health problem is symptomatic of alcohol or drug use. *(p. 582)*

---

[29] There is a consensus among researchers (e.g., Coleman-Cowger, 2012) that WCDs involving MDD among pre- and post-partum women, has particularly *high* rates among those who are either of African continental descent or Hispanic descent. However, these groups, generally, have received the *least* amount of needed therapeutic intervention.

[30] Of the drugs and substances of abuse, alcohol and the other sedative-hypnotics (e.g., benzodiazepines) are those that are the most prominently involved in MDD. Alcohol and the benzodiazepines also happen to be the sedative-hypnotics that are the most commonly abused by women (see Chapter 2, *Women's Alcohol Abuse*, and Chapter 3, *Women's Prescription Sedative-Hypnotic Abuse*).

[31] It also can occur together with an AUD as the result of a shared, underlying *co-factor* (Hasin, Stinson, and Ogburn, 2007, as illustrated in Figure 7.2). For example, the inter-relationship among AUD, MDD, and PTSD (Breslau, Davis, & Peterson, 1997). (Also, see earlier related discussion in the section, *WCDs: Anxiety Disorders*, "PTSD.")

Twenty-five years later, this controversy remains unresolved. As found by Lo, Cheng, and de la Rosa (2015), "empirical evidence," from their study of depression and substance use, "only partially supported the self-medication hypothesis" (p. 1274).

For several decades, many reasons have been suggested for an *antecedent* association. For example, among women who have *not* yet been diagnosed as being depressed, a tendency to *self-medicate* with alcohol is commonly observed as an attempt to temporarily diminish the distressing features, including the signs and symptoms of depression. As described by Boyle and Offord (1991), "The risks for drug and alcohol abuse are high among young adults experiencing depression or anxiety who are not undergoing treatment" (p. 699). Or, as identified by Burke, Burke, and Rae (1994), "Age at onset for drug abuse and dependence ... appears to peak in the age interval of 15 to 19 if there is a pre-existing mood or anxiety disorder" (p. 454).

A large study aimed at disentangling the relationship between alcohol problems and depressive symptoms among adolescent girls and young women was conducted by Marmorstein (2009). Participants for this study were drawn from the *National Longitudinal Study of Adolescent Health* using a sample of over 20,000 adolescents. As reported by Marmorstein:

> The results of this study indicate that alcohol use-related problems and depressive symptoms have reciprocal, positive effects on each other during the period from early adolescence through early adulthood; however, these effects differ somewhat by gender and age. Overall, higher levels of depressive symptoms were associated with higher initial levels of alcohol problems (particularly among females), as well as faster increases in alcohol problems over time among males. Reciprocally, high levels of alcohol problems were associated with higher initial levels of depressive symptoms (particularly among females).
>
> *(p. 49)*

Suggested reasons for a *consequential* association between an AUD and MDD include: "physiological symptoms of withdrawal, the apathy of the alcoholic personality, the state of chronic intoxication, and concomitant drug use" (Gold & Slaby, 1991, p. 1). In this regard, it is important to note that the principal *direct* pharmacologic effect of alcohol, and other psychodepressants, is *depression* of the CNS (Pagliaro & Pagliaro, 1999, 2009). (Also, see related discussion in Chapters 1, 2, and 3, *Women's Opiate Analgesic Abuse*, *Women's Alcohol Abuse*, and *Women's Prescription Sedative-Hypnotic Abuse*, respectively.) Consonant with the expected pharmacological actions associated with alcohol use, Satre, Chi, and Eisendrath (2011) identified that the alcohol-related actions appear to occur along a continuum in the context of contribution to depression. Thus, the researchers could identify and examine "sub-diagnostic alcohol use and related problems among psychiatric outpatients with depression" (p. 695).

Regardless of the nature of the association between AUD and MDD (i.e., as either an *antecedent* or *consequence*), of particular concern is the fact that, this particular contemporaneous diagnosis is all too frequently accompanied by suicide attempts and completed suicides (Grant, Stinson, & Dawson, 2004)—particularly when AUDs are involved (Carballo, Bird, & Giner, 2007; Davis, Uezato, & Newell, 2008; Ruiz, Douglas, & Edens, 2012; Sher, 2006). As suggested by Sher, Sperling, and Stanley (2007), suicide attempts and completed suicides are probably due to both the impaired higher level cognitive control of aggression and increased impulsivity that is mediated by using alcohol.[32]

As noted by Rich and Runeson (1992), "Depressive and substance use disorders predominate in the psychopathological backgrounds of suicides of all ages. In five published studies of consecutive suicides by women, the average reported rates are 41% for major depression and 48% for substance abuse" (p. 335). As further noted by Quinnett (1995): "The most dangerous combination of risk factors [for suicide] for people of any age is untreated depression combined with substance abuse and addiction" (p. 65).[33]

Cannabis Use Disorder (CUD) and MDD

As noted by Aspis, Feingold, and Weiser (2015):

> Cannabis is the *most* widely used illicit substance among individuals with depressive disorders.
>
> *(p. 341)*

The effects of cannabis on mood (e.g., causing or exacerbating depression), appear to be mediated by the actions of the endocannabinoid system on neurotransmitters, particularly serotonin (see Chapter 6, *Women's Psychodelic Abuse*, "Cannabis" section—Pharmacology, Mechanism of Action). Several studies and reports (e.g., Pagliaro & Pagliaro, *Clinical Patient Data Files*) have found that a significant number of cannabis users—perhaps up to one-third—use marijuana to *self-medicate* a variety of disorders, including depression.

However, the use of cannabis can worsen or intensify depression and, thus, significantly *increase* the occurrence of suicidal thoughts and suicide attempts.

---

32 N.B. Both suggested mechanisms are *directly* related to the expected pharmacologic action of alcohol as a psychodepressant that *decreases* executive cognitive functioning (see Chapter 2, *Women's Alcohol Abuse*).

33 Interestingly, among new millennial women of college age, *opiate analgesic* use was found to be significantly associated with depressive symptoms and suicidality (Zullig & Divin, 2012).

Combination pharmacotherapy (e.g., fluoxetine, Prozac®) and psychotherapy, in the form of behavioral therapy, have been demonstrated to be an effective intervention for this contemporaneous diagnosis. Among a large U.S. community cohort of mixed-gendered participants of predominantly African descent (90%), Green, Zebrak, and Fothergill (2012) found that the early onset of cannabis use during adolescence was associated with the development of *both* a CUD and an MDD in adulthood. In addition, Khan, Secades-Villa, and Okuda (2013), in their large nationally representative U.S. sample of adults with a CUD, including 1,217 women, found that over 90% (i.e., 94.1% for women) had a contemporaneous diagnosis. For women with a CUD, anxiety and mood disorders were the most frequently encountered other mental disorders (OMDs). Finally, in their study of over 3,400 patients with a diagnosis of "depressive disorder" associated with cannabis use, Aspis, Feingold, and Weiser (2015, p. 341) found that depression was adversely affected to a significant degree *only* among "women who used cannabis regularly" (i.e., at least weekly).

Cocaine Use Disorder and MDD

Women, who are depressed, and who have *not* yet been diagnosed or otherwise treated for depression, often use cocaine as a means to *self-medicate* their depression (Pagliaro, Jaglalsingh, & Pagliaro, 1992; Pagliaro & Pagliaro, *Clinical Patient Data Files*). (Also, see related discussion in Chapter 5, *Women's Amphetamine and Cocaine Abuse.*)

Nicotine Use Disorder and MDD

Janes, Pedrelli, and Whitton (2015, p. 1940) identified that "major depressive disorder (MDD) and nicotine dependence are highly comorbid, with studies showing that approximately 50% of individuals with MDD smoke." For example, Berg, Wen, and Cummings (2013), in their secondary logistical regression analysis of data from almost 40,000 adult participants in the 2008 *National Survey on Drug Use and Health*, found significant effects related to smoking behavior. Current smokers more frequently reported a major depressive episode, AUD, and *illicit* drug dependence.

Jessup, Dibble, and Cooper (2012), in a study of smoking and behavioral health in women, found that smokers had *higher* rates of concurrent AUDs, SUDs, and OMDs, including: anxiety; depression; and PTSD; as well as childhood abuse, IPV, and suicidality. In addition, one-third of the Jessup, Dibble, and Cooper (2012) sample self-identified as smokers, and the *highest* rates of smoking were reported by bisexual women and women of either African continental descent or American Indian descent. Although not yet demonstrated, it is quite likely that nicotine use among women with depressive disorders is, at least partially, employed as a means of *self-medication* for the management of their depression.

Regarding nicotine use disorder and MDD, the addition of alcohol abuse, or AUD, is correlated with both an *increase* in nicotine use and an *increase* in depression and/or its signs and symptoms. Adding chronic moderate to severe pain[34] to this combination of disorders *increases* the severity of both nicotine use disorder and major depressive disorder. (Also, see related discussion in Chapter 2, *Women's Alcohol Abuse.*)

Successful interventions, in terms of smoking cessation, have been repeatedly associated with adequate clinical attention to comorbid depression, particularly for women who are mothers, and can be measured and monitored by the administration of the Beck Depression Inventory (BDI-II) (Beck, Steer, & Brown, 1996; Berlin & Covey, 2006; Prusakowski, Shofer, & Rhodes, 2011).[35] Others (e.g., Parrott, 2003) have suggested that nicotine use, while appearing to relieve the symptoms of depression, actually only provides "temporary relief of withdrawal symptoms" (p. 49).

Unfortunately, the nature of the present healthcare system tends to *compartmentalize* mental disorders (e.g., SUDs *versus* OMDs—see the introduction and overview of WCDs, including common terms and definitions, at the beginning of this chapter) and, consequently, their treatment (for further discussion, see later section, *Optimal Treatment Approaches for Women's Contemporaneous Diagnoses*). Consequently, all too often the depressive disorders that are involved are *misdiagnosed*. Consider, for example, the findings from an early, seminal study of a sample of "drug-using homicidal adolescents," comprised of both girls and boys, reported by Malmquist (1990):

> Impressive besides the past history connected with drug usage was the finding that only *one*, of the 44 subjects, was ever diagnosed as depressed before the acts that led to their being included in this study. The difficulty is partly explained by where they made contact, such as in a court probation system, a chemical dependency referral, a clinic, or a hospital unit. The few times depression was considered it was viewed as secondary to the primary problem of chemical dependency. A related finding was that 10 of the males and three of the females had previously been through chemical dependency treatment programs.
>
> *(p. 29)*

[34] While pain is most often categorized as a symptom of another disorder, we believe that pain, particularly in certain contexts, also can be identified as a mental disorder that is often involved in contemporaneous diagnoses along with AUDs and SUDs, particularly those involving the use of psychodepressants (Pagliaro & Pagliaro, 1999, 2003; Pagliaro & Pagliaro, *Clinical Patient Data Files*). In addition, as noted by Volkman, DeRycke, and Driscoll (2015), in their study of approximately 51,000 women, who were U.S. veterans, moderate to severe pain intensity was highly associated with current tobacco smoking. (Also, see related discussion in the following section, "WCDs: Pain Disorders.")

[35] Interestingly, some researchers and clinicians (e.g., Janes, Pedrelli, & Whitton, 2015) have noted that high levels of nicotine dependence may remain among women with a history of MDD—even after the clinical signs and symptoms of depression have subsided. Although confirmatory data are

WCDs: Pain Disorders

Pain, whether considered as a distinct clinical disorder or as a symptom of another mental or physical disorder, often is integrally involved in contemporaneous diagnoses involving AUDs and/or SUDs.

Several researchers (e.g., Barry, Pilver, & Hoff, 2013; Beasley, Macfarlane, & Macfarlane, 2016; Brennan, Schutte, & Moos, 2005; NIAAA, 2013) have reported that alcohol is commonly used as a form of "self-medication" to relieve both chronic and severe pain. This behavior is routinely noted among older women—particularly, those who:

- Are depressed
- Are homeless
- Reside alone

(*Pagliaro & Pagliaro,* Clinical Patient Data Files)

In addition, as noted by Brennan, Schutte, and Moos (2005), in their longitudinal survey of 401 community-dwelling adults:

> Among older women, more baseline drinking problems interacted with use of alcohol to manage pain to predict more drinking problems 3 years later. (*p. 777*)

Even more common than the noted relationships between women's pain and alcohol abuse is the relationship between women's *pain and opiate analgesic abuse*. For example, women, who are prescribed opiate analgesics (e.g., methadone; oxycodone) by their physicians for the management of chronic pain, commonly develop *increasingly* harmful patterns of use (e.g., "Habitual Use," "Abuse," and "Compulsive Use"). Unfortunately, when their prescribed opiate analgesic: (1) no longer helps to manage their pain due to the development of tolerance; (2) cannot be refilled; or (3) the prescription is declined, women may resort to illicit opiate analgesics, including street heroin (Kern, Akerman, & Nordstrom, 2014). Also of concern is the finding that the risk for developing harmful patterns of use is significantly *increased* when women with chronic pain also suffer from anxiety or mood disorders (e.g., Howe & Sullivan, 2014; Sehgal, Manchikanti, & Smith, 2012; Wasan, Butler, & Budman, 2007; Wasan, Michna, & Edwards, 2015).[36] (Also, see Chapter 1, *Women's Opiate Analgesic Abuse*, and Chapter 2, *Women's Alcohol Abuse*.)

---

lacking, it appears that this observation is associated with women's genetically-controlled nicotine reward sensitivity mechanisms.

36 For example, in a related study of "500 consecutive adult pain patients," Manchikanti, Giordano, and Boswell (2007) found that 59% had depressive disorders and 64% had anxiety disorders (p. 89). We have, for some time now, noted that chronic medical disorders, including chronic pain, are *typically* accompanied by depression (Pagliaro & Pagliaro, *Clinical Patient Data Files*).

In a related example, Manchikanti, Giordano, and Boswell (2007, p. 89) identified that, among their sample of women with chronic pain, those with depression were significantly *more* likely to have a SUD (22%) than those who did *not* have depression (14%).

Regarding anxiety disorders, PTSD appears to most frequently be associated with chronic pain and SUDs (e.g., Gros, Szafranski, & Brady, 2015; Shorter, Hsieh, & Kosten, 2015; Sofuoglu, Rosenheck, & Petrakis, 2014). It has been suggested that the "stress system" is integrally involved in this relationship (Sofuoglu, Rosenheck, & Petrakis, 2014). (Also, see related discussion in earlier sections, *WCDs: Anxiety Disorders* and *WCDs: Mood Disorders.*)

WCDs: Psychotic Disorders—Schizophrenia

Alcohol and substance use disorders have been identified in a significant number of cohorts of subjects diagnosed with schizophrenia (e.g., Thirthalli & Benegal, 2006; Winklbaur, Ebner, & Sachs, 2006). In addition, women have been found to commonly use drugs and substances of abuse that can *mimic* psychotic disorders, including schizophrenia. For example, women's use of *psychostimulants* (i.e., amphetamines; cocaine) or *psychodelics* (e.g., cannabis; ketamine; lysergic acid diethylamide [LSD]; and phencyclidine [PCP]) has been associated with signs and symptoms that are virtually indistinguishable from those associated with *acute* schizophrenia, including:

- Delusions
- Hallucinations
- Disorganized speech
- Grossly disorganized or catatonic behavior

(Pagliaro & Pagliaro, 2009)

In fact, the psychodelics have been pharmacologically referred to as *psychotomimetics* or *psychotogens*—drugs that mimic or cause psychosis (see Chapter 6, *Women's Psychodelic Abuse*). Fortunately, these effects, often associated with acute intoxication, are usually transitory in nature. (Also, see later in this section, *Cannabis Use Disorder [CUD] and Schizophrenia.*) Consequently, it is not surprising that, regarding the identification of WCDs, many researchers (e.g., Moghaddam, Dickerson, & Yoon, 2014) have found that the *strongest* associations involve psychotic disorders and drug and substance abuse.

Regarding the further identification of WCDs, the prototype psychotic disorder, *schizophrenia*, is often involved with one or more AUDs and/or SUDs, particularly those related to the use of: (1) *alcohol*; (2) *amphetamines*; (3) *cannabis*; (4) *cocaine*; and (5) *nicotine* (e.g., Dervaux, Laquelle, & Bourdel, 2003; Green, Young, & Kavanagh, 2005; Margolese, Malchy, & Negrete, 2004; Pagliaro & Pagliaro, 2009; Winklbaur, Ebner, & Sachs, 2006).

Schizophrenia is usually *first* identified during early adulthood with a worldwide incidence of approximately 1% of the population. In addition to depression and suicide attempts and completion, women who have schizophrenia may be at a particularly *high* risk for AUDs, SUDs, and conduct disorder (CD)—*all* of which appear to be interrelated.

Among both women and men with schizophrenia, the incidence of *concurrent* AUDs and/or SUDs can be up to 3 times *higher* than that found for the general population (Green, 2005; Margolese, Malchy, & Negrete, 2004; Pagliaro & Pagliaro, 2009; Winklbaur, Ebner, & Sachs, 2006).[37] In addition, Aakre, Brown, and Benson (2014) reported that women with *schizophrenia* were 4 times *more* likely to meet the criteria for *PTSD* than were women with severe *non-psychotic depression* (see earlier section, *WCDs: Anxiety Disorders*, "PTSD"). As noted by Green and Brown (2006), the major concerns regarding contemporaneous diagnoses involving schizophrenia and an AUD and/or a SUD, include:

1. Therapeutic complications that require appropriate management of *each* condition
2. Poor short- and long-term therapeutic outcomes in the management of schizophrenia (e.g., significantly *longer* durations of hospitalization and a *higher* incidence of suicide attempts among women, as well as men, who have this contemporaneous diagnosis versus those who do not)

In this regard, it appears that many people who have schizophrenia use drugs and substances of abuse as a means of *self-medication* in an attempt to *decrease* associated undesired signs and symptoms, particularly the *negative* symptoms associated with schizophrenia that include apathy and poor social functioning (e.g., Pagliaro & Pagliaro, *Clinical Patient Data Files*; Potvin, Stip, & Roy, 2003). Although *not* universally accepted, this theory helps to explain, at least in part, the *high* incidence of AUDs and/or SUDs diagnosed among women who have schizophrenia.

Cannabis Use Disorder (CUD) and Schizophrenia

> Popular Notion: Marijuana is a relatively safe and gentle drug that is primarily used to relax and feel good. Its use is *not* associated with any major mental disorders.
>
> NOT TRUE. See following discussion.

[37] In addition, among women with both an AUD and SUD and schizophrenia, Caton, Xie, and Drake (2014) noted a "greater history of abuse and depression in comparison to a matched cohort of men" (p. 177).

In their meta-review of published data obtained from 58 studies examining reported cannabis use among research participants with psychosis/schizophrenia, Green, Young, and Kavanagh (2005, p. 306) found several *significant* summary statistics:

- Current use (23.0%)
- Current *misuse* (11.3%)
- 12-month use (29.2%)
- 12-month *misuse* (18.8%)
- Life-time use (42.1%)
- Life-time *misuse* (22.5%)

Historically, cannabis is the substance of abuse that has the *longest* association with schizophrenia (Pagliaro & Pagliaro, 2004, 2009). (Also, see related discussion in the "Cannabis" section of Chapter 6, *Women's Psychodelic Abuse.*) Consequently, most data related to contemporaneous diagnoses involving SUDs and psychotic disorders are associated with *cannabis*. A review of these data revealed *six* distinct, but *not* mutually exclusive, relationships between cannabis use disorder and the occurrence of psychotic disorders.

First, among cannabis users who are *not* psychotic, the use of cannabis that has a *high* THC concentration can produce symptomatology associated with *transient* psychosis (i.e., positive, negative, and cognitive signs and symptoms of schizophrenia) (Castle, 2013; D'Souza, 2007; D'Souza, Sewell, & Ranganathan, 2009; Linszen & van Amelsvoort, 2007; Verdoux & Tournier, 2004). These signs and symptoms usually occur with *acute* cannabis intoxication and generally resolve: (1) virtually *immediately* with the administration of an antipsychotic tranquilizer (e.g., haloperidol, Haldol®); or (2) in a matter of days following the discontinuation of cannabis use, without intervention (Pagliaro & Pagliaro, 2009).

Second, among users who have a predisposition to developing schizophrenia (i.e., *pre-schizophrenic*, or genetic vulnerability to developing schizophrenia),[38] the use of *cannabis* can produce a *true* psychosis (*Cannabis could increase*, 2007; *Daily pot smoking*, 2009; Degenhardt & Hall, 2006; Di Forti, Morrison, & Butt, 2007; Fernandez-Espejo, Viveros, & Nunez, 2009; Hall & Degenhardt, 2008; Hall, Degenhardt & Teesson, 2004; Henquet, Di Forti, & Morrison, 2008; Le Bec, Fatseas, & Denis, 2009; Muller-Vahl & Emrich, 2008; Tucker, 2009; Verdoux & Tournier, 2004).[39]

[38] This vulnerability is generally suggested by a positive family history of schizophrenia and/or the development of related signs and symptoms (e.g., unusual sensory experiences). Vulnerability also has been associated with specific genetic variables. For example, Radhakrishnan, Wilkinson, and D'Souza (2014, p. 1) identified that women with "polymorphisms of COMT and AKT1 genes" may be at significantly increased risk for the development or exacerbation of psychosis in conjunction with the use of cannabis.

[39] The relationship between *cannabis* use and schizophrenia begins with the heavy use of *cannabis* by women, who are genetically vulnerable, followed by the development of schizophrenia during early

Risk appears to directly *increase* among women in relation to: (1) age at the time of initiating daily marijuana use; and (2) duration of use (*Daily pot smoking*, 2009; *Long-time cannabis*, 2010). In addition, a gender effect has been suggested—with overall risk being *greater* for women than men (*Daily pot smoking*, 2009).

Third, among women who have *untreated*, pre-existing schizophrenia (i.e., those who have schizophrenia, but have *not* been diagnosed with schizophrenia or who are currently in remission), the use of cannabis can *trigger* either: (1) a relapse; or (2) an exacerbation of latent schizophrenia. Both effects are associated with expected signs and symptoms that persist past the period of acute cannabis intoxication and, in some cases, continue indefinitely (D'Souza, 2007; D'Souza, Sewell, & Ranganathan, 2009; Hall, Degenhardt, & Teesson, 2004; van Os, Bak, & Hanssen, 2002).

Fourth, among women who have been diagnosed with schizophrenia, and who are receiving treatment (i.e., antipsychotic pharmacotherapy), the use of cannabis is associated with *increased* rates of non-compliance with, or failure to follow, prescribed antipsychotic pharmacotherapy. Consequently, these effects are generally associated with *increased* rates of relapse (Hides, Dawe, & Kavanagh, 2006; Zammit, Moore, & Lingford-Hughes, 2008).[40]

Fifth, among some women, who have been diagnosed with schizophrenia, the relationship is *bi-directional*. For example, in their prospective, longitudinal study of 229 patients with a diagnosis of schizophrenia, Foti, Kotov, and Guey (2010) noted that: (1) lifetime cannabis use was *directly* associated with an *earlier* onset of psychosis; (2) cannabis use was associated with an adverse course of psychotic symptoms in schizophrenia; and (3) adverse psychotic symptoms were associated with an *increase* in cannabis use.

Sixth, among women, who were diagnosed with active schizophrenia, the use of cannabis was *directly* related to the degree of personal distress experienced as a result of the psychotic disorder (i.e., the amount of cannabis used and its frequency of use are reflected by the women's attempts to ameliorate distressing signs and symptoms of schizophrenia—as a form of *self-medication*) (Castle, 2013; Henquet, van Os, & Kuepper, 2010; Hides, Dawe, & Kavanagh, 2006).

These six relationships do *not* exhaust all possible relationships that can occur between the use of cannabis and schizophrenia. For example, as more is learned about the endogenous cannabinoid, or *endocannabinoid*, system—including its various components, actions on neurotransmitters and receptors, and genetic mediation—other, yet, unidentified factors and co-factors may be discovered that play significant roles regarding cannabis use and the development of schizophrenia. In addition, as posited by Houston, Murphy, and Adamson (2007), the relationship between cannabis use and schizophrenia may be mediated by one

adulthood (Di Forti, Morrison, & Butt, 2007; Rubino & Parolaro, 2008). Young adults, in their early twenties, appear to be particularly vulnerable regarding these deleterious effects because the brain is in the process of completing neuronal maturation that began during the perinatal period (Pagliaro & Pagliaro, 2009; Schneider, 2008).

40 Although the data presented by Zammit, Moore, and Lingford-Hughes (2008) support this observation, they did *not* come to the same conclusion.

or more additional factors or co-factors. The additional factor identified in their study was *childhood sexual abuse*. When present, this factor resulted in an interaction effect that significantly *increased* the correlation between adolescent *cannabis* use and subsequent development of psychosis.

WCDs: Sleep Disorders—Insomnia

Insomnia is the primary sleep disorder associated with WCDs. However, because of the often-concealed nature of the relationship between AUDs and/or SUDs and insomnia, significantly *less* data are available than for the other *more* common WCDs discussed in this chapter. The *concealment* is due to several factors, including: (1) the generally low level of attention given to diagnosing sleep disorders among young women; (2) the interpretation, or classification, of insomnia as a symptom of another disorder rather than a *primary disorder*;[41] and (3) the occurrence of insomnia in association with OMDs, particularly anxiety disorders and mood disorders. The under-diagnosis of insomnia among adults (Edinger & Means, 2005) contributes to both numbers 2 and 3, above.

> Is insomnia a clinical entity or is it simply a symptom of an underlying medical or psychological disorder?
>
> *(p. 1037)*

This question, rhetorically asked by Harvey (2001), over 15 years ago, still resonates in the clinical community (e.g., Mai & Buysse, 2008). Part of the difficulty in answering this question is due to the *significant* association of insomnia with contemporaneous diagnoses.[42]

Insomnia among women, as well as other sleep disorders, is frequently associated with OMDs, including: (1) *anxiety disorders* (e.g., PTSD); and (2) *mood disorders* (i.e., MDD) (e.g., Ivanenko & Gururaj, 2009). Etiologically, the relationship can be bi-directional. For example, Johnson, Roth, and Breslau (2006) found that, among individuals with insomnia and OMDs: (1) "anxiety disorders preceded insomnia 73% of the time"; and (2) "insomnia occurred first in 69% of comorbid insomnia and depression cases" (p. 700). Several other relationships also have been demonstrated that involve AUDs and/or SUDs and insomnia (see Figure 7.2). For example, insomnia is a common symptom of withdrawal from sedative-hypnotic use. It also can be caused, as a direct and expected pharmacologic action, by *psychostimulant* use (e.g., Pagliaro & Pagliaro, 2009; Roehrs & Roth, 2008).

---

41 This philosophical divergence is similar in perspective and context to that involving previous discussions concerning "pain." See, for example, the earlier related discussion in the section, "WCDs: Pain Disorders."

42 It should be noted that insomnia, even when related to another mental disorder, is amenable to specific and appropriate treatment interventions (Pagliaro & Pagliaro, 1999, 2009; Stepanski & Rybarczyk, 2006).

WCDs and Human Immunodeficiency Virus (HIV) Infection

The nature of the relationship among AUDs and/or SUDs, OMDs, and HIV[43] infection is clear, but can be *indirect*. Several early research studies and reports (e.g., Pagliaro, Pagliaro, & Thauberger, 1993) noted that the use of the drugs and substances of abuse is an *antecedent* risk factor that places women at *significant* risk for HIV infection in several specific ways, including: (1) sharing contaminated needles and syringes;[44] (2) decreasing inhibitions and, consequently, increasing the likelihood of engaging in unprotected sex; (3) trading sex for desired drugs or substances of abuse or participating in the sex trade in order to obtain the money needed to buy desired drugs or substances of abuse;[45] and (4) as a consequence of numbers 2 and 3, above, having multiple sexual partners and engaging in high-risk, unprotected anal, oral, and vaginal sex.[46]

In addition, several researchers (e.g., Herbst, Jacobs, & Finlayson, 2008; Rowe, Santos, & McFarland, 2015; Santos, Rapues, & Wilson, 2014) have, more recently, during the new millennium, reported similar findings for trans females. For example, Herbst, Jacobs, and Finlayson (2008), in their meta-analysis of 29 studies focusing on male-to-female (MTF) transgender women in the U.S., found that 27.7% of the MTF women in their study tested positive for HIV infection. In another study, Santos, Rapues, and Wilson (2014) found that the risk of testing *positive* for HIV significantly *increased* for trans women who reported methamphetamine use.

---

[43] We note that a virtually parallel argument can be made for a WCD and hepatitis C virus (HCV) infection. Rates of HCV infection have risen significantly over the new millennium, particularly among young women in the U.S. This *rise* in HCV infection, and that noted among women of various continental descents and other descents or ethnicities, including Native Hawaiians, has been directly related to *increased* intravenous drug use (IVDU) (e.g., Pagliaro & Pagliaro, *Clinical Patient Data Files*; Takeuchi, Pham, & Katz, 2015).

[44] For example, as noted by Davis, Ancis, and Ashby (2015)—citing data from the CDC:

> HIV/AIDS is the leading, third, and fourth cause of death among African American women ages 25–34, 35–44, and 45–54, respectively; and 24% of African American women contract HIV infection through substance use, largely drug injections.
>
> *(p. 126)*

[45] Rash, Burki, and Montezuma-Rusca (2016) identified that trading sex for drugs or money is extremely common with lifetime prevalence ranging from 30% to 50% among women seeking treatment for drug and substance abuse, particularly for cocaine abuse. Women, who participated in their study, and who traded sex for drugs or money, were "*more* likely to be African American, older and less educated, had *more* severe employment problems, and were *more* likely to be HIV positive" (p. 182).

[46] Use of drugs and substances of abuse can also be a response to a diagnosis of HIV (Pagliaro & Pagliaro, *Clinical Patient Data Files*). For example, Galvan, Bing, and Fleishman (2002), in their survey of 2,864 "HIV-infection adults" (including 847 women), found that:

> Alcohol consumption is common among people in care for HIV, with rates of heavy drinking almost twice those found in the general population.
>
> *(p. 179)*

Unfortunately, little, if anything, has improved—even though we,[47] and many others, have repeatedly called for greater attention to this critical situation (as previously stated). As noted by Rondinelli, Ouellet, and Strathdee (2009), commenting on the findings from their large, cross-sectional study of *injection drug users* (IDUs), 15 to 30 years-of-age, who were sampled from *five* large cities across the U.S.:

> More than two decades after injection and sexual practices were identified as risk factors for HIV infection, these behaviors remain common among young IDUs.
>
> *(p. 167)*

This observation, and our concerns, appear to be further substantiated by findings from the *National Survey and Analysis of the Sexual Health of Adolescents in the U.S.*, which was conducted by Gavin, Mackay, and Brown (2009) for the CDC. In this report, they noted that:

> Many young people engage in risky sexual behavior ... In 2006, approximately 22,000 women aged 10 to 24 years in 33 states were living with human immunodeficiency virus/acquired immune deficiency syndrome (HIV/AIDS).
>
> *(p. 2)*

Several researchers, including ourselves, have identified that certain OMDs (e.g., depression; PTSD) have a higher incidence among women (i.e., in the context of WCDs), who also are HIV positive. For example, Kalokhe, Paranjape, and Bell (2012), in their sample of female "HIV-infected crack users," found that the incidence of IPV was 68% (p. 234).

In addition, several other researchers (e.g., Pagliaro & Pagliaro, *Clinical Patient Data Files*; Torchalla, Strehlau, & Li, 2011) report an extremely *high* level of contemporaneous diagnoses (range, 60% to 90%) involving AUDs and/or SUDs, and OMDs among homeless women, particularly women of American Indian descent, living in urban areas, and who support their drug and substance abuse with sex-for-drug exchanges or other sex trade work and, consequently, are often HIV positive. Finally, in their study, which had a sample that was *highly* skewed toward participants of African continental descent (i.e., more than 74%), Majer, Komes, and Jason (2015) found that, "gender [i.e., *women*] and psychiatric severity [i.e., *higher*] were significantly related to *greater* HIV-risk sexual behaviors" (p. 3).

[47] Having co-directed one of the first research groups studying HIV infection and AIDS among intravenous drug users (IVDUs) (e.g., Pagliaro & Pagliaro, 1993a, 1993b, 1994; Pagliaro, Pagliaro, & Thauberger, 1993), we, and our colleagues, concluded with considerable concern, that once the antiretrovirus pharmacotherapy was developed and became widely available, attention to ours and other's recommendations aimed at *preventing* HIV infection among IVDUs and their families and communities would significantly *decrease* as if the problem had been eliminated—when, in fact, it has not. Unfortunately, this conclusion has, 25 years later, been validated.

WCDs and Barriers to Treatment

This section presents an overview of the barriers that have been identified regarding the provision of appropriate and efficacious treatment approaches for women who have contemporaneous diagnoses. It also highlights several effective treatment approaches and programs that have been specifically designed and developed for women.

Popular Notion: Women, in comparison to men, generally present with less severe and less complicated forms of contemporaneous diagnoses that are, consequently, easier to treat.

NOT TRUE.

As identified by Greenfield, Back, and Lawson (2010):

> When women enter substance abuse treatment they typically present with a more severe clinical profile (e.g., more medical, behavioral, psychological, and social problems) than men, despite having used less of the substance and having used the substance for a shorter period compared with men.
>
> *(p. 339)*

This seemingly paradoxical effect is commonly referred to as, "telescoping."[48] Telescoping is characterized by an accelerated progression (i.e., contracted period) from the initiation of drug and substance abuse to the onset of *increasingly* harmful patterns of drug and substance abuse and, subsequently, the first admission to treatment. Primarily occurring among women, who have alcohol, cannabis, and opiate-analgesics use disorders, telescoping can present complex treatment challenges for health and social care professionals, particularly when the involved AUDs and SUDs also involve anxiety disorders (e.g., PTSD) or OMDs in various combinations of WCDs (e.g., Hernandez-Avila, Rounsaville, & Kranzler, 2004; Pagliaro & Pagliaro, *Clinical Patient Data Files*; Piazza, Vrbka, & Yeager, 1989; Randall, Roberts, & Del Boca, 1999).[49]

Although the availability of appropriate treatment services for women, who have a contemporaneous diagnosis, has *increased* significantly during the last 2 decades, it still remains all too common for them to be refused admission to a *drug*

---

48 See the *Index* for a detailed listing of the page locations that address *telescoping*.

49 The literature also includes studies that failed to confirm, or support, significant telescoping effects among women who abuse drugs and substances of abuse (e.g., Holscher, Reissner, & Di Furia, 2010; Keyes, Martins, & Blanco, 2010).

abuse treatment center because of their OMDs (e.g., major depression; schizophrenia) or to be refused admission to a *mental health facility* because of their AUDs (e.g., alcoholism) and/or SUDs (e.g., heroin addiction) (McClean, Anspikian, & Winters, 2014). This *Catch-22* situation reflects a general lack of pertinent education and clinical expertise among health and social care professionals (Carey, Bradizza, & Stasiewicz, 1999; Drake, Essock, & Shaner, 2001; Renner, 2004), particularly those professionals in mental health and treatment settings that provide services for women with contemporaneous diagnoses. As noted almost 30 years ago, by Adger Jr., McDonald, and DeAngelis, in their 1990 survey of drug abuse education during medical school training:

> At the medical student and residency training levels, only 44% and 40% of programs, respectively, required any formal instruction, and only 27% and 34% respectively, offered an elective for medical students or residents. Although most respondents endorsed the inclusion of both required and elective alcohol and drug education in the curriculum, few programs that did not include it already had a future plan for it.
>
> *(p. 555)*

This situation has *not* changed significantly during the almost 30 years since that survey was conducted, although some significant progress has been achieved (e.g., Iannucci, Sanders, & Greenfield, 2009; Polydorou, Gunderson, & Levin, 2008). As noted by Hawkins (2009), regarding treatment services aimed at contemporaneous diagnoses:

> In general, current service systems are inadequately prepared to meet this need due to a variety of clinical, administrative, financial, and policy barriers.
>
> *(p. 197)*

Chen, Strain, and Crum (2013) posit that "attitudinal factors" are the *most* common barriers to effective treatment of WCDs. Studying the *facilitators* and *barriers* to treatment for women with contemporaneous diagnoses, Brunette, Asher, and Whitley (2008) found that the *two* most prevalent barriers were inadequacies in: (1) funding; and (2) staffing. However, even when adequate funding was secured and in place, treatment programs continued to have *severe* staffing problems, particularly a *high* staff turnover.

In addition, treatment services also continue to reflect the widespread and common practice of employing paraprofessionals and people with histories of their own AUDs (e.g., *recovering alcoholics*) and/or SUDs (e.g., *recovering heroin addicts*) as *drug counselors* for the treatment of women who have a contemporaneous diagnosis (e.g., Barlow, Mullany, & Neault, 2013; Doukas & Cullen, 2011). Although these people may have an important role to play in the complex treatment of contemporaneous diagnoses, they are generally *not* qualified, neither academically, nor clinically, as *primary* therapists. For example, as noted by Penick, Nickel, and Cantrell (1990):

> Many of the traditional caregivers in the substance abuse field are, themselves, recovering from chemical dependency; [these individuals, generally,] tend to know and use only one approach to treatment. If they are recovering themselves, the approach taken is usually the one that "worked" for them. When confronted with failure, substance abuse workers typically have no "fall back" position to draw upon, continuing instead to do "more of the same" rather than shift to a different treatment strategy.
>
> *(pp. 7–8)*

From our related professional observations over the decades, as well as a detailed review of related published data and other material, we have concluded that the continued use of *paraprofessionals* and *recovering addicts* in the clinical context of treatment of women with contemporaneous diagnoses is primarily guided by economic/financial concerns (i.e., factors related to limited budgets and maximizing profits). For example, in a study published by the University of Wisconsin School of Medicine and Public Health, it was reported that:

> Expanding the health care team to include [paraprofessional] health educators to handle alcohol and other drug screening is a low-cost option that results in two-year net savings of $782 per Medicaid patient who underwent screening … inpatient days dropped and lower cost outpatient visits increased significantly when Medicaid patients were screened and treated as necessary by paraprofessions.
>
> *(University of Wisconsin, 2016, p. 1)*

Unfortunately, these observations, and associated practices, have *not* changed significantly during the new millennium and must be actively addressed in an open and objective manner with a focus on optimizing therapeutic outcomes for women with contemporaneous diagnoses (e.g., Ayyagari, 2014; Pagliaro & Pagliaro, 2000; Rush & Koegl, 2008; Ziedonis, Smelson, & Rosenthal, 2005).

As a point of departure, we fully endorse and urge others to adopt the following "general approaches" for helping health and social care professionals to optimally meet the unique needs of women, who have contemporaneous diagnoses:

- Provide each woman with individualized, goal-directed treatment that is aimed at the successful resolution of *each* identified AUD, SUD, and OMD
- Be guided by each woman's individual needs, personality, and cognitive abilities
- Provide each woman with a safe and trusting treatment environment

- Provide each woman, as appropriate, with integrated and multimodal approaches to her treatment program that include: family-based therapies; appropriate referrals to other health and social care providers; and integrated outreach services, particularly if she is homeless, living on the street, is pregnant, or has young children (or elderly parents) to care for
- Be sensitive when interacting with each woman
- Involve each woman, as appropriate to her recovery and abilities, in planning and delivering optimal treatment for each AUD and/or SUD and OMD
- Support each woman's abstinence from problematic drugs and substances of abuse
- Provide each woman with insight and management of her OMDs
- Help each woman to build her self-confidence and self-esteem
- Help each woman to develop and use healthy coping styles
- Empower each woman with a sense of control over her life and responsibility for her actions and behaviors
- Encourage each woman's participation, as appropriate, in peer self-help programs
- Assure that each woman is provided with appropriate follow-up, aftercare, and other relapse prevention services

Attention to these "general approaches" for each woman seeking and receiving treatment for her specific contemporaneous diagnosis, will help her to maximize positive therapeutic outcomes. For additional discussion, also see Chapter 8, *Preventing and Treating Women's Drug and Substance Abuse.*

References[50,51,52]

Aakre, J. M., Brown, C. H., & Benson, K. M. (2014). Trauma exposure and PTSD in women with schizophrenia and coexisting substance use disorders: Comparisons to women with severe depression and substance use disorders. *Psychiatry Research*, 220(3), 840–845.

Adger Jr., H., McDonald, E. M., & DeAngelis, C. (1990). Substance abuse education in pediatrics. *Pediatrics*, 86(4), 555–560.

---

[50] As per publisher style, only the first three authors are listed for each reference.

[51] Several times the number of references listed were found, obtained, and analyzed by the authors during the preparation of this chapter. However, only the references that were cited at least once in the body of the text are included in the list. Major reasons for not citing other references, include that they: (1) did not provide any additional unique data; (2) were not well researched or written (i.e., were evaluated as not being valid or reliable); (3) were based predominantly, or exclusively, on animal studies; (4) provided usage statistics from outside the U.S.; and/or (5) were redundant with, or not as recent as, the already cited references.

[52] The reference citation, "Pagliaro & Pagliaro, *Clinical Patient Data Files*," refers to unpublished data collected, with permission, over the last 50 years by the authors, in the formal course of their professional academic roles as clinician scientists and professors—from their patients, research subjects, and students, from the 1970s to date.

Alegria, A. A., Hasin, D. S., & Nunes, E. V. (2010). Comorbidity of generalized anxiety disorder and substance use disorders: Results from the National Epidemiologic Survey on Alcohol and Related Conditions. *The Journal of Clinical Psychiatry*, 71(9), 1187–1195. doi:10.4088/JCP.09m05328gry

Armeli, S., Todd, M., & Conner, T. S. (2008). Drinking to cope with negative moods and the immediacy of drinking within the weekly cycle among college students. *Journal of Studies on Alcohol and Drugs*, 69(2), 313–322.

Aspis, I., Feingold, D., & Weiser, M. (2015, December 15). Cannabis use and mental health-related quality of life among individuals with depressive disorders. *Psychiatry Research*, 230(2), 341–349. doi:10.1016/j.psychres.2015.09.014

Austin, E. L., & Irwin, J. A. (2010). Age differences in the correlates of problematic alcohol use among southern lesbians. *Journal of Studies on Alcohol and Drugs*, 71(2), 295–298.

Ayyagari, A. (2014, May 16). *Exploring the dynamics of high-challenge encounters in residential substance abuse treatment settings.* Retrieved August 13, 2016, from Univeristy of Pennsylvania Scholarly Commons: http://repository-upenn.edu/edissertations_sp2/52

Azorin, J. M., Belzeaux, R., & Kaladjian, A. (2013). Risks associated with gender differences in bipolar 1 disorder. *Journal of Affective Disorders*, 151(3), 1033–1040. doi:10.1016/j.jad.2013.08.031

Azorin, J. M., Bowden, C. L., & Garay, R. P. (2010). Possible new ways in the pharmacological treatment of bipolar disorder and comorbid alcoholism. *Neuropsychiatric Disease and Treatment*, 6, 37–46.

Barlow, A., Mullany, B., & Neault, N. (2013). Effect of a paraprofessional home-visiting intervention on American Indian teen mothers' and infants' behavioral risks: A randomized controlled trial. *American Journal of Psychiatry*, 170(1), 83–93. doi:10.1176/appi.aip.2012.12010121

Barry, D. T., Pilver, C. E., & Hoff, R. A. (2013). Pain interference and incident mood, anxiety, and substance-use disorders: Findings from a representative sample of men and women in the general population. *Journal of Psychiatric Research*, 47(11), 1658–1664. doi:10–1016/j.jpsychires.2013.08.004

BBC (2016, December 6). News: US & Canada. *Lady Gaga says she has PTSD after being raped at 19*, 1–6. BBC News. Retrieved December 6, 2016, from www.bbc.co.uk/news/world-us-canada-38218247

Beasley, M. J., Macfarlane, T. V., & Macfarlane, G. J. (2016, July 19). Is alcohol consumption related to likelihood of reporting chronic widespread pain in people with stable consumption? Results from UK Biobank. *Pain*, 157(11), 2552–2560. doi:10.1097/j.pain.0000000000000675

Beck, A., Steer, R., & Brown, G. (1996). *The Beck Depression Inventory—Second Edition Manual.* San Antonio, TX: The Psychological Corporation.

Becker, D. F., & Grilo, C. M. (2015). Comorbidity of mood and substance use disorders in patients with binge-eating disorder: Associations with personality disorder and eating disorder pathology. *Journal of Psychosomatic Research*, 79(2), 159–164. doi:10.1016/j.jpsychores.2015.01.016

Belfer, M. L. (1993). Substance abuse with psychiatric illness in children and adolescents: Definitions and terminology. *American Journal of Orthopsychiatry*, 63(1), 70–79.

Berg, C. J., Wen, H., & Cummings, J. R. (2013). Depression and substance abuse and dependency in relation to current smoking status and frequency of smoking among nondaily and daily smokers. *American Journal on Addictions*, 22(6), 581–589.

Berlin, I., & Covey, L. S. (2006). Pre-cessation depressive mood predicts failure to quit smoking: The role of coping and personality traits. *Addiction*, 101(12), 1814–1821.

Bolton, J., Cox, B., & Clara, I. (2006). Use of alcohol and drugs to self-medicate anxiety disorders in a nationally representative sample. *The Journal of Nervous and Mental Disease*, 194(11), 818–825. doi:10.1097/01.nmd.0000244481.63148.98

Bolton, J. M., Robinson, J., & Sareen, J. (2009). Self-medication of mood disorders with alcohol and drugs in the National Epidemiologic Survey on Alcohol and Related Conditions. *Journal of Affective Disorders*, 115(3), 367–375. doi:10.1016/j.jad.2008.10.003

Bowe, A., & Rosenheck, R. (2015). PTSD and substance use disorder among veterans: Characteristics, service utilization, and pharmacotherapy. *Journal of Dual Diagnosis*, 11(1), 22–32. doi:10.1080/15504263.2014.989653

Boyle, M. H., & Offord, D. R. (1991). Psychiatric disorder and substance use in adolescence. *The Canadian Journal of Psychiatry*, 36(10), 699–705.

Brady, K. T., Killeen, T. K., & Brewerton, T. (2000). Comorbidity of psychiatric disorders and posttraumatic stress disorder. *Journal of Clinical Psychiatry*, 61(Supplement 7), 22–32.

Brennan, P. L., Schutte, K. K., & Moos, R. H. (2005). Pain and use of alcohol to manage pain: Prevalence and 3-year outcomes among older problem and non-problem drinkers. *Addiction*, 100(6), 777–786.

Breslau, N. (2002, May 9). Post-traumatic stress disorder. *The New England Journal of Medicine*, 346(19), 1495–1498.

Breslau, N., Davis, G. C., & Peterson, E. L. (1997). Psychiatric sequelae of posttraumatic stress disorder in women. *Archives of General Psychiatry*, 54(1), 81–87.

Breslau, N., Davis, G. C., & Schultz, L. R. (2003). Posttraumatic stress disorder and the incidence of nicotine, alcohol, and other drug disorders in persons who have experienced trauma. *Archives of General Psychiatry*, 60(3), 289–294.

Brunette, M. F., Asher, D., & Whitley, R. (2008). Implementation of integrated dual disorders treatment: A qualitative analysis of facilitators and barriers. *Psychiatric Services*, 59(9), 989–995.

Bulik, C. M., Klump, K. L., & Thornton, L. (2004). Alcohol use disorder comorbidity in eating disorders: A multicenter study. *Journal of Clinical Psychiatry*, 65(7), 1000–1006.

Bulik, C. M., Prescott, C. A., & Kendler, K. S. (2001). Features of childhood sexual abuse and the development of psychiatric and substance use disorders. *The British Journal of Psychiatry*, 179, 444–449.

Burgalassi, A., Ramacciotti, C. E., & Bianchi, M. (2009). Caffeine consumption among eating disorder patients: Epidemiology, motivations, and potential of abuse. *Eating & Weight Disorders*, 14(4), e212–e218.

Burke Jr, J. D., Burke, K. C., & Rae, D. S. (1994). Increased rates of drug abuse and dependence after onset of mood or anxiety disorders in adolescence. *Hospital & Community Psychiatry*, 45(5), 451–455.

Cannabis could increase risks of psychotic illness by 40 percent. (2007, August 1). Retrieved from ScienceDaily.com: www.sciencedaily.com/release/2007/07/070731125526.htm

Carballo, J. J., Bird, H., & Giner, L. (2007). Pathological personality traits and suicidal ideation among older adolescents and young adults with alcohol misuse: A pilot case-control study in a primary care setting. *International Journal of Adolescent Medicine and Health*, 19(1), 79–89.

Carey, K. B., Bradizza, C. M., & Stasiewicz, P. R. (1999). The case for enhanced addictions training in graduate programs. *Behavior Therapist*, 22, 27–31.

Carra, G., Bartoli, F., & Crocamo, C. (2014). Attempted suicide in people with co-occurring bipolar and substance use disorders: Systematic review and meta-analysis. *Journal of Affective Disorders*, 167, 125–135. doi:10.1016/j.jad.2014.05.066

Castle, D. J. (2013). Cannabis and psychosis: What causes what? *Faculty of 1000 Medicine Reports*, 5(1), NP. doi:10.3410M5-1

Caton, C. L., Xie, H., & Drake, R. E. (2014). Gender differences in psychotic disorders with concurrent substance use. *Journal of Dual Diagnosis*, 10(4), 177–186. doi:10.1080/15504263.2014.961882

Chen, L. Y., Strain, E. C., & Crum, R. M. (2013). Gender differences in substance abuse treatment and barriers to care among persons with substance use disorders with and without comorbid major depression. *Journal of Addiction Medicine*, 7(5), 325–334. doi:10.1097/ADM.0b013e31829b7afe

Cochran, S. D., Mays, V. M., & Alegria, M. (2007). Mental health and substance use disorders among Latino and Asian American lesbian, gay, and bisexual adults. *Journal of Consulting and Clinical Psychology*, 75(5), 785–794.

Cohen, J. A., Mannarino, A. P., & Zhitova, A. C. (2003). Treating child abuse-related post-traumatic stress and comorbid substance abuse in adolescents. *Child Abuse & Neglect*, 27(12), 1345–1365.

Cohen, L. R., Field, C., & Campbell, A. (2013). Intimate partner violence outcomes in women with PTSD and substance abuse: A secondary analysis of NIDA Clinical Trials Network "Women and Trauma" Multi-site Study. *Addictive Behaviors*, 38(7), 2325–2332. doi:10.1016/jaddbeh.2013.03.006

Cohen, L. R., Greenfield, S. F., & Gordon, S. (2010). Survey of eating disorder symptoms among women in treatment for substance abuse. *The American Journal on Addictions*, 19(3), 245–251. doi:10.1111/j.1521-0391.2010.00038.x

Coleman-Cowger, V. H. (2012). Mental health treatment need among pregnant and post-partum women/girls entering substance abuse treatment. *Psychology of Addictive Behaviors*, 26(2), 345–350. doi:10.1037/a0025355

Conway, K. P., Compton, W., & Stinson, F. S. (2006). Lifetime comorbidity of DSM-IV mood and anxiety disorders and specific drug use disorders: Results from the National Epidemiologic Survey on Alcohol and Related Conditions. *Journal of Clinical Psychiatry*, 67(2), 247–257.

Cumyn, L., French, L., & Hechtman, L. (2009). Comorbidity in adults with attention-deficit hyperactivity disorder. *Canadian Journal of Psychiatry*, 54(10), 673–683.

Czarlinski, J. A., Aase, D. M., & Jason, L. A. (2012). Eating disorders, normative eating self-efficacy and body image self-efficacy: Women in recovery homes. *European Eating Disorders Review*, 20(3), 190–195. doi:10.1002/erv.1116

Daily pot smoking may hasten onset of psychosis. (2009, December 21). Retrieved from ScienceDaily.com: www.sciencedaily.com/releases/2009/12/091220144936.htm

Daley, D. C., Moss, H., & Campbell, F. (1987). *Dual disorders: Counseling clients with chemical dependency and mental illness*. Center City, MN: Hazelden.

Dansky, B. S., Brewerton, T. D., & Kilpatrick, D. G. (2000). Comorbidity of bulimia nervosa and alcohol use disorders: Results from the National Women's Study. *International Journal of Eating Disorders*, 27(2), 180–190.

Davis, L., Uezato, A., & Newell, J. M. (2008). Major depression and comorbid substance use disorders. *Current Opinion in Psychiatry*, 21(1), 14–18. doi:10.1097/YCO.0b013e3282f32408

Davis, T. A., Ancis, J. R., & Ashby, J. S. (2015). Therapist effects, working alliance, and African American women substance users. *Cultural Diversity and Ethnic Minority Psychology*, 21(1), 126–135.

Degenhardt, L., & Hall, W. (2006). Is cannabis use a contributory cause of psychosis? *The Canadian Journal of Psychiatry*, 51(9), 556–565.

Dekker, N., Linszen, D. H., & De Haan, L. (2009). Reasons for cannabis use and effects of cannabis use as reported by patients with psychotic disorders. *Psychopathology*, 42(6), 350–360. doi:10.1159/000236906

Dervaux, A., Laquelle, X., & Bourdel, M. C. (2003). Cannabis and schizophrenia: Demographic and clinical correlates. *Encephale*, 29(1), 11–17.

Di Forte, M., Morrison, P. D., & Butt, A. (2007). Cannabis use and psychiatric and cognitive disorders: The chicken or the egg? *Current Opinion in Psychiatry*, 20(3), 228–234.

Doukas, N., & Cullen, J. (2011). Addiction counselors in recovery: Perceived barriers in the workplace. *Journal of Addiction Research & Therapy*, 2(3), 1–7. doi:10.4172/2155-6105.1000112

Drake, R. E., Essock, S. M., & Shaner, A. (2001). Implementing dual diagnosis services for clients with severe mental illness. *Psychiatric Services*, 52(4), 469–476.

D'Souza, D. C. (2007). Cannabinoids and psychosis. *International Review of Neurobiology*, 78, 289–326.

D'Souza, D. C., Sewell, R. A., & Ranganathan, M. (2009). Cannabis and psychosis/schizophrenia: Human studies. *European Archives of Psychiatry Clinical Neuroscience*, 259(7), 413–431.

Dunlap, E., Golub, A., & Johnson, B. D. (2003). Girls' sexual development in the inner city: From compelled childhood sexual contact to sex-for-drug exchanges. *Journal of Child Sexual Abuse*, 12(2), 73–96. doi:10.1300/J070v12n02_04

Dunn, E. C., Neighbors, C., & Fossos, N. (2009). A cross-lagged evaluation of eating disorder symptomatology and substance-use problems. *Journal of Studies on Alcohol and Drugs*, 70, 106–116.

Edinger, J. D., & Means, M. K. (2005). Overview of insomnia: Definitions, epidemiology, differential diagnosis, and assessment. In M. H. Kryger, T. Roth, & W. C. Dement (Eds.), *Principles and practice of sleep medicine* (4th ed., pp. 702–713). Philadelphia, PA: Elsevier/Saunders.

Eggleston, A. M., Calhoun, P. S., & Svikis, D. S. (2009). Suicidality, aggression, and other treatment considerations among pregnant, substance-dependent women with posttraumatic stress disorder. *Comprehensive Psychiatry*, 50(5), 415–423.

Elmquist, J., Shorey, R. C., & Anderson, S. (2015). Eating disorder symptoms and length of stay in residential treatment for substance use: A brief report. *Journal of Dual Diagnosis*, 11(3–4), 233–237. doi:10.1080/15504263.2015.1104480

Falck, R. S., Carlson, R. G., & Wang, J. (2006). Psychiatric disorders and their correlates among young adult MDMA users in Ohio. *Journal of Psychoactive Drugs*, 38(1), 19–29. doi:10.1080/02791072.2006.10399824

Fernandez-Espejo, E., Viveros, M. P., & Nunez, L. (2009). Role of cannabis and endocannabinoids in the genesis of schizophrenia. *Psychopharmacology (Berlin)*, 206(4), 531–549. doi:10.1007/s00213-009-1612-6

Finseth, P. I., Morken, G., & Andreassen, O. A. (2012). Risk factors related to lifetime suicide attempts in acutely admitted bipolar disorder inpatients. *Bipolar Disorders*, 14(7), 727–734. doi:10.1111/bdi.12004

Foti, D. J., Kotov, R., & Guey, L. T. (2010). Cannabis use and the course of schizophrenia: 10-year follow-up after first hospitalization. *The American Journal of Psychiatry*, 167, 987–993.

Franco, M. (2007). Posttraumatic stress disorder and older women. *Journal of Women & Aging*, 19(1–2), 103–117. doi:10.1300/J074v19n01_07

Franko, D. L., Dorer, D. J., & Keel, P. K. (2008). Interactions between eating disorders and drug abuse. *The Journal of Nervous and Mental Disease*, 196(7), 556–561. doi:10.1097/NMD.0b013e31817d0153

Galvan, F. H., Bing, E. G., & Fleishman, J. A. (2002). The prevalence of alcohol consumption and heavy drinking among people with HIV in the United States: Results from the HIV cost and services utilization study. *Journal of Studies on Alcohol*, 63(2), 179–186.

Gamble, S. A., Talbot, N. L., & Cashman-Brown, S. M. (2013). A pilot study of interpersonal psychotherapy for alcohol-dependent women with co-occurring major depression. *Substance Abuse*, 34(3), 233–241. doi:10.1080/08897077.2012.746950

Gavin, L., MacKay, A. P., & Brown, K. (2009, July 17). Sexual and reproductive health of persons aged 10–24 years—United States, 2002–2007. *MMWR Surveillance Summaries*, 58(SS06), 1–58.

Gilmore, A. K., Walsh, K., & Badour, C. L. (2017, March 6). Suicide ideation, posttraumatic stress, and substance abuse based on forcible and drug- or alcohol-facilitated/incapacitated rape histories in a national sample of women. *Suicide and Life-Threatening Behavior* [Epub ahead of print]. doi: 10.1111/sltb. 12337

Glanton Holzhauer, C., Zenner, A., & Wulfert, E. (2016). Poor body image and alcohol use in women. *Psychology of Addictive Behaviors*, 30(1), 122–127. doi: 10.1037/adb0000115

Gold, M. S., & Slaby, A. E. (1991). *Dual diagnosis in substance abuse*. New York, NY: Dekker.

Goldstein, B. I., & Bukstein, O. G. (2010). Comorbid substance use disorders among youth with bipolar disorder: Opportunities for early identification and prevention. *Journal of Clinical Psychiatry*, 71(3), 348–358.

Goodwin, R. D., Lieb, R., & Hoefler, M. (2004). Panic attack as a risk factor for severe psychopathology. *The American Journal of Psychiatry*, 161(12), 2207–2214.

Grant, B. F., Stinson, F. S., & Dawson, D. A. (2004). Prevalence and co-occurrence of substance use disorders and independent mood and anxiety disorders: Results from the National Epidemiologic Survey on Alcohol and Related Conditions. *Archives of General Psychiatry*, 61(8), 807–816. doi:10.1001/archpsyc.61.8.807

Green, A. I. (2005). Schizophrenia and comorbid substance use disorder: Effects of antipsychotics. *The Journal of Clinical Psychiatry*, 66(Supplement 6), 21–26.

Green, A. I., & Brown, E. S. (2006). Comorbid schizophrenia and substance abuse. *The Journal of Clinical Psychiatry*, 67(9), e08.

Green, B., Young, R., & Kavanagh, D. (2005). Cannabis use and misuse prevalence among people with psychosis. *British Journal of Psychiatry*, 187, 306–313.

Green, K. M., Zebrak, K. A., & Fothergill, K. E. (2012). Childhood and adolescent risk factors for comorbid depression and substance use disorders in adulthood. *Addictive Behaviors*, 37(11), 1240–1247. doi:10.1016/j.addbeh.2012.06.008

Greenbaum, P. E., Prange, M. E., & Friedman, R. M. (1991). Substance abuse prevalence and comorbidity with other psychiatric disorders among adolescents with severe emotional disturbances. *Journal of the American Academy of Child & Adolescent Psychiatry*, 30(4), 575–583. doi:10.1097/00004583-19910700-00008

Greenfield, S. F., Back, S. E., & Lawson, K. (2010). Substance abuse in women. *Psychiatric Clinics of North America*, 33(2), 339–355. doi:10.1016/j.psc.2010.01.004

Gros, D. F., Szafranski, D. D., & Brady, K. T. (2015). Relations between pain, PTSD symptoms, and substance use in veterans. *Psychiatry*, 78(3), 277–287. doi:10.1080/00332747.2015.1069659

Hahm, H. C., Tzu-Han Chang, S., & Tong, H. Q. (2014). Intersection of suicidality and substance abuse among young Asian-American women: Implications for developing interventions in young adulthood. *Advances in Dual Diagnosis*, 7(2), 90–104. doi:10.1108/ADD-03-20140012

Hall, W., & Degenhardt, L. (2008). Cannabis use and the risk of developing a psychotic disorder. *World Psychiatry*, 7(2), 68–71.

Hall, W., Degenhardt, L., & Teesson, M. (2004). Cannabis use and psychotic disorders: An update. *Drug and Alcohol Review*, 23(4), 433–443.

Harvey, A. G. (2001). Insomnia: Symptom or diagnosis. *Clinical Psychology Review*, 21(7), 1037–1059.

Hasin, D. S., Goodwin, R. D., & Stinson, F. S. (2005). Epidemiology of major depressive disorder: Results from the National Epidemiologic Survey on Alcoholism and Related Conditions. *Archives of General Psychiatry*, 62, 1097–1106.

Hasin, D. S., Stinson, F. S., & Ogburn, E. (2007). Prevalence, correlates, disability, and comorbidity of DSM-IV alcohol abuse and dependence in the United States: Results from the National Epidemiologic Survey on Alcohol and Related Conditions. *Archives of General Psychiatry*, 64(7), 830–842.

Hawkins, E. H. (2009). A tale of two systems: Co-occurring mental health and substance abuse disorders treatment for adolescents. *Annual Review of Psychology*, 60, 197–227.

Heffner, J. L., Strawn, J. R., & DelBello, M. P. (2011). The co-occurrence of cigarette smoking and bipolar disorder: Phenomenology and treatment considerations. *Bipolar Disorders*, 13(0), 439–453. doi:10.1111/j.1399-5618.2011.00943.x

Hemingway, E. M. (1929). *A farewell to arms* (1st ed.). New York, NY: Charles Scribner's Sons.

Henquet, C., Di Forti, M., & Morrison, P. (2008). Gene-environment interplay between cannabis and psychosis. *Schizophrenia Bulletin*, 34(6), 1111–1121.

Henquet, C., van Os, J., & Kuepper, R. (2010). Psychosis reactivity to cannabis use in daily life: An experience sampling study. *The British Journal of Psychiatry*, 196, 447–453.

Herbst, J. H., Jacobs, E. D., & Finlayson, T. J. (2008). Estimating HIV prevalence and risk behaviors of transgendered persons in the United States: A systematic review. *AIDS and Behavior*, 12(1), 1–17. doi:10.1007/s10461-007-9299-3

Hernandez-Avila, C. A., Rounsaville, B. J., & Kranzler, H. R. (2004). Opioid-, cannabis-, and alcohol-dependent women show more rapid progression to substance abuse treatment. *Drug and Alcohol Dependence*, 74(3), 265–272.

Hesselbrock, M. N., Hesselbrock, V. M., & Segal, B. (2003). Ethnicity and psychiatric comorbidity among alcohol-dependent persons who receive inpatient treatment: African Americans, Alaska Natives, Caucasians, and Hispanics. *Alcoholism: Clinical and Experimental Research*, 27(8), 1368–1373. doi:10.1097/01.ALC.0000080164.21934.F9

Hides, L., Dawe, S., & Kavanagh, D. J. (2006). Psychotic symptom and cannabis relapse in recent-onset psychosis. *The British Journal of Psychiatry*, 189, 137–143.

Holscher, F., Reissner, V., & Di Furia, L. (2010). Differences between men and women in the course of opiate dependence: Is there a telescoping effect? *European Archives of Psychiatry and Clinical Neuroscience*, 260(3), 235–241. doi:10.1007/s00406-009-0053-x

Houston, J. E., Murphy, J., & Adamson, G. (2007). Childhood sexual abuse, early cannabis use, and psychosis: Testing an interaction model based on the National Comorbidity Survey. *Schizophrenia Bulletin*, 34(3), 580–585.

Howard, J. (2016, December 27). Carrie Fisher was a champion for mental health, too. *Health*. CNN NewSource. Retrieved from www.kion546.com/health/carrie-fisher-was-a-champion-for-mental-health-too/235236766

Howe, C. Q., & Sullivan, M. D. (2014). The missing 'P' in pain manage: How the current opioid epidemic highlights the need for psychiatric services in chronic pain care. *General Hospital Psychiatry*, 36(1), 99–104. doi:10.1016/j.genhosppsych.2013.10.003

Hughes, T. L. (2003). Lesbians' drinking patterns: Beyond the data. *Substance Use & Misuse*, 38(11–13), 1739–1758.

Hughes, T. L. (2005). Alcohol use and alcohol-related problems among lesbians and gay men. *Annual Review of Nursing Research*, 23, 283–325.

Hunt, G. E., Malhi, G. S., & Cleary, M. (2016, June 25). Comorbidity of bipolar and substance use disorders in national surveys of general populations, 1990–2015: Systematic review and meta-analysis. *Journal of Affective Disorders*, 206, 321–330. doi:10.1016.j./jad.2016.06.051

Hussey, J. M., Chang, J. J., & Kotch, K. B. (2006). Child maltreatment in the United States: Prevalence, risk factors, and adolescent health consequences. *Pediatrics*, 118(3), 933–942.

Iannucci, R., Sanders, K., & Greenfield, S. F. (2009). A 4-year curriculum on substance use disorders for psychiatry residents. *Academic Psychiatry*, 33(1), 60–66.

Ivanenko, A., & Gururaj, B. R. (2009). Classification and epidemiology of sleep disorders. *Child and Adolescent Psychiatric Clinics of North America*, 18(4), 839–848.

Janes, A. C., Pedrelli, P., & Whitton, A. E. (2015). Reward responsiveness varies by smoking status in women with a history of major depressive disorder. *Neuropsychopharmacology*, 40(8), 1940–1946. doi:10.1038/npp.2015.43

Jessup, M. A., Dibble, S. L., & Cooper, B. A. (2012). Smoking and behavioral health of women. *Journal of Women's Health*, 21(7), 783–791. doi:10.1089/jwh.2011.2886

Johnson, E. O., Roth, T., & Breslau, N. (2006). The association of insomnia with anxiety disorders and depression: Exploration of the direction of risk. *Journal of Psychiatric Research*, 40(8), 700–708.

Johnson, S. D., Cottier, L. B., & Callahan O'Leary, C. (2010). The association of trauma and PTSD with the substance use profiles of alcohol and cocaine dependent out-of-treatment women. *The American Journal on Addictions*, 19(6), 490–495. doi:10.1011/j.1521-0391.2010.00075.x

Kalokhe, A. S., Paranjape, A., & Bell, C. E. (2012). Intimate partner violence among HIV-infected crack cocaine users. *AIDS Patient Care and STDs*, 26(4), 234–240. doi:10.1089/apc.2011.0275

Keller, M. B., Lavori, P. W., & Beardslee, W. R. (1992). The disruptive behavioral disorder in children and adolescents: Comorbidity and clinical course. *Journal of the American Academy of Child & Adolescent Psychiatry*, 31(2), 204–209. doi:10.1097/00004583-199203000-00005

Kendler, K., Bulik, C. M., & Silberg, J. (2000). Childhood sexual abuse and adult psychiatric and substance use disorders in women: An epidemiological and co-twin control analysis. *Archives of General Psychiatry*, 57(10), 953–959.

Kern, A. M., Akerman, S. C., & Nordstrom, B. R. (2014). Opiate dependence in schizophrenia: Case presentation and literature review. *Journal of Dual Diagnosis*, 10(1), 52–57. doi:10,1080/15504263.2013.867199

Keuroghlian, A. S., Reisner, S. L., & White, J. M. (2015, July 1). Substance use and treatment of substance use disorders in a community sample of transgender adults. *Drug and Alcohol Dependence*, 152, 134–146. doi:10.1016/j.drugalcdep.2015.04.008

Keyes, K. M., Martins, S. S., & Blanco, C. (2010). Telescoping and gender differences in alcohol dependence: New evidence from two national surveys. *The American Journal of Psychiatry*, 167(8), 969–976. doi:10.1176/appi.ajp.2009.09081161

Khan, S. S., Secades-Villa, R., & Okuda, M. (2013). Gender differences in cannabis use disorders: Results from the National Epidemiologic Survey of Alcohol and Related Conditions. *Drug and Alcohol Dependence*, 130(1–3), 101–108. doi:10.1016/j.drugalcdep.2012.10.10.015

Killeen, T., Brewerton, T. D., & Campbell, A. (2015, November). Exploring the relationship between eating disorder symptoms and substance use severity in women with comorbid PTSD and substance use disorders. *The American Journal of Drug and Alcohol Abuse*, 41(6), 547–552. doi:10.3109/00952990.2015.1080263

Kreek, M. J., & Stimmel, B. (Eds.). (1984). *Dual addiction: Pharmacological issues in the treatment of concomitant alcoholism and drug abuse*. Binghamton, NY: Haworth.

Krishnan, K. R. (2005). Psychiatric and medical comorbidities of bipolar disorder. *Psychosomatic Medicine*, 67(1), 1–8.

Krystal, J. H., D'Souza, D. C., & Gallinat, J. (2006). The vulnerability to alcohol and substance abuse in individuals diagnosed with schizophrenia. *Neurotoxicity Research*, 10(3–4), 235–252.

Lai, H. M., Cleary, M., & Sitharthan, T. (2015, September 1). Prevalence of comorbid substance use, anxiety and mood disorders in epidemiological surveys, 1990–2014: A systematic review and meta-analysis. *Drug and Alcohol Dependence*, 154, 1–13. doi:10.1016/j.drugalcdep.2015.05.031

Lala, S. V., & Sajatovic, M. (2012). Medical and psychiatric comorbidities among elderly individuals with bipolar disorder: A literature review. *Journal of Geriatric Psychiatry and Neurology*, 25(1), 20–25. doi:10.1177/0891988712446683

Le Bec, P. Y., Fatseas, M., & Denis, C. (2009). Cannabis and psychosis: Search of a causal link through a critical and systematic review. *L'Encephale*, 35(4), 377–385. doi:10.1016/j.encep.2008.02.012

Leeies, M., Pagura, J., & Sareen, J. (2010). The use of alcohol and drugs to self-medicate symptoms of posttraumatic stress disorder. *Depression and Anxiety*, 27(8), 731–736. doi:10.1002/da.20677

Linszen, D., & van Amelsvoort, T. (2007). Cannabis and psychosis: An update on course and biological plausible mechanisms. *Current Opinion in Psychiatry*, 20(2), 116–120.

Lo, C. C., Cheng, T. C., & de la Rosa, I. A. (2015). Depression and substance use: A temporal-ordered model. *Substance Use & Misuse*, 50(10), 1274–1283. doi:10.3109/10826084.2014.998236

Long-time cannabis use associated with psychosis. (2010, March 2). Retrieved from ScienceDaily.com: www.sciencedaily.com/releases/2010/03/100301165726.htm

Lynch, S. M., Dehart, D. D., & Belknap, J. E. (2014). A multisite study of the prevalence of serious mental illness, PTSD, and substance abuse disorders of women in jail. *Psychiatric Services*, 65(5), 670–674. doi:10.1176/appi.201300172

Ma, L. (2001, November 1). Interview: The Fisher Queen. *Psychology Today*, 1–6. Retrieved from www.psychologytoday.com/articles/200111/interview-the-fisher-queen

Mai, E., & Buysse, D. J. (2008). Insomnia: Prevalence, impact, pathogenesis, differential diagnosis, and evaluation. *Sleep Medicine Clinics*, 3(2), 167–174.

Majer, J. M., Komer, A. C., & Jason, L. A. (2015). Psychiatric severity and HIV-risk sexual behaviors among persons with substance use disorders. *Journal of Dual Diagnosis*, 11(1), 3–11. doi:10.1080/15504263.2014.990802

Malmquist, C. P. (1990). Depression in homicidal adolescents. *The Bulletin of the American Academy of Psychiatry and the Law*, 18(1), 23–36.

Manchikanti, L., Giordano, J., & Boswell, M. V. (2007). Psychological factors as predictors of opioid abuse and illicit drug use in chronic pain patients. *Journal of Opioid Management*, 3(2), 89–100.

Mangweth-Matzek, B., Hoek, H. W., & Pope Jr., H. G. (2014). Pathological eating and body dissatisfaction in middle-aged and older women. *Current Opinion in Psychiatry*, 27(6), 431–435. doi:10.1097/YCO.0000000000000102

Margolese, H. C., Malchy, L., & Negrete, J. C. (2004). Drug and alcohol use among patients with schizophrenia and related psychoses: Levels and consequences. *Schizophrenia Research*, 67(2–3), 157–166.

Marineti, L., & Montgomery, M. A. (2010). The use of GHB to facilitate sexual assault. *Forensic Science Review*, 22(1), 41–59.

Marmorstein, N. R. (2009). Longitudinal associations between alcohol problems and depressive symptoms: Early adolescence through early adulthood. *Alcoholism: Clinical & Experimental Research*, 33(1), 49–59.

McClean, J. M., Anspikian, A., & Winters, B. N. (2014). Factors that affect treatment among individuals with serious mental illness and substance abuse disorder. *Addictive Disorders & Their Treatment*, 13(1), 16–24.

McHugh, R. K., Votaw, V. R., & Bogunovic, O. (2017, February). Anxiety sensitivity and nonmedical benzodiazepine use among adults with opioid use disorder. *Addictive Behaviors*, 65, 283–288. doi:10.1016/j.addbeh.2016.08.020

Miller, L. J., Girgis, C., & Gupta, R. (2009). Depression and related disorders during the female reproductive cycle. *Women's Health (London, England)*, 5(5), 577–587. doi:10.2217/whe.09.44

Miller, N. S., Belkin, B. M., & Gibbons, R. (1994). Clinical diagnosis of substance use disorders in private psychiatric populations. *Journal of Substance Abuse Treatment*, 11(4), 387–392.

Moghaddam, J. F., Dickerson, D. L., & Yoon, G. (2014, November 1). Nicotine dependence and psychiatric and substance use disorder comorbidities among American Indians/Alaska Natives: Findings from the National Epidemiologic Survey on Alcohol and Related Conditions. *Drug and Alcohol Dependence*, 144, 127–133. doi:10.1016/j.drugalcdep.2014.08.017

Morris, E. P., Stewart, S. H., & Ham, L. S. (2005). The relationship between social anxiety disorder and alcohol use disorders: A critical review. *Clinical Psychology Review*, 25(6), 734–760. doi:10.1016/j.cpr.2005.05.004

Muller-Vahl, K. R., & Emrich, H. M. (2008). Cannabis and schizophrenia: Towards a cannabinoid hypothesis of schizophrenia. *Expert Review of Neurotherapeutics*, 8(7), 1037–1048.

Myers, U.S., Browne, K. C., & Norman, S. B. (2015). Treatment engagement: Female survivors of intimate partner violence in treatment for PTSD and alcohol use disorder. *Journal of Dual Diagnosis*, 11(3–4), 238–247. doi:10.1080/15504263.2015.1113762

Najavits, L. M., Weiss, R. D., & Shaw, S. R. (1997). The link between substance abuse and posttraumatic stress disorder in women. *The American Journal on Addictions*, 6(4), 273–283. doi:10.1111/j.1521-0391.1997.tb00408.x

Nauert, R. (2014, June 28). *Severe mental illness ups risk for substance abuse.* Retrieved June 28, 2014, from Psych Central News, pp. 1–2: http://psychcentral.com/news/2014/01/06/severe-mental-illness-ups-risk-for-substance-abuse/64161.html

Nelson, E. C., Heath, A. C., & Lynskey, M. T. (2006). Childhood sexual abuse and risks for licit and illicit drug-related outcomes. *Psychological Medicine*, 36(10), 1473–1483.

NIAAA, National Institute on Alcohol Abuse and Alcoholism. (2013, July). *Using alcohol to relieve your pain: What are the risks?* Retrieved from National Institute on Alcohol Abuse and Alcoholism: www.niaaa.nih.gov

Nivoli, A. M., Pacchiarotti, I., & Rosa, A. R. (2011). Gender differences in a cohort study of 604 bipolar patients: The role of predominant polarity. *Journal of Affective Disorders*, 133(3), 443–449. doi:10.1016/j.jad.2011.04.055

Nurnberger, J. I., Foroud, T., & Flury, L. (2002). Is there a genetic relationship between alcoholism and depression? *Alcohol Research & Health*, 26(3), 233–240.

Ouimette, P., & Brown, P. J. (2003). *Trauma and substance abuse: Causes, consequences, and treatment of comorbid disorders*. Washington, DC: American Psychological Association.

Ouimette, P., Read, J. P., & Wade, M. (2010). Modeling associations between posttraumatic stress symptoms and substance use. *Addictive Behaviors*, 35(1), 64–67. doi:10.1016/j.addbeh.2009.08.009

Padilla, Y. C., Crisp, C., & Rew, D. L. (2010). Parental acceptance and illegal drug use among gay, lesbian, and bisexual adolescents: Results from a national survey. *Social Work*, 55(3), 265–275.

Pagliaro, A. M., & Pagliaro, L. A. (1992). Sentenced to death? HIV infection and AIDS in prisons—current and future concerns. *Canadian Journal of Criminology*, 34, 201–214.

Pagliaro, A. M., & Pagliaro, L. A. (1993a). Knowledge, behaviours, and risk perception of intravenous drug users (IVDUs) in relation to HIV infection and AIDS: Initial results of the PIARG major study (abstract). *Proceedings of the First International Conference on Community Health Nursing Research*, 1, p. 113. Edmonton, Alberta, Canada.

Pagliaro, A. M., & Pagliaro, L. A. (1994). What do 261 "hardcore" intravenous drug using women know and do in relation to HIV infection and AIDS? A report from the PIARG Major Study. *Proceedings of the Eighth Annual Margaret Scott Wright Lectureship and Research Conference (Abstract)*, p. 27. Edmonton, Alberta, Canada.

Pagliaro, A. M., & Pagliaro, L. A. (2000). *Substance use among women: A reference and resource guide*. Philadelphia, PA: Brunner Mazel.

Pagliaro, A. M., & Pagliaro, L. A. (2003). Addictionologists' perspective on catastrophic injury. In K. N. Anchor, J. Shmerling, & J. M. Anchor (Eds.), *The catastrophic injury handbook* (pp. 213–227). Dubuque, IO: Kendall/Hunt.

Pagliaro, A. M., Pagliaro, L. A., & Thauberger, P. C. (1993). Knowledge, behaviours, and risk perception of intravenous drug users in relation to HIV infection and AIDS: The PIARG projects. *Advances in Medical Psychotherapy*, 6, 1–28.

Pagliaro, L. A. (1990). Dual diagnosis. *Alberta Psychology*, 19(5), 23–24.

Pagliaro, L. A., & Pagliaro, A. M. (1993b). What do 1,045 "hard-core" intravenous drug users know and do in relation to HIV infection and AIDS? A report from the PIARG Major Study (abstract). *Canadian Psychology*, 15(2a), p. 181. Toronto: Canadian Psychology Association.

Pagliaro, L. A., & Pagliaro, A. M. (1999). *PPDR: The psychologists' psychotropic drug reference*. Philadelphia, PA: Brunner/Mazel.

Pagliaro, L. A., & Pagliaro, A. M. (2004). *Pagliaros' comprehensive guide to drugs and substances of abuse* (1st ed.). Washington, DC: American Pharmacists Association.

Pagliaro, L. A., & Pagliaro, A. M. (2009). *Pagliaros' comprehensive guide to drugs and substances of abuse* (2nd ed.). Washington, DC: American Pharmacists Association.

Pagliaro, L. A., Jaglalsingh, L. H., & Pagliaro, A. M. (1992). Cocaine use and depression. *Canadian Medical Association Journal*, 147, 1636–1637.

Parrott, A. C. (2003). Cigarette-derived nicotine is not a medicine. *The World Journal of Biological Psychiatry*, 4(2), 49–55.

Pedersen, E. R., Myers, U.S., & Browne, K. C. (2014). The role of alcohol expectancies in drinking behavior among women with alcohol use disorder and comorbid posttraumatic stress disorder. *Journal of Psychoactive Drugs*, 46(3), 178–187. doi:10.1080/02791072.2014.917750

Penick, E. C., Nickel, E. J., & Cantrell, P. F. (1990). The emerging concept of dual diagnosis: An overview and implications. In D. F. O'Connell (Ed.), *Managing the dually diagnosed patient: Current issues and clinical approaches* (pp. 1–54). New York, NY: Haworth.

Piazza, N. J., Vrbka, J. L., & Yeager, R. D. (1989). Telescoping of alcoholism in women alcoholics. *International Journal of Addiction*, 24(1), 19–28.

Polydorou, S., Gunderson, E. W., & Levin, F. R. (2008). Training physicians to treat substance use disorders. *Current Psychiatry Reports*, 10(5), 399–404.

Potvin, S., Stip, E., & Roy, J. Y. (2003). Schizophrenia and addiction: An evaluation of the self-medication hypothesis. *Encephale*, 29(3, Part 1), 193–203.

Prusakowski, M. K., Shofer, F. S., & Rhodes, K. V. (2011). Effect of depression and psychosocial stressors on cessation self-efficacy in mothers who smoke. *Maternal and Child Health Journal*, 15(5), 620–626. doi:10.1007/s10995-010-0640-5

Quinnett, P. G. (1995). *Suicide: The forever decision. For those thinking about suicide, and for those who know, love or counsel them.* New York, NY: Crossroad.

Radhakrishnan, R., Wilkinson, S. T., & D'Souza, D. C. (2014). Gone to pot—A review of the association between cannabis and psychosis. *Frontiers in Psychiatry*, 5(Article 54), 1–24. doi:10.3389/fpsyt.2014.00054

Randall, C. L., Roberts, J. S., & Del Boca, F. K. (1999). Telescoping of landmark events associated with drinking: A gender comparison. *Journal of Studies on Alcohol*, 60(2), 252–260.

Rash, C. J., Burki, M., & Montezuma-Rusca, J. M. (2016). A retrospective and prospective analysis of trading sex for drugs or money in women substance abuse treatment patients. *Drug and Alcohol Dependence*, 162, 182–189.

Rasmussen, H. F., Borelli, J. L., & Decoste, C. (2016). A longitudinal examination of toddlers' behavioral cues as a function of substance-abusing mothers' disengagement. *Infant Mental Health Journal*, 37(2), 140–150. doi:10.1002/imhj.21552

Reed, P. L., Anthony, J. C., & Breslau, N. (2007). Incidence of drug problems in young adults exposed to trauma and posttraumatic stress disorder: Do early life experiences and predispositions matter? *Archives of General Psychiatry*, 64(12), 1435–1442.

Renner, J. A. (2004). How to train residents to identify and treat dual diagnosis patients. *Biological Psychiatry*, 56(10), 810–816.

Rich, C. L., & Runeson, B. S. (1992). Similarities in diagnostic comorbidity between suicide among young people in Sweden and the United States. *Acta Psychiatrica Scandinavica*, 86(5), 335–339.

Robinson, J., Sareen, J., & Cox, B. J. (2009). Self-medication of anxiety disorders with alcohol and drugs: Results from a nationally representative sample. *Journal of Anxiety Disorders*, 23(1), 38–45. doi:10.1016/j.janxdis.2008.03.013

Roehrs, T., & Roth, T. (2008). Caffeine: Sleep and daytime sleepiness. *Sleep Medicine Reviews*, 12(2), 153–162.

Rondinelli, A. J., Ouellet, L. J., & Strathdee, S. A. (2009). Young adult injection drug users in the United States continue to practice HIV risk behaviors. *Drug and Alcohol Dependence*, 104(1–2), 167–174.

Rosario, M. (2008). Elevated substance use among lesbian and bisexual women: Possible explanations and intervention implications for an urgent public health concern. *Substance Use & Misuse*, 43(8–9), 1268–1270. doi:10.1080/10826080802215130

Rosario, M., Schrimshaw, E. W., & Hunter, J. (2004). Predictors of substance use over time among gay, lesbian, and bisexual youths: An examination of three hypotheses. *Addictive Behaviors*, 29(8), 1623–1631.

Rowe, C., Santos, G. M., & McFarland, W. (2015, February 1). Prevalence and correlates of substance use among trans female youth ages 16–24 years in the San Francisco Bay Area. *Drug and Alcohol Dependence*, 147, 160–166. doi:10.1016/j.drugalcdep.2014.11.023

Rubino, T., & Parolaro, D. (2008). Long lasting consequences of cannabis exposure in adolescence. *Molecular and Cellular Endocrinology*, 286(1–2, Supplement 1), S108–S113.

Ruiz, M. A., Douglas, K. S., & Edens, J. F. (2012). Co-occurring mental health and substance use problems in offenders: Implications for risk assessment. *Psychological Assessment*, 24(1), 77–87. doi:10.1037/a0024623

Rush, B., & Koegl, C. J. (2008). Prevalence and profile of people with co-occurring mental and substance use disorders within a comprehensive mental health system. *Canadian Journal of Psychiatry*, 53(12), 810–821.

Ryan, C., Huebner, D., & Diaz, R. (2009). Family rejection as a predictor of negative health outcomes in white and Latino lesbian, gay, and bisexual young adults. *Pediatrics*, 123(1), 346–352.

Ryder, J. A., & Brisgone, R. E. (2013). Cracked perspectives: Reflections of women and girls in the aftermath of the crack cocaine era. *Feminist Criminology*, 8(1), 40–62. doi:10.1177/1557085112444899

Santos, G. M., Rapues, J., & Wilson, E. C. (2014). Alcohol and substance use among transgender women in San Francisco: Prevalence and association with human immunodeficiency virus infection. *Drug and Alcohol Review*, 33(3), 287–295. doi:10.1111/dar.12116

Satre, D. D., Chi, F. W., & Eisendrath, S. (2011). Sub-diagnostic alcohol use by depressed men and women seeking outpatient psychiatric services: Consumption patterns and motivation to reduce drinking. *Alcoholism: Clinical and Experimental Research*, 35(4), 695–702. doi:10.1111/j.1530-0277.2010.01387.x

Satre, D. D., Sterling, S. A., & Mackin, R. S. (2011). Patterns of alcohol and drug use among depressed older adults seeking outpatient psychiatric services. *The American Journal of Geriatric Psychiatry*, 19(8), 695–703. doi:10.1097/JGP.0b013e3181f17f0a

Schaumberg, K., Vinci, C., & Raiker, J. S. (2015, February). PTSD-related alcohol expectancies and impulsivity interact to predict alcohol use severity in a substance dependent sample with PTSD. *Addictive Behaviors*, 41, 41–45. doi:10.1016/j.addbeh.2014.09.022

Schneider, M. (2008). Puberty as a highly vulnerable developmental period for the consequences of cannabis exposure. *Addiction Biology*, 13(2), 253–263.

Schoemaker, C., Smit, F., & Bijl, R. V. (2002). Bulimia nervosa following psychological and multiple child abuse: Support for the self-medication hypothesis in a population-based cohort study. *International Journal of Eating Disorders*, 32(4), 381–388. doi:10.1002/eat.10102

Seay, K. D., & Kohl, P. L. (2015). The comorbid and individual impacts of maternal depression and substance dependence on parenting and child behavior problems. *Journal of Family Violence*, 30(7), 899–910. doi:10.10076/s10896-015-9721-y

Sehgal, N., Manchikanti, L., & Smith, H. S. (2012). Prescription opioid abuse in chronic pain: A review of opioid abuse predictors and strategies to curb opioid abuse. *Pain Physician*, 15(Supplement 3), ES67–ES92.

Sher, L. (2006). Alcohol and suicide: Neurobiological and clinical aspects. *The Scientific World Journal*, 6, 700–706.

Sher, L., Sperling, D., & Stanley, B. H. (2007). Triggers for suicidal behavior in depressed older adolescents and young adults: Do alcohol use disorders make a difference? *International Journal of Adolescent Medicine and Health*, 19(1), 91–98.

Shorter, D., Hsieh, J., & Kosten, T. R. (2015). Pharmacologic management of comorbid post-traumatic stress disorder and addictions. *The American Journal on Addictions*, 24(8), 705–712. doi:10.1111/ajad.12306

Simpson, T. L., & Miller, W. R. (2002). Concomitance between childhood sexual and physical abuse and substance use problems: A review. *Clinical Psychology Review*, 22(1), 27–77.

Slesnick, N., & Prestopnik, J. (2005). Dual and multiple diagnosis among substance using runaway youth. *The American Journal of Drug and Alcohol Abuse*, 31(1), 179–201.

Smink, F. R., van Hoeken, D., & Hoek, H. W. (2013). Epidemiology, course, and outcome of eating disorders. *Current Opinion in Psychiatry*, 26(6), 543–548. doi:10.1097/YCO.0b013e328365a24f

Sofuoglu, M., Rosenheck, R., & Petrakis, I. (2014). Pharmacological treatment of comorbid PTSD and substance use disorder: Recent progress. *Addictive Behaviors*, 39(2), 1–13. doi:10.1016/j.addbeh.2013.08.014

Sonne, S. C., & Brady, K. T. (2002, November). *Bipolar disorder and alcoholism*. Retrieved August 9, 2016, from National Institute on Alcohol Abuse and Alcoholism: http://pubs.niaaa.nih.gov/publications/arh26-2/103–108.htm

Spence, S., & Courbasson, C. (2012). The role of emotional dysregulation in concurrent eating disorders and substance use disorders. *Eating Behaviors*, 382–387. doi:10.1016/j.eatbeh.2012.05.006

Stepanski, E. J., & Rybarczyk, B. (2006). Emerging research on the treatment and etiology of secondary or comorbid insomnia. *Sleep Medicine Reviews*, 10, 7–18.

Stowell, R. J. (1991). Dual diagnosis issues. *Psychiatric Annals*, 21(2), 98–104. doi:10.3928/0048-5713-19910201-09

Strakowski, S. M., DelBello, M. P., & Fleck, D. E. (2000). The impact of substance abuse on the course of bipolar disorder. *Biological Psychiatry*, 48(6), 477–485.

Stromwall, L. K., & Larson, N. C. (2004). Women's experience of co-occurring substance abuse and mental health conditions. *Journal of Social Work Practice in the Addictions*, 4(1), 81–96.

Sublette, M. E., Carballo, J. J., & Moreno, C. (2009). Substance use disorders and suicide attempts in bipolar subtypes. *Journal of Psychiatric Research*, 43(3), 230–238. doi:10.1016/j.jpsychires.2008.05.001

Suchman, N. E., Decoste, C., & Rosenberger, P. (2012). Attachment-based intervention for substance-using mothers: A preliminary test of the proposed mechanisms of change. *Infant Mental Health Journal*, 33(4), 360–371. doi:10.1002/imhj.21311

Sullivan, T. P., Weiss, N. H., & Flanagan, J. C. (2016). PTSD and daily co-occurrence of drug and alcohol use among women experiencing intimate partner violence. *Journal of Dual Diagnosis*, 12(1), 36–42. doi:10.1080/15504263.2016.1146516

Takeuchi, L. C., Pham, T. K., & Katz, A. R. (2015). Hepatitis C virus antibody prevalence, demographics and associated factors among persons screened at Hawai'i community-based health settings, 2010–2013. *Hawaii Journal of Medicine & Public Health*, 74(1), 9–15.

Thirthalli, J., & Benegal, V. (2006). Psychosis among substance users. *Current Opinion in Psychiatry*, 19(3), 239–245.

Thompson-Brenner, H., Eddy, K. T., & Franko, D. L. (2008). Personality pathology and substance abuse in eating disorders: A longitudinal study. *International Journal of Eating Disorders*, 41(3), 203–208. doi:10.1002/eat.20489

Torchalla, I., Strehlau, V., & Li, K. (2011). Substance use and predictors of substance dependence in homeless women. *Drug and Alcohol Dependence*, 118(2–3), 173–179. doi:10.1016/j.drugalcdep.2011.03.016

Tuchman, E. (2010). Women and addiction: The importance of gender issues in substance abuse research. *Journal of Addictive Diseases*, 29(2), 127–138. doi:10.1080/10550881003684582

Tucker, P. (2009). Substance misuse and early psychosis. *Australasian Psychiatry*, 17(4), 291–294.

University of Wisconsin School of Medicine and Public Health. (2016, June 27). *Alcohol and drug screening by paraprofessionals reduces Medicaid costs*. Retrieved August 13, 2016, from University of Wisconsin School of Medicine and Public Health: www.med.wisc.edu/news-events/alcohol-and-drug-screening-reduces-medicaid-costs/48746

Valentiner, D. P., Mounts, N. S., & Deacon, B. J. (2004). Panic attacks, depression and anxiety symptoms, and substance use behaviors during late adolescence. *Journal of Anxiety Disorders*, 18(5), 573–585. doi:10.1016/j.janxdis.2003.04.001

van Os, J., Bak, M., & Hanssen, M. (2002). Cannabis use and psychosis: A longitudinal population-based study. *American Journal of Epidemiology*, 156, 319–327.

Verdoux, H., & Tournier, M. (2004). Cannabis use and risk of psychosis: An etiological link? *Epidemiologia Psichiatria Sociale*, 13(2), 113–119.

Volkman, J. E., DeRycke, E. C., & Driscoll, M. A. (2015). Smoking status and pain intensity among OEF/OIF/OND veterans. *Pain Medicine*, 16(9), 1690–1696. doi:10.1111/pme.12753

Warren, C. S., Lindsay, A. R., & White, E. K. (2013). Weight-related concerns related to drug use for women in substance abuse treatment: Prevalence and relationships with eating pathology. *Journal of Substance Abuse Treatment* 44(5), 494–501. doi:10.1016/j.sat.2012.08.222

Wasan, A. D., Butler, S. F., & Budman, S. H. (2007). Psychiatric history and psychologic adjustment as risk factors for aberrant drug-related behavior among patients with chronic pain. *The Clinical Journal of Pain*, 23(4), 307–315. doi:10.1097/AJP.0b013e3180330dc5

Wasan, A. D., Michna, E., & Edwards, R. R. (2015). Psychiatric comorbidity is associated prospectively with diminished opioid analgesia and increased opioid misuse in patients with chronic low back pain. *Anesthesiology*, 123(4), 861–872. doi:10.1097/ALN.0000000000000768

Westermeyer, J., Wahmanholm, K., & Thuras, P. (2001). Effects of childhood physical abuse on course and severity of substance abuse. *The American Journal on Addictions*, 10(2), 101–110.

White, M. A., & Grilo, C. M. (2006). Psychiatric comorbidity in binge-eating disorder as a function of smoking history. *Journal of Clinical Psychiatry*, 67(4), 594–599.

Wilkinson, S. T., Stefanovics, E., & Rosenheck, R. A. (2015). Marijuana use is associated with worse outcomes in symptom severity and violent behavior in patients with posttraumatic stress disorder. *Journal of Clinical Psychiatry*, 76(9), 1174–1180. doi:10.4088/JCP.14m09475

Williams, J. M., & Gandhi, K. K. (2008, June). Use of caffeine and nicotine in people with schizophrenia. *Current Drug Abuse Reviews*, 1(2), 155–161.

Winklbaur, B., Ebner, N., & Sachs, G. (2006). Substance abuse in patients with schizophrenia. *Dialogues in Clinical Neuroscience*, 8(1), 37–43.

Worley, L. L., Conners, N. A., & Crone, C. C. (2005). Building a residential treatment program for dually diagnosed women with their children. *Archives of Women's Mental Health*, 8(2), 105–111.

Wu, L. T., & Blazer, D. G. (2014). Substance use disorders and psychiatric comorbidity in mid and later life: A review. *International Journal of Epidemiology*, 43(2), 304–317. doi:10.1093/ije/dyt173

Wu, L. T., Gersing, K. R., & Swartz, M. S. (2013). Using electronic health records data to assess comorbidities of substance use and psychiatric diagnoses and treatment settings among adults. *Journal of Psychiatric Research*, 47(4), 555–563. doi:10.1016/j.jpsychires.2012.12.009

Yoon, G., Petrakis, I. L., & Rosenheck, R. A. (2015). Correlates of major depressive disorder with and without comorbid alcohol use disorder nationally in the Veterans Health Administration. *The American Journal on Addictions*, 419–426. doi:10.1111/ajad.12219

Yoon, Y. H., Chen, C. M., & Yi, H. Y. (2011). Effect of comorbid alcohol and drug use disorders on premature death among unipolar and bipolar disorder decedents in the United States, 1999 to 2006. *Comprehensive Psychiatry*, 52(5), 453–464. doi:10.1016/j.comppsych.2010.10.005

Zammit, S., Moore, T. H., & Lingford-Hughes, A. (2008, November). Effects of cannabis use on outcomes of psychotic disorders: Systematic review. *British Journal of Psychiatry*, 193(5), 357–363. doi:10.1192/bjp.bp.107.046375

Ziedonis, D. M., Smelson, D., & Rosenthal, R. N. (2005). Improving the care of individuals with schizophrenia and substance use disorders: Consensus recommendations. *Journal of Psychiatric Practice*, 11(5), 315–339.

Zlotnick, C., Clarke, J. G., & Friedmann, P. D. (2008). Gender differences in comorbid disorders among offenders in prison substance abuse treatment programs. *Behavioral Sciences & Law*, 26(4), 403–412. doi:10.1002/bsl.831

Zukov, I., Ptacek, R., & Raboch, J. (2010). Premenstrual dysphoric disorder—Review of actual findings about mental disorders related to menstrual cycle and possibilities of their therapy. *Prague Medical Report*, 111(1), 12–24.

Zullig, K. J., & Divin, A. L. (2012). The association between non-medical prescription drug use, depressive symptoms, and suicidality among college students. *Addictive Behaviors*, 37(8), 890–899. doi:10.1016/j.addbeh.2012.02.008

8

PREVENTING AND TREATING WOMEN'S DRUG AND SUBSTANCE ABUSE

Popular Notion: The severity and complications of alcohol use disorders (AUDs) and substance use disorders (SUDs) among women, when compared to men, are relatively minor, making prevention and treatment much easier.

NOT TRUE. When compared to men, women are less likely to enter drug and substance abuse treatment and, when they do enter treatment, they are *more* likely to: (1) be younger; (2) have been referred from a community agency (e.g., child welfare; drug court; mental health services); (3) be pregnant; (4) be responsible for one or more minor dependent children; (5) have *more* drug and substance abuse related problems (medical; psychological; and social); (6) have more severe personal problems; (7) have experienced *more* physical, mental, and sexual abuse; and (8) have a greater number of contemporaneous diagnoses that require treatment.[1] (See following chapter sections for additional discussion and documentation.)

Exposure to and use of the drugs and substances of abuse by women during the new millennium in the U.S. are associated with significant physical, mental, and social harm (e.g., Greenfield, Back, & Lawson, 2010; Pagliaro & Pagliaro, *Clinical Patient Data Files*;Tuchman, 2010). Consequently, it is patently obvious that, whenever possible, *increased* attention must be given to preventing, or at least minimizing, women's drug and substance abuse. To assist health and social care professionals

[1] For detailed, related discussion, documentation, and referencing, see the previous chapters in this text. For example, regarding the last factor, "contemporaneous diagnoses," see Chapter 7, *Identifying Women's Contemporaneous Diagnoses*.

in meeting this challenge, we collected, analyzed, and synthesized the available literature that both: (1) addressed specific treatment approaches for women; and (2) was published between 2000 and 2017. We found that many of these approaches were significantly associated with a *decrease* in women's drug and substance abuse. Although challenging, and often difficult to effect,[2] our findings provide strong evidence that, with early and accurate detection of women's harmful use of the drugs and substances of abuse, as well as timely implementation of appropriate treatment approaches, positive treatment outcomes can be both *achievable* and *maintainable*.

As a result of our findings, this chapter focuses on prevention approaches that are concerned with fostering and maintaining patterns of:

1. Nonuse
2. Social Use, once use has begun
3. Controlled Use, including changing method of use or substitution (or replacement) pharmacotherapy, once Habitual Use, Abuse, or Compulsive Use have begun
4. Resumed Nonuse, once abstinence has been achieved, to prevent Relapsed Use, or a return to harmful patterns of drug and substance abuse

Popular Notion: Gender-specific, or "women-only," programs provide *optimal* outcomes for almost all women who seek treatment for harmful patterns of drug and substance abuse.

NOT TRUE, on *many* levels and for *many* reasons (see related discussion in the following sections of this chapter).

As noted in the previous chapters of this text, women's drug and substance abuse is a long-standing, complex, and pervasive concern in the U.S. Therefore, it is *illogical* and *naive* to expect that a single, overly simplistic prevention approach (e.g., increasing a woman's knowledge concerning the dangers associated with the use of the drugs and substances of abuse; increasing a woman's empowerment, self-esteem, or decision-making abilities) will *always*, or even in most cases, be effective for *all* women. In fact, what is needed to achieve *optimal* efficacious treatment outcomes for women is the use of a variety of primary, secondary, and tertiary approaches that have been designed for: (1) *individual* women and *groups* of

[2] "Difficult to effect" because, as demonstrated, documented, and discussed in this chapter, there is no "magic bullet." Amidst this ever growing and worsening problem of drug and substance abuse by women in the U.S. during the new millennium, successful prevention and efficacious treatment is possible. However, what is required is empirically validated treatment approaches, which—because of their very nature—necessitate specialized knowledge and clinical abilities, along with immense attention and dedication, among health and social care professionals.

women—young, middle-aged, and older women; (2) women of various continental and other descents; and (3) women, who are bisexual, heterosexual, lesbian, or trans—and their identified *unique* patterns of drug and substance abuse.[3]

As recommended by Ashley, Marsden, and Brady (2003, p. 19), in addition to women-only and other relatively successful drug and substance abuse treatment programs that have been developed for women over the last 2 decades, for optimal success, attention also must be given to the *specific needs* identified by new millennial women in treatment, including those of women, who are pregnant, or who are mothers of dependent children, including for these women:

1. Prenatal care
2. Child care
3. Supplemental services and workshops that address women-focused topics
4. Mental health programming
5. Comprehensive programming

Since these recommendations were made, many different approaches, programs, and services (e.g., Covington, 2008a, 2008b) have been developed and implemented in an effort to *prevent* women from *initiating* drug and substance use or to *minimize* the associated harmful effects and toxicities associated with increasingly harmful patterns of use. Unfortunately, during the first 2 decades of the new millennium, a large number of these programs and services were *unsuccessful* due to: (1) inadequate attention to the recommendations that were made; and (2) changing mental, physical, and social factors commonly associated with new millennial women's drug and substance abuse.

For example, the significant *increase* in the numbers of homeless women in the U.S. during the new millennium, which has been linked to a corresponding significant increase in the numbers and percentages of women with alcohol use disorders (AUDs) or substance use disorders (SUDs) (Campbell, 2015; Greenfield, Rosa, & Putnins, 2011; Lynch, Roth, & Carroll, 2002; McHugh, Wigderson, & Greenfield, 2014; Roth, Cosgrove, & Carroll, 2004; Shaw, Grant, & Barbosa-Leiker, 2015; Slesnick & Erdem, 2013; Welch-Lazoritz, Whitbeck, & Armenta, 2015).

Consequently, we have taken these, and other similar recommendations, much further in the various sections throughout this chapter as we identify and discuss the following *specific needs* that require increased attention and operationalization in drug and substance abuse treatment programs for women:

- Academic assistance
- Age-appropriate focus (e.g., young women versus older women)

---

[3] See, for example, the section, *New Millennial Interactive Model of Women's Drug and Substance Abuse*, at the end of this chapter.

- Anger and aggression management
- Birthing and neonatal care courses for pregnant women
- Body weight management and reduction[4]
- Building self-esteem
- Child care
- Communication skills
- Conflict resolution
- Dealing with shame and stigma
- Dental care (preventive and restorative dentistry [e.g., caries; cracked teeth due to bruxism; gingivitis; tooth loss]—particularly associated with regular, long-term use of amphetamines [e.g., "meth mouth"], cocaine, and MDMA)
- Drug and substance abuse education
- Employment/vocational counseling or training
- Family therapy
- Financial counseling
- Follow-up (aftercare)
- Group therapy
- HIV and other infection testing (e.g., hepatitis C) and counseling/referral
- Housing assistance (e.g., rental and utility assistance; transitional housing)
- Individual therapy
- Intimate partner violence (IPV)
- Legal services
- Life skills programs
- Maternal-infant bonding
- Medical care
- Mothering courses for young women, including pregnant, new, and other mothers
- Nutritional counseling
- Pharmacotherapy for AUDs and/or SUDs and OMDs
- Prenatal care for pregnant women
- Professional referrals for family members (e.g., children; spouses; or significant others)
- Protective behavioral strategies
- Psychotherapy for women with AUDs and/or SUDs and other mental disorders (OMDs)
- Relapse prevention programs
- Risk reduction strategies for sexual victimization

---

[4] As noted by Warren, Lindsay, and White (2013), women's body weight-related concerns (e.g., weight gain during and after treatment; the potential contribution of weight gain to relapsed use) are often identified by women, who are receiving treatment for AUDs and/or SUDs. (See Chapter 7, *Identifying Women's Contemporaneous Diagnoses*, section "WCDs: Eating Disorders."

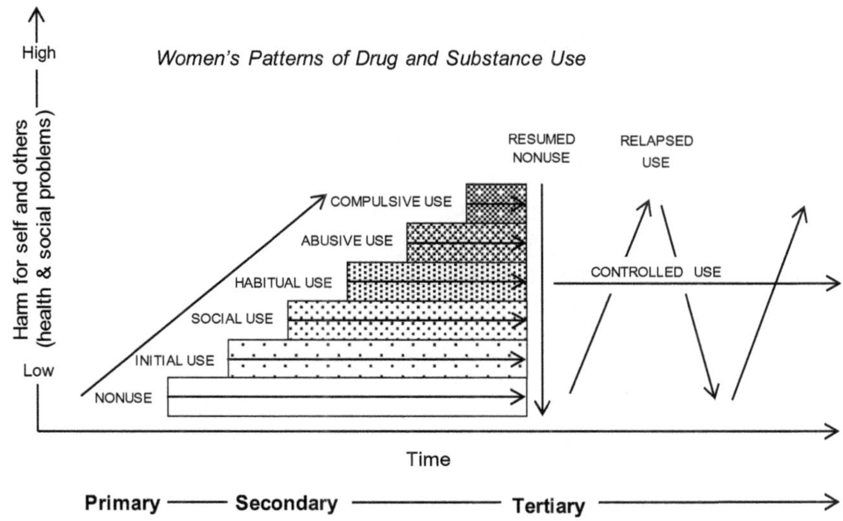

FIGURE 8.1 Women's Patterns of Drug and Substance Use and Levels of Prevention

- Sexual abuse services/counseling
- Stress management programs
- Transportation to and from treatment and work
- Women's contemporaneous diagnoses (including, for example, treatment for mental depression and PTSD)

There are generally *three* levels of prevention: (1) primary; (2) secondary; and (3) tertiary. Each of these levels focuses on specific patterns of women's drug and substance abuse and guides approaches for their treatment (Figure 8.1). These prevention approaches are discussed in the following sections. (For brief topic outlines for these sections, see, respectively, Boxes: 8.1, *Primary and Secondary Prevention*; 8.2, *Tertiary Prevention: Pharmacotherapy*; and 8.3, *Tertiary Prevention: Psychotherapy and Counseling*.) We begin with *primary prevention*.

BOX 8.1: PRIMARY AND SECONDARY PREVENTION

Primary Prevention
- Lack of Appropriate and Sufficient Research-Based Theory
- Lack of Appropriate and Sufficient Focus and Goals
- Lack of Appropriate and Sufficient Political or Social Resolve

Secondary Prevention

Primary Prevention

Primary prevention is aimed at preventing women's *initial use* of a drug or substance of abuse (see Box 8.1). In planning primary prevention programs, it is interesting to note that successful programs, particularly those aimed at preventing women's initiation of drinking alcoholic beverages and smoking tobacco cigarettes, are associated with the implementation of successful programs aimed at preventing the initiation of drinking and smoking among adolescent girls. This observation is particularly important regarding tobacco smoking because, as consistently noted across the U.S., during the new millennium, *new* tobacco smokers primarily comprise increasing numbers of women and smoking *begins* during adolescence (Grucza, Plunk, & Hipp, 2013; NIDA, 2013).

Other approaches include: (1) increasing parental and other *protective* factors associated with *nonuse* of the drugs and substances of abuse among adolescent girls; and (2) reducing childhood and adolescent *vulnerabilities* to using the drugs and substances of abuse, including their availability and parental, or peer group, attitudes and values that support drug and substance use.

Multi-pronged approaches are required to prevent the use of drugs and substances of abuse before it begins among preadolescent and adolescent girls and young women, 10 years-of-age to 30 years-of-age. These approaches, for example, include prenatal programs for adolescent girls and women, who are pregnant or thinking about becoming pregnant, that are aimed at preventing neonatal exposure to, and the harmful effects associated with, the maternal use of alcohol, amphetamines, cocaine, and nicotine in regard to risks for self and the developing embryo or fetus.

In this context, a timely and potentially extremely beneficial area for primary prevention involves strategies aimed at preventing the development of the neonatal abstinence syndrome (NAS) involving the opiate analgesics (see Chapter 1, *Women's Opiate Analgesic Abuse*, for related background discussion). Both professional and public primary prevention educational initiatives, which specifically address the over- and inappropriate prescribing of opiate analgesics for pregnant women and the subsequent risk for NAS, may help to *reduce* this pattern of women's medical use/abuse and, consequently, *reduce* the associated incidence of NAS in the U.S. (Garcia, 2013; Stover & Davis, 2015).

Interdisciplinary action provided in primary healthcare centers, and public health agencies, by way of specialized programs and municipal legislation may also be of benefit regarding the protection of embryos and neonates. For example, the FASD media campaign created by and for American Indian communities in the Northwest Plains, described by Hanson, Winberg, and Elliott (2012) (e.g., alcohol-free American Indian Reservations). Other approaches aimed at protecting mothers and other women include municipal programs that are focused on decreasing the incidence of *drinking and driving* (e.g., police *check stops* during holidays) and industrial workplace programs focused on preventing drug and substance abuse-related accidents in the workplace (e.g., prominent posting of the number of "accident free days" at worksites), where specific drugs, such as alcohol and cannabis, have been documented as significant contributors to major accidents (e.g., railway industries).

However, *primary prevention*—preventing women from *initiating* the use of a drug or substance of abuse—appears to be the *ultimate* ideal goal. Thus, other prevention programs need to be developed specifically for pre-teen girls, adolescent girls, and young women, who are *drug free*, but remain *at risk* for using alcohol, cannabis, cocaine, heroin, MDMA, nicotine, in the form of tobacco cigarettes, and other drugs and substances of abuse that are commonly used during adolescence and young adulthood. For example, just because a 17-year-old girl in high school does *not* drink alcohol, does not mean that she will not drink alcohol as a 20-year-old college co-ed. Conversely, alcohol use as a pre-teen does *not* preclude the use of primary prevention techniques in relation to preventing future use of other drugs and substances of abuse, such as MDMA (*Ecstasy*) that may be introduced to her in her early twenties, while at college or university.

Trait-like variables associated with women's drug and substance abuse (e.g., antisocial personality disorder; external locus of control; genetic predisposition to alcoholism; sensation-seeking personality), place pre-teen and adolescent girls and young women at risk for, or make them more vulnerable to, using the drugs and substances of abuse (see Table 8.1). Primary prevention for these girls and women often involves the strengthening of *protective factors*. Protective factors also may be effectively used with other high-risk or vulnerable women who have experienced: serious early childhood losses; significant neglect; physical and/or sexual abuse; or psychiatric inpatient treatment for selected mental disorders—all of which may be related to alcohol and/or substance use disorders and the development of a contemporaneous diagnosis if preventive treatment is *not* appropriately provided (see related discussion in Chapter 7, *Identifying Women's Contemporaneous Diagnoses*).

Unfortunately, most of the past *attempts* aimed at achieving the goals of primary prevention, in regard to the use of the drugs and substances of abuse, have ended in failure or—at best—in only *partial success* (Anderson, 2010; Erceg-Hurn, 2008; Grimshaw & Stanton, 2006; Pan & Bai, 2009; Sloboda, Stephens, & Stephens, 2009; Thomas & Perera, 2006; Wakefield, Flay, & Nichter, 2003). For example, several national and international tobacco control organizations have, for well over a decade, recommended mandating a reduction in nicotine content in cigarettes to levels that would make physical dependence less likely to occur, on average, among smoking populations. However, as noted by Kozlowski (2015):

> This proposal has been met with significant resistance, particularly from U.S. tobacco cigarette manufacturers, and, thus, has not been generally implemented or even attempted.
>
> *(p. 543)*

TABLE 8.1 Woman Dimension and Societal Dimension Variables Amenable to Primary, Secondary, and Tertiary Prevention of Drug and Substance Abuse[a,b,c]

Woman Dimension & Societal Dimension Variables	*Level of Prevention*		
	Primary	*Secondary*	*Tertiary*
Woman Dimension Variables			
Biological Variables			
Age	X	✓	(✓)
Continental descent/ethnicity/race	X	✓	✓
Female gender	X	✓	✓
Genetic predisposition to AUDs, SUDs, or OMDs (e.g., schizophrenia)	X	✓	✓
Menstrual phase (estrogen and progesterone blood concentrations)	(✓)	✓	✓
Physical impairment or disability	(✓)	✓	✓
Psychological Variables			
Active Mental Disorders			
ANXIETY DISORDER			
panic disorder	X	✓	✓
posttraumatic stress disorder	X	✓	✓
ANTISOCIAL PERSONALITY DISORDER	X	(✓)	(✓)
ATTENTION-DEFICIT/HYPERACTIVITY DISORDER	X	✓	✓
CONDUCT DISORDER	X	✓	(✓)
GENDER DYSPHORIA	(✓)	✓	✓
MAJOR DEPRESSIVE DISORDER	(✓)	✓	✓
PSYCHOTIC DISORDER (SCHIZOPHRENIA)	X	✓	✓
SLEEP DISORDER (INSOMNIA)	✓	✓	✓
Other Psychological Variables			
BOREDOM	✓	✓	✓
CRAVING	X	✓	✓
EXTERNAL LOCUS OF CONTROL	X	✓	✓
HOPELESSNESS	✓	✓	✓
LACK OF MEANING IN LIFE	✓	✓	✓
LONELINESS	✓	✓	✓
LOW EDUCATIONAL LEVEL	(✓)	✓	✓
LOW SELF-ESTEEM	✓	✓	✓
MOTIVATION	(✓)	✓	✓
RESILIENCE	X	(✓)	✓
Psychosocial Variables			
Absence of maternal figure or role model	X	✓	✓
Absence of paternal figure or role model	X	✓	✓
Adult physical and/or sexual abuse, including IPV	(✓)	✓	✓
Early childhood physical and/or sexual abuse or other traumatic experiences	(✓)	✓	✓
Powerlessness	✓	✓	✓

TABLE 8.1 *(cont.)*

Woman Dimension & Societal Dimension Variables	*Level of Prevention*		
	Primary	*Secondary*	*Tertiary*
Previous drug and substance abuse	(✓)	✓	✓
Previous inpatient treatment for mental disorders	(✓)	✓	✓
Serious early childhood losses	X	✓	✓
Sociological Variables			
Dissatisfaction with family relationships	(✓)	✓	✓
Drug and substance abuse by close friends, life partner, or spouse	(✓)	✓	✓
Ethnicity	X	✓	(✓)
Family structure, function	✓	✓	✓
Friends involved in deviant behavior	X	✓	✓
History of neglect by parents/family	X	✓	✓
History of recent arrests	X	✓	✓
Homelessness	(✓)	✓	✓
Parent or sibling use of alcohol or other drugs and substances of abuse	(✓)	✓	✓
Peer pressure	(✓)	✓	✓
Presence of/responsibility for dependent children	(✓)	✓	✓
Religiosity	(✓)	✓	✓
Social labeling	✓	✓	✓
Social ostracism, rejection	✓	✓	✓
Sociocultural influences	✓	✓	✓
Spirituality	(✓)	✓	✓
Stigmatization, social stigma	✓	✓	✓
Societal Dimension Variables			
Availability of drugs and substances of abuse	✓	✓	✓
Availability of accessible drug and substance abuse programs and treatment services	✓	✓	✓
Availability of resources, programs, and other services for poor, homeless, and other groups in need	(✓)	✓	✓
Ethnicity, or social group with membership that shares a common national or cultural tradition	✓	✓	✓
Formal, dominant religions	✓	✓	✓
Laws of the Land, or legal statutes and sanctions, for possession, use, production, or trafficking of drugs and substances of abuse	✓	✓	✓
Media messages	✓	✓	✓
Women's gender roles	✓	✓	✓

[a] Key: amenable: ✓; *partially* amenable (✓); *not* amenable X

[b] Also, see Figure 8.2. *New Millennial Interactive Model of Women's Drug and Substance Abuse.*

[c] N.B. In specific contexts, several of the listed variables may act as "protective variables" for some women.

Another example of primary prevention is the policy to reduce, particularly for youth, repeated, heavy exposure to advertisements on television that promote the consumption of alcohol, mainly, "hard liquor." This attempt has been virtually *neutralized* by the concomitant *increase* in the advertising of alcoholic beverages on cable television. For example, researchers from Johns Hopkins Bloomberg School of Public Health found that:

> From October 2012 through September 2015, underage viewers saw an alcohol advertisement on a cable TV program that violated alcohol industry voluntary guidelines 5.8 billion times.
>
> *(Johns Hopkins, 2015, p. 2)*

Three major reasons for the *failure* of these and other primary prevention programs have been suggested, including a lack of appropriate and sufficient: (1) research-based theory to develop and guide treatment strategies; (2) focus and goals; and (3) political commitment or social resolve. Each of these reasons for failure are briefly discussed in the following sections.

Lack of Appropriate and Sufficient Research-Based Theory

None of the strategies associated with primary prevention has uniformly demonstrated widespread, long-lasting effectiveness. A clue to their general *lack* of success may be gleaned by a quick perusal of the variables listed in Table 8.1. For example, "lack of knowledge about the substances of abuse" is *not* identified as an important variable, or risk factor. It is no wonder, then, that the *information-only model*, which focused on knowledge acquisition *alone*, has virtually *no* significant lasting therapeutic effect. Similarly, the appearance of "low self-esteem" as an important variable, or risk factor, helps to explain the *limited* success of the "alternatives" and the "affective educational/social competency" models, both of which have self-esteem as a major focus.

A similar analysis of future prevention models using the *New Millennial Interactive Model of Women's Drug and Substance Abuse* would be expected to predict, *a priori*, their propensity for success—or lack thereof. (Also, see related discussion of the model in the section preceding, *References*, at the end of this chapter.)

As governments continue to reduce spending following the world economic crash of 2008, it appears likely that less and less funding will be available for preventing women's use of the drugs and substances of abuse. In this context, ineffective, or marginally effective, programs that waste time and money have *no* place in an increasingly stressed environment and budget (i.e., with increasing problems of women's drug and substance abuse in a context in which generally less funding is available).[5] With some indication of the prevention strategies that

[5] This concern is *not* new. In fact, it was voiced over 25 years ago, by Becker, Agopian, and Yeh (1992). Unfortunately, the concern has *not* yet been adequately addressed.

work, and the ones that do not, we can begin to develop more effective programs. However, answers to many pressing questions remain—questions that echo those paraphrased from Norman and Turner (1993), approximately 25 years ago:

1. Do we target high-risk women or the general population? Some researchers contend that the prevention programs currently most widely used may be affecting prevalence of alcohol and other drug use in the general population, but they are failing to reach the 5% to 15% of the population who are at greatest risk for becoming substance abusers.[6] Although high-risk women are in the minority, they may account for the *majority* of those involved in both: (a) the criminal justice system; and (b) drug-related harm to self or others (e.g., DUI-related automobile crashes).
2. Do we focus on primary or secondary prevention? For example, currently, many New York State prevention resources are allocated for secondary prevention or counseling youth and young adults, who already have problems related to substance use. Some experts believe that, if we continue to do secondary prevention, we will never have any significant impact on overall substance use and abuse, and that we will be continuing to put Band-Aids® on problems that already exist, as opposed to trying to eliminate the problems through primary prevention strategies.
3. Do we concentrate on first order or second order change? Most of the prevention efforts of the 1980s and 1990s were aimed at trying to change the behavior of individuals (second order change). An increasing number of prevention planners believe that the emphasis should be on first order change—that is, addressing the societal problems that are influencing individuals to become substance abusers. Increasing the price of legal substances, banning cigarette and alcohol advertising, and raising the legal drinking age are examples of first order change (p. 17).

Lack of Appropriate and Sufficient Focus and Goals

Generally, the purpose of programs and services, which are aimed at preventing women's drug and substance abuse, is to: (1) *increase* related awareness and understanding among women, significant others, communities, and other significant stakeholders; (2) provide accurate information regarding the nature and extent of the use of the drugs and substances of abuse—as well as the harm associated with their use; and (3) positively change the related attitudes and values of targeted groups of women. However, the focus and priorities of these, primarily government-sponsored programs and services, are sensitive to public opinion and pressure. Hence, they are often educationally unsound and short-lived. For example, the programs directed toward the burgeoning problem of methamphetamine

[6] These women may be at high risk because of biological (i.e., genetic), psychological (e.g., personality), or sociological (e.g., socioeconomic status) risk factors—many of which are identifiable.

abuse in the 1990s, including the use of posters and highway bulletin board signs warning that "Speed Kills," as funding "dried up," and interest in their novelty waned, these largely *ineffective* programs slowly disappeared.

Subsequently, the first 2 decades of the new millennium witnessed a general return to the more permissive, or liberal, views of the 1970s regarding issues related to the use of the drugs and substances of abuse. These issues included a concomitant primary focus on *harm reduction*[7] and the decriminalization, and/or legalization, of marijuana and other drugs and substances of abuse (see related discussion in the *cannabis* section of Chapter 6, *Women's Psychodelic Abuse*).

Another area of focus, which is receiving increased attention, is to *increase* the monetary cost of drugs and substances of abuse. As noted by Smith, Sved, and Hatsukami (2014, p. 23), the underlying theoretical basis for "taxing" resides in the principles and practices of behavioral economics. Behavioral economics uses principles from the field of microeconomics to characterize how consumption of a *reinforcer* changes as a function of the unit price of that reinforcer (i.e., "unit price" *equals* "cost" divided by "reinforcement magnitude").[8] Several studies (e.g., Krause, Cavazos-Rehg, & Plunk, 2014; Wagenaar, Salois, & Komro, 2009; Young-Wolff, Kasza, & Hyland, 2014) have demonstrated an *inverse* relationship between *increasing* the overall cost of alcohol and tobacco cigarettes (i.e., increasing related consumer taxes)[9] and the amount of their use (i.e., as costs *increase*, drinking alcohol and smoking tobacco cigarettes *decrease*). In fact, most would agree that "taxing" is one of the most, if not the most, effective primary intervention strategy for *decreasing* drug and substance abuse—at least for *legal* drugs and substances of abuse, like alcohol and tobacco cigarettes.

The published literature is filled with both theories and accounts of attempts to deal with the problems of drug and substance abuse *without* adequate attention to related focus and goals. Major examples include programs that basically, at their core, are simply requests for funding—generally in the form of community, state, or federal grants—without any specific plan or goals. In addition, these programs often claim that sexism and/or racism, is the underlying major contributory factor responsible for drug and substance abuse among new millennial women in the U.S. without providing any definitive supportive data or other objective evidence.

---

[7] We have always tended to view harm reduction as a *last resort*. However, in terms of reducing alcohol-related motor vehicle crashes (MVCs) and the transmission of infections associated with the use of contaminated needles and syringes, there exists strong evidence to support its use (e.g., Ritter & Cameron, 2006). For example, we strongly endorse "designated driver" programs. See related discussion in the later section, *Secondary Prevention*.

[8] However, as noted throughout this text, the effectiveness of "high cost" alone, as a prevention strategy, can be circumvented or significantly diminished by women's involvement in "sex-for-drugs" exchanges.

[9] During the last century, these taxes were often commonly referred to as "sin taxes."

Lack of Appropriate and Sufficient Political or Social Resolve

Popular Notion: The "War on Drugs," which has been fought over the past 50 years by the U.S. government, has been well-executed and largely successful.

NOT TRUE. The "war," for the most part, has been feckless and, consequently, is more accurately described as an unmitigated and abject failure. Reasons for this failure can be largely ascribed to the "lack of appropriate and sufficient political and social resolve."

Examples of the lack of appropriate and sufficient political or social resolve abound,[10] but are probably best illustrated in the context of nicotine use in the form of tobacco smoking. As noted in Chapter 4, *Women's Caffeine and Nicotine Abuse*, and formally recognized by the WHO for over half a century, tobacco smoke has *no* defined safe level of use and, singularly, causes more deaths in the U.S. than any other drug or substance of abuse.[11] However, despite these readily verifiable facts, the use of nicotine—a so-called "*soft*" *drug*—remains legal.

Popular Notion: Society would be much improved if "soft" drugs were ignored and political and social resolve were, instead, directly focused on the use and abuse of "hard drugs."

NOT TRUE. (See following discussion in the body of this chapter.)[12]

---

10 The lack of resolve also includes the generally chronic underfunding of public sector programs aimed at preventing women's drug and substance abuse over the past 3 decades (e.g., McAuliffe, 1990; Meara & Frank, 2005).

11 In addition, tobacco farmers continue to receive government subsidies and export tobacco as a *cash crop* to China and other countries, such as India, where use continues to be on the rise (Pagliaro & Pagliaro, 2004).

12 N.B. We have refrained from using the term "soft drug" in this text, or elsewhere, because, in its general context of use, we find it misleading, oxymoronic, pharmacologically meaningless, and scientifically inaccurate. For example, more harm accrues annually among women in the U.S. from the use of so-called "soft" drugs than from the use of so-called "hard" drugs (see related discussion in the preceding chapters for specific examples and documentation).

Interestingly, from a historical view, the descriptive term, "soft drinks," was originally coined, and appropriately used, during the late 19th/early 20th centuries, in the context of carbonated, soda fountain drinks that did *not* contain alcohol (i.e., "hard liquor") from those that did contain alcohol (Pagliaro & Pagliaro, 2004).

However, proactive community involvement, extended to communities across the U.S., can be a significant factor for reducing women's harmful patterns of drug and substance use. One such program, the *Vermont Anti-Smoking Campaign*, significantly reduced the prevalence of smoking and did so with a *low* per capita cost (Pechmann & Reibling, 2000). Similar programs have involved the use of local, state, and federal billboard advertisements and radio and television public service announcements (PSAs) directed at adolescent girls and young women regarding the dangers of *drinking and driving.* Unfortunately, most programs have *not* been as successful. For example, formal analysis of the well-funded, multi-year *Montana Meth Project* (MMP), found that it had "no discernable impact … on methamphetamine use among Montana's youth" (Anderson, 2010, p. 732).

The legal age for purchasing tobacco products differs from state to state and, sometimes, among different jurisdictions (e.g., cities/counties) within states. There is general agreement that *raising* the minimum legal sale age (MLSA) for tobacco products to 21 years-of-age would significantly reduce tobacco use (Knox, 2016). For example, the Institute of Medicine (2015) has predicted that this change would *reduce* the rate of tobacco use in the U.S. by approximately 12%.

Despite the general agreement regarding harm reduction associated with the implementation of this primary prevention strategy, progress over the past 30 years has been very slow. In 2015, Hawaii became the first state to increase the MLSA to 21 years-of-age. In addition, a number of local jurisdictions (e.g., New York City) have similarly raised the MLSA (Hartocollis, 2013). However, resistance has been well-established and well-funded by tobacco lobbyists—both in Congress and in various state assemblies. This should be of no surprise when a report from the major cigarette/tobacco producer, Philip Morris, noted back in 1986 is considered:

> Raising the legal minimum age for cigarette purchase to 21 could gut our key young adult market (17–20) where we sell about 25 billion cigarettes and enjoy a 70 percent market share.
>
> *(p. 1)*

Subsequently, over the years, members of legislatures (both at state and federal levels) have consistently rejected efforts to raise the MLSA to 21 years-of-age. For example, in 2014, Maryland lawmakers defeated a related bill (Winter, 2014) and in 2016 New Jersey governor Chris Christie *vetoed* a bill passed by the state legislature to *increase* the MLSA to 21 years-of-age (Morain, Winickoff, & Mello, 2016). Despite these setbacks, and resultant slowed progress, we believe that a MLSA of 21 years will, eventually, become the "law of the land" in the U.S.[13]

13 However, considering current trends, by that time 18-year-olds will probably be able to *legally* purchase cannabis in the U.S.—as they already can in several states (see Chapter 6, *Women's Psychodelic Abuse*) and several countries (e.g., Canada; Columbia; Netherlands; Portugal; Spain; Switzerland; and Uruguay).

Some similar discussions concerning the implementation of primary prevention approaches regarding the use of electronic nicotine delivery systems (ENDS) has occurred since these products were developed and introduced for use in the U.S. during the new millennium. Related progress has been made, but has been *constrained*. Marynak, Holmes, and King (2014), in their *Morbidity and Mortality Weekly Report* review for the CDC reported that:

> As of November 30, 2014, 40 states have enacted laws prohibiting ENDS sales to minors, but only three of the 27 states with comprehensive smoke-free air laws have incorporated ENDS.
>
> *(p. 1145)*

In addition, an analysis of related state laws for these 40 states reveals that the MLSA for ENDS is almost always set at 18 years-of-age (in a few cases, 19 years-of-age). In *no* states has it been set at 21 years-of-age.

Regarding electronic cigarettes (ECS), Dobbs, Hammig, and Sudduth (2016) noted that 17 states passed laws requiring child-safety packaging for e-cigarettes—an additional primary prevention strategy that has been implemented to prevent or minimize unintentional poisoning among children of women who smoke ECS (p. 1).

Drug and substance abuse among *older* women has become a significant and growing problem over the first 2 decades of the new millennium. As noted by Wu and Blazer (2011), among others (e.g., Culberson & Ziska, 2008; Pagliaro & Pagliaro, 1992b, 2000), *older* women are *less* likely than *younger* women to: (1) perceive their own drug or substance use to be harmful; and, consequently, (2) seek and use related treatment services. This is obviously a situation in which the appropriate application of primary prevention techniques could yield significant positive results, particularly as increasing numbers of "baby-boomers" join this age-cohort on an annual basis. Yet, relatively little has been done in this regard.

It should be recognized that attempts aimed at preventing the use of the drugs and substances of abuse by women, although potentially of tremendous benefit, have *failed* more often than they have succeeded. However, the failures are rarely reported in the published literature and, when they are reported, the "failure" is often *hidden*, *disguised*, or *minimized* by misleading and, often, meaningless phrases. For example, we quickly sampled the following phrases from a number of recently published research studies that were available on our work desks: "a fairly consistent magnitude of program effects..."; "may be warranted..."; "iatrogenic effect..."; "considerable consensus indicates..."; "inconclusive..."; "more effective than a similar intensity of..."; "no main effects..."; "offer promise..."' "positive point-in-time differences..."; "positively associated with..."; "the vast majority of..."; "variation of the heterogeneous effects..."; "positive trend...";

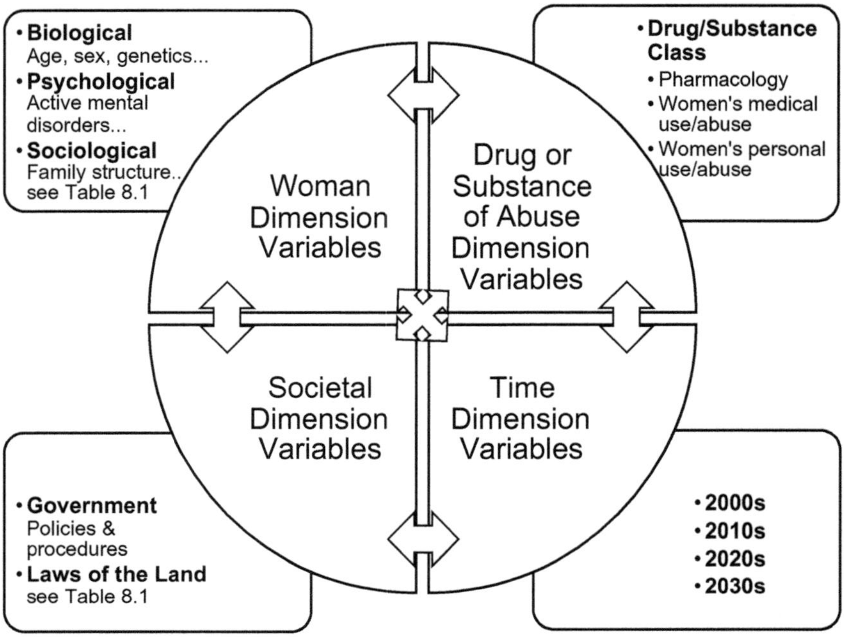

FIGURE 8.2 New Millennial Interactive Model of Women's Drug and Substance Abuse

"incomplete outcome data…"; "may suggest…"; "correlated with …"[14] etc.; etc.; etc… Although each of these phrases can be appropriately used, in most cases in which they have been used, they tend more to obscure or make unintelligible, rather than clarify, the generally *insignificant* research results.

Thus, to avoid *past mistakes* or endlessly *reinventing the wheel*, the development of efficacious prevention programs and services must openly and fully address strategies and approaches to treatment that have failed in the past as well as those that have been found to be successful with a particular group of women (e.g., women of Hispanic descent in the U.S.; young women). The *New Millennial Interactive Model of Women's Drug and Substance Abuse* (Figure 8.2) was developed as a comprehensive, integrative model to facilitate this endeavor (see related discussion at the end of this chapter).

Finally, regarding primary prevention, we remind health and social care professionals, that this technique should be part of a constantly renewing, or repeated, process. It should *not* be "done once" and, then, relegated to history, but can—and

[14] N.B. Virtually everything can correlate with everything else (i.e., correlations can range from −1 to +1). However, only significant positive correlations are generally of clinical relevance. In addition, even then, many clinicians and researchers appear to *forget* the single most crucial fact—that correlation can, and often does, occur *without* any relationship to causation.

commonly must—be renewed/reapplied with: (1) new successive generations of women; (2) new drugs and substances of abuse; and (3) new methods of use or delivery. For example, successful primary prevention programs should be reformulated, as necessary, to provide optimal prevention exposure and then repeated with new generations of women, such as women who may be of different ages, continental descents, or ethnic cohorts. Successful programs also can be developed to target *new* drugs and substances of abuse or *new* methods of using commonly used drugs and substances of abuse. An example of the latter, is the development, or extension, of primary prevention strategies aimed at preventing hookah use by new millennial women in the U.S. (Also, see related sections dealing with hookah use in Chapter 4, *Women's Caffeine and Nicotine Abuse*, and Chapter 6, *Women's Psychodelic Abuse*.)

Whenever public interest in the use of a *new* drug or substance of abuse, or a *new* method of use, is introduced, researchers and clinicians, who are aware of potential related risks to health and social harm, must quickly respond with the implementation of efficacious primary prevention strategies. For example, the strategies aimed at preventing new millennial women's increasing hookah use in the U.S. suggested by the American Lung Association (2016) and several researchers and clinicians (e.g., Morris, Fiala, & Pawlak, 2012; Pagliaro & Pagliaro, *Clinical Patient Data Files*):

- Development and implementation of education campaigns for health and social care professionals addressing health risks associated with hookah use of tobacco and or marijuana, particularly for new millennial and other women who are at high risk for use
- Application of specific warning labels for all hookahs and hookah tobacco products, such as the labels used for tobacco cigarettes
- FDA approval for supported claims of safety or harm associated with hookah use
- Prohibition of hookah use in areas where tobacco smoking or cannabis use are typically prohibited
- Designation and implementation of smoke-free area laws for hookah use—such as those designated for cigarette or marijuana smoking
- Closure of hookah lounges pending safety studies concerning hazards associated with sidestream smoke and other environmental exposure, for both smokers and non-smokers, to hookah smoke
- Extension of tobacco flavoring bans for all commercially available hookah tobacco brands
- Increasing federal and state taxation on both hookahs and hookah tobacco products

Secondary Prevention

Secondary prevention is concerned with the *early* detection of women's use of the drugs and substances of abuse *before* associated harmful effects develop or begin to significantly escalate. Early and accurate detection of women's harmful use of the drugs and substances of abuse and the ready implementation of appropriate treatment approaches, including those for women who have concurrent mental disorders (see Chapter 7, *Identifying Women's Contemporaneous Diagnoses*), are required to achieve optimal treatment outcomes with secondary prevention techniques. In this regard, and as identified and reported by several researchers (e.g., Harris and Knight, 2014; Pagliaro & Pagliaro, 2000), many popular psychometric screening tests have demonstrated clinical value regarding identifying harmful patterns of drug and substance abuse and promoting successful treatment and positive outcomes for a variety of women (e.g., older women; pregnant women; younger women).

Examples of effective secondary prevention approaches include: *employee alcohol assistance programs* and many *harm reduction strategies* (Ritter & Cameron, 2006), such as: (1) needle exchange programs aimed at reducing HIV transmission from infected intravenous drug users to non-infected intravenous drug users; and (2) methadone maintenance programs for heroin users, which allow them to lead more productive lives (e.g., care for their children and families; maintain employment) while decreasing the risk for continued health problems (e.g., progression of malnutrition or untreated tuberculosis) associated with: *living on the street*; the harm related to injecting heroin several times a day; and the daily *hustle* required in order to get a *fix* (e.g., additional personal injuries, such as violent beatings or falls; progression of infections to gangrene infection and need for limb amputation; septicemia; or death). (Also, see later section, *Pharmacotherapy*, "Methadone," for additional related discussion.)

Secondary prevention approaches could be used with *all* the risk factors identified in Table 8.1. For example, if a woman was depressed and was using alcohol to *self-medicate* her depression, perhaps in relation to a gender dysphoria, then the provision of, or a referral to, an appropriate counselor, physician, or psychologist for needed psychotherapy, or other necessary therapy (e.g., antidepressant pharmacotherapy; gender specific program for lesbians who have alcoholism) should be made to help her manage her depression and gender dysphoria. This intervention may help her to: resolve her gender dysphoria; rectify the accompanying depression; and, consequently, prevent the development of increasingly harmful patterns of alcohol and other drug and substance abuse—patterns that are often seen among lesbians who suffer from depression.

Secondary prevention also is concerned with early intervention for women who have already begun to use one or more of the drugs and substances of abuse, but for whom serious related harmful effects have *not* yet developed. For example, secondary prevention strategies may include: (1) programs aimed at convincing women, most of whom drink alcohol, *not* to drink and drive (e.g., designated driver programs); (2) programs aimed at helping pregnant women, many of whom drink alcohol, *not* to drink while pregnant;[15,16] and (3) programs (e.g., needle exchange programs; safe injection site programs) that provide sterile injection equipment to women, who intravenously abuse drugs, in order to avoid, or to decrease, the risk for being infected with, or spreading, the HIV or other blood-borne infections, including hepatitis C.[17]

In addition to the early detection of harmful patterns of drug and substance abuse among women, secondary prevention also involves the provision of *immediate* therapeutic efforts aimed at:

1. Discontinuing the use of the drugs and substances of abuse
2. Reducing the possibility that others in contact with the user will begin to use the drugs and substances of abuse
3. Limiting any harm associated with the use of the drugs and substances of abuse

For example, several studies (e.g., Braitman, Henson, & Carey, 2015; LaBrie, Lac, & Kenney, 2011; Linden, Kite, & Braitman, 2014; Napper, Kenney, & Lac, 2014; Pearson, D'Lima, & Kelley, 2013) examined the effectiveness of utilizing *protective behavioral strategies* (PBSs) as a secondary prevention technique (i.e., harm reduction strategy). The majority of the related published literature has focused

[15] From the perspective of the fetus, this program may be considered to be a form of "primary prevention." In a similar manner, the therapeutic intervention to promote the healthy attachment of mothers and neonates, particularly mothers who abuse drugs and substances of abuse (e.g., Rasmussen, Borelli, & Decoste, 2016; Suchman, Decoste, & Rosenberger, 2012), and, consequently, prevent or minimize related problems (e.g., anaclitic depression; disengagement; poor maternal-infant bonding; future drug and substance abuse among female offspring), may be considered to be a form of either primary or secondary prevention depending upon one's perspective.

[16] For example, FAS/FASD has been, and continues to be, a particularly prominent concern identified in American Indian communities and Reservations across the U.S. (see related discussion in Chapter 2, *Women's Alcohol Abuse*) and, accordingly, related specific prevention strategies have been developed and implemented. One such program, "CHOICES," was developed by the Oglala Sioux Tribe. In this prevention program, American Indian women who are at risk for alcohol abuse while pregnant: (1) set goals for drinking behavior; (2) complete daily diaries; (3) work with a tribal interventionist; and (4) identify social support (e.g., female Elder, mother, or younger female relative, such as a sister or cousin) (Hanson & Pourier, 2016).

[17] To reiterate an important point made several times earlier in this text, we believe that it is our job, as authors, to provide a comprehensive, unbiased, and factually correct overview and evaluation of the published data regarding the use of the drugs and substances of abuse by women in the U.S. However, we must also recognize our own biases and, when they arise, make them explicit to the reader. This example is one such case: based on the results of our own research involving women participants, we do *not* generally favor the use of *needle exchange programs* or *safe injection sites* for women (Pagliaro & Pagliaro, 1993; Pagliaro, Pagliaro, & Thauberger, 1993). Alternatively, we recommend that every effort and strategy available be used to assist women to *discontinue* intravenous drug use (i.e., in the context of our clinical practice and related research, we find these programs [e.g., safe injection sites], on balance, to function *more* as "enablers" than as "harm reducers").

on alcohol consumption, particularly heavy drinking among young women, who were college/university undergraduate students.

Protective behavioral strategies typically include a diverse number of cognitively-rehearsed behaviors, including:

- Alternating the consumption of alcoholic and non-alcoholic drinks
- Asking a friend to let you know when you start to appear intoxicated
- Avoiding deliberate heavy-drinking situations (e.g., participating in drinking games)
- Avoiding heavy-drinking behaviors (e.g., "chugging down drinks"; drinking "shots")
- Avoiding drinks that contain different types of alcoholic beverages
- Avoiding drinking situations/locations where alcohol is the focus (e.g., beer parties; cocktail parties)
- Avoiding trying to "keep up with" or "outdrink" others
- Drinking alcoholic beverages more slowly (i.e., spacing drinks over a longer period of time)
- Drinking alcohol-reduced drinks (e.g., low-alcohol beer or cider)
- Drinking non-alcoholic, "look-alike" drinks (e.g., cola drinks *without rum*; tonic water *without gin*; margarita *without tequila*)
- Eating prior to, or while, drinking
- Holding onto a drink without drinking it
- Knowing where your drink is always (i.e., *never* leaving your drink unattended)
- Leaving a party, or other drinking situation, at a predetermined time
- Limiting the number of drinks consumed per drinking episode
- Making sure to go home with a friend instead of staying behind at a party or drinking location (e.g., bar; dance club)
- Putting, or requesting, extra ice or mixer in drinks
- Secretly emptying alcoholic beverages instead of drinking them
- Using a designated driver or taxi service

These strategies have been repeatedly demonstrated to be effective—to varying degrees—with different groups of drinkers. For example, LaBrie, Lac, and Kenney (2011) found that these strategies were both *more* often used and, consequently, *more* effective among their sample of undergraduate college/university women. In addition, they noted that:[18]

> Equipping women with PBS then, may be especially warranted to minimize alcohol-related harm including deleterious sexual consequences.
>
> *(p. 354)*

[18] In a similar study, Napper, Kenney, and Lac (2014) came to the same general conclusion.

Pearson (2013), in a critical review of the use of PBS among college students, supported the use of PBS and reiterated that women are: (1) *more* likely to use PBS; and (2) likely to have PBS-related positive outcomes, including reduced alcohol use and reduced negative consequences from drinking. However, as noted by Litt, Lewis, and Blayney (2013), these positive outcomes do *not* appear to be generalizable to bisexual and lesbian women.

While most available data concerning the use of PBS among college students have noted variance in the efficacy of PBS, we have consistently observed the general success of these measures among *all* women. Consequently, we highly recommend the use of this form of secondary prevention, as appropriate, for *all* women and urge health and social care professionals to encourage *all* women who drink to learn about and appropriately use these strategies.

Secondary prevention programs for women also have been directed at reducing or quitting tobacco smoking. These programs are aimed at improving the health of women who smoke, and the health of their family members by reducing their exposure to the toxicities associated with secondhand tobacco smoke—smoke that often remains suspended in the air, as well as "hangs around" in the home environment on tables, floors, and other surfaces (i.e., *thirdhand exposure*). In terms of harm reduction theory, reducing or terminating tobacco smoking by women will reduce their chances of developing COPD, cardiovascular disease, and both breast and lung cancers (see related discussion in Chapter 4, *Women's Caffeine and Nicotine Abuse*).

Similarly, at risk for resuming her use of the drugs and substances of abuse and for the development of increasingly harmful patterns of use (e.g., abuse or compulsive use), is, for example, a young woman, who lives on the streets because of family discord associated with her past "promiscuity" and "drug using lifestyle." She is now "living on her own" and is "clean and sober." However, she recently moved back home with her aging alcoholic father to "look after" him as a result of her mother's recent death in a motor vehicle crash (MVC) (see Figure 8.1).

Recognizing that she is at increased risk for returning to her drug and substance abuse, this young woman should be regularly assessed for normal grieving and referred to, for example, a bereavement group for women who have lost loved ones as a result of MVCs, monitored for grief resolution, and provided, along with her father, appropriate: psychotherapy or counseling to address their father-daughter relationship; pharmacotherapy; and other required treatment together with referral to effective self-help programs (e.g., Alcoholics Anonymous; a women's 12-step program, Al-Anon), as needed.

Tertiary Prevention

Tertiary prevention is aimed at limiting the degree of harm associated with the active use of the drugs and substances of abuse and promoting optimal health and social functioning when harmful *effects* have already occurred, including those that are largely *irreversible* (e.g., cirrhosis of the liver; FASD; HIV infection). Interventions include instruction regarding the management of the associated conditions and diseases with the end goal of maintaining: (1) optimal personal functioning; and (2) prevention of further deterioration or loss of function—physical, mental, and social.

Although researchers have been largely successful in accumulating knowledge regarding the pharmacology, toxicology, abuse potential, and addiction liability of the drugs and substances of abuse for adults, in general, increased attention must be specifically directed at women's drug and substance abuse. To this end, it should be recognized that:

- *Women*, because certain drugs and substances of abuse (e.g., alcohol; cannabis; prescription sedative-hypnotics; tobacco [nicotine]) are particularly attractive to them, may preferentially use these drugs and substance of abuse for many different reasons (e.g., availability and cost; desired effects; peer pressure; sociocultural norms)
- *Women*, because of their unique stages of physical, psychological, and social development, may be at particular risk for personal and social problems associated with their use of drugs and substances of abuse (e.g., family discord, including violence, such as IPV, and incest; incarceration for possession of, or dealing, illicit drugs and substances of abuse; infection with STDs, including gonorrhea, syphilis, and HIV; sex-for-drug exchanges; unplanned pregnancy; and morbidity and mortality related to home accidents or automobile crashes, overdosage death, and suicide attempts and completions)
- *Women*, because of the variable influence of endogenous ovarian hormones, reproductive cycle phases, and hormone replacement (e.g., use of birth control pills), respond differently than men in regard to outcomes associated with several of the drugs and substances of abuse (e.g., Moran-Santa Maria, Flanagan, & Brady, 2014; Pagliaro & Pagliaro, 1986, 2000). For example, Esterlis, McKee, and Kirk (2013) reported a *higher* availability of $GABA_A$-benzodiazepine receptor among women than men. In a related review, Moran-Santa Maria, Flanagan, and Brady (2014) found a *significant* relationship between systemic ovarian hormone levels and the use of several drugs and substances of abuse, including: alcohol; cocaine; marijuana; methamphetamine; nicotine; and opiate analgesics (see related discussion in Table 8.3, "Menstrual Phase Effects on Women's Nicotine Withdrawal and Therapy for Tobacco Smoking Cessation")
- *Women*, because of their biological ability to become pregnant, may enter a drug and substance abuse program at any time during their pregnancy. These women may be: *unaware* they are pregnant; in denial regarding their pregnancy; or *aware* of their pregnancy, which may be their reason for seeking

treatment. In addition to the treatment needs of other groups of women, pregnant women have additional unique and specific needs that require attention, including:

- Knowledge regarding the effects of drug and substance abuse upon: pregnancy; fetal development; neonates (e.g., neonatal withdrawal syndrome); and nursing infants (e.g., undesired, or harmful, effects and toxicities)
- Maintaining a healthy pregnancy (e.g., diet, exercise, rest; routine physician visits; prenatal vitamins with folic acid)
- Childbirth classes (e.g., anesthetic or natural birth; possible complications, such as preterm labor, breech birth, preeclampsia; plans for managing early labor and delivery)
- Early signs of labor; labor coaches; pain management; options for delivery, such as use of anesthesia or natural; preparation for selected method of delivery
- What to pack and have ready to bring to the hospital
- What to have ready when the newborn is discharged home with her/his mother
- Plans for getting to the hospital safely for delivery
- Plans and techniques for optimizing maternal-infant bonding, infant safety, bathing, feeding, diapering, and other care; provision of safe living arrangements and support systems

- *Women*, because of a variety of sociocultural factors are *more* likely than men to be the head of a homeless, single-parent family in the U.S., and—embedded within this specific sociocultural context—extremely likely to have significant drug and substance abuse problems (e.g., Pagliaro & Pagliaro, *Clinical Patient Data Files*; Slesnick, Glassman, & Katafiasz, 2012; Sun, 2012). Consequently, these women may have a particular need for treatment approaches that are firmly rooted in social work. For example, Slesnick and her colleagues (e.g., Slesnick & Erdem, 2012, 2013; Slesnick, Glassman, & Katafiasz, 2012) have recommended "ecologically based treatment," in which, "housing [for homeless women and their children] is the first focus of therapists" (Slesnick, Glassman, & Katafiasz, 2012, p. 343).
- *Women*, including mothers, aunts, and grandmothers, because of a variety of sociocultural influences associated with their continental descent or ethnicity, are more likely than men to have primary responsibilities for mothering and care of neonates, infants, and young children, as well as, particularly over the new millennium, older children, adolescents, and young adults. In this context, unaddressed issues of drug and substance abuse, including abandonment, abuse, and neglect, among mothers has been associated with such care and mothering deficits as: (1) poor neonate-, infant-, and child-attachment, or bonding; and (2) separation or loss of dependent children to child protective

services (CPS), due to deficits in mothering or incarceration related to drug and substance abuse (Nair, Black, & Schuler, 1997; Neger & Prinz, 2015; Pagliaro & Pagliaro, *Clinical Patient Data Files*).

In a related study of the factors that *increase* the potential for abuse and neglect of offspring by mothers who abuse drugs and substances of abuse, Nair, Schuler, and Black (2003) identified and evaluated *ten* related maternal risk factors:

1. Absence of significant or intimate other in the home
2. Domestic violence
3. Family size
4. Homelessness
5. Incarceration
6. Maternal depression
7. Negative life events
8. Non-domestic violence
9. Psychiatric problems
10. Severity of drug use

In addition, they found that:

> Parenting stress and child abuse potential were higher for women with five risks or more compared with women (i.e., drug abusing mothers) who had four or fewer risks.
>
> *(p. 997)*

Since this time, others (e.g., Paris, Herriott, & Holt, 2015) also have identified both a differential need and a differential response to parenting interventions for mothers in drug and substance abuse treatment depending primarily on other concurrent mental health concerns (e.g., depression). Regarding treatment programs for mothers, who abuse drugs and substances of abuse, over 20 years ago, Nair, Black, and Schuler (1997) recommended that:

> Intervention programs should be comprehensive, theoretically based on adaptive models of parenting, focus on maternal needs, and provide psychosocial support and parenting skills to women and their families, *not* just referral to drug treatment. In addition, interventions must involve the family, as defined by the mother, because the support provided by the family is often crucial for the well-being of both mothers and children and should be well coordinated with other service systems to ensure access to medical care and social services.
>
> *(p. 8)*

- *Women*, because of sociocultural and gender factors, are *more* likely than men to be emotionally, physically, or sexually assaulted/abused. As noted by Covington (2008b):

> In one of the first studies on addicted women and trauma, 74% of the addicted women reported emotional abuse. Moreover, the addicted women were found to have been abused sexually, physically, and emotionally by more perpetrators, more frequently, and for longer periods of time than their non-addicted counterparts. The addicted women also reported more incidents of incest and rape.
>
> *(p. 377)*

Several researchers (e.g., Boyd, Mackey, & Phillips, 2006; Nehls & Sallmann, 2005; Pagliaro & Pagliaro, *Clinical Patient Data Files*) also have noted this association and suggest that the physical and sexual abuse often contribute to major depressive disorder and/or PTSD and that women, in response, commonly use the drugs and substances of abuse in an attempt to "self-medicate" these mental disorders. (For additional discussion, see related sections in Chapter 7, *Identifying Women's Contemporaneous Diagnoses.*)

What is known, for certain, is that multi-modal prevention and treatment approaches have the *greatest* potential for success.[19] For example, in addition to psychotherapy, adjunctive pharmacotherapy and participation in AA, or another 12-step program, when deemed appropriate and potentially beneficial, we also often encourage our patients to participate in therapeutic *story-telling*, or the use of narratives, art therapy, and bibliotherapy as part of their individual or group therapy. The narratives can be written diary entries, poems, or stories that are written and shared orally. They also can be songs, drawings, collages, paintings, or musical renditions that are presented and shared. It is interesting to note that several of the narratives have been later published by our former patients as autobiographies and short stories. Over the years, we have found that to be optimally effective, multi-modal therapy approaches must consider both the needs of a particular woman and the properties of selected approaches.[20] The importance of this recommendation is highlighted throughout the remainder of this chapter and is incorporated in the

---

19 Several researchers (e.g., Laniado-Laborin, 2010; Ranney, Melvin, & Lux, 2006) have identified the need for multiple therapeutic approaches to effectively deal with the varied nature of the problems encountered among women, who have developed harmful effects associated with their drug and substance abuse. In this regard, we recommend that the individual approaches to treatment, noted in this chapter, be considered and applied in the context of the *New Millennial Interactive Model of Women's Drug and Substance Abuse* (Figure 8.2). (See both earlier and later related discussion.)

20 Of course, there must be a *goodness of fit*, or congruence, between the selected preventive interventions and the attributes, needs, and abilities of one woman or a group of women—as noted for some time (e.g., Project Match, 1993).

following general treatment guidelines for health and social care professionals who are providing services for women.

For example, regarding *assessment*:

- Conduct a comprehensive assessment prior to planning and initiating treatment
- Maintain an appropriate level of confidentiality during all aspects of the assessment and treatment processes
- Assess women who have AUDs and/or SUDs for any accompanying other mental disorders (see Chapter 7, *Identifying Women's Contemporaneous Diagnoses*)

For example, regarding *treatment planning*:

- Remember that reasons for using drugs and substances of abuse may differ from one woman to another woman, and may also differ for the *same* woman over time or with the use of different drugs and substances of abuse
- Recognize that different types of treatment may be required (i.e., the type of treatment that works best for one woman may not necessarily work best for another)
- Be willing to consider all available and appropriate treatment approaches and strategies (e.g., AA; cognitive therapy; pharmacotherapy) that may be efficacious for a particular woman

For example, regarding *treatment delivery*:

- Provide individualized treatment
- Be non-judgmental in approaching treatment
- Break the denial of problems associated with the use of drugs and substances of abuse
- Respect women who have problems associated with the use of drugs and substances of abuse, including those women who have contemporaneous diagnoses (i.e., AUDs and/or SUDs and other mental disorders [OMDs])
- Provide drug and substance abuse education in a straightforward, non-biased manner that is appropriately tailored to each woman's cognitive and developmental abilities, learning needs, and social needs
- Work toward realistic and achievable goals that have been mutually developed and agreed upon
- Appropriately address underlying problems (e.g., lack of self-esteem; poor coping skills; previous sexual abuse)
- Involve family, friends, and others—as appropriate—in confrontation, treatment planning, and program implementation
- Develop women's therapeutic groups according to specific age, continental descent, ethnicity, primary language, socioeconomic status, sexual orientation,

or other specific grouping as deemed appropriate and beneficial for group members and their optimal treatment and recovery
- Use community social agencies designed for women (e.g., women's health center)
- Provide appropriate home child care services for mothers in treatment
- Make referrals to other appropriate health and social care professionals and agencies, when needed
- Develop and use procedures and techniques that help to minimize treatment attrition, or drop-out rates, and to maximize treatment compliance and completion of treatment programs

For example, regarding *treatment evaluation*:

- Provide appropriate follow-up, or aftercare, services
- Remember that success or failure is ultimately the woman's responsibility (i.e., do not become co-dependent or over-responsible)

(Pagliaro & Pagliaro, Clinical Patient Data Files*)*

Tertiary prevention involves *minimizing* the harm related to a history of regular, long-term harmful patterns of using the drugs and substances of abuse among women, who have developed *abusive* or *compulsive* patterns of drug or substance use (see Chapters 1 through 6) (also see Figure 8.1). Aspects of tertiary prevention typically involve active medical or psychological treatment, including residential treatment and rehabilitation focusing on the achievement of abstinence and attention to relapse prevention. As such, this section provides an overview of the various treatment approaches that have been specifically developed and used in this regard for women. Attention also is given to reported outcomes, particularly in relation to success or failure. Although many such programs exist, they can be conveniently grouped into four major treatment categories:[21,22] (1) drug courts; (2) pharmacotherapy; (3) psychotherapy and

---

21 Other therapeutic modalities exist. However, they generally lack sufficient empirical evidence of efficacy. An example is acupuncture, which has been used for the treatment of various drug and substance use disorders, but with unsubstantiated or extremely variable reports of efficacy (e.g., Cui, Wu, & Luo, 2008; D'Alberto, 2004; Gates, Smith, & Foxcroft, 2006; Janssen, Demorest, & Kelly, 2012; Margolin, Avants, & Holford, 2002).

22 N.B. As theoretically effective as these various interventions and programs may be, it is imperative to keep in mind—as advised by numerous researchers, including ourselves—that *access* to treatment is often the *first*, and *most* formidable, barrier for women. For example, as found by Fisher, Reynolds, and D'Anna (2017), sexual minority women are "significantly more likely than heterosexuals to have tried, but been unable, to get into treatment" (p. 55). In addition, they identified the following typical barriers often encountered by women accessing drug and substance abuse treatment: (1) no room in the program or long waiting lists; (2) lack of funding (adequate insurance coverage); (3) no detoxification services for managing active drug and substance abuse or recidivism at the time of

counseling; and (4) Alcoholics Anonymous and other spiritually-based, 12-step programs. These *four* major treatment categories are discussed in the following sections.

Drug Courts

Popular Notion: Drug courts are just like other courts (e.g., municipal courts, superior courts), except that they only deal with criminal charges involving the illicit use and/or distribution of drugs and substances of abuse.

NOT TRUE, as described in the following section.

A significant number of women with tertiary drug and substance abuse problems in the U.S. are increasingly being referred for treatment by "drug courts."[23,24] These courts were originally developed to "address the poor outcomes derived from family reunification programs for substance-abusing parents" (Marlowe & Carey, 2012, p. 1). Introduced in 1994, and expanded by the U.S. Department of Justice during the new millennium, they deal primarily with civil or criminal cases that involve parental rights as related to a parent's drug and substance abuse. Currently, over 300 drug courts are in operation across the U.S. (U.S. Department of Justice, 2016).[25]

Thus, drug courts are commonly utilized in cases involving child protective services (CPS) and child welfare (CW). For example, Donohue, Azrin, and Bradshaw (2014) noted that "approximately 50% of CPS referrals" involve parental drug and substance abuse (p. 706). Oliveros and Kaufman (2011), in a similar context, noted that:

> It is estimated that 60%–70% of all substantiated child welfare cases, and 80% or more of parents whose children are placed in foster care, have SUDs. *(p. 25)*

their request for admission; and (4) arrest or incarceration prior to start of treatment with *no* treatment programs available in jail or prison.

23 These courts also are referred to in the published literature as, "dependency drug courts," "family dependency treatment courts," "family drug and alcohol courts," "family drug courts," "family drug treatment courts," "family treatment courts," and "family treatment drug courts."

24 Currently, over 250,000 children are placed into protective custody and, subsequently, into foster care annually in the U.S. The largest contributing factor to this situation is parental drug and substance abuse (Gold, 2016).

25 Drug courts also increased significantly in numbers and in use by the end of the 20th century as a response to all-time *high* rates of incarceration in the U.S. Inherent in this response, "the criminal justice system made a paradigm shift, from a punishment-based paradigm of incarceration to a restorative justice approach" (Bates, 2009, p. 4873).

Mothers, in these cases, are commonly involved in the neglect and physical, mental, and sexual abuse of their dependent children (Oliveros & Kaufman, 2011; Pagliaro & Pagliaro, *Clinical Patient Data Files*; Testa & Smith, 2009). As identified by Oliveros and Kaufman (2011, p. 25), in their related review of the literature, the need for intervention in these situations, including drug court ordered interventions, is further supported by the observations that the lack of appropriate intervention, generally, results in:

- *Higher* rates of child re-victimization
- *Greater* likelihood of out-of-home placement[26]
- *Longer* stays in care
- *Higher* rates of termination of parental rights
- *Higher* rates of child adoption

The standard mandated requirements for women, who attend drug courts, are to: (1) refrain from drug and substance abuse; (2) regularly attend court hearings, often weekly, to review and monitor their progress and compliance; (3) undergo random urine drug testing; and (4) complete proscribed drug and substance abuse treatment. However, the actual tertiary prevention approaches that are implemented in a particular case depend on the agency/healthcare professional selected to provide the court-mandated therapeutic intervention.[27] In addition, drug courts in different states, or within different judicial districts in the same state, often specify requirements for participant referral. For example, in Florida, the 11th Circuit Judicial Juvenile Court, mandates that parents must:

1. Be 18 years-of-age or older
2. Be with at least one child adjudicated dependent
3. Have a diagnosis of substance abuse or dependence
4. Have a potential for family reunification
5. After consultation with their attorney, "voluntarily enroll in drug court"

(Cohen, Dakof, & Duarte, 2011, p. 252)

---

[26] As noted by Kenny, Barrington, and Green (2015), in their thematic narrative analysis of in-depth interviews of mothers in the context of loss of child custody, this loss can have a devastating psychological effect. As shared by one of the mothers in their study, "I felt for a long time like everything beautiful in me had been taken out" (p. 1158).

[27] Some cases are referred to available government sponsored agencies, whereas other cases are referred to private therapists. For example, when cases are referred to us, they are usually referred in conjunction with a specific planned approach proposed to the court by the defense—with our case-specific analyses and recommendations. In this context, we, and so many others (e.g., Donohue, Azrin, & Bradshaw, 2014; Schaeffer, Swenson, & Tuerk, 2013), commonly use some form of cognitive-behavioral psychotherapy or family therapy, including couple's therapy. (See related discussion later in this chapter, *Psychotherapy and Counseling*.)

The theoretical rationale for these courts and their success is based largely on the social psychological *theory of procedural justice*. This theory, with its gender sensitivity, reportedly can "predict and explain outcomes in treatment courts better than therapeutic jurisprudence" (Lloyd, 2015, p. 113). A number of studies (e.g., Somers, Currie, & Moniruzzaman, 2012) have demonstrated the efficacy of drug courts, particularly in regard to significantly reducing recidivism related to drug-involved crime (e.g., driving while intoxicated, or driving under the influence, DUI; drug possession; drug trafficking) and—by inference—associated personal drug and substance abuse. As reported by Gardner (2007), women, particularly mothers, who are formally involved in drug courts, have, on average, significantly *less* criminal recidivism and significantly *less* subsequent involvement with children's protective services (CPS). In addition, other researchers (e.g., Boles, Young, & Moore, 2007; Brown, 2011; Powell, Stevens, & Lo Dolce, 2012; Worcel, Furrer, & Green, 2008; York, Lamis, & Garfinkel, 2012) have reported that women, who have been formally involved in drug courts:

- Enter AUD/SUD treatment more rapidly
- Have fewer days in out-of-home placement for their children
- Participate in more treatment episodes
- Stay in treatment longer
- Have a higher treatment completion rate
- Have a higher rate of family reunification
- Have a greater reduction in recidivism rates

In addition, as reported by Bates (2009), the drug courts were well-evaluated by most women who participated:

> 96% spoke of drug court as "saving them." Acceptance, caring, and genuine positive regard trumped everything else the drug court was doing.
>
> *(p. 4873)*

Women, particularly those of European descent, who have contemporaneous diagnoses, have reported *higher* levels of both problem recognition and positive response to involvement in drug courts (Brown, 2010; Webster, Rosen, & Krietemeyer, 2006; Wittouck, Dekkers, & De Ruyver, 2013).

Pharmacotherapy

Pharmacotherapy has been, and continues to be, the mainstay of the medical management of both: (1) acute overdosages involving the various drugs and substances of abuse; and (2) their respective withdrawal syndromes. Pharmacotherapy also has been shown to be useful for: cessation (i.e., drug-assisted abstinence); maintenance (i.e., drug substitution or replacement); and relapse prevention programs. In addition, pharmacotherapy is often a necessary and integral component of the treatment of women who have alcohol and/or substance use disorders along with other mental disorders (see Chapter 7, *Identifying Women's Contemporaneous Diagnoses*).

Past advances regarding the pharmacologic treatment of substance use disorders are quite diverse. For example, regarding the opiate analgesics: the use of methadone (Dolophine®) for opiate addiction maintenance (i.e., methadone maintenance) (Fareed, Casarella, & Amar, 2010); naltrexone (Trexan®) for the treatment of alcohol dependence (Garbutt, 2009, 2010); buprenorphine (Buprenex®) as an aid for opiate analgesic detoxification (Flassing, 2010; Kovas, McFarland, & McCarty, 2007); and naloxone (Narcan®) for the treatment of opiate analgesic overdosage. Other examples of pharmacologic intervention include the use of flumazenil (Anexate®) for the treatment of benzodiazepine overdosage (Seger, 2004) and disulfiram (Antabuse®) for the prevention of resumed drinking among people who are abstinent alcoholics (i.e., to prevent *relapsed use* of alcohol) (Barth & Malcolm, 2010). See Box 8.2.

Pharmaceutical Alterations

<u>Popular Notion</u>: Newer drug formulations have been developed that totally *prevent* the abuse of opiate analgesics without interfering with their desired effects.

NOT TRUE. None of the pharmaceutical alternatives, which have been developed and implemented for use in the U.S. (i.e., received FDA approval), consistently *prevent* opiate analgesic abuse. However, there is growing evidence that supports their efficacy in terms of *deterring* or *reducing* opiate analgesic abuse.

Another area of attention in pharmacotherapy is the active development of dosage formulations and drug delivery systems (i.e., *pharmaceutical alterations*) that can help to deter or to lessen the harm associated with a method of using a drug or substance of abuse (Table 8.2). (Also, see the discussion of *naltrexone injection* [Vivitrol®] later in this chapter.) These formulations, which differ significantly, are often referred to as *abuse-deterrent formulations*, or ADFs (Schaeffer, 2012). As noted by the FDA, "most abuse deterrent technologies developed to date are intended to make manipulation more difficult or to make abuse of the manipulated product less attractive or less rewarding" (U.S. Department of Health and Human Services, 2015, p. 3). That is to say that these technologies, or formulations, *deter* abuse by making it *more* difficult for the user, not by making it impossible (i.e., *not* by fully preventing abuse). This is currently an active focus of pharmaceutical research and development.

BOX 8.2: TERTIARY PREVENTION: *PHARMACOTHERAPY*

- Pharmaceutical Alterations
  - Embeda®
  - Oxycodone CR/ER
- Electronic Cigarettes
- Vaccines
- Managing Acute Overdosages
  - Flumazenil (Anexate®)
  - Naloxone (Narcan®)
- Managing Women's Contemporaneous Diagnoses
- Managing Specific Withdrawal Syndromes
  - Alcohol Withdrawal Syndrome
  - Cocaine Withdrawal Syndrome
  - Nicotine Withdrawal Syndrome
    - Ovarian cycle effects on nicotine treatment outcomes
    - Other co-variable effects on nicotine treatment outcomes
  - Opiate Analgesic Withdrawal Syndrome
- Abstinence Maintenance
  - Alcohol Abstinence Maintenance
    - Acamprosate (Campral®)
    - Disulfiram (Antabuse®)
    - Naltrexone (Revia®)
    - Topiramate (Topamax®)
  - Opiate Analgesic Abstinence Maintenance
    - Naltrexone (Vivitrol®)
- Maintenance, Replacement, or Substitution
  - Methadone
  - Buprenorphine/Naloxone Combination
  - Nicotine and Varenicline
    - Nicotine
    - Varenicline

Because of the "steep increase in abuse, misuse, and both fatal and non-fatal overdoses involving prescription opioids" in the U.S. over the new millennium (Bannwarth, 2012, p. 1713), the focus of developmental research within the area of "abuse-deterrent" formulations has been primarily directed at opiate analgesic abuse, including the preparation of "tamper-resistant" formulations (Passik, 2014). In addition, as noted by Passik, Hays, and Eisner (2006), in their study sample of adults who abused prescription drugs and who were entering drug rehabilitation, 80% reported tampering with prescription opiate analgesic tablets by chewing

TABLE 8.2 Examples of Drug Formulations Aimed at Deterring Women's Opiate Analgesic Abuse[a]

Abuse-Deterrent Drug Formulation	*Description*
Injectable	
Depot delivery system	Once-monthly, extended-release intramuscular injectable formulation deters *rapid* achievement of *high* blood concentrations and desired effects
Oral Capsules/Caplets & Tablets	
Controlled-, extended-, or sustained-release	Deters *rapid* achievement of *high* blood concentrations and desired effects by *slowing* drug release and, consequently, absorption
Crush-resistant	Deters nasal insufflation of crushed, or ground, capsule contents or tablets
Gelling agents, e.g., Arymo ER®; Hysingla ER®; OxyContin®	Deters intravenous injection and nasal insufflation of crushed or ground capsule contents or tablets due to the addition of gelling agents that form a viscous gel when moistened or mixed with water
Prevention of drug extraction	Deters intravenous injection or nasal insufflation of crushed or ground capsule contents or tablets
Increased particle size with attempts to crush or grind	Deters nasal insufflation due to poor absorption of drug from large particles
Local nasal mucosal irritant	Deters nasal insufflation due to irritation of nostrils
Reduced vaporized drug availability	Deters *vaping* when capsule contents or tablets are crushed or ground and then heated for vaporization
Sequestered opiate analgesic combination agonist and antagonist capsule or tablet, e.g., Targiniq ER®	Deters intranasal and intravenous use due to a hidden antagonist pellet core that, unlike the agonist that dissolves following oral ingestion and is absorbed into the blood stream during passage through the GI tract, does *not* dissolve. However, if crushed or dissolved for intravenous injection or intranasal insufflation, the antagonist is released along with the agonist, thus, preventing agonistic effects

[a] It is common for a particular product to be formulated using a combination of these abuse-deterrent formulations.

them or administering them by intranasal or intravenous routes.[28] For example, a *highly* successful approach involves the development of the combination buprenorphine/naloxone sublingual tablets (Bunavail®; Suboxone®) to prevent

[28] Interestingly, in their laboratory observational study and survey of adults, who abused prescription opiate analgesics, and were tasked with attempting to modify "crush-resistant" opiate analgesic

the illicit intravenous use of buprenorphine. Because of this pharmacologic/pharmaceutical strategy, the illicit intravenous use of buprenorphine has been *significantly* reduced in the U.S.

The addition of naloxone to the buprenorphine sublingual tablet formulation prevents illicit intravenous use of buprenorphine by an interesting mechanism. The naloxone is *poorly* absorbed from the oral cavity following sublingual placement and, thus, has virtually *no* effect—as intended—on the analgesic action of buprenorphine, when used sublingually. However, if the combination tablet is illicitly crushed, dissolved, and injected intravenously, the naloxone is *immediately* absorbed, blocking the desired action of the buprenorphine at the endogenous CNS opiate analgesic receptors (Connery, 2015; Hard, 2014). (Also, see later related discussion in the section, *Buprenorphine/Naloxone Combination.*) Other examples include EMBEDA®, as well as oxycodone (e.g., OxyContin®), in controlled-release/extended release (CR/ER) formulations. See following sections.

EMBEDA®. EMBEDA® is an extended-release combination of morphine and naltrexone in capsular form. It contains morphine pellets that have a core of sequestered naltrexone. The analysis of post-marketing data regarding undesired, or harmful, effects, and toxicities associated with approximately 97,000 prescriptions for EMBEDA®, indicated a *significant* reduction in abuse (Badalamenti, Buckley, & Smith, 2012). This finding is consistent with the results from a related naltrexone bioavailability study by Johnson and Setnik (2011), who found that, when the capsules are crushed, the naltrexone is immediately released and becomes available to "mitigate morphine-induced effects" and related "drug liking" scores were significantly reduced (p. 391). However, as noted by Smith (2011) in a related review: "No product is likely to be abuse-proof in the hands of clever and determined abusers" (p. 1111).

Oxycodone CR/ER (Continuous Release/Extended Release Formulations). In the U.S., Oxycodone CR/ER—including OxyContin®—was reformulated to replace the original product in August of 2010. The reformulated tablets, intended to *reduce* non-oral methods of abuse, have a polymer coating that makes the tablets difficult to crush into a fine powder and dissolve in water. When mixed in water, the polymer coating turns into a gel that deters intranasal and intravenous use.

Preliminary analysis of "a sentinel surveillance sample of 140,496 individuals assessed for substance abuse treatment at 357 U.S. centers" indicated that the

---

prescription formulations to enable self-administration by either the intranasal or intravenous routes, Vosburg, Jones, and Manubay (2012) found that:

> No particularly unique tools were requested for tampering purposes. Intranasal abusers worked primarily with a hammer, razor, and wax paper; while intravenous abusers primarily employed a razor, spoon, lighter, hammer, syringe and cotton, cookers, and water.
>
> *(p. 206)*

reformulated product was associated with a *significant* (i.e., 41%) reduction in abuse when compared to the original oxycodone product (Butler, Cassidy, & Chilcoat, 2013, p. 351). However, in a subsequent study involving "232,874 adults, at 437 facilities," the same research group *failed* to detect a significant reduction in the abuse of reformulated oxycodone CR/ER (Cassidy, DasMahapatra, & Black, 2014, p. 440).

In a later study, Havens, Leukefeld, and DeVeaugh-Geiss (2014), utilizing structured interviews of 189 adults with a history of opiate analgesic abuse, reported "mixed" results regarding the abuse of the CR/ER formulations (e.g., OxyContin® CR/ER)—*significant* amounts of abuse, but significantly *lower* than that reported for the original, immediate-release (IR) formulations. Others (e.g., Michna, Kirson, & Shei, 2014; Sellers, Perrino, & Colucci, 2013) reported similar findings.

Electronic Cigarettes

Electronic cigarettes (e-cigarettes; ECs) are the *most* prevalent form of electronic nicotine delivery systems (ENDS). (Also, see related discussion in Chapter 4, *Women's Caffeine and Nicotine Abuse*.) Electronic cigarettes are, in fact, battery-operated nicotine-delivery devices. Resembling a typical cigarette, on a quick glance, they are used in much the same manner as tobacco cigarettes and for much of the same purpose. Depending on smoking technique (i.e., number of puffs per unit time; depth and length of inhalation), electronic cigarettes can: (1) deliver approximately the same amount of nicotine to the lungs; and, consequently, (2) achieve blood nicotine concentrations that are comparable to smoking tobacco cigarettes. They were developed and introduced in the U.S. during the first decade of the new millennium in order to deliver *liquid* nicotine in an aerosolized form that, by avoiding *pyrolysis*, was *less* harmful than smoking standard tobacco cigarettes (Brandon, Goniewicz, & Hanna, 2015). The act of "smoking" an EC is generally referred to as "vaping," and women, as well as men, who use "ECs," are commonly referred to as "vapers."

Harrell, Marquinez, and Correa (2015) conducted an interesting study of the *expectancies* of vapers regarding the use of both e-cigarettes and standard tobacco cigarettes. Participants believed that *e-cigarettes*: (1) had fewer health risks; (2) tasted better; (3) were more satisfying; and (4) were associated with less addiction, craving, and withdrawal. In comparison, they also believed that *standard, or conventional, tobacco cigarettes*: (1) were better for controlling appetite and body weight; (2) provided more mental and physical stimulation; (3) were better for reducing stress and depression; and (4) cost less.

Many women, who choose to smoke tobacco cigarettes, as well as women who are unable to successfully quit smoking tobacco cigarettes, have been encouraged to switch to ECs (Bullen, Howe, & Laugesen, 2013). However, results are mixed with some women reporting *higher* and other women reporting *lower* associated rates of smoking cessation (e.g., Harrell, Simmons, & Correa, 2014; Kalkhoran & Glantz, 2016; McRobbie, Bullen, & Hartmann-Boyce, 2014). In addition, several studies and reports (e.g., E-cigarettes, 2015; Orr & Asal, 2014) have suggested that, following tobacco smoking cessation, continued abstinence is of *shorter* duration when the use of ECs is compared to other tobacco smoking cessation products, including placebo and nicotine transdermal delivery systems, or "patches."

Despite over a decade of e-cigarette availability, their use as part of formal tobacco smoking cessation programs has *not* yet received FDA approval (Callahan-Lyon, 2014; Postolache, Nemes, & Serban, 2015). Primary reasons for this lack of formal approval include concerns regarding the:

- Lack of consistency of therapeutic results in terms of tobacco smoking cessation[29]
- Significant variance in manufacturing designs and practice among various producers of e-cigarettes
- Presence of carcinogens in EC vapor (Odum, O'Dell, & Schepers, 2012).

Looking to the future, several groups have made related recommendations in regard to ECs. For example, in 2015, the U.S. Preventive Services Task Force (USPSTF) made the following recommendation:

> That clinicians ask all adults about tobacco use, advise them to stop using tobacco, and provide behavioral interventions and U.S. Food and Drug Administration-approved pharmacotherapy for cessation to adults who use tobacco ... The USPSTF concludes that the current evidence is insufficient to recommend electronic nicotine delivery systems for tobacco cessation in adults, including pregnant women.
>
> *(Siu, 2015, p. 622)*

Similarly, also in 2015, the American Association for Cancer Research (AACR) and the American Society of Clinical Oncology (ASCO) issued a policy statement regarding ENDS, including ECs:

> Key policy recommendations include supporting federal, state, and local regulation of ENDS; requiring childproof caps on ENDS liquids and including warning labels on products and their advertisements; prohibiting

[29] For example, in a randomized, controlled study evaluating the effectiveness of nicotine e-cigarettes, nicotine patches, and placebo e-cigarettes, Bullen, Howe, and Laugesen (2013) found the highest rate of abstinence 6 months after quitting was associated with the use of the nicotine e-cigarette. However, because the abstinence rates were all very low (i.e., ranging from 4.1% to 7.3%) there was insufficient statistical power to determine the superiority of one "quitting method" versus the others.

youth-oriented marketing and sales; prohibiting child-friendly ENDS flavors; and prohibiting ENDS use in places where cigarette smoking is prohibited.

(Brandon, Goniewicz, & Hanna, 2015, p. 952)

On the horizon are many promising developments in pharmacology, including several aimed at the pharmacologic prevention and treatment of cocaine addiction. As poly-use of the drugs and substances of abuse becomes even more prominent in the U.S., clinically significant interactions involving the drugs and substances of abuse, and their methods of use, will need to be adequately addressed (Pagliaro & Pagliaro, 1999, 2009, 2012). Future developments in the area of pharmacotherapy for the treatment of drug and substance use disorders will involve new strategies,[30] including the use of *vaccines*.

Vaccines

Vaccines aimed at protecting women against drug and substance abuse largely work—at least on a molecular level—in a manner similar to that of vaccines used to protect against a number of infectious diseases. However, most drugs, including many of the drugs and substances of abuse, are *not* readily amenable to having an effective anti-drug vaccine created. For example, the alcohol molecule (i.e., ethyl alcohol) is too *small* and the molecular structure of the cannabinoids is too *large* and *unstable* (Kinsey, 2014). For others (e.g., nicotine), the development of a vaccine has progressed to clinical trials.

Preliminary research in this area has involved the development and testing of vaccines for preventing nicotine use (Cerny & Cerny, 2009). The vaccines work by inducing the development of specific antibodies that bind to nicotine once it is absorbed into the blood stream. Consequently, the nicotine that is bound in the blood stream, is *unable* to cross the "blood-brain barrier" and, thus, is *prevented* from: (1) binding to its receptor sites in the CNS; and consequently, (2) eliciting its desired actions (Maurer & Bachmann, 2006, 2007). Unable to achieve the desired and reinforcing nicotine effects, it is expected that smokers will *decrease* or *cease* tobacco cigarette smoking, or other sources of nicotine use (e.g., chewing tobacco; applying nicotine transdermal delivery systems).[31] Thus, the nicotine vaccines have

---

[30] Some related research for these new strategies, although *not* yet yielding new therapeutic modalities, appears to have future promise. For example, given the reported interaction between nicotine and the endocannabinoid system, research has looked at CB1 receptor antagonists (e.g., rimonabant) as potential alternatives, or adjuvants, to current nicotine withdrawal cessation modalities (Cohen, Kodas, & Griebel, 2005).

[31] The associated mechanism of action involves the blockade of the experience of reinforcement, which is typically associated with nicotine use by tobacco smokers. Consequently, continued subsequent attempted use of nicotine in this context facilitates the process of extinction (i.e., fading) of the desired, and once positive, reinforcing effects of nicotine.

the potential to reduce tobacco smoking among two principal groups of smokers: (1) current smokers who are trying to quit smoking; and (2) former smokers who want to prevent relapse (Vocci & Chiang, 2001). Unfortunately, clinical trial results to date have failed to produce significant improvements in maintaining long-term smoking cessation (Kinsey, 2014).

Hartmann-Boyce, Cahill, and Hatsukami (2012) conducted a meta-analysis of drug development clinical trials by pharmaceutical companies that had attempted to demonstrate the efficacy of nicotine vaccines in comparison to a placebo. In four separate studies, involving a total of 2,642 participants, the researchers found that, although the vaccines were generally well-tolerated (i.e., associated adverse effects that were reported by participants were classified as *mild or moderate*), the overall smoking cessation rate was only about 1% (i.e., *not* significantly different from placebo results). However, research in this area continues.

Other drugs and substances of abuse for which vaccines are being evaluated include cocaine, fentanyl, heroin, and methamphetamine (Alving, Matyas, & Torres, 2014; Bremer, Kimishima, & Schlosburg, 2016; Orson, Wang, & Brimijoin, 2014). The application of other more recent vaccine technologies (e.g., gene transfer of highly optimized monoclonal antibodies [Brimijoin, Shen, & Orson, 2013]) is expected to improve the therapeutic efficacy of vaccines in the future.

As previously noted, the major clinical indications for pharmacotherapy, in regard to actual or potential harmful use of the drugs and substances of abuse, include: (1) management of acute overdosages involving benzodiazepines and the opiate analgesics; (2) management of specific withdrawal syndromes; (3) *abstinence maintenance*, or prevention of relapsed use; (4) *substitution* or *replacement* pharmacotherapy (i.e., substituting or replacing a particular drug or substance of abuse with a less harmful one) for opiate analgesics and nicotine (tobacco smoking); and (5) management of contemporaneous diagnoses. Each of these areas of pharmacotherapy is presented and briefly discussed.

Managing Acute Overdosages

Specific pharmacologic antagonists are available for two groups of the drugs and substances of abuse classified as psychodepressants (i.e., benzodiazepine sedative-hypnotics and opiate analgesics) (see Chapter 1, *Women's Opiate Analgesic Abuse*; and Chapter 3, *Women's Prescription Sedative-Hypnotic Abuse*). These antagonists are, respectively, flumazenil (Anexate®, Romazicon®) and naloxone (Narcan®). Both of these antagonists reverse—to a significant degree, if not completely—the acute toxicities and other effects associated with these drugs and substances of abuse.

Flumazenil (Anexate®). Flumazenil is an essentially pure benzodiazepine receptor antagonist. Flumazenil elicits its antagonistic effects within the CNS by means of competitive inhibition. The onset of action for flumazenil is generally within 2 minutes of intravenous injection with effects lasting for approximately 1 hour. Although flumazenil effectively antagonizes the sedative and hypnotic effects (i.e., conscious sedation or general anesthesia) produced by the benzodiazepines, it is less effective in regard to reversing associated respiratory depression. The use of flumazenil for a person who is physiologically dependent (i.e., addicted) on the benzodiazepines may sometimes precipitate convulsions (i.e., in association with the onset of the acute benzodiazepine withdrawal syndrome) (Karavokiros & Tsipis, 1990; Pagliaro & Pagliaro, 1998, 1999).

Naloxone (Narcan®). Naloxone is an essentially pure opiate analgesic antagonist that has virtually *no* direct observable effects other than its antagonistic effects. These effects are elicited within the CNS by competitive inhibition (i.e., it selectively competes with opiate analgesics for binding sites on endogenous endorphin receptors). By displacing the opiate from its binding sites, naloxone immediately inhibits the pharmacologic activity of the opiates, including, in cases of severe overdose, life-threatening respiratory depression.[32] In addition, when administered to a person who is physiologically dependent (i.e., addicted) to the opiates, naloxone can precipitate an acute opiate withdrawal syndrome with the usual associated signs and symptoms (e.g., increased blood pressure; nausea; tachycardia; and vomiting). The onset of action for naloxone is generally within 2 minutes of administration. Effects last for approximately 1 to 2 hours. Consequently, naloxone may need to be periodically re-administered in cases of overdoses involving the long-acting opiates (e.g., methadone) (Pagliaro & Pagliaro, 1998, 1999).

Managing Women's Contemporaneous Diagnoses

Appropriate pharmacotherapy for the symptomatic management of concurrent alcohol and/or substance use disorders (AUDs/SUDs) that occur with other mental disorders (OMDs) is a common and integral component of the medical, psychological, and other health and social care services required by women who have contemporaneous diagnoses (see the following section, *Psychotherapy and Counseling*; also, see Chapter 7, *Identifying Women's Contemporaneous Diagnoses*). In addition, as noted by several researchers (e.g., McCarthy, Tomlinson, & Anderson, 2005), failure to *adequately* treat the other mental disorders involved may significantly contribute, following successful treatment outcomes regarding the AUDs/SUDs, to relapsed use of the drug or substance of abuse that was of initial concern. (Also, see later related discussion in the section, *Relapse Prevention*.)

[32] Increasingly, in response to the rapid and significant escalation of opiate analgesic overdosage deaths in the U.S. over the second decade of the new millennium, first responders (e.g., paramedics; police officers) are being equipped with Narcan (naloxone) nasal spray (4 mg) in a preloaded, easily administered disposable single use nasal spray unit. In some jurisdictions, these units also are supplied to the relatives of known opiate analgesic addicts—or to the addicts, themselves (Lim, Bratberg, & Davis, 2016; Pagliaro & Pagliaro, *Clinical Patient Data Files*).

Consider, for example, women with both an AUD, a SUD, and PTSD. Several researchers have noted the frequent concurrence of these mental disorders among women (e.g., Pagliaro & Pagliaro, *Clinical Patient Data Files*; Roberts, Roberts, & Jones, 2016). (For specific discussion, also see Chapter 7, *Identifying Women's Contemporaneous Diagnoses*, *Anxiety Disorders*, "PTSD" section.) Some researchers (e.g., Hien, Campbell, & Ruglass, 2010) have identified that *AUDs*, specifically, are associated with a *more* severe form of PTSD, which, in general, is *more* resistant to treatment and has a poorer clinical prognosis than other forms of PTSD.

Regarding SUDs, Roberts, Roberts, and Jones (2016) conducted a retrospective meta-analysis of 14 studies with over 1,500 participants who had PTSD and comorbid SUDs. The researchers *failed* to find significant results in terms of cognitive-behavioral therapy for PTSD, SUDs, or both. In a related study involving 353 women, with both a SUD and a PTSD, enrolled in an outpatient substance abuse treatment program, Hien, Jiang, and Campbell (2010) found that:

> PTSD severity reductions were more likely to be associated with substance use improvement, with minimal evidence of substance use symptoms reduction improving PTSD symptoms. Results support the self-medication model of coping with PTSD symptoms and an empirical basis for integrated interventions for improved substance use outcomes in patients with severe symptoms.
>
> *(p. 95)*

In a subsequent re-analysis of their data from the "Women and Trauma" study, Hien and colleagues focused on a subset of 141 women who reported amphetamine or cocaine use in the context of PTSD (Ruglass, Hien, & Hu, 2014). Heavy psychostimulant users, at baseline, reported significantly *more* PTSD symptoms in comparison to light psychostimulant users. However, *all* women, who were psychostimulant users, achieved *improvements* in PTSD symptoms and *reduced* psychostimulant use. In addition, their findings are supportive of "the growing body of research indicating that when individuals achieve relief from PTSD symptoms, they are then able to reduce substance use" (p. 5). Further, their findings "support treatment models that address PTSD *concurrently* with substance use disorder treatment" (p. 6).

Three major approaches are commonly used in the treatment of women with contemporaneous diagnoses. These approaches have been categorized by Smith and Randall (2012) as: (1) *sequential*; (2) *parallel*; and (3) *integrated*. In the *sequential* approach, *one* disorder is selected[33] and treated first based largely on the hypotheses

---

33 Unfortunately, in this situation, the order of treatment is almost always chosen on an "ad hoc" basis predicated primarily on the background, knowledge, and clinical strengths of the clinician as opposed to the individual needs of the woman seeking treatment and the relationship between, or among, the presenting concurrent disorders.

that a single clinician can optimally treat the other mental disorders a woman may have, while *ignoring* the treatment of the concurrent AUD or SUD. A second related hypothesis asserts that once the woman's other mental disorder is treated and is in control/remission, the AUD/SUD can be successfully treated.

In the *parallel* approach, specific treatment approaches are separately delivered simultaneously for a woman. The treatments (e.g., for an AUD and/or a SUD and an OMD) are usually delivered by different clinicians in different facilities. Coordination and communication among the patient and the clinicians involved in this approach are of critical importance for optimal therapeutic success—given that significant deficits in coordination and communication are the major reasons for the failures associated with the parallel approach. For example, when one clinician says one thing to a patient and the other clinician(s) says something else in terms of the cause of her condition, the preferred therapeutic approach, and the necessary length of treatment. Inadequate coordination and communication between and among the treating clinicians, as is particularly apt to occur when they are *not* part of the same clinic or treatment unit/site (e.g., university hospitals), is another major area of concern that can lead to therapeutic failures when utilizing the "parallel approach."

In the *integrated* approach, treatment is delivered in a similar way to the parallel approach, but by a single healthcare professional. This is our preferred approach for the treatment of women with contemporaneous diagnoses. We have consistently used this approach with great success over the decades as well as recommending its use to others. However, it is the most difficult approach to successfully employ because of the absolute requirements for a skilled, knowledgeable, and clinically experienced clinician or therapist. It also is important to note that, when needed, appropriate consultation, collaboration, and referral are extremely beneficial to the treatment outcomes. In the majority of *failed* cases that have been referred to us over the years, the most common problem has been the use of non-professionally educated para-professional therapists, usually recovering from their own drug or substance abuse, who have experience and strengths in group therapy and other related skills, but are ill-prepared to plan and deliver complex therapeutic treatment that tends to be far beyond their abilities when confronted with contemporaneous disorders involving AUDs, SUDs, and often multiple OMDs (Pagliaro & Pagliaro, *Clinical Patient Data Files*).

An example of the application of these approaches can be illustrated in the context of the treatment of women who smoke tobacco while pregnant, or during the perinatal period, who also have a history of current or past mental depression. This cohort of women has been found to:

- Have a *higher* incidence of nicotine dependence than cohorts of women without depression (e.g., van der Meer, Willemsen, & Smit, 2013)
- Be able, with or without formal therapeutic treatment, to significantly reduce their tobacco use, particularly during the third trimester of pregnancy (e.g., El-Mohandes, El-Khorazaty, & Kiely, 2011)

- Have a significant smoking relapse rate postpartum (e.g., Forray, Gotman, & Kershaw, 2014)
- Respond inadequately to cognitive therapy (i.e., counseling), when provided as the only therapeutic treatment (e.g., Chamberlain, O'Mara-Eves, & Oliver, 2013)[34]

In their sample of pregnant women with depression and concurrent substance abuse, Forray, Gotman, and Kershaw (2014) found that "66% of women smoked in the three months before pregnancy, 42% of pre-pregnancy smokers achieved abstinence before delivery, and 60% of the baseline cohort smoked postpartum" (p. 749).[35]

Managing Specific Withdrawal Syndromes

Several types of pharmacotherapy have been used, with varying degrees of success, to reduce the unpleasant physiological and psychological signs and symptoms of withdrawal associated with the abrupt discontinuation of the regular, long-term use of various drugs and substances of abuse, including alcohol, cocaine, nicotine, and the opiate analgesics.

Alcohol Withdrawal Syndrome. Acute alcohol withdrawal is often managed quite successfully with a long-acting benzodiazepine—usually chlordiazepoxide (Librium®) or diazepam (Valium®) (Pagliaro & Pagliaro, 2009). As noted by Amato, Minozzi, and Vecchi (2010), in their comprehensive review of 64 studies on the use of benzodiazepines for the management of the alcohol withdrawal syndrome:

> Benzodiazepines showed a protective benefit against alcohol withdrawal symptoms, in particular seizures.
>
> *(p. 1)*

Benzodiazepine pharmacotherapy for the management of alcohol withdrawal requires a gradual reduction of dosage over a 1 to 2 week period and, when appropriately used, can make the alcohol withdrawal syndrome virtually *symptomless* (Pagliaro & Pagliaro, 1999). Although less efficacious, clonidine (Catapres®), an alpha-adrenergic agonist, which also is clinically used for its antihypertensive effects, has been used as an adjunct for the management of both the alcohol (Bayard, McIntyre,

34 As noted by Chamberlain, O'Mara-Eves, and Oliver (2013) "a significant effect was only seen in subjects where counseling was provided in conjunction with other strategies" (p. 1). El-Mohandes, El-Korazaty, and Kiely (2011) also noted a similar effect in their study of smoking cessation among women of African descent (i.e., "*no* response to a CBT intervention during pregnancy" [p. S96]).

35 In this regard, it also is worth noting that Gaalema, Higgins, and Pepin (2013) noted that—in their study of pregnant women primarily of European descent, *younger* than 25 years-of-age, and who smoked, on average, one package of cigarettes daily and were enrolled in a smoking cessation program—approximately one-third had *illicit* substances of abuse detected in their urine samples. The researchers further noted that, "The most common drug detected was marijuana (90% of positive specimens), followed by opioids (18%), cocaine (5%), benzodiazepines (3%), and methadone (3%)" (p. 987).

& Hill, 2004; Stanley, Worrall, & Lunsford, 2005) and opiate analgesic (e.g., heroin; methadone) withdrawal syndromes (Gold & Dackis, 1984; Gowing, Farrell, & Ali, 2002, 2009; Washton & Resnick, 1981). The signs and symptoms of withdrawal are effectively managed by gradually decreasing the clonidine dosage over a 1 to 2 week period. (See related discussion in later section, *Opiate Analgesic Withdrawal Syndrome.*)

Cocaine Withdrawal Syndrome. The cocaine withdrawal syndrome (see Chapter 5, *Women's Amphetamine and Cocaine Abuse*), particularly its associated psychologic symptom of craving, has been a significant contributor to the relapsed use of cocaine. Consequently, a number of different drugs, including the: amphetamine, dextroamphetamine (Dexedrine®); anticonvulsant, topiramate (Topamax®); anti-convulsant/mood-stabilizing drug, valproate (Depakene®, Depakote®); antidepressant, bupropion (Wellbutrin®, Zyban®); antipsychotic tranquilizers; antiepileptic, carbamazepine (Tegretol®); anti-parkinsonians, bromocriptine (Parlodel®), carbidopa/levodopa (Sinemet®), and pergolide mesylate (Permax®); anti-viral, amantadine (Symmetrel®); and wakefulness promoting drug, modafinil (Alertec®, Provigil®) have been used, *off-label*,[36] for the management of cocaine withdrawal, as well as, cocaine dependence.

However, the general clinical efficacy associated with these various forms of pharmacotherapy for the management of cocaine withdrawal have been reported—in a wide number of studies and reviews—to be *poor* and *disappointing* (e.g., Amato, Minozzi, & Pani, 2007; Ballon & Feifel, 2006; de Lima, de Oliveira Soares, & Reisser, 2002; de Lima, Farrell, & Lima Reisser, 2010; Dursteler & Vogel, 2016; Kumar, 2008; Lima, Lima, & Soares, 2002; Lima, Reisser, & Soares, 2003; Martinez-Raga, Knecht, & Cepeda, 2008; Nuijten, Blanken, & van de Wetering, 2016; Reid & Thakkar, 2009; Shinn & Greenfield, 2010; Soares, Lima, & Reisser, 2003; Soares, Lima Reisser, & Farrell, 2010; Stoops & Rush, 2013). Because of the lack of supportive evidence regarding the efficacy of the pharmacologic management of the cocaine withdrawal syndrome, we do not, at this time, recommend any specific pharmacologic interventions. Instead, women should be closely clinically monitored when going through cocaine withdrawal and be provided with appropriate individual treatment, both pharmacotherapy and psychotherapy, as indicated, to effectively deal with problematic signs and symptoms.

Nicotine Withdrawal Syndrome. Two decades ago, bupropion (Wellbutrin SR®, Zyban®), an antidepressant, was approved for the management of the nicotine withdrawal syndrome associated with cessation of tobacco smoking (Corelli & Hudmon, 2006; Pagliaro & Pagliaro, 1999). Bupropion pharmacotherapy was continued for 2 to 3 months while monitoring patient response and progress in terms of smoking cessation. Studies and reviews of approaches for tobacco smoking cessation/withdrawal (e.g., Anthenelli, Benowitz, & West, 2016; Cahill, Stevens,

---

[36] "Off-label" indicates legitimate prescription use that is for an indication that has *not* been specifically evaluated and approved by the FDA and, consequently, is *not* found on the list of indications included in the official drug package insert.

& Perera, 2013) have generally found bupropion pharmacotherapy and nicotine replacement pharmacotherapy (NRT) to be *equally* efficacious.

However, several studies (e.g., Cox, Nollen, & Mayo, 2012; Robles, Singh-Franco, & Ghin, 2008) have *failed* to demonstrate long-term smoking cessation with bupropion use among smokers of African continental descent, particularly those who smoke: (1) menthol cigarettes; (2) fewer than 10 cigarettes per day; and/or (3) within 30 minutes of waking. (Also, see the later section, *Nicotine Replacement Therapy*.)

As briefly discussed in previous chapters of this text (e.g., Chapter 4, *Women's Caffeine and Nicotine Abuse*), several researchers have examined the relationship between menstrual phase and signs and symptoms of the nicotine withdrawal syndrome among premenopausal women (see Table 8.3). In addition, several other researchers have recognized relationships among various treatment outcomes and the follicular and luteal menstrual phases. These findings are briefly presented and discussed in the following section.

OVARIAN CYCLE EFFECTS ON NICOTINE TREATMENT OUTCOMES. In terms of ovarian effects, the normal menstrual cycle consists of three phases:

1. *Follicular phase* (days 0 to 14);
2. *Ovulatory phase* (days 13 to 15); and
3. *Luteal phase* (days 15 to 28).

Uterine effects also occur in three distinct phases:

1. *Menstrual phase* (days 0 to 6);
2. *Proliferative phase* (days 6 to 14); and
3. *Secretory phase* (days 14 to 28).

Both estrogens, primarily estradiol, and progestins, primarily progesterone, are present throughout the 28 days of the menstrual cycle. Estrogens predominate, in terms of hormone levels, during the first half of the menstrual cycle and progestins, during the second half (i.e., estradiol is predominant during the follicular, or pre-ovulation, phase, while progesterone is dominant during the luteal, or premenstrual phase).[37] The normal menstrual cycle is significantly changed when women are either pregnant or are using oral contraceptives (Pagliaro & Pagliaro, 1986). In numerous studies (for examples, see, Table 8.3), the menstrual cycle has been demonstrated to *significantly* impact the efficacy of pharmacological prevention and treatment efforts.

[37] Allopregnanolone, a metabolite of progesterone, also is noted to naturally occur in high concentration during the luteal phase among premenopausal women and has been associated with depressive symptomatology and may be associated with a blunted response to nicotine from smoking (Allen, al'Absi, & Lando, 2015).

TABLE 8.3 Menstrual Phase Effects on Women's Nicotine Withdrawal and Therapy for Tobacco Smoking Cessation

Menstrual Phase	*Outcome*	*Reference*
Follicular Phase	*Less* favorable outcome in relation to tobacco smoking cessation	Allen, Bade, & Center, 2008
	Greater success in tobacco smoking cessation when initiated during this phase	Franklin, Ehrman, & Lynch, 2008
	Greater nicotine *craving* upon awakening that may contribute to "smoking first thing in the morning"	Allen, Allen, & Widenmier, 2009
	Increased stress and arousal	Saladin, Wray, & Carpenter, 2015
Luteal Phase	Greater success in tobacco smoking cessation and continued abstinence with bupropion sustained release formulation (Wellbutrin SR®) when initiated during this phase	Mazure, Toll, & McKee, 2011
	Decreased subjective effects of nicotine and *increased* cognition	DeVito, Herman, & Waters, 2014
	Greater *increase* in stimulation and greater *decrease* in urge to smoke following use of nicotine nasal spray (Nicotrol NS®)	Allen, Lunos, & Heishman, 2015
	Improved nicotine tobacco smoking cessation outcomes following nicotine or varenicline (Chantix®) pharmacotherapy	Saladin, McClure, & Baker, 2015
	Greater craving for nicotine among women during this phase when compared to men	Saladin, Wray, & Carpenter, 2015
	Greater nicotine withdrawal symptomatology	Weinberger, Smith, & Allen, 2015

Regarding women's nicotine tobacco smoking prevention and treatment, *estradiol* may *enhance* drug reward and *increase* tobacco smoking behavior while *progesterone* may *decrease* drug reward, nicotine craving, and tobacco smoking behavior (Saladin, McClure, & Baker, 2015).[38] Among *premenopausal* women, the *luteal* phase is generally associated with a blunted response to nicotine and, consequently:

[38] Recognizing: (1) the noted effects of progesterone; (2) "pregnancy is a strong motivator to quit smoking, yet postpartum relapse rates are high" (p. 2145); and (3) that "in pregnancy, progesterone increases by more than tenfold … then within the first few hours, postpartum levels drop to near

1. *Better* smoking cessation outcomes
2. A *longer* period of smoking cessation with a *decreased* craving for nicotine and an associated *decreased* urge to smoke

(e.g., Allen, Allen, & Widenmier, 2009; Allen, Lunos, & Heishman, 2015; Allen, Bade, & Center, 2008; Franklin, Ehrman, & Lynch, 2008)

While the reported relationships are significant, they are *not* universal.

OTHER CO-VARIABLE EFFECTS ON NICOTINE TREATMENT OUTCOMES. Other co-variables may play a major contributory role, such as *mental depression* (e.g., Allen, al'Absi, & Lando, 2013; Pang, Bello, & Stone, 2016)—particularly the premenstrual dysphoric disorder (PMDD), which is most specific to the *luteal* phase of the menstrual cycle (Pinkerton, Guico-Pabia, & Taylor, 2010; Steiner, 2000). Others (e.g., Huttlin, Allen, & Tosun, 2015) posited a significant role for related endogenous adrenocortical activity. When, for example, nicotine nasal spray was administered to women smokers during the follicular phase, *higher* morning cortisol levels were associated with *decreases* in negative affect and withdrawal symptomatology coincident with *increases* in reported feelings of relaxation. Conversely, when nicotine nasal spray was administered during the luteal phase, *higher* morning cortisol levels were associated with *decreases* in reported "head rush" and "urge to smoke."

Opiate Analgesic Withdrawal Syndrome. Women's long-term, regular use of pure opiate analgesic agonists (e.g., morphine) or mixed opiate analgesic agonists/antagonists (e.g., pentazocine, Talwin®) are associated with the development of physical (and psychological) dependence. Thus, among women, who are physically dependent on opiate analgesics, abrupt discontinuation of regular, long-term use, or the use of an opiate analgesic antagonist (e.g., naloxone, Narcan®), may result in the opiate analgesic withdrawal syndrome.

Signs and symptoms of the acute opiate analgesic withdrawal syndrome, include: abdominal cramps and pain; anorexia; anxiety; backache and other body aches; chills; diarrhea; dysphoria; hypertension; insomnia; increased respiratory rate; irritability; nausea; nervousness; piloerection (gooseflesh); restlessness; rhinitis; rhinorrhea; sensitivity to pain (increased); shivering; sneezing; sweating (excessive); tachycardia; tremors; unexplained fever; weakness; and yawning. Although the opiate analgesic withdrawal syndrome is *not* usually life threatening, the appropriate use of opiate analgesic withdrawal pharmacotherapy and monitoring is generally indicated in its management. Gradual discontinuation of the regular, long-term

---

pre-pregnancy levels" (p. 2146)—Allen, Allen, and Lunos (2016) explored the feasibility of utilizing exogenous progesterone as an active pharmacotherapeutic approach to prevent smoking relapse during the postpartum period. Participants, in their 12-week, double-blind, placebo-controlled, randomized pilot study, were 46 cigarette-smoking women, who were initially abstinent postpartum. Although the study lacked sufficient statistical power, results demonstrated a *higher* rate of abstinence maintenance in the progesterone treatment group.

use of the opiate analgesics will prevent or minimize related signs and symptoms of withdrawal. Relapse to resumed use of the opiate analgesics during opiate analgesic withdrawal is common (see Chapter 1, *Women's Opiate Analgesic Abuse*, for additional related discussion).

We generally would *not* recommend pharmacological adjuncts for the management of the heroin withdrawal syndrome because it is generally relatively mild and can *usually* be handled "cold turkey" (i.e., signs and symptoms of the heroin withdrawal syndrome typically resemble those of a bad case of influenza—dependent, of course, on both the amount of heroin used daily and the length of time it has been used). In contrast, the methadone withdrawal syndrome may be quite severe with convulsions and other physiological effects that require appropriate treatment under direct medical supervision. Even when not required medically, we strongly recommend that patients undergo methadone withdrawal in an inpatient setting, particularly patients with concomitant histories of long-standing or high-dose use of alcohol or another drug or substance of abuse, in order to provide appropriate psychological support and significantly improve compliance (i.e., ensure that the patient successfully completes the withdrawal process). The average stay for people in detoxification units or centers in these situations is typically approximately 3 days (Pagliaro & Pagliaro, *Clinical Patient Data Files*).

Following a woman's successful opiate analgesic withdrawal, we strongly recommend that she be immediately started on long-term, relapse prevention treatment, including, if deemed clinically appropriate, abstinence maintenance (see related discussion in the following section, *Abstinence Maintenance*, "Opiate Analgesics").

Abstinence Maintenance

Several drugs have been developed to help to ensure continued abstinence among people who have discontinued their regular, long-term abusive or compulsive use of alcohol or opiate analgesics, particularly heroin.[39] Abstinence maintenance pharmacotherapy generally involves either: (1) *pairing* unpleasant effects with the use of a drug or substance of abuse (e.g., use of disulfiram [Antabuse®]); or (2) *blocking* desired effects when the drug or substance of abuse is used (e.g., use of naltrexone [Vivitrol®]). Thus, abstinence maintenance pharmacotherapy helps to ensure abstinence by means of either association with *aversive* stimuli or blocking of *rewarding* stimuli. These actions are discussed in the following sections in the context of pharmacotherapy for alcohol abstinence maintenance.

Alcohol Abstinence Maintenance. The FDA has approved *three* drugs for alcohol abstinence maintenance: (1) *acamprosate* (Campral®); (2) *disulfiram* (Antabuse®); and

[39] Abstinence, in this context, is actually a form of relapse prevention (see *Relapse Prevention* section later in this chapter).

(3) *naltrexone* (ReVia®). In addition, *topiramate* (Topamax®) has been clinically used, *off-label*, for this indication and has demonstrated some noted clinical efficacy.

ACAMPROSATE (CAMPRAL®). Acamprosate (Campral®) was approved for use by the FDA in 2004 and has since been demonstrated to be safe and effective for the prevention of relapse among abstinent drinkers (Higuchi, 2015; Jung & Namkoong, 2006; Kennedy, Leloux, & Kutscher, 2010; Kranzler & Gage, 2008; Rosner, Hackl-Herrwerth, & Leucht, 2010). The exact mechanism of action for acamprosate has *not* been fully determined (Kiefer & Mann, 2010). The regular, long-term use of alcohol increases the production of N-Methyl-D-aspartate (NMDA) receptors. During periods of alcohol withdrawal, these receptors are stimulated by a surge in the release of neurotransmitters, such as glutamate. Acamprosate appears to work by reducing this surge of glutamate (i.e., restoring glutamatergic neurotransmission to normal) (De Witte, Littleton, & Parot, 2005; Mason & Heyser, 2010).

Available from the manufacturer as a delayed-release oral tablet, acamprosate is ingested daily in three divided doses. To increase GI absorption, because of its low oral bioavailability (i.e., approximately 11%), it should be ingested on an empty stomach. Although a variety of adverse effects have been associated with its use, diarrhea is the most commonly reported adverse effect (Boothby & Doering, 2005; Diehl, Ulmer, & Mutschler, 2010). Combination pharmacotherapy for alcohol abstinence maintenance (e.g., acamprosate and naltrexone), as well as adjunctive psychotherapy (e.g., acamprosate and cognitive-behavioral therapy) have been found to significantly increase efficacy (Boothby & Doering, 2005; Kennedy, Leloux, & Kutscher, 2010; Mason, 2001, 2003).

DISULFIRAM (ANTABUSE®). Disulfiram (Antabuse®) *blocks* the metabolism of alcohol at the acetaldehyde stage by means of inhibition of the enzyme, acetaldehyde dehydrogenase. Consequently, when alcohol is consumed, even in small quantities, acetaldehyde accumulates in the blood stream and elicits a number of unpleasant effects, including: blurred vision; chest pain; confusion; copious vomiting; dyspnea; flushing; hyperventilation; hypotension; nausea; respiratory difficulty; syncope; tachycardia; throbbing headache; vertigo; and weakness. The intensity of this reaction, which is known as the disulfiram-alcohol-reaction (or more commonly as the Antabuse® reaction or disulfiram flush), is generally proportional to the amount of disulfiram used as a component of the alcohol abstinence maintenance program and to the amount of alcohol consumed at a particular drinking session (Pagliaro & Pagliaro, 1999).

Disulfiram pharmacotherapy is begun following at least 1 day of abstinence from alcohol use in order to avoid precipitating the disulfiram reaction. Subsequently, disulfiram is orally ingested daily each morning for a period of months to years until abstinence can be maintained without the aid of the drug.[40]

---

[40] Although controlled studies have *not* demonstrated significant efficacy for disulfiram pharmacotherapy when used alone (largely due to noncompliance), we have found it to be effective for highly

Daytime tiredness and night-time sleep disturbances are the most commonly reported adverse effects (Diehl, Ulmer, & Mutschler, 2010).

NALTREXONE (REVIA®). Another FDA approved form of pharmacotherapy for promoting alcohol abstinence maintenance is naltrexone (ReVia®) pharmacotherapy. Naltrexone, a long-acting oral opiate antagonist, was originally developed and marketed in the U.S. in 1984 under the brand name, Trexan®, for the treatment of compulsive patterns of opiate analgesic use (i.e., *physical and psychological dependence*)—particularly among practicing physicians and other healthcare professionals (e.g., Greenstein, Arndt, & McLellan, 1984; Kirchmayer, Davoli, & Verster, 2000). In addition, an injectable, extended-release formulation of naltrexone (Vivitrol®) has been approved by the FDA for abstinence maintenance (Gastfriend, 2014).

Largely by serendipity, it was discovered that naltrexone also *blocked* the disinhibitory euphoria associated with alcohol use.[41] Subsequently, in 1994, it was approved by the FDA for this use. The oral form of naltrexone is usually ingested on a daily basis without the need for attention to meals, or the ingestion of other foods and beverages. An injectable form of naltrexone also is available and is considered a major pharmaceutical advancement regarding naltrexone pharmacotherapy for alcohol abstinence maintenance (Garbutt, Kranzler, & O'Malley, 2005). The naltrexone injection (Vivitrol®), an extended release injectable suspension formulation, is injected intramuscularly[42] by a healthcare provider once a month, which significantly increases compliance with alcohol abstinence maintenance pharmacotherapy (Naltrexone Injection, 2010; SAMHSA, 2015; Swift, 2007).

The endogenous opiate system (see Chapter 1, *Women's Opiate Analgesic Abuse*), plays a significant role in the mediation of the disinhibitory euphoria and other desired effects associated with alcohol use, particularly those associated with the modulation of dopaminergic neurotransmission in the mesolimbic area of the brain (Jung & Namkoong, 2006; Soyka & Rosner, 2010). Consequently, when the receptors are blocked by naltrexone, the associated *urge* to drink is reduced, thus, strengthening the ability to cease drinking. Although additional research is required, it appears that carriers of a variant of the *mu*-opiate receptor gene may be particularly receptive to the efficacious effects of naltrexone pharmacotherapy for promoting abstinence among women who are regular, long-term users of alcohol (Mann & Hermann, 2010).

motivated, compliant women when used as an initial adjunct to Alcoholics Anonymous, or another 12-Step program, and weekly psychotherapy (Pagliaro & Pagliaro, *Clinical Patient Data Files*). (See related discussion later in this chapter.)

41 The CNS depressant effects, including alcohol-related effects on cognition, do *not* appear to be significantly affected by naltrexone ("Naltrexone," 2009). Thus, it is *not* a "sobriety pill."

42 Intramuscular injection of naltrexone has been associated with *severe* injection site reactions, including: dark scabbing; intense pain; lumps; open wounds; and swelling. On occasion, these reactions can be severe enough to warrant surgical or other therapeutic intervention. Thus, appropriate routine monitoring of injection sites is indicated.

To better address two perennial problems associated with naltrexone pharmacotherapy—(1) *low motivation* to begin naltrexone pharmacotherapy; and (2) *non-compliance* in terms of continuing pharmacotherapy—pharmaceutical companies in the U.S. have specifically developed and are testing several diverse formulations, including:

- Depot injectable formulations (e.g.,Vivitrol®)
- Extended-release formulations (e.g., Naltrexone XR®)
- Implantable polymers or systems

In contrast to the oral dosage form of naltrexone, which is dosed on a daily basis, these formulations are designed to be administered once every 1 to 12 months (Goonoo, Bhaw-Luximon, & Ujoodha, 2014; Kunoe, Lobmaier, & Ngo, 2014; Larney, Gowing, & Mattick, 2014; Syed & Keating, 2013).

When used as an adjunct to effective psychotherapy, naltrexone pharmacotherapy demonstrates significant clinical utility with reports of less craving for alcohol, a *lower* rate of relapse, and, when drinking, the consumption of fewer drinks per occasion (Naltrexone, 2009; Volpicelli, Clay, & Watson, 1995). The most common undesired effect associated with the use of naltrexone is nausea. However, its long-term safety and efficacy have *not* yet been clearly established and the FDA has added a *box* warning to its official monograph stating that:

> Naltrexone may cause liver damage when taken in large doses [i.e., several times the normal recommended daily dose for an extended period].
>
> *(Naltrexone, 2009, p. 1)*

In addition, as a potent opiate analgesic antagonist, naltrexone can precipitate the opiate analgesic withdrawal syndrome among women who are regular, long-term users of the opiate analgesics, including those who are being medically managed for chronic pain (e.g., chronic cancer pain). Thus, caution must be exercised when naltrexone abstinence maintenance pharmacotherapy is implemented for these women, who also would require alternative pain relief measures (e.g., non-opiate analgesics, such as acetaminophen [Tylenol®]; non-steroidal anti-inflammatory drugs [NSAIDs, e.g., aspirin, ibuprofen]; regional nerve block, or other related procedures) (Pagliaro & Pagliaro, 1999; Volpicelli, Clay, & Watson, 1995).

The National Institutes of Health (NIH) recommends that oral naltrexone pharmacotherapy is most appropriate for women who are:

1. Highly motivated or monitored for compliance by family members or close friends
2. Abstinent from opiate analgesics
3. Identified as having intense cravings for alcohol

(Center for Substance Abuse Treatment, 2009, p. 11)

TOPIRAMATE (TOPAMAX®). Topiramate (Topamax®) is an anticonvulsant that has been used in the U.S. for over 30 years to symptomatically manage various seizure disorders (Maryanoff, Nortey, & Gardocki, 1987). While *not* FDA approved for alcohol abstinence maintenance, its *off-label* use for this indication has been reported for over a decade (e.g., Johnson, Ait-Daoud, & Bowden, 2003; Johnson, Rosenthal, & Capece, 2007). Several published studies and reviews (e.g., Arbaizar, Diersen-Sotos, & Gomez-Acebo, 2010; De Sousa, 2010; Florez, Saiz, & Garcia-Portilla, 2010; Garbutt, 2009; Johnson & Ait-Daoud, 2010; Johnson, Ait-Daoud, & Bowden, 2003; Kenna, Lomastro, & Schiesl, 2009) have indicated that, when compared to either placebo or naltrexone abstinence maintenance for alcohol, topiramate abstinence maintenance resulted in: (1) *fewer* drinks per day; (2) *fewer* drinks per drinking episode; (3) *fewer* heavy drinking days; (4) more abstinent days; and (5) *increased* reduction in reports of craving.

The mechanism of action for topiramate in regard to alcohol abstinence maintenance has *not* yet been determined. However, topiramate appears to modulate dopaminergic neurotransmission in the mesolimbic area of the brain by decreasing the changes in NMDA receptor activity that have been associated with damage caused by regular, long-term alcohol use—or *heavy drinking*. Consequently, dopamine release is *inhibited* and GABA function is *enhanced* (Johnson, Ait-Daoud, & Bowden, 2003; Olmsted & Kockler, 2008).

Following ingestion, topiramate is rapidly and well-absorbed from the GI tract with approximately 70% excreted in unchanged form in the urine. The most common reported undesired effects associated with its use, include: cognitive impairment (e.g., memory impairment); dizziness; GI distress; paresthesia, or a sensation of burning, pricking, or tingling of the skin; psychomotor slowing; and weight loss. These undesired effects may significantly limit its use regarding alcohol abstinence maintenance (Arbaizar, Diersen-Sotos, & Gomez-Acebo, 2010; Shinn & Greenfield, 2010).

Opiate Analgesics. Naltrexone is FDA approved for opiate analgesic abstinence maintenance, as well as for *alcohol* abstinence maintenance (see earlier related discussion in the section, "Abstinence Maintenance, Alcohol, Naltrexone"). Also, see related discussion in the following section, "Naltrexone (Vivitrol®)."

NALTREXONE (VIVITROL®). The clinical use of naltrexone for alcohol abstinence maintenance pharmacotherapy, or to prevent opiate analgesic relapse, has been severely limited by *poor* patient compliance and *low* treatment retention rates (e.g., Minozzi, Amato, & Vecchi, 2011). For example, among a sample of over 300 community-living ex-prisoners, who had limited use of heroin within the 30 days *prior* to the commencement of the research study, monthly injections of extended-release naltrexone (Vivitrol®), used in combination with relapse-prevention counseling and community support, demonstrated significant efficacy *only* during the first 6 months of therapy (Lee, Friedmann, & Kinlock, 2016). In addition, as expected, based on the pharmacologic action of naltrexone, rates of cocaine use and other injectable drug use was *not* significantly reduced—even within the first 6 months of treatment.

Efficacy has been demonstrated when used among limited samples of prison inmates. After demonstrating that they are "opiate analgesic free" for a minimum of 7 days to avoid precipitating acute opiate analgesic withdrawal, inmates begin once-monthly intramuscular injections of long-acting naltrexone (i.e., Vivitrol®). For optimal outcomes, an active counseling program also is recommended. Cautions include risks for hepatotoxicity and blocking of the potential therapeutic effects of the opiate analgesics (i.e., in terms of their use to relieve pain, cough, and diarrhea) (Pagliaro & Pagliaro, *Clinical Patient Data Files*).

However, during the second decade of the new millennium, the use of naltrexone extended-release injections for the maintenance of opiate-analgesic abstinence received renewed interest. The transition of opiate analgesic dependent patients to naltrexone extended-release injection therapy may be problematic because it typically requires a 7-day period of abstinence from opiate analgesic use in order to avoid precipitating the acute opiate analgesic withdrawal syndrome. In addition, risk for resumed use, or relapse, is *very* high during this 7-day period of abstinence.

To deal with this problem, several related protocols involving both naltrexone and buprenorphine, as well as adjunctive pharmacotherapy for the management of the signs and symptoms of opiate analgesic withdrawal, have been developed. The protocol,[43] which appears to be *most* promising, is the *rapid* naltrexone induction procedure that begins with a single "drug free" day, followed by an oral dosage of buprenorphine, 7 days of *increasing* oral dosages of naltrexone, and, finally, the initiation of naltrexone extended-release injectable pharmacotherapy (Sullivan, Bisaga, & Pavlicova, 2017). Reportedly, women (and men), who respond *best* to the *rapid* naltrexone induction procedure with buprenorphine, followed by long-term abstinence management with naltrexone extended-release injectable pharmacotherapy, generally: (1) are older in age; and (2) used *less* than 10 bags of heroin daily, or an equivalent amount (Mogali, Khan, & Drill, 2015).

Maintenance, Replacement, or Substitution[44]

Maintenance, replacement, or substitution (MRS) pharmacotherapy is based on the principle of harm reduction—an integral component of tertiary prevention (see earlier discussion). As such, MRS pharmacotherapy does *not* attempt to cease

[43] An alternative outpatient approach for initiating naltrexone extended-release injectable abstinence pharmacotherapy involves simultaneously *increasing* oral dosages of naltrexone and *decreasing* oral dosages of buprenorphine for 7 days—followed by the initiation of naltrexone extended-release injectable pharmacotherapy (Mannelli, Wu, & Peindl, 2014).

[44] N.B. Several factors have been noted among women, who abuse opiate analgesics, that may significantly adversely affect/complicate the efficacy of related pharmacotherapy. For example, Back, Payne, and Wahlquist (2011), in their sample of 892 adults screened for the National Institute on Drug Abuse *Clinical Trials Network*, found that significantly *more* women than men: (1) tested

the use of a drug or substance of abuse. Rather, it attempts to change the *level* of harm associated with its use, including the harm associated with its *method of use*. In the U.S., the *two* major examples of MRS pharmacotherapy are: (1) for heroin abuse, the substitution of methadone; and (2) for nicotine abuse in the form of tobacco smoking, the substitution of less harmful methods of use (e.g., e-cigarettes; nicotine chewing gum, nasal sprays, or "patches").

Methadone Maintenance. Methadone (Dolophine®), a long-acting opiate analgesic, has been used for over 50 years in the U.S. as a *legal* form of pharmacotherapy for *opiate analgesic maintenance*, particularly for women, who are addicted to heroin, and who have been unable to successfully complete opiate analgesic detoxification. We generally recommend that methadone maintenance be reserved for women: (1) who fail to respond to naltrexone with or without buprenorphine combination pharmacotherapy (see related discussion in the earlier section, "Naltrexone," and the following section, "Buprenorphine/Naloxone combination"); or (2) for whom naltrexone/buprenorphine is determined to be inappropriate (e.g., contraindicated).

Over the last decade, methadone maintenance also has been associated with a disproportionate number of deaths related to opiate analgesic overdosages, particularly among *older* women who have been prescribed methadone in place of oxycodone for the management of chronic pain (Pagliaro & Pagliaro, *Clinical Patient Data Files*; Webster, Cochella, & Dasgupta, 2011). (Also, see Chapter 1, *Women's Opiate Analgesic Abuse*, for additional discussion.) As reported by Collins (2010), many of these deaths, believed to be iatrogenic, specifically involved: (1) inappropriate use of conversion tables for dosing methadone; and (2) initiating methadone maintenance at too *high* a dosage (i.e., 80 mg/day as opposed to 30 mg/day). Despite its associated limitations and problems, methadone remains the "gold standard" for opiate analgesic maintenance pharmacotherapy (Connery, 2015, p. 63).

The goals of methadone maintenance pharmacotherapy for opiate addiction are to allow women, who are addicted to heroin, to: (1) discontinue their *illicit* use of heroin while legally using methadone to *ward off* the signs and symptoms of the opiate analgesic withdrawal syndrome; and (2) return to more *normal* and, consequently, less harmful lifestyles. For example, opiate analgesic maintenance with methadone has been associated with a significant reduction in *hustling* and other related behaviors (e.g., *breaks and entries*; *child neglect*; *imprisonment*; *overdosage*

positive for amphetamines, methamphetamine, and phencyclidine; (2) reported *more* current and past medical problems; and (3) had *greater* craving for opiate analgesics (p. 313).

Conversely, several factors have been identified among women, who abuse opiate analgesics, that may significantly *enhance* the efficacy of related pharmacotherapy (e.g., appropriate psychotherapy and/or residential treatment [Pagliaro & Pagliaro, *Clinical Patient Data Files*]). (Also, see related discussion in later section, *Psychotherapy and Counseling*.)

death; *prostitution*) that are commonly associated with women's heroin addiction (Pagliaro & Pagliaro, *Clinical Patient Data Files*).

While prescribed in dosages[45] that, generally, do *not* produce euphoria or other desired psychotropic effects, opiate analgesic maintenance with methadone *keeps the edge off* for these women and enables them to maintain effective parenting, work, and other social responsibilities, as well as participate in psychotherapy and other tertiary prevention approaches. Although continuing a woman's physical and psychological dependence on an opiate analgesic, methadone maintenance pharmacotherapy offers several benefits: (1) ingested once daily, it eliminates the hazards associated with obtaining illegal heroin for injection at least 4, or more, times a day; (2) prevents associated harmful effects associated with intravenous heroin injection (e.g., HIV infection; overdosage); (3) decreases *craving* for heroin; (4) avoids the occurrence of both euphoria and excessive sedation; (5) relatively inexpensive; (6) legally available; and (7) conveniently and safely obtained, at licensed neighborhood pharmacies. (Also, see Chapter 1, *Women's Opiate Analgesic Abuse*, for additional related discussion.)

Although methadone pharmacotherapy for opiate analgesic maintenance has many benefits, it also has some *drawbacks*. For example, the withdrawal syndrome associated with methadone use is much more *severe* than that associated with heroin use.[46] Thus, many women, who enroll in methadone maintenance programs, remain in these programs for several years. During this time, they often begin, or continue, to abuse other drugs and substances of abuse, such as alcohol and cocaine that are *not* deterred by methadone use (Pagliaro & Pagliaro, 1999, 2009; Pagliaro & Pagliaro, *Clinical Patient Data Files*).[47] Women, who decide to discontinue their methadone maintenance programs, often *resume* their heroin use. Other potential disadvantages of methadone use, when compared to, for example, buprenorphine (see following section), include a *higher* risk for: (1) overdosage, particularly during treatment initiation; (2) *increased* severity of undesired effects (e.g., cognitive impairment; sedation; weight gain); (3) cardiac dysrhythmias related to QTc-prolongation; (4) abuse; and (5) diminished analgesic effects with concurrent opiate-analgesic administration.

---

[45] Dosages must be individually adjusted for each woman, who abuses opiate analgesics, based on several factors, including: age; concurrent pharmacotherapy; hepatic function; physical health; and the specific opiate analgesic to which she is addicted, the length of time she has used it, and the current dosage used (Pagliaro & Pagliaro, *Clinical Patient Data Files*). We recommend that, initially, dosages start low (e.g., 20 to 30 mg/day) and, depending on a woman's individual response, are slowly *increased* to an optimal daily dose ranging from 60 mg to 120 mg (Donny, Walsh, & Bigelow, 2002; Faggiano, Vigna-Taglianti, & Versino, 2003).

[46] This problem is often related to unidentified or untreated contemporaneous diagnoses (Wu & Blazer, 2014). (See Chapter 7, *Identifying Women's Contemporaneous Diagnoses*, for additional related discussion, including treatment approaches.)

[47] Random urine testing is a standard of care in this clinical context and is of benefit regarding: (1) validation of self-reported use/nonuse of opiate analgesics; (2) adherence to treatment (i.e., daily methadone dosing); (3) detection of other drug or substance use (e.g., benzodiazepines; cocaine); and (4) evaluation of treatment response.

Finally, for women who are pregnant and addicted to opiate analgesics, methadone generally is *not* the first drug of choice. However, attrition (i.e., the treatment drop-out rate) is generally significantly *lower* for methadone treatment versus buprenorphine treatment among opiate-dependent pregnant women. Thus, some researchers (e.g., Jumah, Graves, & Kahan, 2015) recommend methadone use for pregnant women who are opiate analgesic-dependent. In addition, when compared to the continued use of heroin, or detoxification, among pregnant heroin-dependent women, methadone—over the years—has been associated with several positive outcomes, including: *higher* birth weights; *longer* periods of gestation; *lower* risk for HIV infection; and *more* visits for antenatal healthcare.

However, the preponderance of available data suggest that buprenorphine pharmacotherapy: (1) is *equally* efficacious as methadone pharmacotherapy for women, who are pregnant and heroin-dependent; (2) presents *no* greater risk in terms of fetal growth measures; and (3) offers *three* unique benefits for embryos/fetuses/neonates:

1. Reduced embryo/fetal cardiac suppression
2. Reduced fetal movement suppression
3. Less severe neonatal abstinence syndrome

(Jones, Finnegan, & Kaltenbach, 2012; Minozzi, Amato, & Bellisario, 2013; Pagliaro & Pagliaro, 2012; Sutter, Leeman, & Hsi, 2014; Zedler, Mann, & Kim, 2016)

In regard to the latter benefit, Pritham (2013) noted that both buprenorphine and methadone are excreted in breast milk and, consequently, breast-feeding by mothers maintained on either buprenorphine or methadone *decreased* the severity of the neonatal abstinence syndrome among their neonates.

Buprenorphine/Naloxone Combination. Buprenorphine, like methadone, has been found to be effective for both the: (1) management of acute opiate analgesic detoxification; and (2) long-term opiate analgesic maintenance pharmacotherapy in a number of studies (Kovas, McFarland, & McCarty, 2007; Nielsen, Larance, & Degenhardt, 2016; Pagliaro & Pagliaro, 2009). It also has been found to be *safer* than methadone in cases of overdosage and is associated with a *less* severe opiate analgesic withdrawal syndrome experience when regular, long-term use is abruptly discontinued (Raisch, Fye, & Boardman, 2002).

In an effort to curtail the widespread abuse of buprenorphine associated with the increasing opiate analgesic epidemic occurring across the U.S. during the new millennium, the FDA endorsed the marketing of combination drug products that contained *both* buprenorphine and naloxone.

Buprenorphine, a *mixed opiate analgesic agonist/antagonist* (i.e., partial mu-receptor *agonist* and full kappa-receptor *antagonist*), is preferentially administered *sublingually* (absorption F = 0.5; half-life of elimination, approximately 30 hours). Naloxone, an *opiate analgesic antagonist*, also can be administered sublingually (absorption $F = 0.1$; half-life of elimination, approximately 1 hour) (Chiang & Hawks, 2003; Pagliaro & Pagliaro, 2009; Robinson, 2006). Thus, the pharmacokinetics of these two drugs, particularly their difference in "*F*," allows their combination as a *mixed opiate analgesic agonist/antagonist* in different buccal or sublingual formulations that could be dosed once daily:

- Buccal film (Bunavail®)
- Sublingual film (Suboxone®)
- Sublingual tablet (SubSolv®)

However, when the combined product is administered intravenously, absorption is 100% for *both* drugs (i.e., F = 1) and, consequently, results in the *desired* euphoric and analgesic effects of buprenorphine being totally *blocked* by the naloxone. (For further related discussion, see Chapter 1, *Women's Opiate Analgesic Abuse.*) In addition to the expected undesired effects and toxicities associated with the use of buprenorphine, the buccal/sublingual formulations have been associated with mouth numbness, redness, and tongue pain. Since 2000 in the U.S., physicians have been required to: (1) undergo a training course; and (2) apply for a license to prescribe combination buprenorphine/naloxone opiate analgesic MRS pharmacotherapy on an outpatient basis. However, as noted by Williams and Bisaga (2016), in their editorial regarding the "vast epidemic of opioid-related deaths" facing the U.S.:

> In 40% of U.S. counties there is currently no physician authorized to prescribe buprenorphine, and the majority of authorized providers actually treat few or no patients.
>
> *(p. 814)*

Nicotine and Varenicline (Chantix®). Both nicotine and varenicline are used for MRS pharmacotherapy for achieving tobacco smoking abstinence. (Also, see related discussion of bupropion in the earlier section, *Nicotine Withdrawal Syndrome.*)

NICOTINE. The widest application of MRS pharmacotherapy in the U.S. has been the use of nicotine in the forms of chewing gum, inhalers, lozenges, nasal and oral sprays, sublingual tablets, and transdermal drug delivery systems, or "patches," to manage the nicotine withdrawal syndrome associated with the cessation of tobacco smoking among regular, long-term smokers (Crain & Bhat, 2010; Fant, Buchhalter, & Buchman, 2009). Whereas methadone maintenance is just that, *maintenance* (i.e., maintained on a "semi-permanent" basis), it is generally expected that nicotine substitutes be used for *short* periods of time (e.g., up to 12 weeks).[48]

[48] However, in reality, many women continue to use nicotine substitutes beyond this recommended time frame.

The nicotine substitutes help women to *slowly* discontinue their regular, long-term nicotine use while experiencing diminished signs and symptoms of the nicotine withdrawal syndrome (Cahill, Stevens, & Perera, 2013; Frishman, 2007). The transdermal nicotine delivery systems (e.g., Habitrol®; Nicoderm®) and nicotine nasal sprays (Nicotrol NS®) have become important adjuncts to smoking cessation programs and have demonstrated positive effects in relation to decreasing tobacco smoking among women.

While potentially beneficial, studies over the last 25 years (e.g., Grimshaw & Stanton, 2006) have repeatedly demonstrated that the use of nicotine substitutes is, in most cases, only significantly effective when *combined* with appropriate counseling or other psychotherapeutic approaches.[49] For example, as noted by Covey and Glassman (1991):

> Evidence of the addictive nature of chronic tobacco use suggests that pharmacologic interventions, in conjunction with behaviorally oriented therapy, may present the best hope for achieving smoking cessation in refractory smokers.
>
> *(p. 69)*

Or, as noted by Generali (1992):

> Smoking cessation rates associated with nicotine transdermal patch therapy have varied in clinical trials. However, appropriate patient instruction and an extensive behavioral modification program ensure optimal response to transdermal nicotine therapy.
>
> *(p. 34)*

As noted by Laniado-Laborin (2010):

> The rate of successful smoking cessation at 1 year is 3% to 5% when the patient simply tries to stop, 7% to 16% if the smoker undergoes behavioral intervention, and up to 25% when receiving pharmacologic treatment and behavioral support.
>
> *(p. 74)*

---

49 Several researchers, including Bowker, Lewis, and Coleman (2014), have suggested possible explanations related to *increased* metabolism during pregnancy:

> Our findings are significant and consistent with the hypothesis that NRT (Nicotine Replacement Therapy) patches deliver an inadequate dose of nicotine to aid smoking cessation during pregnancy.
>
> *(p. 895)*

And, finally, as noted by Stead, Koilpillai, and Fanshawe (2016), in their retrospective meta-analysis of 53 studies including a total of over 25,000 participants:

> Interventions that combine pharmacotherapy and behavioral support increase smoking cessation success.
>
> *(p. 1)*

VARENICLINE. Varenicline (Chantix®) was approved by the FDA in 2006 for first-line pharmacotherapy aimed at facilitating smoking cessation. An alternative to NRT (Fant, Buchhalter, & Buchman, 2009; Frishman, 2009), it also is associated with, on average, a 1.5 times greater efficacy in smoking cessation success (Cahill, Stevens, & Perera, 2013). A *partial* nicotine antagonist, varenicline competitively binds to the nicotinic acetylcholine receptors (nAChRs), particularly the $\alpha_4\beta_2$ subtype (see related discussion in Chapter 4, *Women's Caffeine and Nicotine Abuse*) where it helps to stop smoking by its actions as a:

1. *Partial agonist*, reducing the signs and symptoms of nicotine withdrawal by maintaining moderate levels of dopamine
2. *Partial antagonist*, blocking nicotine from binding to the receptor sites and reducing its desired actions, including smoking satisfaction

Consequently, the ability of nicotine to stimulate the mesolimbic dopamine system is significantly reduced.

Varenicline is available as an oral tablet that is ingested once or twice daily, after meals, for generally 3 to 6 months (FDA, 2006). The most common *undesired* effect associated with varenicline pharmacotherapy is nausea, which is usually *mild to moderate* and subsides over time (Cahill, Stead, & Lancaster, 2012; Garrison & Dugan, 2009; Hays, Croghan, & Schroeder, 2010). It also can *lower* the seizure threshold. The FDA required a *black box* warning for the official labeling of Chantix® that includes the statement, "some people have had changes in behavior, hostility, agitation, depressed mood, and suicidal thoughts" (FDA, 2009; Varenicline, 2009, p. 1). The risk for these less common undesired, or harmful, effects and toxicities is reportedly *greater* for women who have a positive history of mental disorders (Ahmed, Ali, & Kramers, 2013). However, in late 2016, the FDA officially removed this "black box" warning from varenicline's official labeling (FDA, 2016).

Women also are cautioned to limit their alcohol consumption until they have monitored the effects of varenicline use (and the associated decreased tobacco smoking) on their drinking patterns. However, the results from a large-scale, double-blind, triple-dummy, placebo-controlled study indicate that varenicline's associated risk for *undesired* neuropsychiatric effects and toxicities was *not* significantly greater than that associated with the use of a placebo (Anthenelli, Benowitz, & West, 2016).

Serious cardiovascular events also have been reported to be related to varenicline pharmacotherapy, including congestive heart failure, dysrhythmias, and myocardial infarction (Singh, Loke, & Spangler, 2011). However, a comprehensive meta-analysis *failed* to substantiate either the clinical or statistical significance of these concerns (Prochaska & Hilton, 2012).

Although generally associated with nausea and a need for cautious use, varenicline pharmacotherapy for tobacco smoking cessation is well established as a suitable alternative to NRT, particularly for women who smoke tobacco and who have been unsuccessful in achieving smoking cessation with NRT. Several studies (e.g., Anthenelli, Benowitz, & West, 2016; Baker, Piper, & Stein, 2016; Gonzales, Rennard, & Nides, 2006; Jorenby, Hays, & Rigotti, 2006; Nides, Oncken, & Gonzales, 2006; Oncken, Gonzales, & Nides, 2006; Tonstad, Tonnesen, & Hajek, 2006) have demonstrated significant *increases* in abstinence with the use of varenicline when compared to placebo and/or bupropion pharmacotherapy. For example, Jorenby, Hays, and Rigotti (2006) found that, after 1 year, the rate of continuous abstinence for varenicline was 23% in comparison to 15% for bupropion and 10% for placebo. Cahill, Lindson-Hawley, and Thomas (2016), in their meta-analysis of 39 trials that tested varenicline, found that:

> Varenicline at standard dose increased the chances of successful long-term smoking cessation between two- and three-fold compared with pharmacologically unassisted quit attempts.
>
> *(p. 1)*

Chang, Chiang, and Ho (2015) found that combined varenicline and nicotine replacement therapy has been recommended and touted as being more efficacious than varenicline alone. For example, it has been found that the efficacy of varenicline can be *increased* significantly with combination varenicline pharmacotherapy and appropriate cognitive-behavioral psychotherapy (Ebbert, Wyatt, & Hays, 2010; Ebbert, Wyatt, & Zirakzadeh, 2009; Hays, Croghan, & Schroeder, 2010). A systematic review of approximately 20 randomized, controlled studies that compared varenicline pharmacotherapy with placebo, bupropion, nicotine replacement therapy, or counseling, found that varenicline pharmacotherapy had superior efficacy and increased the overall chances of long-term smoking cessation by two to threefold (Cahill, Stead, & Lancaster, 2012). (Also, see the following related discussion in this chapter.)

Regardless of which therapeutic intervention(s) is chosen for a specific woman who wants to quit smoking, it should be generally noted that: (1) combination therapeutic interventions, as previously discussed, usually provide the *most* favorable results; and (2) although the optimal duration of therapy must be individually determined for each woman, based on experience with *most* smokers, it should be maintained for a minimal period of 3 to 6 months.

In addition, as identified by Babb, Malarcher, and Schauer (2017), in their comprehensive report on behalf of the CDC, although currently available therapeutic interventions designed to assist adults to stop smoking cigarettes clearly can provide significant assistance/success, these strategies, such as those previously presented in this chapter, generally have considerable "room for improvement." As noted in the report, which was based upon data received from the *National Health Interview Surveys* (NHIS), for *women*, who were current cigarette smokers in the U.S. during 2015, *approximately*:

1. 70% expressed an interest in "quitting" smoking
2. 60% reported receiving advice to quit smoking from a healthcare professional
3. 10% used/received counseling
4. 30% used/received adjunctive pharmacotherapy
5. 35% used/received a *combination* of counseling and adjunctive pharmacotherapy
6. 8%, using #2, #3, or #4, were able to successfully quit smoking

Psychotherapy and Counseling

Both individual and group psychotherapeutic and counseling approaches can be used for women, alone, or as an adjunct to pharmacotherapy in the treatment of AUDs and SUDs (Azorin, Bowden, & Garay, 2010; Miller & Roache, 2009; Patnode, Henderson, & Thompson, 2015). (Also, see previous section, *Pharmacotherapy*.) These approaches include: (1) cognitive therapy; (2) group therapy; (3) family therapy; (4) couples therapy; (5) social skills training; (6) alternative psychotherapeutic delivery modalities; (7) residential treatment (i.e., therapeutic communities; short-term residential treatment); (8) continental descent-specific (e.g., African; Asian; European descent) and other descent-specific (e.g., Aboriginal, or American Indian; Alaska Native; Hispanic, or Latin American) approaches; (9) bisexual-, lesbian-, and trans woman-specific approaches; (10) 12-step programs; and (11) relapse prevention. Each of these approaches is briefly discussed in the following sections (see Box 8.3).[50]

Cognitive Therapy

Cognitive therapy, empirically supported by many researchers (e.g., McHugh, Hearon, & Otto, 2010; Waldron & Kaminer, 2004),[51] is one of the most commonly used forms of psychotherapy for women who have developed harmful patterns of

[50] Although pharmacotherapy, psychotherapy, and counseling approaches are discussed separately, optimal therapeutic outcomes for women, generally involve combination, or multimodal, therapy as demonstrated by many studies (e.g., Clarke, Mun, & Kelly, 2013; Hudman, Corelli, & Prokhorov, 2010; McCaul & Petry, 2003; Swift, 2007)—as well as our own extensive clinical practice experience.

[51] N.B. *However*, several studies and reviews (e.g., Gates, Sabioni, & Copeland, 2016; Minozzi, Saulle, & De Crescenzo, 2016) have suggested that the efficacy of cognitive therapy, as well as other forms of psychotherapy and counseling, may be limited in the therapeutic context of drug and substance abuse treatment. In this regard, we have consistently argued that the efficacy of psychotherapy

BOX 8.3: TERTIARY PREVENTION: *PSYCHOTHERAPY AND COUNSELING*

- Cognitive Therapy
- Group Therapy
  - Cognitive-Behavioral (Problem-Solving) Groups
  - Interpersonal Processes, or Psychotherapy, Groups
  - Peer Group Therapy
  - Psychoeducational Groups
  - Skills Development Groups
  - Support Groups
- Family Therapy
  - Boundaries
  - Feedback
  - Homeostasis
  - Validation
- Couples Therapy
- Social Skills Training
- Alternative Psychotherapeutic Delivery Modalities
  - Computer-Based Brief Interventions
  - E-mail
  - Teleconferencing
  - Telephone Support
  - Texting or Text Messaging
  - Videoconferencing
- Residential Programs
  - Therapeutic Communities
  - Short-Term Residential Programs
- Continental and Other Descent-Specific Treatment Programs
- Lesbian-Specific Treatment Programs
- Transgender-Specific Treatment Programs
- 12-Step Programs
  - Alcoholics Anonymous (AA)
  - Women's 12-Step Programs
  - Abstinence-Based Self/Mutual Help Groups
- Relapse Prevention Programs

---

and counseling for the treatment of drug and substance abuse disorders among women *primarily* depends on the: (1) multiple clinical characteristics of women, *individually*, including their *unique* personalities and *specific* drug and substance abuse problems; (2) *specific* type of psychotherapy/counseling selected and duration of treatment; and (3) *individual* knowledge and abilities of selected professional therapists in clinical counseling, psychotherapy, and/or addiction medicine or nursing.

drug and substance abuse. This form of psychotherapy assumes that harmful patterns of drug and substance abuse are indicative of maladaptive coping (i.e., that a woman has *not* learned effective ways to cope with her problems or to meet certain needs, often including developmental needs). Cognitive therapy is, therefore, directed at the correction, or modification, of:

- Maladaptive or deficient coping skills
- Irrational belief systems
- Faulty thinking patterns or styles

In addition, focus also is on strengthening specific intrapersonal and interpersonal skills (e.g., Kadden, 1994, p. 281).

Intrapersonal skills include:

- Anger control/management
- Conflict resolution
- Decision making
- Effective coping
- Increasing self-involvement in pleasurable activities
- Managing negative thinking, including managing thoughts about using alcohol or other drugs and substances of abuse
- Leisure time management
- Planning for emergencies
- Problem solving
- Relaxation training
- Resistance training

Interpersonal skills include:

- Assertiveness training
- Communication skills training
    - Communicating in intimate relationships
    - Communicating at work and in public
    - Giving and receiving criticism
    - Giving and receiving compliments
    - Initiating conversations
    - Refusing offers to use drugs and substances of abuse
    - Enhancing social support networks
    - Refusing requests
    - Using body language effectively

Thus, psychotherapeutic techniques include: (1) cognitive training in self-observation; (2) the sharing of thoughts and emotions with the therapist; (3) the systematic analysis of the validity of negative and irrational self-statements; and (4) the gradual substitution of positive logical thinking patterns based on rational belief systems. Through this process, women gradually become more aware of their problems, which, in the past, may have been avoided, denied, or repressed, and begin to develop the strategies, skills, and abilities they need to effectively deal with these problems.

Cognitive therapy is often applied in the context of *relapse prevention* in order to help to assure that the positive gains achieved during early abstinence are maintained. A central component to the achievement of this goal involves teaching women how to identify high-risk situations that may lead to patterns of relapsed use and to apply previously learned and rehearsed techniques to effectively avoid or deal with these high-risk situations. (Also, see related discussion in the earlier section, *Secondary Prevention*, "Protective Behavioral Strategies.")

Group Therapy

As noted by the Center for Substance Abuse Treatment (2005):

> The natural propensity of human beings to congregate makes group therapy a powerful therapeutic tool for treating substance abuse, one that is as helpful as individual therapy, and sometimes more successful.
>
> *(p. 1)*

In the U.S., therapeutic groups,[52] alone or in various combinations, have been found to provide effective outcomes for many women with alcohol use disorder (AUD) and other substance use disorders (SUDs) and include the following groups identified by the Center for Substance Abuse Treatment (2005, p. 6):[53]

- Cognitive-behavioral (problem-solving) groups
- Interpersonal process groups

---

52 The therapeutic groups can be *single-gendered*, in which all of the members, including the group leader or therapist, are women, or can be *mixed-gendered*. Although women may have a personal preference for single-gendered or mixed-gendered therapeutic groups, and may do better in their preferred group, research studies (e.g., Greenfield, Sugarman, & Freid, 2014; Hser, Evans, & Huang, 2011; Hser, Hunt, & Evans, 2012) have demonstrated comparable effectiveness with *no* significant differences generally found between the single-gendered and the mixed-gendered therapeutic groups. However, Evans, Li, and Pierce (2013) *did* note that the women-only programs were generally more likely than mixed-gendered programs for drug and substance abuse treatment to:

> offer special services such as pregnancy care, assistance with housing, transportation, job training, practical skills training, and on-site child care and child developmental services.
>
> *(p. 293)*

53 In the U.S., most of these therapeutic groups for women who, have AUDs and SUDs, are comprised of a *mixture* of several of these types of groups. The groups are often designed by treatment center

- Peer groups
- Psychoeducational groups
- Skills development groups
- Support groups

Cognitive-Behavioral (Problem-Solving) Groups. Cognitive-behavioral groups are based upon the assumption that drug and substance abuse is primarily a learned behavior that can be modified through various cognitive interventions. Consequently, effort is directed at changing harmful learned behavior by changing contributory thinking patterns, beliefs, and perceptions. A variety of approaches, which are grounded in the theory of cognitive-behavioral change, are used to teach group members about self-destructive drug and substance abuse behaviors and to help them to learn and develop more effective problem-solving abilities.

Interpersonal Process, or Psychotherapy, Groups. Utilizing psychodynamic processes, these groups delve into *major* developmental issues, both genetically and environmentally based, that may consciously or subconsciously contribute to members' drug and substance abuse and adverse treatment recovery outcomes. This form of group therapy is largely predicated upon *two* major assumptions: (1) that drug and substance abuse is a medical disease/mental disorder; and (2) that disturbing life events (e.g., complicated bereavement or role transition) can significantly compromise interpersonal functioning and, subsequently, significantly contribute to the development of drug and substance use disorders.

In order to function optimally, interpersonal process, or psychotherapy, groups have a well-defined hierarchical leadership structure in which group leaders are required to have a *high* degree of understanding and insight into group dynamics and individual behavior. These characteristics help to enable and support each group member to recreate and rethink her past in the context of the present and address relational and other life problems that have heretofore been avoided or suppressed—often with the assistance of drug and substance abuse.

Peer Group Therapy. Peer group psychotherapy for women also can be extremely effective. For example, Stead and Lancaster (2005), in their meta-analysis of group behavioral therapy programs for smoking cessation, found that group participants could: (1) learn behavioral techniques for smoking cessation; and (2) provide each other with mutual support. In terms of smoking cessation, they also found that outcomes were: (1) superior to those achieved with self-help; and (2) similar to those achieved with individual counseling.

---

staff without, we believe, adequate attention to incompatible theoretical underpinnings or assumptions that affect treatment approaches. Consequently, these individually designed treatment groups may work well for some women and *not* at all for others. Attention to consistencies of these group approaches, in terms of research and practice outcomes, should help to formally identify approaches that work *best* for specific groups of women and help to assure increasingly positive outcomes.

Psychoeducational Groups. Psychoeducational groups are often highly structured groups that use a formal manual or "course outline" (i.e., structured curriculum) to help group members learn about their drug and substance abuse. To achieve optimal therapeutic outcomes, psychoeducational group leaders and therapists require competent teaching and counseling skills. In addition, women who are members of psychoeducation groups, and their family members, are encouraged to assume responsibility for their own learning. Often incorporated in therapy is the "Stages of Change Model" (e.g., DiClemente, Schlundt, & Gemmell, 2004) that emphasizes *seven* stages of change (i.e., *pre-contemplation*; *contemplation*; *preparation*; *action*; *maintenance*; *termination*; and *relapse*)[54] and provides therapists with "providers tasks" to address during each stage to help patients move along the change process and to help to assure optimal learning and resultant therapeutic outcomes.[55]

Skills Development Groups. Skills development groups vary according to the behavioral and cognitive skills required by the members of the group to achieve and maintain member abstinence/recovery regarding drug and substance abuse. Deficits in, for example, life skills are assessed and members are then taught deficit skills, which they can practice or rehearse during group therapy sessions. In addition to group therapy knowledge, group leaders are required to have knowledge concerning various specific life-skills deficits, and the ability to teach these life-skills to individual group members.

Support Groups. Support groups attempt to build and promote positive supportive connections among members and draw attention to what they have in common. Leaders facilitate open communications that foster group development and improve the self-esteem and self-confidence of members. Open discussion involving peer feedback, with appropriate accountability, is encouraged.

As identified by the Center for Substance Abuse Treatment (2005), "There are many advantages to using group therapy in substance abuse treatment." For example, therapeutic groups can:

- Provide information to women who are *new* to recovery
- Allow a single treatment professional to help several women at the same time
- Provide positive peer support and pressure for achieving abstinence regarding personal drug and substance abuse
- Help members to learn to cope with problems related to their drug and substance abuse by allowing them to see how others cope with similar problems

---

[54] *Relapse* is often *not* considered to be a formal stage in the noted process/stages of change model. Instead it simply signifies the return to the problem behavior (e.g., alcohol, drug, or substance abuse) following the successful completion of the other six stages.

[55] This model also shares principles with motivational interviewing (e.g., patient's ambivalence to change; often *nonlinear* change process; and waxing and waning of readiness to change).

- Provide feedback concerning the values and abilities of group members
- Help members overcome past, harmful family experiences
- Encourage, coach, support, and reinforce members as they undertake difficult or anxiety-provoking tasks
- Offer members the opportunity to learn or relearn the social skills they need to cope with everyday life instead of resorting to the use of drugs and substances of abuse
- Effectively confront individual members about drug and substance abuse and other harmful behaviors
- Add needed structure and discipline to the lives of group members with drug and substance use disorders, who often enter treatment with their lives in chaos
- Instill hope, and a sense that, "If they can make it, so can I"
- Support and provide encouragement to one another outside the group setting

(pp. 4–5)

Regardless of the type of group therapy that is provided, a competent and effective group leader is central to maximizing the success achieved by the group members. The Center for Substance Abuse Treatment (2005, pp. 39–40) identified specific personal qualities of group counselors as leaders that have been associated with individual group member success and optimal therapeutic outcomes:

- *Constancy*, the group leader's ability to promote an environment with small, infrequent changes that are helpful to women in recovery
- *Active listening*, or the group leader's ability to use strong listening skills that are the keystone of any effective therapy
- *Firm identity*, or the group leader's ability to demonstrate a firm sense of her own identity, together with a clear reflection on experiences in group, that enables her to understand and manage her own emotional life
- *Confidence*, or the group leader's ability to model the consistency that comes from self-knowledge and clarity of intent while remaining attentive to each woman's experiences. The secure grounding enables the leader to model stability for the group
- *Spontaneity*, or the group leader being creative and flexible as a leader
- *Integrity*, the group leader being aware of ethical issues that arise
- *Trust*, or the ability of the group leader to be able to trust others, and vice versa
- *Humor*, the ability of the group leader to use humor appropriately
- *Empathy*, the ability of the group leader to project empathy, an essential skill for the counselor/leader

Additional details of *group therapy* will be discussed within the contexts of the following sections: *Family Therapy*; *Social Skills Training*; *Therapeutic Communities*; and *Residential Programs*.

Family Therapy[56]

The family often plays a significant role in the etiology and maintenance of drug and substance abuse among women—as has been identified throughout the various chapters of this text. As noted by Lander, Howsare, and Byrne (2013):

> Each family and each family member is uniquely affected by the individual using substances including but not limited to having unmet developmental needs, impaired attachment, economic hardship, legal problems, emotional distress, and sometimes violence being perpetrated against him or her. For children, there is also an increased risk of developing an SUD themselves.
> *(p. 194)*

Thus, various forms of family therapy, which are generally based on the basic principles of family systems therapy, have been developed and utilized to treat substance use disorders among women—women, who as family members, also have a role as aunts, daughters, grandmothers and great grandmothers, life partners, mothers, significant others, sisters, and wives. For example, *Ecologically-Based Family Therapy* (EBFT) is based on the social, ecological theoretical perspective initially developed by Bronfenbrenner (1979) and further extended in the therapeutic context of drug and substance abuse by Slesnick and her colleagues (e.g., Slesnick & Prestopnik, 2005; Slesnick & Zhang, 2016). A 12-session form of family therapy, EBFT focuses on helping families to identify and address specific dysfunctional interactions that contribute to the development and maintenance of harmful drug and substance abuse behaviors among family members. Specific therapeutic strategies and techniques include: (1) cognitive-behavioral skills training; (2) communication and problem-solving skills training; (3) obtaining necessary services (e.g., health and medical services; job training); (4) reframing techniques; and (5) role playing.

Some general guidelines for family therapists that can assist family and other therapists, regardless of their specific theoretical orientations, are presented in the following list that we modified from the earlier work of Frankel (1990, p. 47):

- Respect the hierarchical structure of the family, or, if needed, try to help the family re-establish a functional hierarchy
- Listen to what is being said—and not said, asking relevant questions for both
- Don't interrupt a family member while he or she is speaking to ask for clarification. Wait until they have finished
- Closely observe non-verbal behavior as a basis for understanding family relationships and for possible intervention (e.g., attending behaviors, or lack thereof; crossed arms and legs; seating placement close to or away from certain family members)
- Give equal attention to each family member
- Do not attempt to minimize problems to the family

[56] Also referred to as *Marital and Family Therapy* (MFT) or *Multisystemic Therapy* (MST).

- Be honest and open
- Empathize with the stated family issues
- Be non-judgmental so that the family feels free to discuss problems without fear of censure
- Establish open communication patterns early in therapy
- Be aware of your own biases (and countertransference tendencies)
- Be flexible enough to shift your approach—if you find that it is not working
- Do *not* give advice, only suggestions as they fit the therapeutic plan
- Do *not* allow yourself to be triangulated or manipulated; you are the therapist
- Evaluate each individual member of the family in terms of, for example, anxiety, depression, guilt, hostility, PTSD, and self-esteem
- When you sense that the family feels that it has failed, attempt to bring up past successful experiences as reinforcement
- Become a role model for the family
- Allow the family to see you as a person who can make mistakes and own up to these mistakes
- Allow the family to see you as a person with feelings
- Try to have a purpose and reason for all your actions or lack of action
- Do not copy another therapist's style. Be yourself. Act in a manner that is comfortable for you and fits your personality
- Your role is to provide options for the family to select and pursue.You can plant a seed for growth that will enable the therapeutic process to bring about a change

Family therapy[57] attempts to correct the dysfunctional behavior of family members, both individually and as a group (e.g., Kaufman, 1990; Szapocznik & Williams, 2000). Behavioral and strategic-structural family therapies are the most commonly used, excluding mixed therapies. These systemic approaches will be briefly discussed in the context of their application to the treatment of harmful patterns of women's drug and substance abuse.

Lewis, Piercy, and Sprenkle (1990, p. 88) described the *Purdue Brief Family Therapy Model*, a "mixed" family therapy model with *seven* major goals that we believe are still applicable to many types of family therapy:

1. To decrease a family's resistance to treatment
2. To redefine drug and substance use as a family problem

---

57 When the concept of circular or reciprocal causality is applied, this approach also is commonly referred to as a systemic (i.e., family systems oriented) approach or model (Lewis, Piercy, & Sprenkle, 1990). This approach or model should *not* be confused with "systemic family therapy," a particular model of family therapy that uses a cybernetic process. Systemic intervention or treatment differs from psychologic and pharmacologic approaches because of the inherent focus of these intervention strategies. Whereas the focus of the latter is on the woman, as an individual, the focus of the former is on the entire family, as a group, that includes member(s) (e.g., the woman) who display harmful patterns of using drugs and substances of abuse. In this regard, the woman member is often identified as the "thermostat" of family health and functioning. Thus, therapists attempt (optimally) to assess and treat *all* the members of the family, including nuclear and extended family members, or significant others, as a group.

3. To re-establish appropriate family member influence
4. To interrupt dysfunctional family sequences of behavior
5. To assess the interpersonal function of drug and substance abuse
6. To implement change strategies consistent with the family's interpersonal functioning
7. To provide assertive training skills for family members so that they will be better able to resist pressures to engage in drug and substance use

To facilitate communication among family members, various techniques are taught and used during family therapy sessions. For example, individual family members may be taught to use the expression "I feel" as opposed to "you feel." This communication technique helps to avoid casting blame based on "mind-reading" and allows other family members to clarify their own feelings. It also allows them to state for themselves what *they* feel as opposed to responding to what a family member *thinks* they feel. As such, the "I feel" communications tend to engender more empathetic responses than do "you feel" communications, which tend to elicit decidedly more defensive responses.

Several terms have been commonly used in the context of family therapy. These terms include "boundaries," "feedback," "homeostasis," and "validation." Each of these terms will be briefly defined and discussed.

Boundaries. Boundaries refer to the limits, both internal and external, of the family system. Boundaries generally serve a protective, although *not* necessarily therapeutic, function (e.g., maintaining a "family secret" involving drug and substance abuse). Boundaries also facilitate and regulate family function by helping to separate, for example, maternal/parental and child subsystems within the family.

Feedback. "Feedback" refers to the circular, or reciprocal, manner in which communication typically occurs within the family system. For example, a woman may recognize that she drinks and overuses her prescription for sedative-hypnotics because her significant other is having an affair with a younger woman. In turn, her lesbian partner may state that she turned to another woman because of her partner's alcoholism and related chronic state of depression. Thus, within the family system, the actions of one member of the family system may directly affect the actions of another member of the family. In this context, verbal and non-verbal feedback in large part, also accounts for, or contributes to, the process of maternal-child attachment.

Homeostasis. "Homeostasis" refers to the tendency of a system, including a family system, to seek and maintain equilibrium and stability. Although generally a necessary and healthy process in both biologic and sociologic systems, this process can become destructive or unhealthy—even when used with the "best of intentions." For example, when a child calls into work for her mother and reports that she is ill today and won't be able to come into work when, in fact, her mother is home drunk or hungover. These "enabling" behaviors commonly occur in "addicted families" almost always with the very best of intentions (e.g., to protect the family member and, consequently, the family), but also, almost always, are accompanied by the unintended consequence of furthering the harmful effects of drug and substance abuse for the individual family member (e.g., mother), as well as other family members. Thus, although equilibrium/homeostasis is maintained over the short term, for the family, it perpetrates drug and substance abuse behavior within the individual family member—to the eventual detriment of the affected member and the entire family.

Another commonly encountered example, is an older woman, who has abused alcohol throughout her entire adult life and is now living in a near-by extended care facility. During her daily visits with her adult daughter, she incessantly requests that her daughter bring her a bottle of her favorite apricot brandy, "a small bottle that can fit in my purse," which she keeps close-by with her in her wheel chair all day. Reluctantly, in order to keep her mother happy (and quiet), the daughter brings the alcohol as requested to her mother—against explicit extended care facility policies—replacing it, as needed.

Validation. "Validation" refers to the process by which the family therapist, while acting as a role model for family members, acknowledges and expresses an understanding of each family member's concerns, desires, and feelings. This approach encourages each family member to listen to, or *hear out*, the concerns, desires, and feelings of other family members before reacting to or judging them.

Couples Therapy

Couples therapy[58] can be considered to be a subset, or special case, of family therapy that involves a variety of approaches that always include the participation of an *intimate* significant other (e.g., partner; spouse) in an active treatment program.[59,60]

---

58 Couples therapy also is known as *Behavioral Couples Therapy* (BCT) and *Alcohol Behavioral Couples Therapy* (ABCT) (e.g., Fischer, Baucom, & Cohen, 2016; Hallgren, Crotwell, & Munoz, 2016; McCrady, Wilson, & Munoz, 2016).

59 A subset, or special case, of couples therapy is used when the "couple" comprises a woman with an AUD and/or SUD and resides with one or more dependent school-aged children (e.g., Kelley, Bravo, & Braitman, 2016a). In this context, "couples family therapy" also has been applied with homeless mothers with AUDs and/or SUDs (e.g., Slesnick & Erdem, 2013). This treatment approach can be used either in lieu of, or in conjunction with, drug courts (see earlier section, *Drug Courts*). The importance of these therapeutic interventions cannot be overstated because, in addition to the effects of drug and substance abuse on the "couple," as noted by Lander, Howsare, and Byrne (2013)—and noted in several of the earlier chapters in this text:

> A parent with a SUD is 3 times more likely to physically or sexually abuse her child.
>
> *(p. 194)*

This deplorable situation, in turn, can be a major contributing factor to the subsequent development of AUDs and SUDs among abused children when they subsequently become adults (see, for example, the related discussion in Chapter 7, *Identifying Women's Contemporaneous Diagnoses*).

60 We, and many other health and social care professionals, who provide therapeutic services to women—who both abuse drugs and substances of abuse and are currently in a personal relationship with a significant or intimate other (i.e., spouse; life partner)—have long noted that effective

Thus, the couples may be comprised of: (1) a non-drinker/non-alcoholic and a drinker/alcoholic; or (2) both drinkers/alcoholics. As explained by Ruff, McComb, and Coker (2010, p. 439):

> Behavioral couples therapy (BCT) is an evidence-based couple therapy intervention for married or cohabitating substance abusers and their partners.

Couples therapy is grounded in both social learning theory and the family systems model. As such, it assumes a reciprocal relationship between drug and substance abuse, particularly alcohol abuse, and couple/family functioning with a major focus on partner satisfaction in regard to the nature and quality of the relationship (Epstein & McCrady, 1998).

Couples therapy assumes that, because the two domains of interest are *interconnected* as opposed to being *independent*, improvement in a couple's relationship will: (1) *decrease* drug or substance abuse; which, in turn, (2) will *improve* the couple's relationship. In the Alcohol Behavioral Couples Therapy (ABCT) model, the alcohol-focused interventions center on the involvement of spouses or significant partners. For example, it involves teaching the spouse or partner specific skills to deal with problems and situations that are commonly encountered,[61] such as how to *decrease* behaviors that "trigger" drinking and how to maintain and reinforce abstinence (Noel & McCrady, 1993).

Consequently, the primary objectives of BCT, as identified by Fals-Stewart, O'Farrell, and Birchler (2004), are to:

1. Eliminate abusive drinking and drug abuse
2. Engage the family's support for the patient's efforts to change
3. Restructure couple and family interaction patterns in ways conducive to long-term stable abstinence

---

intervention is extremely difficult, if not virtually impossible, without the understanding, engagement, and support of the significant, or intimate, other. The major contributing factor regarding this observation is that, as noted by McCrady, Epstein, and Hallgren (2016):

> Intimate partners have an integral role in the development, maintenance, and resolution of AUDs in women.
>
> *(p. 287)*

In this context, Desrosiers, Thompson, and Divney (2016), in their study of romantic partner influences on drug and substance use/abuse by mothers during pregnancy and during the postnatal period, found that fathers, who used drugs and substances of abuse during the *prenatal* period, significantly influenced drug and substance use/abuse among mothers during the *postnatal* period.

In addition, as noted by Braitman and Kelley (2016):

> Couples in which men reported more depressive symptoms, less hostility, and less phobic anxiety were more likely to initiate treatment.
>
> *(p. 182)*

61 These "situations and problems" often include "poor communication and problem solving, habitual arguing, and financial stressors" (Fals-Stewart, O'Farrell, & Birchler, 2004, p. 31).

The overwhelming preponderance of empirical data available to date (e.g., Fischer, Baucom, & Cohen, 2016; Hallgren, Crotwell, & Munoz, 2016; McCrady, Wilson, & Munoz, 2016) demonstrates the efficacy of BCT and its general therapeutic superiority to individual therapy, or individually-based therapy (IBT) (e.g., O'Farrell, 2012 ; O'Farrell, Schumm, & Murphy, 2017).[62] Moreover, the addition of CBT to BCT, for individual women, has resulted in further optimism regarding therapeutic results, particularly for women who express a specific desire for individual counseling sessions (McCrady, Epstein, & Hallgren, 2016).

As emphasized by Fals-Stewart, O'Farrell, and Birchler (2004, pp. 31–32), to maximize the potential for therapeutic success, BCT requires:

- A competent therapist, generally minimally a bachelor's level counselor who is versed in BCT
- Use of standardized BCT manuals and behavioral assignments (e.g., "homework" for couples)
- Commitment of couples/partners to maintaining and improving their relationship
- Commitment of couples/partners to abstain from drug and substance use
- Completion of prescribed number of sessions (i.e., generally, 12 to 24 sessions over 5 to 6 months)
- Concurrent individual psychotherapy, as indicated

In their meta-analysis of 12 randomized controlled studies evaluating couples therapy, Powers, Vedel, and Emmelkamp (2008) found that, on average, couples therapy:

1. Produced better outcomes than individual-based treatment interventions for couples affected by alcoholism and drug abuse problems
2. Was *superior* to individual-based treatment specifically in regard to frequency of use, consequences of use, and relationship satisfaction at follow-up[63]
3. Was *ineffective* for couples with a *low* severity index of alcohol-related disorders[64]

In a comprehensive review of couple's therapy, O'Farrell (2012, p. 122) identified that, for couples:

[62] In addition, when comparing BCT combined with IBT versus IBT alone, O'Farrell, Schuum, and Murphy (2017) found that the combined approach "was more efficacious than IBT in improving relationship satisfaction and preventing relationship breakups" (p. 309).

[63] Further, regarding "relationship satisfaction," Kelley, Bravo, and Braitman (2016b) noted that this outcome: (1) was related to the number of BCT sessions attended; and (2) for mothers, contributed *to decreases* in their children's depressive symptoms post-intervention.

[64] In this regard, Fals-Stewart, O'Farrell, and Birchler (2004) suggested that BCT is "most-effective when only one partner has a problem with drugs or alcohol" (p. 32).

1. *Alcohol*-focused interventions directly *build* support for abstinence
2. *Relationship*-focused interventions *increase* positive feelings, shared activities, and constructive communication

In addition, Ruff, McComb, and Coker (2010), in their review of 23 related studies, found that BCT was efficacious regarding, "improving substance use behavior, dyadic adjustment, child psychosocial outcomes, and reducing partner violence" (p. 439).

Social Skills Training

Social skills training attempts to help women who have insufficient social skills to interact more effectively with their family members, friends, peers, and employers. Social skills training involves detailed, focused training sessions that deal with common problems related to a woman's poor social skills. Thus, training focuses on such skills as: (1) understanding non-verbal expression; (2) refusing unreasonable requests; (3) making difficult requests; (4) expressing and receiving positive emotions; (5) replying appropriately to criticism; and (6) initiating social conversations (Oei & Jackson, 1980).

Alternative Psychotherapeutic Delivery Modalities

A variety of digital technologies[65] have been developed and utilized to deliver counseling and psychotherapy to women with AUDs and/or SUDs and OMDs (Hilty, Luo, & Morache, 2002; Molfenter, Boyle, & Holloway, 2015; Muench, 2014; Nair, Newton, & Shakeshaft, 2015; White, Kavanagh, & Stallman, 2010). In general, these technologies allow the delivery of various types of psychotherapy to women, particularly those living in remote or rural areas—as well as those women who live in areas that do not have an adequate number of available, qualified mental health professionals. In so doing, these technologies greatly increase accessibility for these traditionally underserved women by significantly reducing or eliminating the barriers of time and distance—for both the women, who require professional care assistance, and for the clinician/therapist, who provides the therapeutic intervention (Molfenter, Boyle, & Holloway, 2015). Consequently, the appropriate use of digital technologies, in the context of alternative therapeutic

---

[65] N.B. We make these observations and comments regarding the digital technologies, both current and under future development, in the context of some degree of reflective historical nostalgia. This is due to having, ourselves, been integrally involved in the seminal development and application of computer assisted instruction (CAI) to teach clinical pharmacology to medical students and the use of business computers for the long-distance rural continuing drug education of pharmacists at a time before the development of personal computers or the Internet (e.g., Pagliaro, 1981; Pagliaro & Burkhalter, 1979; Pagliaro, Cook, & Bidwell, 1979; Pagliaro & Kline, 1978).

delivery modalities, can significantly enhance patient care and related clinical outcomes (Muench, 2014).

Several of these technologies have been used in relation to treating women's drug and substance abuse, including:

- Computer-Based Brief Interventions
- E-mail
- Teleconferencing
- Telephone Support (i.e., "Quitlines")
- Texting (Text Messaging)
- Videoconferencing

Each of these technologies is briefly discussed in the following sections.

Computer-Based Brief Interventions. Computer-based brief interventions, generally commercially available, have been demonstrated to be effective, particularly in the context of *alcohol misuse* (e.g., Nair, Newton, & Shakeshaft, 2015). In their systematic review of 17 studies involving online alcohol interventions, White, Kavanagh, and Stallman (2010) found that they were particularly useful for women and young adults. In their secondary analysis of data from the NIDA's multi-site effectiveness trial of a computer-assisted behavioral intervention, Campbell, Nunes, and Pavlicova (2015) found that "men and women derived similar benefits" (p. 9). However—largely due to a "high risk of bias" they identified in the representative studies, Civljak, Stead, and Hartmann-Boyce (2013) *failed* to demonstrate clear support for the effectiveness of these interventions in their review and statistical analysis of 28 studies, involving over 45,000 participants, which evaluated the effectiveness of internet-based intervention strategies for smoking cessation (also see sections, "E-mail" and "Videoconferencing").

E-mail. E-mail, as well as texting, is used to provide appointment reminders and brief notes of encouragement and support (e.g., motivational enhancement). These technologies are currently: ubiquitous; well accepted—by both therapists and patients; easy to use (i.e., familiar to virtually all); and inexpensive (Quanbeck, Chih, & Isham, 2016).

Teleconferencing (see *Videoconferencing*).

Telephone Support. Telephone support, commonly known as "quitlines," involves programs most frequently used to assist tobacco users to quit smoking. These programs have increased significantly across the U.S. over the new millennium and are now available in *all* 50 states (Fildes, Wilson, & Crawford, 2012; Keller, Feltracco, & Bailey, 2010). Quitlines, depending upon the approach or program that they have selected to implement and follow, generally have nurses, or other healthcare providers: (1) assist with the selection and use of NRT (see related discussion in the earlier section of this chapter, *Pharmacotherapy*); (2) refer patients after discussion, to various professional smoking cessation programs; (3) monitor progress and success with maintenance of smoking cessation; (4) answer patient/client questions; and (5) provide short-term smoking-related counseling sessions (Richter, Shireman, & Ellerbeck, 2015; Pagliaro & Pagliaro, *Clinical Patient Data Files*). Integration with medication support for smoking cessation/maintenance, as well as other digital technologies (e.g., e-mail) have been utilized (McAfee, 2007).

Telephone support is used with over 1% of adult tobacco smokers annually in the U.S., particularly in rural areas (Keller, Feltracco, & Bailey, 2010; McAfee, 2007). It has been demonstrated to be both potentially beneficial, depending upon the approach utilized and the context of use, and generally easier to use and more cost effective than other currently available digital technologies (Richter, Shireman, & Ellerbeck, 2015). (Also, see "E-mail," "Texting," and "Videoconferencing" sections.)

Texting or Text Messaging. Texting, or text messaging, to cellular/mobile telephones, has the potential to support discontinuation and subsequent abstinence from drug and substance abuse. As noted in reviews on the topic (e.g., Keoleian, Polcin, & Galloway, 2015; Kong, Ells, & Camenga, 2014), numerous studies have been conducted among adults in regard to reducing or ceasing the use of various drugs and substances of abuse, including: alcohol; cannabis; methamphetamine; and nicotine. Although associated results have been reported to be "encouraging" or "positive," definitive supportive data, including replicative studies, are currently insufficient to *confirm* the suggested benefits of this approach.

To advance the use and the potential success of texting, Muench, Weiss, and Kuerbis (2013) worked on developing a theory-driven text messaging intervention for addiction care. Working with 50 adults enrolled in intensive outpatient substance abuse treatment, they found that: (1) virtually 100% of the participants (i.e., 98%) expressed interest in utilizing texting as a continuing care strategy; and (2) most preferred "benefit driven" over "consequence driven" text messages. These findings should help the future development and further success in this area of patient care delivery.

In addition, this finding is consistent with and supported by other research aimed at evaluating text messaging as a behavioral intervention—although not specifically in relation to AUDs or SUDs. For example, Muench, van Stolk-Cooke, and Morgenstern (2014) examined participant preferences for messages in the broad context of use as an intervention for medical and behavioral problems. They discovered that participants were sensitive to variations in the linguistic content of text messages. Thus, for example, changing, "Try to…" to "You might want to try to…" can positively affect message choice.

Videoconferencing. Videoconferencing, as well as teleconferencing, is among the *earliest* of the distant technologies used for substance abuse prevention and treatment—actually, originally predating the "digital age" and initially utilized in the late 1970s (Pagliaro & Pagliaro, *Clinical Patient Data Files*), but now included among the digital technologies and commonly denoted as part of telemedicine or telepsychiatry (e.g., Hilty, Luo, & Morache, 2002).

Videoconferencing was originally provided with the use of dedicated equipment in centralized or dedicated delivery locations. Increasingly, video interfaces are: (1) found and used on individual personal computers (PCs), laptops, or tablets; and (2) utilize specialized software "apps," and webcams (e.g., Mussulman, Ellerbeck, & Cupertino, 2014). This technology appears to work best in academic healthcare environments (and/or business environments) in which the presenters are *more* adept at using this "educational" technology and in which funding is less of an issue or concern.

Several significant issues are commonly encountered in regard to the development and implementation of the alternative delivery modalities. These include: (1) lack of experience with optimal use of the technologies; (2) limited funding for start-up costs, delivery expenses, and reimbursement of healthcare professionals for their healthcare services; and (3) professional regulatory and jurisdictional issues when, for example, the clinical therapist is in one state and the patient/client is in another state (in which the clinician/therapist is *not* licensed or insured).

Residential Programs

Residential programs include therapeutic communities and short-term residential programs. Each of these treatment approaches for women is discussed in the following sections.[66]

Therapeutic Communities. Therapeutic communities (TCs) assume that harmful patterns of drug and substance use are primarily symptomatic of psychosocial maladaptation to society, often as a result of incompetence in dealing with stress or social privation and alienation. Originally reflecting the growing egalitarian, anti-establishment movements of the 1960s, TCs were developed to operate more democratically and less rigidly than were the more traditional and authoritarian mental health and psychiatric residential facilities, which predominated at that time. Residents are generally viewed as active and equal co-participants with staff in dealing with their own, and each other's, issues in regard to the use of the drugs and substances of abuse (i.e., providing self-help and mutual self-help, respectively) (Hanson, 2002).

Treatment programs within the context of therapeutic communities is based on theories of social control. Consequently, TCs typically are designed and function as hierarchical systems with strict rules and prohibitions. Established rules and

[66] This discussion includes relevant, and interesting, data from several older, classic studies/reports, because of the relative dearth of more recent data (i.e., studies conducted and published during the new millennium).

associated consequences (i.e., of following or breaking these rules), including punishments and rewards, are explicitly defined and enforced. As noted by O'Brien and Biase (1984), the three major goals of TC programs are to:

1. Eliminate drug-taking behavior
2. Promote learning to respond to distress (personal and environmental) in a healthier manner
3. Foster readjustment and return to the outside community as a functioning, independent person (p. 16)

These goals are achieved by providing residential care for women who have *abusive* or *compulsive* patterns of drug and substance use. The residential care is usually provided for 3 to 12 months and gives women the opportunity, often mandated in the context of the criminal justice system (also see related earlier discussion in the section *Drug Courts*), to live with others who have similar problems in a highly-structured home-like environment.[67] As such, the TC provides a setting where everyone shares in the work and responsibility to ensure that community problems are minimized. Ideally, during their residential treatment, women increasingly assume skills and responsibilities that, upon completion of the program, they can transfer to the *larger* community.

Therapeutic communities also require regular meetings *throughout* the day in *informal* settings (e.g., sitting around the kitchen table). These meetings serve to facilitate the operation of the TC (e.g., division of work; provision of feedback on the quality of residents' work performance) and provide a format for decision-making processes. A significant amount of therapy also occurs *informally* throughout the day during which residents learn to take responsibility for and perform their tasks while interacting with the other residents. Recreational and leisure activities also provide a means for socializing and learning to interact more positively with others. As noted by Finfgeld-Connett (2011):

> Within therapeutic communities, women are frequently expected to monitor each other's behavior and to notify staff members when peers do *not* follow the rules. Deviant behavior is commonly addressed in encounter-groups, where "rule breakers" are publicly censured.[68]
>
> *(p. 462)*

---

[67] For example, in their Cochrane review of therapeutic interventions for women offenders, who used drugs and substances of abuse, Perry, Neilson, and Martyn-St. James (2014) found that TCs demonstrate a statistically significant reduction in re-incarceration of women participants.

[68] Although generally effective, even for women, when appropriately designed and implemented, the approaches commonly utilized in TCs (e.g., confrontation; encounter groups; feeling groups; milieu therapy; self-disclosure seminars) are considered by many women to be "un-feminine" or *not* particularly "women-centered."

Most TCs practice a form of egalitarianism. For example, regarding deciding how to handle a resident who is having difficulty *getting on the program* or in dealing with settling a program policy dispute, all residents have an equal opportunity to share input and have an equal vote with the staff members.[69] All TCs require total abstinence from the use of alcohol, cocaine, heroin, LSD, and marijuana, but may still allow caffeine (i.e., coffee) and nicotine (i.e., tobacco) use.

Although TC programs have been widely used across the U.S. for the last 50 years, research studies demonstrating their superior efficacy over other treatment approaches are lacking. As noted by Smith, Gates, and Foxcroft (2006), in their review of randomized controlled studies of the use of TC programs for the Cochrane Database, "There is little evidence that TCs offer significant benefits in comparison with other residential treatment, or that one type of TC is better than another." However, research has demonstrated that some modifications of traditional TCs (e.g., outpatient TCs; short-term residential TCs) can have deleterious results, including significant *reductions* in efficacy outcomes (Dye, Ducharme, & Johnson, 2009).

Residential programs, including TCs, generally have *low* program completion rates because of their failure to adequately address several *specific issues* for women, particularly, mothering.[70] In this regard, Knight, Logan, and Simpson (2001) studied 87 women who were either pregnant and/or entering a residential treatment program with their children. The related issues of parenting and childcare were directly addressed in the program. Upon completion of the study, they found that the three *most* significant predictors of treatment completion by participants were:

1. Educational level[71]
2. History of recent arrest
3. Peer deviance

Short-Term Residential Programs. In comparison to TCs, *short-term* residential treatment programs (e.g., Hazelden) began to develop during the early 1970s

[69] The primary clinical and custodial staff members who are employed by TCs are generally paraprofessionals who have successfully rehabilitated themselves from previous abusive or compulsive use of various drugs and substances of abuse with the assistance of a TC program. Ancillary staff members include professionals from various disciplines (e.g., law; medicine; psychology; social work), who are generally used on a contractual basis (De Leon, 1985). Although this staffing pattern is beginning to change with the use of more certified addiction counselors and social workers, the utilization of clinical psychologists and other university educated social and healthcare professionals generally remains low in these programs (Dye, Ducharme, & Johnson, 2009).

[70] These observations are particularly relevant considering the observation that length of stay within treatment (i.e., generally more than 7 weeks) is *positively* correlated with successful residential treatment intervention (e.g., Gossop, Stewart, & Browne, 2002; Hser, Evans, & Huang, 2004).

[71] Interestingly, Griese and Mack (2016), in their study of maternal-child health post-substance abuse residential treatment, for which participants were primarily mother-child dyads of American Indian descent (i.e., 60%), found that positive results post-treatment, were significantly associated with maternal educational level (i.e., high school degree or *higher* versus *less* than a high school degree).

(Laundergan & Williams, 1993) in response to several identified needs. These needs included: (1) a growing need for services, particularly for women who had problems related to cocaine use; (2) a desire among patients for treatment services other than those where they may be "institutionalized" for months; and (3) limitations placed by third-party insurance carriers for the reimbursement of fees paid for provided treatment services (i.e., often with a 30-day limit).

Following, is a listing of the program objectives and key elements that comprise a "typical" short-term residential treatment program—as modified from Laundergan & Williams (1993, p. 148):

- Key Program Elements
  - Personal inventory and plan
  - Daily schedule of program activities
  - Educational component
  - Group therapy sessions
  - Provision of safe and supportive environment
- Program Objectives
  - Learn about drug and substance abuse and the process of recovery
  - Maintain "sobriety" or "stay clean"
  - Recognize the effects of drug and substance abuse on self and others (e.g., family; friends; co-workers)
  - Develop strategies to maintain "sobriety" or "stay clean"
  - Share thoughts with others in group therapy sessions
  - Utilize the basics of AA or other 12-step programs

Various specific factors have been related to effective or successful outcomes for women who have completed short-term residential treatment programs. For example, Chou, Beeler-Stinn, and Diamond (2014), in their study of women in a residential treatment facility, who were heroin dependent and had co-occurring posttraumatic stress disorder (PTSD), found that treatment engagement and positive outcomes were related to a history of previous treatment and to having their children in care with them. However, as noted earlier, *short-term residential treatment programs*, when compared to *therapeutic communities*, generally have poorer therapeutic outcomes in terms of the attainment and duration of abstinence (Dye, Ducharme, & Johnson, 2009).

Continental- and Other Descent-Specific Treatment Programs

Popular Notion: That the implementation of continental descent- or ethnic-specific treatment approaches for women's drug and substance abuse in the U.S. is limited by systemic racism.

NOT TRUE. Quite simply, despite related voiced concerns involving cultural imperialism and hegemony,[72] these programs have *not* been implemented because they, in fact, do *not* exist (i.e., they, generally, have *not* been formally developed, objectively tested, nor otherwise demonstrated to be clinically efficacious in terms of superiority to placebo interventions or standard therapeutic approaches).

Women's drug and substance abuse treatment programs that reflect specific continental descent, or other descent (e.g., American Indian, Alaska Native, or Hawaiian Native descent), and ethnicity, or sociocultural beliefs and practices, ideally should begin with an understanding of the demographics and significant, self-identified *specific needs* of women in these U.S. population groups. For example, risk for, and incidence of, the fetal alcohol spectrum disorder (FASD) is significantly *higher* among women of American Indian and Alaska Native descent than among other groups of women in the U.S. (e.g., Hanson, Winberg, & Elliott, 2012; Montag, Clapp, & Calac, 2012). This sad statistic has been associated with the general cultural acceptance of alcohol use among women from these demographic groups. Conversely, FASD is *less* commonly reported among young women of Hispanic descent in the U.S., who are culturally restrained regarding alcohol use, as are traditional young Muslim women of *South Asian* and other descent. In another example, Native Hawaiian women have significantly *higher* rates of daily tobacco use and related nicotine dependence than do women of East Asian descent who reside in Hawaii (Herzog & Pokhrel, 2012). Further, as an example among women in the U.S. of African continental descent, AIDS is one of the leading causes of death and is largely associated with drug and substance abuse, particularly intravenous drug use (CDC, 2008).

At the beginning of the new millennium, several researchers (e.g., Roberts, Jackson, & Carlton-LaNey, 2000) advocated for, and suggested the use of various specific approaches for the treatment of drug and substance abuse among women of various specific continental descents in the U.S. In this regard, Morelli and Fong (2000) noted that the utilization of "Kupunas" can play a vital part in facilitating Native Hawaiian women's participation in drug and substance abuse treatment programs. As they explained, this approach is valuable and "especially important to Native Hawaiians who have experienced the cumulative effects of cultural imperialism" (p. 33).

Further, as part of a demonstration grant funded by the Center for Substance Abuse Prevention (CSAP) for Hawaiian women, who abused drugs and substances

[72] For example, the related arguments and opinions expressed by Creswell (2016), Peralta and Jauk (2011), and Stevens-Watkins, Knighton, and Allen (2016).

of abuse and were pregnant or post-partum, Morelli, Fong, and Oliveira (2001) developed the *Na Wahine Makalapua* (NWM), or "Women to Blossom Forth," treatment program. As they noted:

> The heart of the substance abuse treatment was Hawaiian deep cultural therapy, which incorporated Hawaiian values and traditional healing practices. NWM Hawaiian deep cultural therapy consisted of *ho'oponopono* (conflict resolution), deep culture (storytelling), *Lo'i* (taro patch), and *Lomilomi* (massage therapy).
>
> *(p. 268)*

However, even when researchers find significant results, the results are *not* often universal, even for the specific group of women studied. For example, Morelli, Fong, and Oliveira (2001), in their study of "culturally competent substance abuse treatment for Asian/Pacific Islander women," found that:

> [20%] of Hawaiian women did not find deep cultural therapy of benefit to them because it did not seem relevant to their [treatment] process.
>
> *(p. 277)*

More recently, regarding providing drug and substance abuse treatment services for Native Hawaiian women with SUDs, Ta and Chen (2008) recommended the formal involvement of "*Kupunas*, or Elders, in the design and implementation of culturally appropriate programs in order to better serve the [specific] needs of Native Hawaiian women" (p. 411). In another example specifically related to Native Hawaiian women, Herzog and Pokhrel (2012) suggested that treatment interventions for Hawaiian women, who smoke tobacco, should include a "motivational enhancement component" because "Native Hawaiian smokers reported significantly *lower* motivation to quit smoking than Caucasians" (p. 1226).

In addition to research on drug and substance abuse treatment approaches for Native Hawaiian women, most of the other published research articles during the new millennium have focused on women of African continental descent. Included in these articles are several *qualitative* studies concerning "black women's experiences in drug abuse" (e.g., Jones, Hopson, & Warner, 2015). These studies: (1) inform our understanding of the unique experiences of women of African continental descent in the U.S. who use the drugs and substances of abuse; and (2) provide rich descriptive narratives concerning their attitudes, experiences, and opinions in regard to women's drug and substance abuse treatment programs.

Stevens-Watkins, Knighton, and Allen (2016), noted that: "the rates of illicit drug use among African American women are increasing, yet African American women are least likely to participate in treatment for substance use disorders when compared to women of other racial groups" (p. 54). In response to this observation, they conducted a secondary analysis of extant data involving 206 "drug-using" African American women. Contrary to expectations, they found that:

> Women on probation, had children, and had a family history of substance abuse were significantly more likely to report participating in substance abuse treatment. Perceived family support and active coping were significant *negative* correlates of participating in treatment.
>
> *(p. 54)*

Stevens-Watkins, Knighton, and Allen (2016) posited that the *John Henryism Active Coping Theory*,[73] the "cultural correlate," or belief, that "hard work and self-determination are required to cope with and overcome adversities," contributed to an understanding of their observations, but was insufficient, in and of itself, to fully explain them (p. 54).

Thus, while the various available studies tend to provide evidence to support the need for new, continental descent- and ethnic-specific treatment programs for particular groups of women, they are rarely developed into formal theories that explain why these women use or do not use the drugs and substances of abuse nor do they identify explicit structures or guidelines for the development and implementation of related new treatment approaches and programs.[74]

Similarly, a few other studies have addressed the need for specific drug and substance abuse treatment approaches for women of Hispanic or Latin American descent. For example, De La Rosa and White (2001), in their review of studies examining the "drug using behavior of Hispanics," found that familial factors, peer influences, and involvement with religious institutions appeared to play a significant role. Thus, they recommended that:

> Drug prevention and treatment programs within Hispanic communities will be more successful if they incorporate social support systems into their programs.
>
> *(p. 233)*

However, in fact, very *little* related *high*-quality empirical or qualitative data exist regarding the factors of continental descent and ethnicity in regard to drug and substance abuse treatment outcomes for new millennial women in the U.S.

---

73 This theory is a variant of "rugged individualism," or self-sufficiency, and derives its name from the folk song about John Henry—a "steel drivin' man."

74 Regarding the variance in results specifically related to the associated continental descent of women with respect to tertiary prevention of women's harmful patterns of drug and substance abuse, objective, meaningful data are sparse. One theme that has been purported by several researchers (e.g., Roberts, Jackson, & Carlton-LaNey, 2000) is the *lack* of appropriate application of "black feminist theory and black family theoretical perspectives" (p. 901) to therapeutic drug and substance abuse programs for women of African continental descent.

For example, a paucity of research exists regarding "replicative" or "confirmatory" studies regarding the few examples of continental descent- and ethnic-specific treatment approaches just presented. Thus, in the absence of specific treatment programs, *all* women should receive caring, competent, and ethical professional treatment, as requested and agreed upon by the women seeking treatment, with whatever individual adjustments are required to optimize treatment outcomes.

Lesbian-Specific Treatment Programs

As noted by several new millennial researchers (e.g., Drabble & Trocki, 2005; Green & Feinstein, 2012; Koh & Ross, 2006; Pagliaro & Pagliaro, 2000), and identified in the previous chapters of this text, lesbians, as well as bisexual and transgender (LBT) women, when compared to heterosexual women, are significantly *more* likely to display harmful patterns of drug and substance abuse. In addition, Stevens (2012), in her review of the related published literature, found that, in comparison to other women, "less is known about effective models of care [in regard to drug and substance abuse] for LBT women" (p. 32). She also noted that "there are no theoretically guided or evidence-based substance abuse treatment programs based on queer or transgender theory" (p. 27). Consequently, quantitative research studies and findings concerning efficacious treatment approaches aimed at better meeting the needs of LBT women is urgently needed. Unfortunately, such research is *not* available. As noted by Green and Feinstein (2012):

> Research on the efficacy and effectiveness of treatment programs for SUD in LGB populations is limited.
>
> *(p. 265)*

Until these data become available, attention should be given to various factors that have been identified as being particularly relevant to initiating and maintaining harmful patterns of drug and substance abuse among lesbian women.[75] These factors have included, for example, the following:[76]

---

[75] These factors have generally also been ascribed to bisexual women in the related published research literature. However, it is our clinical observation that there is a significant difference between the needs and behaviors of lesbian and bisexual women in very many regards including drug and substance abuse. Further, we have identified that lesbian and bisexual women have been generally grouped together in the published literature for what we believe as convenience, as well as to *normalize* the combined group when these data are published in journals that are specifically identified by title as, "lesbian focused." This observation is most often embodied using the labels, "LBT" or "LGBT," when referring *specifically* to lesbian women.

[76] N.B. It is extremely important to note that: (1) this list is not exhaustive; and (2) many more factors (e.g., anxiety; depression; homelessness; IPV; PTSD) are commonly associated with drug

- Rejection by family and friends
- Feelings of worthlessness
- Self-hatred
- Target of sexual jokes and slurs
- Social isolation
- Stigmatization

Consequently, rates of AUDs and SUDs are significantly *higher* among lesbians in comparison to heterosexual women (see related discussion in the previous chapter of this text—the index also can be used to readily identify the location of this information). For example, even as noted in relation to the life of one of the most famous lesbian soccer stars in the U.S., Abby Wambach:

> She tells of her bouts with vodka and pills, which included Vicodin [prescription combination hydrocodone and acetaminophen product], Ambien [prescription sedative-hypnotic, zolpidem], and Adderall [prescription mixed amphetamines].
>
> *(Associated Press, 2016, p. 2)*

Transgender-Specific Treatment Programs

> <u>Popular Notion</u>: As women, cisgender and transgender women share essentially the same risk and treatment variables regarding drug and substance abuse.
>
> NOT TRUE. See discussion in following sections.

As reported by Flentje, Heck, and Sorensen (2014), in their study of transgender women entering substance abuse treatment:

> This study identified multiple differences between transgender and cisgender persons in basic demographics, psychosocial characteristics, health risk behaviors, health and mental healthcare utilization, and substance use behaviors.
>
> *(p. 969)*

For example, trans women (i.e., male to female, or *MTF*) have been noted by several researchers (e.g., Benotsch, Zimmerman, & Cathers, 2013; Flentje, Heck,

---

and substance abuse among *all* women—including lesbians (see Chapter 7, *Identifying Women's Contemporaneous Diagnoses*, for additional related discussion).

& Sorensen, 2014; Klein & Golub, 2016; Lyons, Shannon, & Pierre, 2015; Pagliaro & Pagliaro, *Clinical Patient Data Files*; Reback & Fletcher, 2014; Santos, Rapues, & Wilson, 2014; White Hughto, Reisner, & Pachankis, 2015) to:

- Be *more* likely than trans men (i.e., female to male, or *FTM*) to identify methamphetamine as their "drug of first choice" (reportedly, generally more than 20%)
- Report *greater* intravenous (IV) drug use
- Have *higher* HIV-positive rates than the general population
- Be *less* likely to have minor dependent children than *cis* women
- Have *higher* rates of contemporaneous diagnoses than other women and men
- Be *more* likely than others to "self" refer for drug and substance abuse treatment
- Have *higher* rates of alcoholism than the general population (reportedly, up to 60%)
- When compared to lesbians or homosexuals, experience *more* stigma and rejection in treatment settings (mostly from others enrolled in treatment)
- Be *more* likely than members of other sexual minority populations to work in the sex trade (reportedly, 75%)—which is both facilitated by methamphetamine use and significantly *increases* the risk for HIV infection
- Have *higher* rates of suicide attempts than cis women or men, which often involves the use of drugs and substances of abuse (e.g., alcohol and other sedative hypnotics or heroin)
- Suffer *more* family rejection than cis women, which significantly contributes to drug and substance abuse

While *no* empirically validated drug and substance abuse treatment approaches currently exist for trans women that are based on the *characteristics* of trans women—as presented in the bullet list, and our related clinical experience—we would generally recommend, as is recommended for *all* women in treatment, as appropriate, for health and social care professionals to:

1. Provide optimal treatment settings for trans women
2. Adapt programs to specific voiced needs of trans women
3. Involve the trans community in program treatment planning revisions
4. Encourage and support ethical academic and governmental trans research at treatment sites

In addition, as a primary prevention strategy (see related discussion earlier in this chapter), Wilson, Chen, and Arayasirikul (2014) suggest that the:

> Utilization of transition-related medical care (i.e., breast augmentation; genital surgery; utilization of hormones) may reduce risk for mental health

problems, especially suicidal ideations, and substance use (particularly binge drinking and non-injection drug use) among transwomen.

(p. 182)

12-Step Programs

The 12-step programs that are commonly used by women in the U.S. are: (1) *Alcoholics Anonymous* (AA); and (2) *Women's 12-step programs*. Each of these programs is described in the following sections. We begin with the *12 Steps of Alcoholics Anonymous* from the *Alcoholics Anonymous* (2001)—"Big Book":

1. We admitted that we were powerless over alcohol, that our lives had become unmanageable.
2. We came to believe that a Power greater than ourselves could restore us to sanity.
3. We decided to turn our will and our lives over to the care of God as we understood Him.
4. We made a searching and fearless moral inventory of ourselves.
5. We admitted to God, to ourselves, and to another human being the exact nature of our wrongs.
6. We were entirely ready to have God remove all these defects of character.
7. We humbly asked him to remove our shortcomings.
8. We made a list of all persons we had harmed, and became willing to make amends to them all.
9. We made direct amends to such people wherever possible, except when to do so would injure them or others.
10. We continue to take personal inventory and when we were wrong promptly admitted it.
11. We sought through prayer and meditation to improve our conscious contact with God as we understood Him, praying only for knowledge of His will for us and the power to carry that out.
12. Having had a spiritual awakening because of these steps, we tried to carry this message to alcoholics and to practice these principles in all our affairs.

Alcoholics Anonymous. Alcoholics Anonymous was started in 1935 in Akron, Ohio by Bill W. (a stockbroker) and Bob S. (a physician), who were its first two members. Alcoholics Anonymous has since spread across North America and now holds meetings worldwide. AA has become, particularly in North America, the most frequently used form of alcohol treatment with over one million recovering members (Laudet, 2008). According to several researchers and therapists (e.g., Room & Greenfield, 1993; Weisner, Greenfield, & Room, 1995), the popularity of AA is due in large part to its *American* themes of individualism, equality, and spirituality, which are embodied in the 12 Steps.[77] As noted by Kurtz (1988, 1993), the organizational structure of AA also supports these themes in that: there is *no* central authority or hierarchy; the only officer in AA groups is a secretary; and members avoid the use of last names.

Alcoholics Anonymous is regarded as *neither* a medical nor a psychological approach for the treatment of alcoholism (Borkman, 2008). As such, the organization maintains that *alcoholism is a disease without cure* and that treatment is social[78] or *spiritual* (McGee, 2000). As noted by Vaillant (2005):

> The suggested mechanism of action of AA is that it employs four factors widely shown to be effective in relapse prevention in addictions: 1) external supervision; 2) substitute dependency; 3) new caring relationships; and 4) increased spirituality.
>
> *(p. 431)*

In this context, women in AA are encouraged to "take one day at a time" and to gain encouragement, guidance, and strength by reciting the "Serenity Prayer":

> God grant me the serenity
> To accept the things I cannot change,
> Courage to change the things I can,
> And wisdom to know the difference.
>
> *(Reinhold Niebuhr, 1892–1971)*

Alcoholics Anonymous relies on a rather informal form of "group" therapy and social support (i.e., frequent meetings with other *fellow* recovering members who maintain total abstinence from alcohol use) and a "buddy" system (i.e., the use of *sponsors* who have remained sober for a period by *working* the 12 steps and who can, thus, show "newcomers" the way to sobriety). As part of the "group therapy," members hear from other members that they are not alone and that they share common,

---

77 These same themes that account for much of the success attributed to AA, also make it an inappropriate treatment approach for some women. The spiritual characteristics of AA are reflected by the wording in the *12 Steps*, and in both the generally accepted moto, *Let Go and Let God*, and the *Serenity Prayer* (see text on following pages), which is often used to conclude group meetings.

Our clinical experience indicates that regardless of gender, ethnicity, or sexual orientation, most women who have alcoholism and other problems related to using the drugs and substances of abuse, can generally derive significant benefit from AA. However, we also have found, over the last two decades, that an increasing number of women, who identify themselves as *agnostic*, generally reject AA as a component of their therapy because they generally find the tenets of AA to be *philosophically incompatible* with their own personal views of the world (i.e., lack of strong belief in God; this observation appears to be particularly relevant for younger women) (Pagliaro & Pagliaro, *Clinical Patient Data Files*).

78 Because of this, AA has often been labeled as a *social* form of treatment.

painful experiences in relation to their alcohol use. In addition, in conjunction with Step 1, members learn to overcome their strong denial of their own drinking problem. The confrontation of denial is both clearly and directly reflected in the members' introductions of themselves at AA group meetings, "Hello, my name is ____ and I'm an alcoholic."

Members are encouraged to work through and practice the "12 steps" daily and, because the AA model purports that there is no cure for alcoholism,[79] maintain life-long abstinence by continued membership in the "fellowship" (i.e., AA) and by regular attendance at meetings. For many alcoholics, AA provides both the social support necessary to maintain abstinence and an effective surrogate for their previously patterned "drinking time" or "familiar bar scene" (i.e., AA meetings serve as a place to go on evenings, weekends, and holidays for socialization with "friends" who, in addition to other benefits, provide understanding and help to alleviate social isolation and loneliness).[80]

The overall effectiveness of AA is difficult to ascertain because:

- AA maintains *no* formal records
- Very *few* scientific studies have been conducted to formally measure its success
- Available data are primarily observational and suffer from an inherent self-selection bias
- Lack of sufficient theory to explain the inherent mechanisms of AA; research is not an AA mandate
- The amount of time that members remain active in AA is extremely variable
- Drop-out rates are high

(Fingarette, 1988; Kelly & Hoeppner, 2013; Miller & McCrady, 1993)

Obviously, the approach used by AA will *not* be suitable for all women and we would *not* recommend it as the sole approach to therapy. However, for women

---

[79] This AA belief would be consonant with what we describe as *compulsive use* (see Figure 8.1). (Also, see Chapters 1 through 6, for additional details.) In this regard, we would concur with the AA philosophy that, once the compulsive level of use has been achieved, treatment, to have optimal opportunity for success, must include a lifetime of *total abstinence*.

[80] The number of AA meetings that a current member regularly attends generally ranges from one daily to one weekly. The number of meetings attended on a regular basis is dictated, in large part, by factors such as: the amount of time that a member has been sober (e.g., 1 day versus 1 year); the personality of the member (e.g., avoidant, dependent, or compulsive); and accessibility (e.g., is the scheduled meeting nearby; does the member require and have available transportation; is the style of the meeting compatible with the member's needs?). However, in some cases an individual member will develop a "cult-like" relationship with AA (i.e., will become obsessive and compulsive regarding AA doctrine; will limit social interaction to AA meetings and members; will increasingly become estranged from other social groups—including family and colleagues) (Pagliaro & Pagliaro, 1992b; Pagliaro, 2002; Pagliaro & Pagliaro, *Clinical Patient Data Files*). These situations, although relatively infrequently encountered, should be appropriately monitored for and dealt with as part of the patient's program of psychotherapy or counseling.

who are willing to attend the AA meetings,[81] we have found it to be an effective and useful *adjunct* to individual psychotherapy, as have others (e.g., Banerjee, Howard, & Mansheim, 2007; Ferri, Amato, & Davoli, 2006), and we can *highly* recommend its use in this context.

The major determinant for success with AA (i.e., as indirectly measured by the total absence of drinking alcohol) has consistently been related to consistency and length of attendance at AA meetings (Humphreys, Blodgett, & Wagner, 2014). Kaskutas, Ye, and Greenfield (2008) noted that "fully one-half of those completing AA's most recent membership survey reported that they had been abstinent for more than 5 years" (p. 261). However, the related observation by Witbrodt and Delucchi (2011) that "relative to men, women with higher drug severity were less likely to participate in AA" (p. 2331) supports our earlier recommendation to use AA for women with AUDs *only* as an adjunct to psychotherapy and/or appropriately selected pharmacotherapy.

In addition, the efficacy of AA programs appears to be substantiated *de facto* by the large number of members who speak positively about it and the use of the AA approach by similar groups (e.g., Cocaine Anonymous [CA], Crystal Meth Anonymous [CMA], Gamblers Anonymous [GA], and Narcotics Anonymous (NA]). It also has been extended to other 12-step self-help groups[82] for families with parents or other family members, who have harmful patterns of drug and substance abuse (e.g., Al-ATEEN; Al-ANON; Families of Alcoholics [FA]) (Laudet, 2008). In addition, AA has consistently been rated highly by health and social care professionals (e.g., Tusa & Burgholzer, 2013).

Women's "12-Step" Programs. During the 1970s, women's concerns with basic concepts integral to AA programs and philosophy, particularly the notions of "powerlessness" (Matheson & McCollum, 2008) and "surrender to God (He)," led to the development of "feminist" interpretations of AA. These reactionary programs have largely disappeared, but some related concerns remain. Donovan, Ingalsbe, and Benbow (2013, p. 332) identified several factors that are likely to present *barriers* to a woman's involvement in traditional 12-step programs:

- A need to surrender
- A sense of powerlessness
- Fluctuations in readiness and commitment to change
- High degree of spirituality or perceived religiosity, especially for individuals who are atheist or agnostic

---

[81] In their review of 12-step programs, based upon a 2007 survey of over 9,000 AA members, Donovan, Ingalsbe, and Benbow (2013) reported that 33% of participants were women.

[82] Also referred to as *Twelve Step Facilitation* (TSF) programs. Over the course of several individual and/or group sessions, participants learn about the 12-step concepts and process. The goal of the TSF programs, by means of education and engagement, is to *increase* the likelihood of personal engagement in formal 12-step programs, such as AA.

- Lack of comfort or perceived support in the group, due to membership, or lack of membership, of a special population (e.g., ethnic minorities; members with contemporaneous diagnoses; men; sexual orientation; youth)
- Lack of compatibility between personal and treatment belief systems and philosophies
- Social anxiety or social phobia

However, as also noted by Donovan, Ingalsbe, and Benbow (2013, p. 318) in response to these concerns:

> A number of 12-step programs, including AA and NA, have women's only groups that may be seen by many women as more welcoming and supportive and, thus, are more likely to be attended than mixed gender groups.

In addition, over the past 20 years, several feminist researchers and therapists have addressed "women's issues with AA" in a variety of compelling manners that actively confront and largely alleviate virtually *all* of the concerns that were originally expressed. For example, Stephanie Covington[83] (1994), in her early work on this topic, *A Woman's Way Through the Twelve Steps*, shared that:

> I have found that a number of issues unique to women are overlooked in most Twelve Step programs. Some of these issues include the effects on women of the language of the Twelve Steps, the psychological development of women as it relates to addiction and recovery, and the social and cultural factors that affect us as women—both in general as females in a male-dominated society and specifically as women living through addiction and recovery.
>
> *(p. 1)*
>
> Rather than rewrite the Steps in a way that attempt to fit all women, we can instead work with the original Steps—paying close attention to the spirit and meaning—and reinterpret the language to support our own recovery. As Ruth, a recovering alcoholic and bulimic says, "The program defies the language."
>
> *(p. 5)*

Abstinence-Based Self/Mutual Help Groups. A related group of therapeutic programs/interventions that use some of the features of 12-step programs, but without the incorporation of a religious component (i.e., "surrender to God"), include: *LifeRing*; *SMART Recovery*; and *Women for Sobriety*. Based upon data

[83] Stephanie S. Covington, a psychotherapist, is well-known for her evidence-based techniques and other work in women's recovery, including her more recent treatment program guides and workbooks, *A Woman's Journal: Helping Women Recover*, 2008; and *Beyond Anger and Violence*, 2014.

obtained from web-based surveys, Zemore, Kaskutas, and Mericle (2017) found that:

> Compared to 12-step members, members of the mutual help alternatives were less religious and generally higher on education and income.
>
> *(p. 16)*

Most of these programs (e.g., *SMART Recovery*) are based on cognitive-behavioral approaches, such as the use of related homework assignments (Kelly, Deane, & Baker, 2015). Reportedly, the efficacy of these programs is equivalent to that for traditional 12-Step programs. However, necessary supporting research findings are *not* available.

Relapse Prevention Programs

The rate of relapse, or recidivism, following "successful" treatment of problematic patterns of substance use among women is quite *high* (see Figure 8.3). Although much research has examined treatment factors, including: (1) the involvement of family in treatment; (2) provision of special services; (3) staff characteristics; and (4) time in treatment. These factors have *not* been found to account for the large variance in post-treatment recidivism regarding problematic patterns of drug and substance use. For example, Davis, Ancis, and Ashby (2015) identified that, when compared to other drug and substance abusers, women of African continental descent, who have substance use disorders, have *lower* rates of treatment retention. They further identified that specific therapist characteristics (i.e., egalitarian, or democratic, leader; willingness to empower others; and multiculturally competent) were significantly correlated with *improved* treatment retention rates for women of African continental descent in their study. Unfortunately, the contribution of these factors, while both interesting and informative, did *not* account for the majority variance associated with treatment retention.

Obviously, much more research is required in this area. Factors implicated as causative or contributory to relapse include: cognitive factors ("Stinkin' Thinkin"); increased craving; interpersonal problems; lack of coping abilities; and negative affective states (McKay, 1999). In addition, it has been noted that a "complicated and dynamic interplay of distal and proximal factors" plays a major role in the relapse process (McKay, Franklin, & Patapis, 2006). In this regard, several researchers (e.g., Panebianco, Gallupe, & Carrington, 2016; Pagliaro & Pagliaro, *Clinical Patient Data Files*; Tracy, Min, & Park, 2016) have found that women's personal social networks play a major role in relapse prevention—that the more women associate post-treatment with family, friends, and other women, who do *not* use or abuse drugs and substances of abuse, the *lower* their risk for relapse. Conversely, the more that women associate post-treatment with family, friends, and other women who use or abuse drugs and substances of abuse, the *higher* their risk for relapse. (Also, see related discussion in Chapter 7, *Identifying Women's Contemporaneous Diagnoses.*)

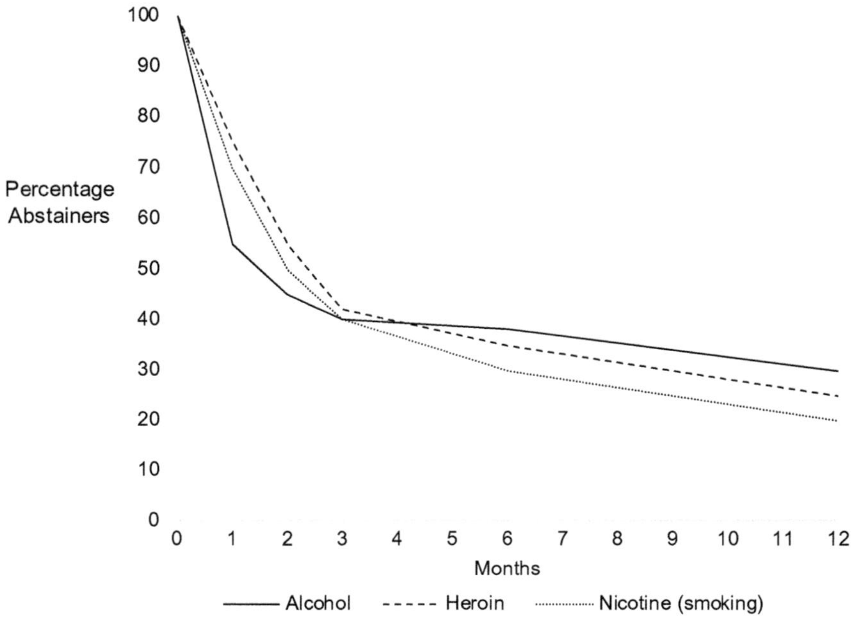

FIGURE 8.3 Typical Relapse Rates (Recidivism) Following Successful Treatment of Women's Compulsive Drug and Substance Abuse

Our own clinical experience, and the currently available research data, would suggest that the use of the following *three* recommendations would, at least, *minimize* the potential for *relapsed use*:

1. Individualize treatment to the specific needs and characteristics of each woman (i.e., *cut the shoe to fit the foot*);[84,85]

---

[84] The use of *patient-treatment matching* has been known and used for over 25 years (e.g., Mattson, 1994; "Project MATCH," 1993). However, usually due to economic and/or time constraints, patient-treatment matching remains the *exception to the rule*.

[85] This advice also extends to promoting enrolment in drug and substance abuse treatment programs. For example, as noted by Green (2006, p. 55):

> Limited research suggests that gender-specific treatment is *no* more effective than mixed-gender treatment, though certain women may only seek treatment in women-only programs.

Several others (e.g., Greenfield, Brooks, & Gordon, 2007; Greenfield, Rosa, & Putnins, 2011) shared this same observation. However, some limited success also has been noted. For example, Greenfield, Trucco, and McHugh (2007) noted, in their study that contrasted results from a women-only counseling treatment group with results from a mixed-gendered group, that while efficacy during the 12-week treatment phase was found to be equal, the women-only group demonstrated greater abstinence in post-treatment follow-up.

2. Employ specific indicators, or performance goals, to objectively evaluate the success of treatment outcomes and, subsequently, the degree of relapse, or efficacy, of relapse prevention (see listing below)
3. Periodically, as individually indicated, re-assess women and proactively intervene to prevent relapse

More specifically, regarding number *2*, above, areas of performance criteria for evaluation of treatment success and relapse prevention, may include:

- Interviewer clinical evaluations of improvement
- Self-report of reduction in, or discontinuation of, drug and substance abuse (e.g., achievement and maintenance of abstinence—*resumed nonuse*)
- Reduction in sociopathy (e.g., discontinuation of criminal behavior, such as drug dealing and engagement in prostitution or "sex-for-drug" exchanges)
- Intrapersonal adjustment with family, friends, co-workers, and peers
- Social adjustment, including regular attendance and/or improved performance in daily activities involving home, college/university, and work
- Social involvement (e.g., membership in church choir, bowling club, or softball team; school parents program; volunteer work for social/charitable agencies)

Some of this periodic monitoring is addressed, for example, in "aftercare" programs and in continued attendance at AA meetings, both of which have been positively correlated with significantly *higher* rates or duration of post-treatment abstinence (Pagliaro & Pagliaro, *Clinical Patient Data Files*). We would suggest, particularly for women, who have engaged in abusive or compulsive patterns of using the drug or substances of abuse, that the propensity for relapsed use—returning to compulsive use of drugs and substances of abuse—be considered a *life-long* concern.

Whenever possible, once a woman is abstinent, we gradually decrease the frequency and length of her psychotherapy sessions (e.g., from bi-weekly, to weekly, to every other week, to monthly, to every other month, to telephone and/or e-mail contact every 6 months). This strategy helps to maintain a communication linkage and "help-line" for each patient. This strategy also demonstrates continued concern and provides an opportunity for the early detection of problems by the therapist and for patients to request needed assistance *before* problems get *out of control*. In our practice, this strategy has resulted in a long-term (i.e., if we can maintain patient contact, generally in excess of 5 years) relapse rate of less than 20% (Pagliaro & Pagliaro, *Clinical Patient Data Files*).

In the context of monitoring women's response to treatment for AUDs and SUDs, as well as the subsequent maintenance of abstinence or related compliance with maintenance pharmacological treatment protocols, Hilton and Pilkonis (2015) developed the following 10 guidelines aimed at minimizing common monitoring measurement deficiencies:

1. Measures should be obtainable at regular intervals to establish baseline status and enable meaningful indicators of change
2. Measures should be brief enough to not be viewed as burdensome to the patient, address a broad enough spectrum of symptoms to seem relevant to the patient's experience with recovery, and therefore sustain engagement over the many years of recovery
3. Precision and sensitivity should not be sacrificed for the sake of brevity
4. Ideally, measures should enable patients in recovery to complete them on their own, at a place and time of their convenience without the need for administration by a trained service provider
5. Measures should not require a significant training burden to recovery support staff to administer and interpret results, as training costs can exclude staff not yet trained, and weaken outreach and support decisions when intervention is indicated by scores
6. Measures should be self-scoring in the sense that results would be instantly recorded and converted to easily-understood trend results for each variable monitored
7. Measures should be broad enough to be sensitive to changes in general physical and mental health as well as social functioning
8. Measures should be modifiable or expandable without a significant increase in burden to address the individualization needs of patients in recovery such as addressing exacerbating conditions like physical health or disability, significant chronic psychiatric conditions, or housing needs
9. Measures should be valid for all patients regardless of race, gender, age, or disease
10. The cost of monitoring should be limited to initial integration with existing record systems, and staff time to examine and interpret trends for sustained improvement or lapse. (pp. 477–479)

New Millennial Interactive Model of Women's Drug and Substance Abuse

The *New Millennial Interactive Model of Women's Drug and Substance Abuse* (Figure 8.2) can serve as a particularly helpful model for considering primary, secondary, and tertiary prevention regarding specific characteristics (e.g., age and developmental level) or patterns of women's drug and substance abuse (nonuse and compulsive use)—and serve as a framework for monitoring. (Also, see the discussion in the previous section, *Relapse Prevention Programs.*) As such, the model consists of *four* interacting dimensions: (1) *Women's Dimension*; (2) *Drug or Substance of Abuse Dimension*; (3) *Societal Dimension*; and (4) *Time Dimension*. The milieu associated with women's use of the drugs and substances of abuse is uniquely characterized for each woman as the complete set of interacting variables, from each of the four dimensions, at a particular point in time. As such, the model helps to account for the multidimensional etiology and context of women's use of the drugs and substances of abuse and serves as a useful heuristic device, providing an orderly and logical approach for understanding these complex interacting phenomena.

The model can help to plan specific, individual treatment strategies by identifying the presenting antecedent, or consequential, variables in each dimension that appear to: (1) contribute to use; (2) are amenable to change; and (3) require attention. For example, if specific stresses and maladaptive coping mechanisms are identified among the psychological variables in the *Woman Dimension*, techniques for stress reduction and the development of better coping abilities would be an integral component of the treatment plan. If a lack of family support is identified as a major contributing factor to drug and substance use among the social variables in the *Woman Dimension*, intervention might include attempts to increase family support (i.e., family therapy might be considered).

If a lack of adequate healthcare resources (e.g., specifically designed programs aimed at providing appropriate services to women, including appropriately trained and qualified staff) is identified as a major factor contributing to the use of the drugs and substances of abuse in the *Societal Dimension*, intervention may include attempts to increase social assistance (i.e., develop and provide specific social programs for women) and the training of clinical psychiatrists and psychologists, counselors, family therapists, social workers, and other health and social care professionals in regard to the specific approaches needed for delivering optimal treatment approaches for women who have an AUD and/or a SUD.

Evaluation of treatment is one of the most crucial, yet perhaps the most frequently overlooked, steps in the treatment process. It is useless to prescribe treatment, or for a woman to rigorously follow a plan of treatment, if the treatment is ineffective. Evaluation can be readily performed by using *The Model* to compare specific variables of interest before treatment (i.e., baseline assessment), during treatment (i.e., formative evaluation), and at a predetermined interval(s) after treatment is completed (i.e., summative evaluation). Although program evaluators and researchers are often particularly interested in the summative evaluation in terms of program success and recidivism rates, others (e.g., counselors; therapists) may be more interested in the formative evaluation because an ineffective treatment plan can be modified *mid-stream* in order to optimize therapy for an individual woman.

For example, if unemployment is a social variable in the *Woman Dimension* that is identified, for a particular woman, as a major contributory factor to her use of a drug or substance of abuse and, if sufficient attention is *not* given to appropriate educational (e.g., GED programs; tutoring for math or reading deficits), job training (e.g., vocational educational programs), and employment strategies (e.g., resume development; subsidized job work programs for single mothers), then the prognosis is *bleak*—despite other treatment interventions.

The Model also is useful because it can reveal factors that may, for a particular woman, contribute to *relapsed use* if not addressed. Such factors may include inadequate coping abilities when the woman is faced with significant stressors such as the death of a parent, a diagnosis of cancer, or a police arrest. In addition, the Model can be useful as a framework for helping women better understand the factors affecting their own use of the drugs and substances of abuse and, thus, enable them to become active participants in their own treatment planning and implementation.

Thus, the *New Millennial Interactive Model of Women's Drug and Substance Abuse* can serve as a particularly useful heuristic device for the primary, secondary, and tertiary prevention of women's use of the drugs and substances of abuse. With the use of this model to identify related variables that require attention, and with knowledge of successful and unsuccessful programs, we can begin to develop more effective prevention and treatment programs for women—both those: (1) who have not yet initiated the use of a drug or substance of abuse; and (2) who have already begun to use and are developing increasingly harmful patterns of use.

References[86,87,88]

Ahmed, A., Ali, A. N., & Kramers, C. (2013). Neuropsychiatric adverse events of varenicline: A systematic review of published reports. *Journal of Clinical Psychopharmacology*, 33(1), 55–62. doi:10.1097/JCP.0b013e31827c0117

Alcoholics Anonymous. (2001). *Alcoholics Anonymous (aka Big Book)* (4th ed.). New York, NY: Alcoholics Anonymous World Services, Inc.

Allen, A. M., al'Absi, M., & Lando, H. (2013). Menstrual phase, depressive symptoms, and allopregnanolone during short-term smoking cessation. *Experimental and Clinical Psychopharmacology*, 21(6), 427–433. doi:10.1037/a0034075

Allen, A. M., al'Absi, M., & Lando, H. (2015). Allopregnanolone association with psychophysiological and cognitive functions during acute smoking abstinence in premenopausal women. *Experimental and Clinical Psychopharmacology*, 23(1), 22–28.

Allen, A. M., Allen, S. S., & Widenmier, J. (2009). Patterns of cortisol and craving by menstrual phase in women attempting to quit smoking. *Addictive Behaviors*, 34(8), 632–635. doi:10.1016/j.addbeh.2009.03.024

Allen, A. M., Lunos, S., & Heishman, S. J. (2015, April). Subjective response to nicotine by menstrual phase. *Addictive Behaviors*, 43, 50–53. doi:10.1016/j.addbeh.2014.12.008

---

86 As per publisher style, only the first three authors are listed for each reference.

87 Several times the number of references listed were found, obtained, and analyzed by the authors during the preparation of this chapter. However, only the references that were cited at least once in the body of the text are included in the list. Major reasons for not citing other references, include that they: (1) did not provide any additional unique data; (2) were not well researched or written (i.e., were evaluated as not being valid or reliable); (3) were based predominantly, or exclusively, on animal studies; (4) provided usage statistics from outside the U.S.; and/or (5) were redundant with, or not as recent as, the already cited references.

88 The reference citation, "Pagliaro & Pagliaro, *Clinical Patient Data Files*," refers to unpublished data collected, with permission, over the last 50 years by the authors, in the formal course of their professional academic roles as clinician scientists and professors—from their patients, research subjects, and students, from the 1970s to date.

Allen, S. S., Allen, A. M., & Lunos, S. (2016). Progesterone and postpartum smoking relapse: A pilot double-blind placebo-controlled randomized trial. *Nicotine & Tobacco Research*, 2145–2153. doi:10.1093/ntr/ntw156

Allen, S. S., Bade, T., & Center, B. (2008). Menstrual phase effects on smoking relapse. *Addiction*, 103(5), 809–821. doi:10.1111/j.1360-0443.2008.02146.x

Alving, C. R., Matyas, G. R., & Torres, O. (2014). Adjuvants for vaccines to drugs of abuse and addiction. *Vaccine*, 32(42), 5382–5389. doi:10.1016/j.vaccine.2014.07.085

Amato, L., Minozzi, S., & Pani, P. P. (2007). Antipsychotic medications for cocaine dependence. *Cochrane Database of Systemic Reviews*, 18(3), CD006306. Retrieved from www.ncbi.nlm.nih.gov/pubmed/17636840

Amato, L., Minozzi, S., & Vecchi, S. (2010, March 17). Benzodiazepines for alcohol withdrawal. *Cochrane Database of Systematic Reviews*, (3), CD005063. doi:10.1002/14651858.CD005063

American Lung Association. (2016). *Hookah smoking: A growing threat to public health*. 1–7. Washington, DC: American Lung Association.

Anderson, D. M. (2010, September). Does information matter? The effect of the Meth Project on meth use among youths. *Journal of Health Economics*, 29(5), 732–742. doi:10.1016/j.healeco.2010.06.005

Anthenelli, R. M., Benowitz, N. L., & West, R. (2016). Neuropsychiatric safety and efficacy of varenicline, bupropion, and nicotine patch in smokers with and without psychiatric disorders (EAGLES): A double-blind, randomised, placebo-controlled clinical trial. *The Lancet*. doi:PIISO140-6736(16)30272-0

Arbaizar, B., Diersen-Sotos, T., & Gomez-Acebo, I. (2010). Topiramate in the treatment of alcohol dependence: A meta-analysis. *Actas Espanolas de Psiquiatria*, 38(1), 8–12.

Ashley, O. S., Marsden, M. E., & Brady, T. M. (2003). Effectiveness of substance abuse treatment programming for women: A review. *American Journal of Drug and Alcohol Abuse*, 29(1), 19–53.

Associated Press. (2016, September 12). *Abby Wambach reveals years-long alcohol, drug abuse*. Retrieved from Associated Press, pp. 1–2.

Azorin, J. M., Bowden, C. L., & Garay, R. P. (2010). Possible new ways in the pharmacological treatment of bipolar disorder and comorbid alcoholism. *Neuropsychiatric Disease and Treatment*, 6, 37–46.

Babb, S., Malarcher, A., & Schauer, G. (2017, January 6). Quitting smoking among adults—United States, 2000–2015. *MMWR, Morbidity and Mortality Weekly Report*, 65(52), 1457–1464.

Back, S. E., Payne, R. L., & Wahlquist, A. H. (2011). Comparative profiles of men and women with opioid dependence: Results from a national multisite effectiveness trial. *The American Journal of Drug and Alcohol Abuse*, 37(5), 313–323. doi:10.3109/00952990

Badalamenti, V. C., Buckley, J. W., & Smith, E. T. (2012). Safety of EMBEda (morphine sulfate and naltrexone hydrochloride) extended-release capsules: Review of postmarketing adverse events during the first year. *Journal of Opioid Management*, 8(2), 115–125.

Baker, T. B., Piper, M. E., & Stein, J. H. (2016). Effects of nicotine patch vs varenicline vs combination nicotine replacement therapy on smoking cessation at 26 weeks: A randomized clinical trial. *JAMA, Journal of the American Medical Association*, 315(4), 371–379. doi:10.1001/jama.2015.19284

Ballon, J. S., & Feifel, D. (2006). A systematic review of modafinil: Potential clinical users and mechanisms of action. *The Journal of Clinical Psychiatry*, 67(4), 554–566.

Banerjee, K., Howard, M., & Mansheim, K. (2007). Comparison of health realization and 12-step treatment in women's residential substance abuse treatment programs. *American Journal of Drug and Alcohol Abuse*, 33(2), 207–215.

Bannwarth, B. (2012). Will abuse-deterrent formulations of opioid analgesics be successful in achieving their purpose? *Drugs*, 72(13), 1713–1723. doi:10.2165/11635860-000000000-00000

Barth, K. S., & Malcolm, R. J. (2010). Disulfiram: An old therapeutic with new applications. *CNS Neurological Disorders—Drug Targets*, 9(1), 5–12.

Bates, T. J. (2009). Drug Court: Breaking the black magic spell of drug addiction for women: A qualitative study. *Dissertation Abstracts International Section A: Humanities and Social Sciences*, 69(12-A), 4873.

Bayard, M., McIntyre, J., & Hill, K. R. (2004, March 15). Alcohol withdrawal syndrome. *American Family Physician*, 69(5), 1443–1450.

Becker, H. K., Agopian, M. W., & Yeh, S. (1992). Impact evaluation of Drug Abuse Resistance Education (DARE). *Journal of Drug Education*, 22(4), 283–291.

Benotsch, E. G., Zimmerman, R., & Cathers, L. (2013). Non-medical use of prescription drugs, polysubstance use, and mental health in transgender adults. *Drug and Alcohol Dependence*, 132(1–2), 391–394. doi:10.1016/j.drugalcdep.2013.02.027

Boles, S., Young, N., & Moore, T. (2007). The Sacramento Dependency Drug Court: Development and outcomes. *Child Maltreatment*, 12(2), 161–171.

Boothby, L. A., & Doering, P. L. (2005). Acamprosate for the treatment of alcohol dependence. *Clinical Therapeutics*, 27(6), 695–714.

Borkman, T. (2008). The twelve-step recovery model of AA: A voluntary mutual help association. *Recent Developments in Alcoholism*, 18, 9–35.

Bowker, K. A., Lewis, S., & Coleman, T. (2014). Comparison of cotinine levels in pregnant women while smoking and when using nicotine replacement therapy. *Nicotine & Tobacco Research*, 16(6), 895–898. doi:10.1093/ntr/ntu029

Boyd, M. B., Mackey, M. C., & Phillips, K. D. (2006). Alcohol and other drug disorders, comorbidity and violence in rural African American women. *Issues in Mental Health Nursing*, 27, 1017–1036. doi:10.1080/01612840600943622

Braitman, A. L., Henson, J. M., & Carey, K. B. (2015). Clarifying observed relationships between protective behavioral strategies and alcohol outcomes: The importance of response options. *Psychology of Addictive Behaviors*, 29(2), 455–466. doi:10.1037/adb0000024

Braitman, A. L., & Kelley, M. L. (2016). Initiation and retention in couples outpatient treatment for parents with drug and alcohol use disorders. *Experimental and Clinical Psychopharmacology*, 3, 174–184.

Brandon, T. H., Goniewicz, M. L., & Hanna, N. H. (2015). Electronic nicotine delivery systems: A policy statement from the American Association for Cancer Research and the American Society of Clinical Oncology. *Journal of Clinical Oncology*, 33(8), 952–963. doi:10.1200/JCO.2014.59.4465

Bremer, P. T., Kimishima, A., & Schlosburg, J. E. (2016, February 16). Combatting synthetic designer opioids: A conjugate vaccine ablates lethal doses of fentanyl class drugs. *Angewandte Chemie International Edition in English*. doi:10.1002/anie.201511654

Brimijoin, S., Shen, X., & Orson, F. (2013). Prospects, promise and problems on the road to effective vaccines and related therapies for substance abuse. *Expert Review of Vaccines*, 12(3), 323–332. doi:10.1586/erv.13.1

Bronfenbrenner, U. (1979). *The ecology of human development: Experiments by nature and design*. Cambridge, MA: Harvard University Press.

Brown, R. (2011). Drug court effectiveness: A matched cohort study in the Dane County drug treatment court. *Journal of Offender Rehabilitation*, 50(4), 191–201. doi:10.1080/10509674.2011.571347

Brown, R. T. (2010). Systematic review of the impact of adult drug treatment courts. *Translational Research*, 155(6), 263–274. doi:10.1016/j.trsl.2010.03.001

Bullen, C., Howe, C., & Laugesen, M. (2013). Electronic cigarettes for smoking cessation: A randomised controlled trial. *Lancet*, 382(9905), 1629–1637. doi:10.1016/S140-6736(13)61842–5

Butler, S. F., Cassidy, T. A., & Chilcoat, H. (2013). Abuse rates and routes of administration of reformulated extended-release oxycodone: Initial findings from a sentinel surveillance sample of individuals assessed for substance abuse treatment. *The Journal of Pain*, 14(4), 351–358. doi:10.1016/j.jpain.2012.08.008

Cahill, K., Lindson-Hawley, N., & Thomas, K. H. (2016, May 9). Nicotine receptor partial agonists for smoking cessation. *Cochrane Database of Systematic Reviews*, 0(5), CD006103. doi:10.1002/14651858.CD006103.pub7

Cahill, K., Stead, L. F., & Lancaster, T. (2012, April 18). Nicotine receptor partial agonists for smoking cessation. *Cochrane Database of Systematic Reviews*, 0(4), CD006103. doi:10.1002/14651858.CD006103.pub6

Cahill, K., Stevens, S., & Perera, R. (2013, May 31). Pharmacological interventions for smoking cessation: An overview and network meta-analysis. *Cochrane Database of Systematic Reviews*, 0(5), CD009329. doi:10.1002/14651858.CD009329.pub2

Callahan-Lyon, P. (2014). Electronic cigarettes: Human health effects. *Tobacco Control—BMJ Journals*, 23(Suppl 2), iii36–40. doi:10.1136/tobaccocontrol-2013–051470

Campbell, A. N., Nunes, E. V., & Pavlicova, M. (2015, June). Gender-based outcomes and acceptability of a computer-assisted psychosocial intervention for substance use disorders. *Journal of Substance Abuse Treatment*, 53, 9–15. doi:10.1016/j.jsat.2014.12.006

Campbell, N. D. (2015). "What would my life look like under a magnifying glass?" Reading "feminist standpoint epistemology" into substance use and misuse. *Substance Use and Misuse*, 50(6), 806–809.

Cassidy, T. A., DasMahapatra, P., & Black, R. A. (2014). Changes in prevalence of prescription opioid abuse after introduction of an abuse-deterrent opioid formulation. *Pain Medicine*, 15(3), 440–451. doi:10.1111/pme.12295

CDC, Centers for Disease Control and Prevention. (2008). HIV/AIDS among women. *HIV/AIDS Fact Sheet*. Retrieved from www.cdc.gov/hiv/topics/women/resources/factsheets/women.htm

Center for Substance Abuse Treatment. (2005). *Substance abuse treatment: Group therapy (Treatment Improvement Protocol [TIP] Series, No. 41)*. Rockville, MD: SAMHSA, Substance Abuse and Mental Health Services Administration.

Center for Substance Abuse Treatment. (2009). *Incorporating alcohol pharmacotherapeutics into medical practice (Treatment Improvement Protocol (TIP) Series, No. 49)*. Rockville, MD: SAMHSA, Substance Abuse and Mental Health Services Administration. Retrieved March 28, 2016, from Chapter 4–Oral naltrexone: www.ncbi.nlm.nih.gov/books/NBK64042/

Cerny, E. H., & Cerny, T. (2009). Vaccines against nicotine. *Human Vaccines*, 5(4), 200–205.

Chamberlain, C., O'Mara-Eves, A., & Oliver, S. (2013, October 23). Psychosocial interventions for supporting women to stop smoking in pregnancy. *Cochrane Database of Systematic Reviews*, (10), CD001055. doi:10.1002/14651858

Chang, P. H., Chiang, C. H., & Ho, W. C. (2015). Combination therapy of varenicline with nicotine replacement therapy is better than varenicline alone: A systematic review and meta-analysis of randomized controlled trials. *BMC Public Health*, 15, 689. doi:10.1186/s12889-015-2055-?

Chiang, C. N., & Hawks, R. L. (2003). Pharmacokinetics of the combination tablet of buprenorphine and naloxone. *Drug and Alcohol Dependence*, 70(2 Supplement), S39–S47.

Chou, J. L., Beeler-Stinn, S., & Diamond, R. M. (2014). Heroin and post-traumatic stress disorder in a women's treatment facility: An exploratory study. *Journal of Feminist Family Therapy: An International Forum*, 26(3), 138–162. doi:10.1080/08952833.2014.933696

Civljak, M., Stead, L. F., & Hartmann-Boyce, J. (2013). Internet-based interventions for smoking cessation. *Cochrane Database of Systematic Reviews*, CD007078. doi:10.1002/14651858.CD007078.pub4

Clarke, N., Mun, E. Y., & Kelly, S. (2013). Treatment outcomes of a combined cognitive behavior therapy and pharmacotherapy for a sample of women with and without substance abuse histories on an acute psychiatric unit: Do therapeutic alliance and motivation matter? *The American Journal on Addictions*, 22(6), 566–573. doi:10.1111/j.1521-0391.2013.12013.x

Cohen, C., Kodas, E., & Griebel, G. (2005). CB1 receptor antagonists for the treatment of nicotine addiction. *Pharmacology Biochemistry and Behavior*, 81(2), 387–395.

Cohen, J. B., Dakof, G. A., & Duarte, E. (2011). Dependency Drug Court. In J. D. Osofsky (Ed.), *Clinical work with traumatized young children* (pp. 252–266). New York, NY: Guilford.

Collins, T. R. (2010, February 8). Deaths from methadone overdose disproportionate to number of prescriptions. *Medscape Medical News*. Retrieved from www.medscape.com/viewarticle/716603_print

Connery, H. S. (2015). Medication-assisted treatment of opioid use disorder: Review of the evidence and future directions. *Harvard Review of Psychiatry*, 23(2), 63–75. doi:10.1097/HRP.0000000000000075

Corelli, R. L., & Hudmon, K. S. (2006). Pharmacologic interventions for smoking cessation. *Critical Care Nursing Clinics of North America*, 18(1), 39–51.

Covey, L. S., & Glassman, A. H. (1991). New approaches to smoking cessation. *Physician Assistant*, 15, 69, 70, 73, 74, 77.

Covington, S. S. (1994). *A woman's way through the twelve steps*. Center City, MN: Hazelden.

Covington, S. S. (2008a). *A woman's journal: A program for treating addiction (helping women recover)* (revised ed.). San Francisco, CA: Jossey-Bass.

Covington, S. S. (2008b, November). Women and addiction: A trauma-informed approach. *Journal of Psychoactive Drugs, SARC*(Supplement 5), 377–385.

Covington, S. S. (2014). *Beyond anger and violence: A program for women participant workbook*. Hoboken, NJ: Wiley.

Cox, L. S., Nollen, N. L., & Mayo, M. S. (2012). Bupropion for smoking cessation in African American light smokers: A randomized controlled study. *Journal of the National Cancer Institute*, 104(4), 290–298. doi:10.1093/jnci/djr513

Crain, D., & Bhat, A. (2010). Current treatment options in smoking cessation. *Hospital Practice (Minneapolis)*, 38(1), 53–61.

Creswell, L. (2016). Review of literature of women with co-occurring disorders through the feminist and black feminist perspective. *Addiction Research & Therapy*, 7(1), 1–7. doi:10.4172/2155–6105.1000267

Cui, C. L., Wu, L. Z., & Luo, F. (2008). Acupuncture for the treatment of drug addiction. *Neurochemical Research*, 33(10), 2013–2022. doi:10.1007/s11064-008-9784-8

Culberson, J. W., & Ziska, M. (2008). Prescription drug misuse/abuse in the elderly. *Geriatrics*, 63(9), 22–31.

D'Alberto, A. (2004). Auricular acupuncture in the treatment of cocaine/crack abuse: A review of the efficacy of the use of the National Acupuncture Detoxification Association protocol, and the selection of sham points. *Journal of Alternative & Contemporary Medicine*, 10(6), 985–1000.

Davis, T. A., Ancis, J. R., & Ashby, J. S. (2015). Therapist effects, working alliance, and African American women substance users. *Cultural Diversity and Ethnic Minority Psychology*, 21(1), 126–135.

De La Rosa, M. R., & White, M. S. (2001). A review of the role of social support systems in the drug use behavior of Hispanics. *Journal of Psychoactive Drugs*, 33(3), 233–240.

De Leon, G. (1985). The therapeutic community: Status and evolution. *The International Journal of the Addictions*, 20, 823–844.

de Lima, M. S., de Oliveira Soares, B. G., & Reisser, A. A. (2002). Pharmacological treatment of cocaine dependence: A systematic review. *Addiction*, 97(8), 931–949.

de Lima, M., Farrell, M., & Lima Reisser, A. A. (2010). WITHDRAWN: Antidepressants for cocaine dependence. *Cochrane Database of Systematic Reviews*, 2, CD002950.

De Sousa, A. (2010). The role of topiramate and other anticonvulsants in the treatment of alcohol dependence: A clinical review. *CNS Neurological Disorders—Drug Targets*, 9(1), 45–49.

De Witte, P., Littleton, J., & Parot, P. (2005). Neuroprotective and abstinence-promoting effects of acamprosate: Elucidating the mechanism of action. *CNS Drugs*, 19(6), 517–537.

Desrosiers, A., Thompson, A., & Divney, A. (2016). Romantic partner influences on prenatal and postnatal substance use in young couples. *Journal of Public Health (Oxford, England)*, 38(2), 300–307. doi:10.1093/pubmed/fdv039

DeVito, E. E., Herman, A. I., & Waters, A. J. (2014). Subjective, physiological, and cognitive responses to intravenous nicotine: Effects of sex and menstrual cycle phase. *Neuropsychopharmacology*, 39(6), 1431–1440. doi:10.1038/npp.2013.339

DiClemente, C. C., Schlundt, D., & Gemmell, L. (2004, March–April). Readiness and stages of change in addiction treatment. *The American Journal on Addictions*, 13(2), 103–119. doi:10.1080/10550490490435777

Diehl, A., Ulmer, L., & Mutschler, J. (2010). Why is disulfiram superior to acamprosate in the routine clinical setting? A retrospective long-term study in 353 alcohol-dependent patients. *Alcohol and Addiction*, 45(3), 271–277.

Dobbs, P. D., Hammig, B., & Sudduth, A. (2016, March 19). 2015 Legislative update of E-cigarettes youth access and exposure laws. *Preventive Medicine*, 1–2. doi:10.1016/j.ypmed.2016.03.010

Donny, E. C., Walsh, S. L., & Bigelow, G. E. (2002). High-dose methadone produces superior opioid blockade and comparable withdrawal suppression to lower doses in opioid-dependent humans. *Psychopharmacology (Berlin)*, 161(2), 202–212.

Donohue, B., Azrin, N. H., & Bradshaw, K. (2014). A controlled evaluation of family behavior therapy in concurrent child neglect and drug abuse. *Journal of Consulting and Clinical Psychology*, 82(4), 706–720. doi:10.1037/a0036920

Donovan, D. M., Ingalsbe, M. H., & Benbow, J. (2013). 12-step interventions and mutual support programs for substance use disorders: An overview. *Social Work in Public Health*, 28(3–4), 313–332. doi:10.1080/19371918.2013.774663

Drabble, L., & Trocki, K. (2005). Alcohol consumption, alcohol-related problems, and other substance use among lesbian and bisexual women. *Journal of Lesbian Studies*, 9(3), 19–30.

Dursteler, K. M., & Vogel, M. (2016, March 22). Effective drug therapy for cocaine dependence: A milestone. *The Lancet*, 1. doi:10.1016/S0140-6736(16)00563-8

Dye, M. H., Ducharme, L. J., & Johnson, J. A. (2009). Modified therapeutic communities and adherence to traditional elements. *Journal of Psychoactive Drugs*, 41(3), 275–283.

Ebbert, J. O., Wyatt, K. D., & Hays, J. T. (2010). Varenicline for smoking cessation: Efficacy, safety, and treatment recommendations. *Patient Preference and Adherence*, 4, 355–362.

Ebbert, J. O., Wyatt, K. D., & Zirakzadeh, A. (2009). Clinical utility of varenicline for smokers with medical and psychiatric comorbidity. *International Journal of Chronic Obstructive Pulmonary Disease*, 4, 421–430.

E-cigarettes and smoking cessation. Similar efficacy to other nicotine delivery devices, but many uncertainties. (2015). *Prescrire International*, 24(165), 271–276.

El-Mohandes, A. A., El-Khorazaty, M. N., & Kiely, M. (2011). Smoking cessation and relapse among pregnant African-American smokers in Washington, DC. *Maternal and Child Health Journal*, 15(Suppl 1), S96–S105. doi:10.1007/s10995-011-0825

Epstein, E. E., & McCrady, B. S. (1998). Behavioral couples treatment of alcohol and drug use disorders: Current status and innovations. *Clinical Psychology Review*, 18(6), 689–711.

Erceg-Hurn, D. M. (2008, December). Drugs, money, and graphic ads: A critical review of the Montana Meth Project. *Prevention Science*, 9(4), 256–263. doi:10.1007/s1121-008-0098-5

Esterlis, I., McKee, S. A., & Kirk, K. (2013). Sex-specific differences in GABA(A)-benzodiazepine receptor availability: Relationship with sensitivity to pain and tobacco smoking craving. *Addiction Biology*, 18(2), 370–378. doi:10.1111/j.1369-1600.2011.00403.x

Evans, E., Li, L., & Pierce, J. (2013). Explaining long-term outcomes among drug dependent mothers treated in women-only versus mixed-gender programs. *Journal of Substance Abuse Treatment*, 45(3), 293–301. doi:10.1016/j.jsat.2013.04.003

Faggiano, F., Vigna-Taglianti, F., & Versino, E. (2003). Methadone maintenance at different dosages for opioid dependence. *Cochrane Database of Systematic Reviews*, 3, CD002208.

Fals-Stewart, W., O'Farrell, T. J., & Birchler, G. R. (2004). Behavioral couples therapy for substance abuse: Rationale, methods, and findings. *Science & Practice Perspectives*, 2(2), 30–41.

Fant, R. V., Buchhalter, A. R., & Buchman, A. C. (2009). Pharmacotherapy for tobacco dependence. *Handbook of Experimental Pharmacology*, (192), 487–510.

Fareed, A., Casarella, J., & Amar, R. (2010). Methadone maintenance dosing guideline for opioid dependence: A literature review. *Journal of Addictive Diseases*, 29(1), 1–14.

FDA, U.S. Food and Drug Administration. (2006, May 11). FDA approves novel medication for smoking cessation. *FDA News Release*. Retrieved from www.fda.gov/NewsEvents/Newsroom/PressAnnouncements/2006/ucm108651.htm

FDA, U.S. Food and Drug Administration. (2009, July 1). FDA requires new boxed warnings for the smoking cessation drugs Chantix and Zyban. *Public Health Advisory*. Retrieved from www.fda.gov/Drugs/DrugSafety/DrugSafetyPodcasts/ucm170906.htm

FDA, U.S. Food and Drug Administration. (2016, December 16). Chantix (varenicline) and Zyban (bupropion): Drug safety communication—Mental health side effects revised. *Safety Alerts for Human Medical Products*, 1–12. Silver Spring, MD: U.S. Food and Drug Administration.

Ferri, M., Amato, L., & Davoli, M. (2006, July 19). Alcoholics Anonymous and other 12-step programmes for alcohol dependence. *Cochrane Database of Systematic Reviews*, 3, CD005032.

Fildes, E. E., Wilson, M. A., & Crawford, B. J. (2012). Tobacco quitlines in the United States. *Nursing Clinics of North America*, 47(1), 97–107. doi:10.1016/j.cnur.2011.10.009

Finfgeld-Connett, D. (2011). Therapeutic substance abuse treatment for incarcerated women. *Clinical Nursing Research*, 20(4), 462–481. doi:10.1177/1054773811415844

Fingarette, H. (1988). *Heavy drinking: The myth of alcoholism as a disease*. Berkeley, CA: University of California.

Fischer, M. S., Baucom, D. H., & Cohen, M. J. (2016, September). Cognitive-behavioral couple therapies: Review of the evidence for the treatment of relationship distress, psychopathology, and chronic health conditions. *Family Process*, 55(3), 423–442. doi:10.1111/famp.12227

Fisher, D. G., Reynolds, G. L., & D'Anna, L. H. (2017, February). Failure to get into substance abuse treatment. *Journal of Substance Abuse Treatment*, 73, 55–62. doi:10.1016/j.jsat.2016.11.004

Flassing, J. (2010). Buprenorphine: A more accessible treatment for opioid dependence. *Journal of the American Academy of Physician Assistants*, 23(9), 40–43.

Flentje, A., Heck, N. C., & Sorensen, J. L. (2014). Characteristics of transgender individuals entering substance abuse treatment. *Addictive Behaviors*, 39(5), 969–975. doi:10.1016/j.addbeh.2014.01.011

Florez, G., Saiz, P. A., & Garcia-Portilla, P. (2010). Topiramate for the treatment of alcohol dependence: Comparison with naltrexone. *European Addiction Research*, 17(1), 29–36.

Forray, A., Gotman, N., & Kershaw, T. (2014). Perinatal smoking and depression in women with concurrent substance use. *Addictive Behaviors*, 39(4), 749–756. doi:10.1016/j.addbeh.2013.12.008

Frankel, L. (1990). Structural family therapy for adolescent substance abusers and their families. In A. S. Friedman, & S. Granick (Eds.), *Family therapy for adolescent drug abuse* (pp. 47–61). New York, NY: Lexington.

Franklin, T. R., Ehrman, R., & Lynch, K. G. (2008). Menstrual cycle phase at quit date predicts smoking status in an NRT treatment trial: A retrospective analysis. *Journal of Women's Health*, 17(2), 287–292. doi:10.1089/jwh.2007.0423

Frishman, W. H. (2007). Smoking cessation pharmacotherapy—Nicotine and non-nicotine preparations. *Preventive Cardiology*, 10(2 (Supplement 1)), 10–22.

Frishman, W. H. (2009). Smoking cessation pharmacotherapy. *Therapeutic Advances in Cardiovascular Disease*, 3(4), 287–308.

Gaalema, D. E., Higgins, S. T., & Pepin, C. S. (2013). Illicit drug use among pregnant women enrolled in treatment for cigarette smoking cessation. *Nicotine & Tobacco Research*, 15(5), 987–991. doi:10.1093/ntr/nts220

Garbutt, J. C. (2009). The state of pharmacotherapy for the treatment of alcohol dependence. *Journal of Substance Abuse Treatment*, 36(1), S15–S23.

Garbutt, J. C. (2010). Efficacy and tolerability of naltrexone in the management of alcohol dependence. *Current Pharmaceutical Design*, 16(19), 2091–2097.

Garbutt, J. C., Kranzler, H. R., & O'Malley, S. S. (2005). Efficacy and tolerability of long-acting injectable naltrexone for alcohol dependence: A randomized controlled study. *JAMA, The Journal of the American Medical Association*, 293, 1617–1625.

Garcia, A. M. (2013). State laws regulating prescribing of controlled substances: Balancing the public health problems of chronic pain and prescription painkiller abuse and overdose. *Journal of Law and Medical Ethics*, 41(Supplement 1), 42–45.

Gardner, S. (2007, May 22). Presentation—San Francisco Dependency Drug Court: Options and Issues. *Children and Family Futures/National Center on Substance Abuse and Child Welfare*. Washington, DC.

Garrison, G. D., & Dugan, S. E. (2009). Varenicline: A first-line treatment option for smoking cessation. *Clinical Therapeutics*, 31(3), 463–491.

Gastfriend, D. R. (2014). A pharmaceutical industry perspective on the economics of treatments for alcohol and opioid use disorders. *Annals of the New York Academy of Sciences*, 1327, 112–130. doi:10.1111/nyas.12538

Gates, P. J., Sabioni, P., & Copeland, J. (2016, May 5). Psychosocial interventions for cannabis use disorder. *The Cochrane Database of Systematic Reviews*, 5, CD005336. doi:10.1002/14651858.CD005336.pub4

Gates, S., Smith, L. A., & Foxcroft, D. R. (2006, January 25). Auricular acupuncture for cocaine dependence. *Cochrane Database of Systematic Reviews*, 1, CD005192. doi:10.1002/14651858.CD005192.pub2

Generali, J. A. (1992). Nicotine transdermal patches. *Facts and Comparisons Drug Newsletter*, 11, 33–34.

Gold, J. (2016, August 16). *California court helps kids by healing parents' addictions: Shots—Health News: NPR*. Retrieved August 16, 2016, from National Public Radio (NPR), pp. 1–7: www.npr.org/sections/health-shots/2016/08/16/48096022/california-court-helps-kids-by-healing-parents-addictions

Gold, M. S., & Dackis, C. A. (1984). New insights and treatments: Opiate withdrawal and cocaine addiction. *Clinical Therapeutics*, 7(1), 6–21.

Gonzales, D., Rennard, S. I., & Nides, M. (2006). Varenicline: An alpha4beta2 nicotine acetylcholine receptor partial agonist vs. sustained-release bupropion and placebo for smoking cessation. *JAMA, The Journal of the American Medical Association*, 296(1), 47–55.

Goonoo, N., Bhaw-Luximon, A., & Ujoodha, R. (2014). Naltrexone: A review of existing sustained drug delivery systems and emerging nano-based systems. *Journal of Controlled Release*, 183, 154–166. doi:10.1016/j.jconrel.2014.03.046

Gossop, M., Stewart, D., & Browne, N. (2002). Factors associated with abstinence, lapse or relapse to heroin use after residential treatment: Protective effect of coping responses. *Addiction*, 97(10), 1259–1267.

Gowing, L. R., Farrell, M., & Ali, R. L. (2002). Alpha2-adrenergic agonists in opioid withdrawal. *Addiction*, 97(1), 49–58.

Gowing, L., Farrell, M., & Ali, R. (2009, April 15). Alpha2-adrenergic agonists for the management of opioid withdrawal. *The Cochrane Database of Systematic Reviews*, 2, CD002024. doi:10.1002/14651858.CD002024.pub3

Green, C. A. (2006). Gender and use of substance abuse treatment services. *Alcohol Research & Health*, 29(1), 55–62.

Green, K. E., & Feinstein, B. A. (2012). Substance use in lesbian, gay, and bisexual populations: An update on empirical research and implications for treatment. *Psychology of Addictive Behaviors*, 26(2), 265–278. doi:10.1037/a0025424

Greenfield, S. F., Back, S. E., & Lawson, K. (2010). Substance abuse in women. *Psychiatric Clinics of North America*, 33(2), 339–355. doi:10.1016/j.psc.2010.01.004

Greenfield, S. F., Brooks, A. J., & Gordon, S. M. (2007). Substance abuse treatment entry, retention, and outcome in women: A review of the literature. *Drug and Alcohol Dependence*, 86(1), 1–21. doi:10.1016/j.drugalcdep.2006.05.012

Greenfield, S. F., Rosa, C., & Putnins, S. I. (2011). Gender research in the National Institute on Drug Abuse National Treatment Clinical Trials Network: A summary of findings. *The American Journal of Drug and Alcohol Abuse*, 37(5), 301–312. doi:10.3109/00952990.2011.596875

Greenfield, S. F., Sugarman, D. E., & Freid, C. M. (2014, September 1). Group therapy for women with substance use disorders: Results from the women's recovery group study. *Drug and Alcohol Dependence*, 142, 245–253. doi:10.1016/j.drugalcdep.2014.06.035

Greenfield, S. F., Trucco, E. M., & McHugh, R. K. (2007). The women's recovery group study: A State 1 trial of women-focused group therapy for substance use disorders versus mixed-gender group drug counseling. *Drug and Alcohol Dependence*, 90(1), 39–47. doi:10.1016/j.drugalcdep.2007.02.009

Greenstein, R. A., Arndt, I. C., & McLellan, A. T. (1984). Naltrexone: A clinical perspective. *The Journal of Clinical Psychiatry*, 45(9, part 2), 25–28.

Griese, E. R., & Mack, L. (2016). Examining American Indian maternal-child health post-substance abuse residential treatment. *American Psychological Association 2016 Conference Presentations, Topic: 76 Substance Abuse*. American Psychological Association.

Grimshaw, G. M., & Stanton, A. (2006, October 18). Tobacco cessation intervention for young people. *Cochrane Database of Systematic Reviews*, 4, CD003289.

Grucza, R. A., Plunk, A. D., & Hipp, P. R. (2013). Long-term effects of laws governing youth access to tobacco. *American Journal of Public Health*, 103(8), 1493–1499. doi:10.2105/AJPH.2012.301123

Hallgren, K. A., Crotwell, S. M., & Munoz, R. E. (2016, June). Assessing treatment integrity in alcohol behavioral couple therapy. *Addictive Disorders & Their Treatment*, 15(2), 74–84.

Hanson, G. R. (2002). Therapeutic community. *National Institute on Drug Abuse Research Report Series*. Rockville, MD: National Institute on Drug Abuse.

Hanson, J. D., & Pourier, S. (2016). The Oglala Sioux Tribe CHOICES Program: Modifying an existing alcohol-exposed pregnancy intervention for use in an American Indian community. *International Journal of Environmental Research and Public Health*, 13, 1–10. doi:10.3390/ijerph13010001

Hanson, J. D., Winberg, A., & Elliott, A. (2012). Development of a media campaign on fetal alcohol spectrum disorders for Northern Plains American Indian communities. *Health Promotion Practice*, 13(6), 842–847. doi:10.1177/1524839911404232

Hard, B. (2014, November 26). Management of opioid painkiller dependence in primary care: Ongoing recovery with buprenorphine/naloxone. *BMJ Case Reports*. doi:10.1136/bcr-2014–207308

Harrell, P. T., Marquinez, N. S., & Correa, J. B. (2015). Expectancies for cigarettes, e-cigarettes, and nicotine replacement therapies among e-cigarette users (aka vapers). *Nicotine & Tobacco Research*, 17(2), 193–200. doi:10.1093/ntr/ntu149

Harrell, P. T., Simmons, V. N., & Correa, J. B. (2014). Electric nicotine delivery systems ("e-cigarettes"): Review of safety and smoking cessation efficacy. *Otolaryngology—Head and Neck Surgery*, 151(3), 381–393. doi:10.1177/0194599814536847

Harris, S. K., & Knight, J. R. (2014). Putting the screen in screening: Technology-based alcohol screening and brief interventions in medical settings. *Alcohol Research*, 36(1), 63–79.

Hartmann-Boyce, J., Cahill, K., & Hatsukami, D. (2012, August 15). Nicotine vaccines for smoking cessation. *Cochrane Database of Systematic Reviews*, 8, CD007072. doi:10.1002/14651858.CD007072

Hartocollis, A. (2013, October 30). *New York raising age to buy cigarettes to 21.* Retrieved from The New York Times: www.nytimes.com/2013/10/31/nyregion/new-york-approves-law-to-raise-tobacco-purchasing-age-to-21.html?_r=0

Havens, J. R., Leukefeld, C. G., & DeVeaugh-Geiss, A. M. (2014, June 1). The impact of a reformulation of extended-release oxycodone designed to deter abuse in a sample of prescription opioid abusers. *Drug and Alcohol Dependence*, 139, 9–17. doi:10.1016/j.drugalcdep.2014.02.018

Hays, J. T., Croghan, I. T., & Schroeder, D. R. (2010, October 12). Varenicline for tobacco dependence treatment in recovering alcohol-dependent smokers: An open-label pilot study. *Journal of Substance Abuse Treatment*, 40(1), 102–107.

Herzog, T. A., & Pokhrel, P. (2012). Ethnic differences in smoking rate, nicotine dependence, and cessation-related variables among adult smokers in Hawaii. *Journal of Community Health*, 37(6), 1226–1233. doi:10.1007/s10900-012-9558-8

Hien, D. A., Campbell, A. N., & Ruglass, L. M. (2010). The role of alcohol misuse in PTSD outcomes for women in community treatment: A secondary analysis of NIDA's Women and Trauma Study. *Drug and Alcohol Dependence*, 111(1–2), 114–119. doi:10.1016/j.drugalcdep.2010.04.011

Hien, D. A., Jiang, H., & Campbell, A. N. (2010). Do treatment improvements in PTSD severity affect substance use outcomes? A secondary analysis from a randomized clinical trial in NIDA's Clinical Trials Network. *American Journal of Psychiatry*, 167(1), 95–101. doi:10.1176/appi.ajp.2009.09091261

Higuchi, S. (2015). Efficacy of acamprosate for the treatment of alcohol dependence long after recovery from withdrawal syndrome: A randomized, double-blind, placebo-controlled study conducted in Japan (Sunrise Study). *Journal of Clinical Psychiatry*, 181–188. doi:10.4088/JCP.13m08940

Hilton, T. F., & Pilkonis, P. A. (2015). The key to individualized addiction treatment is comprehensive assessment and monitoring symptoms and behavioral change. *Behavioral Science*, 5, 477–495. doi:10.3390/bsd.5040477

Hilty, D. M., Luo, J. S., & Morache, C. (2002). Telepsychiatry: An overview for psychiatrists. *CNS Drugs*, 16(8), 527–548.

Hser, Y. I., Evans, E., & Huang, D. (2004). Relationship between drug treatment services, retention, and outcomes. *Psychiatric Services*, 55(7), 767–774.

Hser, Y. I., Evans, E., & Huang, D. (2011). Long-term outcomes among drug-dependent mothers treated in women-only versus mixed-gender programs. *Journal of Substance Abuse Treatment*, 41(2), 115–123. doi:10.1016/j.jsat.2011.02.004

Hser, Y. I., Hunt, S. A., & Evans, E. (2012). Hispanic parenting women in women-only versus mixed-gender drug treatment: A 10-year prospective study. *Addictive Behaviors*, 729–735. doi:10.1016/j.addbeh.2012.02.009

Hudmon, K. S., Corelli, R. L., & Prokhorov, A. V. (2010, February). Current approaches to pharmacotherapy for smoking cessation. *Therapeutic Advances in Respiratory Disease*, 4(1), 35–47. doi:10.1177/1753465809353768

Humphreys, K., Blodgett, J. C., & Wagner, T. H. (2014). Estimating the efficacy of Alcoholics Anonymous without self-selection bias: An instrumental variables re-analysis of randomized clinical trials. *Alcoholism: Clinical and Experimental Research*, 2688–2694. doi:10.1111/acer.12557

Huttlin, E. A., Allen, A. M., & Tosun, N. L. (2015, November). Associations between adrenocortical activity and nicotine response in female smokers by menstrual phase. *Addictive Behaviors*, 50, 135–139. doi:10.1016/j.addbeh.2015.06.026

Institute of Medicine. (2015). *Public health implications of raising the minimum age of legal access to tobacco products*. pp. 1–7. Washington DC: The National Academies Press. Retrieved from www.nationalacademies.org/hmd/Reports/2015/TobaccoMinimumAgeReport.aspx

Janssen, P. A., Demorest, L. C., & Kelly, A. (2012). Auricular acupuncture for chemically dependent pregnant women: A randomized controlled trial of the NADA protocol. *Substance Abuse Treatment, Prevention, and Policy*, 7, 48. doi:10.1186/1747-597X-7–48

Johns Hopkins Bloomberg School of Public Health. (2015). Alcohol advertising on cable TV: Q4 2015. *Report*, 1–3. Center on Alcohol Marketing and Youth. Retrieved from www.camy.org/resources/infographics/alcohol-advertising-on-cable-tv-q4-2015/

Johnson, B. A., & Ait-Daoud, N. (2010). Topiramate in the new generation of drugs: Efficacy in the treatment of alcoholic patients. *Current Pharmaceutical Design*, 16(19), 2103–2112.

Johnson, B. A., Ait-Daoud, N., & Bowden, C. L. (2003). Oral topiramate for treatment of alcohol dependence: A randomized controlled study. *Lancet*, 361(9370), 1677–1685.

Johnson, B. A., Rosenthal, N., & Capece, J. A. (2007). Topiramate for treating alcohol dependence: A randomized controlled study. *JAMA, The Journal of the American Medical Association*, 298(14), 1641–1685.

Johnson, F., & Setnik, B. (2011). Morphine sulfate and naltrexone hydrochloride extended-release capsules: Naltrexone release, pharmacodynamics, and tolerability. *Pain Physician*, 14(4), 391–406.

Jones, H. E., Finnegan, L. P., & Kaltenbach, K. (2012). Methadone and buprenorphine for the management of opioid dependence in pregnancy. *Drugs*, 72(6), 747–757. doi:10.2165/11632820-000000000-00000

Jones, L. V., Hopson, L., & Warner, L. (2015). A qualitative study of black women's experiences in drug abuse and mental health services. *Journal of Women and Social Work*, 30(1), 68–82. doi:10.1177/0886109914531957

Jorenby, D. E., Hays, J. T., & Rigotti, N. A. (2006). Efficacy of varenicline, an alpha4beta2 nicotinic acetylcholine receptor partial agonist, vs. placebo or sustained-release bupropion for smoking cessation: A randomized controlled study. *JAMA, The Journal of the American Medical Association*, 296(1), 56–63.

Jumah, N. A., Graves, L., & Kahan, M. (2015, January 6). The management of opioid dependence during pregnancy in rural and remote settings. *CMAJ, Canadian Medical Association Journal*, 187(1), E41–E46. doi:10.1503/cmaj.131723

Jung, Y. C., & Namkoong, K. (2006). Pharmacotherapy for alcohol dependence: Anticraving medications for relapse prevention. *Yonsei Medical Journal*, 47(2), 167–178.

Kadden, R. M. (1994). Cognitive-behavioral approaches to alcoholism treatment. *Alcohol Health & Research World*, 18, 279–286.

Kalkhoran, S., & Glantz, S. A. (2016). E-cigarettes and smoking cessation in real-world and clinical settings: A systematic review and meta-analysis. *The Lancet Respiratory Medicine*, 4(2), 116–128. doi:10.1016/S2213-2600(15)00521-4

Karavokiros, K. A., & Tsipis, G. B. (1990). Flumazenil: A benzodiazepine antagonist. *Drug Intelligence and Clinical Pharmacy*, 24(10), 976–981.

Kaskutas, L. A., Ye, Y., & Greenfield, T. K. (2008). Epidemiology of Alcoholics Anonymous participation. *Recent Developments in Alcoholism*, 18, 261–282.

Kaufman, E. (1990). Adolescent substance abusers and family therapy. In A. S. Friedman, & S. Granick (Eds.), *Family therapy for adolescent drug abuse* (pp. 47–61). New York, NY: Lexington.

Keller, P. A., Feltracco, A., & Bailey, L. A. (2010). Changes in tobacco quitlines in the United States, 2005–2006. *Preventing Chronic Disease*, 7(2), A36.

Kelley, M. L., Bravo, A. J., & Braitman, A. L. (2016a, March). Behavioral couples treatment for substance use disorder: Secondary effects on the reduction of risk for child abuse. *Journal of Substance Abuse Treatment*, 62, 10–19. doi:10.1016/j.jsat.2015.11.008

Kelley, M. L., Bravo, A. J., & Braitman, A. L. (2016b). Behavioral couples treatment for substance use disorder: Secondary effects on the reduction of youth internalizing symptoms. *Journal of Abnormal Child Psychology*. doi:10.1007/s10802-016-0197-x

Kelly, J. F., & Hoeppner, B. B. (2013). Does Alcoholics Anonymous work differently for men and women? A moderated multiple-mediation analysis in a large clinical sample. *Drug and Alcohol Dependence*, 130(1–3), 186–193. doi:10 1016/j.drugalcdep.2012.11.005

Kelly, P. J., Deane, F. P., & Baker, A. L. (2015, April). Group cohesion and between session homework activities predict self-reported cognitive-behavioral skill use amongst participants of SMART Recovery groups. *Journal of Substance Abuse Treatment*, 51, 53–58. doi:10.1016/j.jsat.2014.10.008

Kenna, G. A., Lomastro, T. L., & Schiesl, A. (2009). Review of topiramate: An antiepileptic for the treatment of alcohol dependence. *Current Drug Abuse Reviews*, 2(2), 135–142.

Kennedy, W. K., Leloux, M., & Kutscher, E. C. (2010). Acamprosate. *Expert Opinion on Drug Metabolism & Toxicology*, 6(3), 363–380.

Kenny, K. S., Barrington, C., & Green, S. L. (2015). "I felt for a long time like everything beautiful in me had been taken out": Women's suffering, remembering, and survival following the loss of child custody. *The International Journal on Drug Policy*, 26(11), 1158–1166. doi:10.1016/j.drugpo.2015.05.024

Keoleian, V., Polcin, D., & Galloway, G. P. (2015). Text messaging for addiction: A review. *Journal of Psychoactive Drugs*, 47(2), 158–176. doi:10.1080/02791072.2015.1009200

Kiefer, F., & Mann, K. (2010). Acamprosate: How, when, and for whom does it work? Mechanisms of action, treatment targets, and individualized therapy. *Current Pharmaceutical Design*, 16(19), 2098–2102.

Kinsey, B. (2014). Vaccines against drugs of abuse: Where are we now? *Therapeutic Advances in Vaccines*, 2(4), 106–117. doi:10.1177/2051013614537818

Kirchmayer, U., Davoli, M., & Verster, A. (2000). Naltrexone maintenance treatment for opioid dependence. *Cochrane Database of Systematic Reviews*, 2, CD001333.

Klein, A., & Golub, S. A. (2016). Family rejection as a predictor of suicide attempts and substance misuse among transgender and gender nonconforming adults. *LGBT Health*, 3(3), 193–199. doi:10.1089/lgbt.2015.0111

Knight, D. K., Logan, S. M., & Simpson, D. D. (2001). Predictors of program completion for women in residential substance abuse treatment. *The American Journal of Drug and Alcohol Abuse*, 27(1), 1–18.

Knox, B. (2016, March 18). *Increasing the minimum legal sale age for tobacco products to 21*, pp. 1–7. Retrieved March 18, 2016, from Campaign for Tobacco-Free Kids: www.tobaccofreekids.org

Koh, A. S., & Ross, L. K. (2006). Mental health issues: A comparison of lesbian, bisexual, and heterosexual women. *Journal of Homosexuality*, 51(1), 33–57.

Kong, G., Ells, D. M., & Camenga, D. R. (2014). Text messaging-based smoking cessation intervention: A narrative review. *Addictive Behaviors*, 39(5), 907–917. doi:10.1016/j.addbeh.2013.11.024

Kovas, A. E., McFarland, B. H., & McCarty, D. J. (2007). Buprenorphine for acute heroin detoxification: Diffusion of research into practice. *Journal of Substance Abuse Treatment*, 32(2), 199–206.

Kozlowski, L. T. (2015). Prospects for a nicotine-reduction strategy in the cigarette endgame: Alternative tobacco harm reduction scenarios. *International Journal of Drug Policy*, 26(6), 543–547. doi:10.1016/j.drugpo.2015.02.001

Kranzler, H. R., & Gage, A. (2008). Acamprosate efficacy in alcohol-dependent patients: Summary of results from three pivotal trials. *The American Journal of Addictions*, 17(1), 70–76. doi:10.1080/10550490701756120

Krauss, M. J., Cavazos-Rehg, P. A., & Plunk, A. D. (2014). Effects of state cigarette excise taxes and smoke-free air policies on state per capita alcohol consumption in the United States, 1980 to 2009. *Alcoholism: Clinical and Experimental Research*, 38(10), 2630–2638. doi:10.1111/acer.12533

Kumar, R. (2008). Approved and investigational uses of modafinil: An evidence-based review. *Drugs*, 68(3), 1803–1839.

Kunoe, N., Lobmaier, P., & Ngo, H. (2014). Injectable and implantable sustained release naltrexone in the treatment of opioid addiction. *British Journal of Clinical Pharmacology*, 77(2), 264–271. doi:10.1111/bcp.12011

Kurtz, E. (1988). *AA: The story*. San Francisco, CA: Harper & Row.

Kurtz, E. (1993). Research on Alcoholics Anonymous: The historical context. In B. S. McCrady, & W. R. Miller (Eds.), *Research on Alcoholics Anonymous* (pp. 13–26). New Brunswick, NJ: Rutgers Center of Alcohol Studies.

LaBrie, J. W., Lac, A., & Kenney, S. R. (2011). Protective behavioral strategies mediate the effect of drinking motives on alcohol use among heavy drinking college students: Gender and race differences. *Addictive Behaviors*, 36(4), 354–361. doi:10.1016/j.addbeh.2010.12.013

Lander, L., Howsare, J., & Byrne, M. (2013). The impact of substance use disorders on families and children: From theory to practice. *Social Work in Public Health*, 28(0), 194–205. doi:10.1080/19371918.2013.759005

Laniado-Laborin, R. (2010). Smoking cessation intervention: An evidence-based approach. *Postgraduate Medicine*, 122(2), 74–82. doi:10.3810/pgm.2010.03.2124

Larney, S., Gowing, L., & Mattick, R. P. (2014). A systematic review and meta-analysis of naltrexone implants for the treatment of opioid dependence. *Drug and Alcohol Review*, 33(2), 115–128. doi:10.1111/dar.12095

Laudet, A. B. (2008). The impact of alcoholics anonymous on other substance abuse-related twelve-step programs. *Recent Developments in Alcoholism*, 18, 71–89.

Laundergan, J. C., & Williams, T. (1993). The Hazelden Residential Family Program: A combined systems and disease model approach. In T. J. O'Farrell (Ed.), *Treating alcohol problems: Marital and family interventions*. New York, NY: Guilford.

Lee, J. D., Friedmann, P. D., & Kinlock, T. W. (2016). Extended-release naltrexone to prevent opioid relapse in criminal justice offenders. *New England Journal of Medicine*, 374(13), 1232–1242. doi:10.1056/NEJMoa1505409

Lewis, R. A., Piercy, F. P., & Sprenkle, D. H. (1990). Family-based interventions for helping drug-abusing adolescents. *Journal of Adolescent Research*, 5(1), 82–95.

Lim, J. K., Bratberg, J. P., & Davis, C. S. (2016, June 3). Prescribe to prevent: Overdose prevention and naloxone rescue kits for prescribers and pharmacists. *Journal of Addiction Medicine*, 10(5), 300–308. doi:10.1097/ADM.0000000000000223

Lima, A. R., Lima, M. S., & Soares, B. G. (2002). Carbamazepine for cocaine dependence. *Cochrane Database of Systematic Reviews*, 2, CD002023.

Lima, M. S., Reisser, A. A., & Soares, B. G. (2003). Antidepressants for cocaine dependence. *Cochrane Database of Systematic Reviews*, 2, CD002950.

Linden, A. N., Kite, B. A., & Braitman, A. L. (2014). Protective behavioral strategy use and motivations for drinking: Exploring alternatives to drinking strategies. *Addictive Behaviors*, 39(2), 469–472. doi:10.1016/j.addbeh.2013.10.008

Litt, D. M., Lewis, M. A., & Blayney, J. A. (2013). Protective behavioral strategies as a mediator of the generalized anxiety and alcohol use relationship among lesbian and bisexual women. *Journal of Studies on Alcohol and Drugs*, 74(1), 168–174.

Lloyd, M. H. (2015). Relationship-based justice for gender-responsive specialty courts. *Journal of Sociology & Social Welfare*, 42(3), 113–135.

Lynch, W. J., Roth, M. E., & Carroll, M. E. (2002). Biological basis of sex differences in drug abuse: Preclinical and clinical studies. *Psychopharmacology (Berlin)*, 164(2), 121–137.

Lyons, T., Shannon, K., & Pierre, L. (2015). A qualitative study of transgender individuals' experiences in residential addiction treatment settings: Stigma and inclusivity. *Substance Abuse Treatment, Prevention, and Policy*, 10(17), 1–6. doi:10.1186/s13011-015-0015-4

Mann, K., & Hermann, D. (2010). Individualised treatment in alcohol-dependent patients. *European Archives of Psychiatry & Clinical Neuroscience*, 260(Supplement 2), S116–S120.

Mannelli, P., Wu, L.-T., & Peindl, K. S. (2014, May 1). Extended release naltrexone injection is performed in the majority of opioid dependent patients receiving outpatient induction: A very low dose naltrexone and buprenorphine open label trial. *Drug and Alcohol Dependence*, 83–88. doi:10.1016/j.drugalcdep.20124.02.002

Margolin, A., Avants, S. K., & Holford, T. R. (2002, April). Interpreting conflicting findings from clinical trials of auricular acupuncture for cocaine addiction: Does treatment context influence outcome? *Journal of Alternative and Complementary Medicine*, 8(2), 111–121. doi:10.1089/107555302317371398

Marlowe, D. B., & Carey, S. M. (2012, May). Research update on family drug courts. *Need to Know*, 1–10. National Association of Drug Court Professionals.

Martinez-Raga, J., Knecht, C., & Cepeda, S. (2008). Modafinil: A useful medication for cocaine addiction? Review of the evidence from neuropharmacological, experimental and clinical studies. *Current Drug Abuse*, 1(2), 213–221.

Maryanoff, B., Nortey, O., & Gardocki, J. (1987). Anticonvulsant O-alkyl sulfamates. 2,3:4,5-Bis-O-(1-methyethylidene)-beta-D-fructopyranose sulfamate and related compounds. *Journal of Medicinal Chemistry*, 30(5), 880–887.

Marynak, K., Holmes, C. B., & King, B. A. (2014, December 12). State laws prohibiting sales to minors and indoor use of electronic nicotine delivery systems—United States, November 2014. *MMWR, Morbidity and Mortality Weekly Report*, 63(49), 1145–1150.

Mason, B. J. (2001). Treatment of alcohol-dependent outpatients with acamprosate: A clinical review. *The Journal of Clinical Psychiatry*, 62(Supplement 20), 42–48.

Mason, B. J. (2003). Acamprosate. *Recent Developments in Alcoholism*, 16, 203–215.

Mason, B. J., & Heyser, C. J. (2010). The neurobiology, clinical efficacy and safety of acamprosate in the treatment of alcohol dependence. *Expert Opinion on Drug Safety*, 9(1), 177–188.

Matheson, J. L., & McCollum, E. E. (2008). Using metaphors to explore the experiences of powerlessness among women in 12-step recovery. *Substance Use & Misuse*, 43(8–9), 1027–1044. doi:10.1080/10826080801914287

Matson, M. E. (1994). Patient-treatment matching: Rationale and results. *Alcohol, Health & Research World*, 18, 287–295.

Maurer, P., & Bachmann, M. F. (2006). Therapeutic vaccines for nicotine dependence. *Current Opinion in Molecular Therapeutics*, 8(1), 11–16.

Maurer, P., & Bachmann, M. F. (2007). Vaccination against nicotine: An emerging therapy for tobacco dependence. *Expert Opinion on Investigational Drugs*, 16(11), 1775–1783. doi:10.1517/13543784.16.11.1775

Mazure, C. M., Toll, B., & McKee, S. A. (2011). Menstrual cycle phase at quit date and smoking abstinence at 6 weeks in an open label trial of bupropion. *Drug and Alcohol Dependence*, 114(1), 68–72. doi:10.1016/j.drugalcdep.2010.07.024

McAfee, T. A. (2007). Quitlines: a tool for research and dissemination of evidence-based cessation practices. *American Journal of Preventive Medicine*, 33(Suppl 6), S357–S367. doi:10.1016/j.amepre.2007.09.011

McAuliffe, W. E. (1990, Summer). Health care policy issues in the drug abuser treatment field. *Journal of Health Politics, Policy and Law*, 15(2), 357–385.

McCarthy, D. M., Tomlinson, K. L., & Anderson, K. G. (2005). Relapse in alcohol and drug disordered adolescents with comorbid psychopathology: Changes in psychiatric symptoms. *Psychology of Addictive Behaviors*, 19(1), 28–34.

McCaul, M. E., & Petry, N. M. (2003). The role of psychosocial treatments in pharmacotherapy for alcoholism. *The American Journal on Addictions*, 12(Supplement 1), S41–S52.

McCrady, B. S., Epstein, E. E., & Hallgren, K. A. (2016). Women with alcohol dependence: A randomized trial of couple versus individual plus couple therapy. *Psychology of Addictive Behaviors*, 30(3), 287–299.

McCrady, B. S., Wilson, A. D., & Munoz, R. E. (2016, September). Alcohol-focused behavioral couple therapy. *Family Process*, 55(3), 443–459. doi:10.1111/famp.12231

McGee, E. M. (2000). Alcoholics Anonymous and nursing: Lessons in holism and spiritual care. *Journal of Holistic Nursing*, 18(1), 11–26.

McHugh, R. K., Hearon, B. A., & Otto, M. W. (2010). Cognitive behavioral therapy for substance use disorders. *Psychiatric Clinics of North America*, 33(3), 511–525.

McHugh, R. K., Wigderson, S., & Greenfield, S. F. (2014). Epidemiology of substance use in reproductive-age women. *Obstetrics & Gynecology Clinics of North America*, 41(2), 177–189. doi:10.1016/j.ogc.2014.02.001

McKay, J. R. (1999). Studies of factors in relapse to alcohol, drug and nicotine use: A critical review of methodologies and findings. *Journal of Studies on Alcohol*, 60(4), 566–576.

McKay, J. R., Franklin, T. R., & Patapis, N. (2006). Conceptual, methodological, and analytical issues in the study of relapse. *Clinical Psychology Reviews*, 26(2), 109–127.

McRobbie, H., Bullen, C., & Hartmann-Boyce, J. (2014). Electronic cigarettes for smoking cessation and reduction. *Cochrane Database of Systematic Reviews*, 12, CD010216. doi:10.1002/14651858.CD010216.pub2

Meara, E., & Frank, R. G. (2005). Spending on substance abuse treatment: How much is enough? *Addiction*, 100(9), 1240–1248. doi:10.1111/j.1360-0443.2005.01227.x

Michna, E., Kirson, N. Y., & Shei, A. (2014). Use of prescription opioids with abuse-deterrent technology to address opioid abuse. *Current Medical Research and Opinion*, 30(8), 1589–1598. doi:10.1185/03007995.2014.915803

Miller, J., & Roache, J. (2009). Benefits of topiramate treatment in a dual-diagnosis patient. *Psychosomatics*, 50(4), 426–427.

Miller, W. R., & McCrady, B. S. (1993). The importance of research on Alcoholics Anonymous. In B. S. McCrady, & W. R. Miller (Eds.), *Research on Alcoholics Anonymous* (pp. 3–11). New Brunswick, NJ: Rutgers Center of Alcohol Studies.

Minozzi, S., Amato, L., & Bellisario, C. (2013, December 23). Maintenance agonist treatments for opiate-dependent pregnant women. *Cochrane Database of Systematic Reviews*, 12, CD006318. doi:10.1002/14651858.CD006318.pub3

Minozzi, S., Amato, L., & Vecchi, S. (2011). Oral naltrexone maintenance treatment for opioid dependence. *Cochrane Database of Systematic Reviews*, 4, CD001333. doi:10,1002/14651858.CD001333.pub4

Minozzi, S., Saulle, R., & De Crescenzo, F. (2016, September 29). Psychosocial interventions for psychostimulant misuse. *The Cochrane Database of Systematic Reviews*, 9, CD011866. doi:10.1002/14651858.CD011866.pub2

Mogali, S., Khan, N. A., & Drill, E. S. (2015, April). Baseline characteristics of patients predicting suitability for rapid naltrexone induction. *American Journal on Addictions*, 24(3), 258–264. doi:10.1111/ajad.12180

Molfenter, T., Boyle, M., & Holloway, D. (2015). Trends in telemedicine use in addiction treatment. *Addiction Science & Clinical Practice*, 10(14), 1–9. doi:10.1186/s13722-015-0035-4

Montag, A., Clapp, J. D., & Calac, D. (2012). A review of evidence-based approaches for reduction of alcohol consumption in Native women who are pregnant or of reproductive age. *The American Journal of Drug and Alcohol Abuse*, 38(5), 436–443. doi:10.3109/00952990.2012.694521

Morain, S. R., Winickoff, J. P., & Mello, M. M. (2016, March 29). Have tobacco 21 laws come of age? *New England Journal of Medicine*. doi:10.1056/NEJMp1603294

Moran-Santa Maria, M. M., Flanagan, J., & Brady, K. (2014). Ovarian hormones and drug abuse. *Current Psychiatry Reports*, 16(11), 511. doi:10.1007/s11920-014-0511-7

Morelli, P. T., & Fong, R. (2000). The role of Hawaiian Elders in substance abuse treatment among Asian/Pacific Islander women. *Journal of Family Social Work*, 4(4), 33–44.

Morelli, P. T., Fong, R., & Oliveira, J. (2001). Culturally competent substance abuse treatment for Asian/Pacific Islander women. *Journal of Human Behavior in the Social Environment*, 3(3/4), 263–280.

Morris, D. S., Fiala, S. C., & Pawlak, R. (2012). Opportunities for policy interventions to reduce youth hookah smoking in the United States. *Preventing Chronic Disease*, 9(120082), 1–4. doi:http://dx.doi.org/10.5888/pcd9.120082

Muench, F. (2014). The promises and pitfalls of digital technology in its application to alcohol treatment. *Alcohol Research: Current Reviews*, 36(1), 131–142.

Muench, F., van Stolk-Cooke, K., & Morgenstern, J. (2014). Understanding messaging preferences to inform development of mobile goal-directed behavioral interventions. *Journal of Medical Internet Research*, 16(2), 1–19. doi:10.2196/jmir.2945

Muench, F., Weiss, R. A., & Kuerbis, A. (2013). Developing a theory driven text messaging intervention for addiction care with user driven content. *Psychology of Addictive Behaviors*, 27(1), 315–321. doi:10.1037/a0029963

Mussulman, L., Ellerbeck, E. F., & Cupertino, P. (2014). Design and participant characteristics of a randomized-controlled trial of telemedicine for smoking cessation among rural smokers. *Contemporary Clinical Trials*, 38(2), 173–181. doi:10.1016/j.cct.2014.04.008

Nair, N. K., Newton, N. C., & Shakeshaft, A. (2015). A systematic review of digital and computer-based alcohol intervention programs in primary care. *Current Drug Abuse Reviews*, 8(2), 111–118.

Nair, P., Black, M., & Schuler, M. (1997). Risk factors for disruption in primary caregiving among infants of substance abusing women. *Child Abuse & Neglect*, 21(11), 1039–1051.

Nair, P., Schuler, M. E., & Black, M. M. (2003). Cumulative environmental risk in substance abusing women: Early intervention, parenting stress, child abuse potential and child development. *Child Abuse & Neglect*, 27(9), 997–1017.

Naltrexone. (2009, February 1). *Medline Plus*, 1–4. Retrieved from www.nlm.nih.gov/medlineplus/druginfo/meds/a685041.html

Naltrexone Injection. (2010, May 1). *Medline Plus*, 1–4. Retrieved from www.nlm.nih.gov/medlineplus/druginfo/meds/a609007.html

Napper, L. E., Kenney, S. R., & Lac, A. (2014). A cross-lagged panel model examining protective behavioral strategies: Are types of strategies differentially related to alcohol use and consequences? *Addictive Behaviors*, 39(2), 480–486. doi:10.1016/j.addbeh.2013.10.020

Neger, E. N., & Prinz, R. J. (2015). Interventions to address parenting and parental substance abuse: Conceptual and methodological considerations. *Clinical Psychology Review*, 39, 71–82. doi:10.120126/j.cpr.2015.04.004

Nehls, N., & Sallmann, J. (2005). Women living with a history of physical and/or sexual abuse, substance use, and mental health problems. *Qualitative Health Research*, 15(3), 365–381. doi:10.1177/1049732304272917

NIDA, National Institute on Drug Abuse. (2013, November 6). *Women benefit from policies to prevent teens from buying tobacco*. Retrieved from National Institute on Drug Abuse, pp. 1–5: www.drugabuse.gov/news-events/nida-notes/2013/10/women-benefit-policies-to-prevent-teens-buying-tobacco

Nides, M., Oncken, C., & Gonzales, D. (2006). Smoking cessation with varenicline, a selective alpha-4 beta-2 nicotinic receptor partial agonist: Results from a 7-week, randomized, placebo- and bupropion-controlled trial with 1-year follow-up. *Archives of Internal Medicine*, 166, 1561–1568.

Nielsen, S., Larance, B., & Degenhardt, L. (2016, May 9). Opioid agonist treatment for pharmaceutical opioid dependent people. *Cochrane Database of Systematic Reviews*, CD011117. doi:10.1002/14651858.CD011117.pub2

Noel, N. E., & McCrady, B. S. (1993). Alcohol-focused spouse involvement with behavioral marital therapy. In T. J. O'Farrell (Ed.), *Treating alcohol problems: Marital and family interventions* (pp. 210–235). New York, NY: Guilford.

Norman, E., & Turner, S. (1993, September). Adolescent substance abuse prevention programs: Theories, models, and research in the encouraging 80's. *The Journal of Primary Prevention*, 14(1), 3–20. doi:10.1007/BF01324652

Nuijten, M., Blanken, P., & van de Wetering, B. (2016, March 22). Sustained-release dexamfetamine in the treatment of chronic cocaine-dependent patients on heroin-assisted treatment: A randomised, double-blind, placebo-controlled trial. *The Lancet*. doi:10.1016/S0140-6736(16)00205-1

O'Brien, W., & Biase, D. V. (1984). The therapeutic community: A current perspective. *Journal of Psychoactive Drugs*, 16, 9–21.

Odum, L. E., O'Dell, K. A., & Schepers, J. S. (2012). Electronic cigarettes: Do they have a role in smoking cessation? *Journal of Pharmacy Practice*, 25(6), 611–614. doi:10.1177/0897190012451909

Oei, T., & Jackson, P. (1980). Long-term effects of group and individual social skills training with alcoholics. *Addictive Behavior*, 5, 129–136.

O'Farrell, T. J. (2012). Review of outcome research on marital and family therapy in treatment of alcoholism. *Journal of Marital and Family Therapy*, 38(1), 122–144. doi:10.1111/j.1752-0606.2011.00242.x

O'Farrell, T. J., Schumm, J. A., & Murphy, M. M. (2017). A randomized clinical trial of Behavioral Couples Therapy versus Individualy-Based Treatment for drug-abusing women. *Journal of Consulting and Clinical Psychology*, 85(4), 309–322. doi:10/1037/ccp0000185

Oliveros, A., & Kaufman, J. (2011). Addressing substance abuse treatment needs of parents involved with the child welfare system. *Child Welfare*, 90(1), 25–41.

Olmsted, C. L., & Kockler, D. R. (2008). Topiramate for alcohol dependence. *Annals of Pharmacotherapy*, 42(10), 1475–1480.

Oncken, C., Gonzales, D., & Nides, M. (2006). Efficacy and safety of the novel selective nicotinic acetylcholine receptor partial agonist, varenicline, for smoking cessation. *Archives of Internal Medicine*, 166, 1571–1577.

Orr, K. K., & Asal, N. J. (2014). Efficacy of electronic cigarettes for smoking cessation. *Annals of Pharmacotherapy*, 48(11), 1502–1506. doi:10.1177/1060028014547076

Orson, F. M., Wang, R., & Brimijoin, S. (2014). The future potential for cocaine vaccines. *Expert Opinion on Biological Therapy*, 14(9), 1271–1283. doi:10.1517/14712598.2014.920319

Pagliaro, A. M., & Pagliaro, L. A. (1986). Chapter 63, Estrogens, Progestins, and Antiestrogens. In A. M. Pagliaro, & L. A. Pagliaro (Eds.), *Pharmacologic aspects of nursing* (pp. 1450–1472). St. Louis, MO: CV Mosby.

Pagliaro, A. M., & Pagliaro, L. A. (1992a). Phenomenon of drug and substance abuse among the elderly. Part 2: The Mega Interactive Model. *Journal of Pharmacy Technology*, 8, 111–118.

Pagliaro, A. M., & Pagliaro, L. A. (1993). Knowledge, behaviours, and risk perception of intravenous drug users in relation to HIV infection and AIDS: The PIARG projects. *Advances in Medical Psychotherapy*, 6, 1–28.

Pagliaro, A. M., & Pagliaro, L. A. (2000). *Substance use among women: A reference and research guide*. Philadelphia, PA: Brunner/Mazel.

Pagliaro, A. M., Pagliaro, L. A., & Thauberger, P. C. (1993). Knowledge, behaviours, and risk perception of intravenous drug users in relation to HIV infection and AIDS: The PIARG projects. *Advances in Medical Psychotherapy*, 6, 1–28.

Pagliaro, L. A. (1981). Analysis of computer assisted instruction in pharmacology. *Proceedings: Western Pharmacology Society*, 24, pp. 113–115.

Pagliaro, L. A. (2002). Foreword in Edwards, B., *The bottle hopper: Surviving ethyl alcohol*. Pittsburgh, PA: Sterling House.

Pagliaro, L. A., & Burkhalter, A. (1979). Application and testing of computer aided instruction in pharmacology. *Association for the Development of Computer Based Instructional Systems Proceedings*, 2, pp. 711–727.

Pagliaro, L. A., Cook, D. A., & Bidwell, C. M. (1979). CAI in pharmacology at the University of Alberta (Summary). *Association for the Development of Computer-Based Instructional Systems Proceedings*, 1, p. 316.

Pagliaro, L. A., & Kline, L. W. (1978). Dental students to learn pharmacology with computer aided instruction. *Association of Canadian Faculties of Dentistry Newsletter*, 11, pp. 18–20.

Pagliaro, L. A., & Pagliaro, A. M. (1986). Estrogens, progestins, and antiestrogens. In A. M. Pagliaro, & L. A. Pagliaro (Eds.), *Pharmacologic aspects of nursing* (pp. 1450–1472). St. Louis, MO: CV Mosby.

Pagliaro, L. A., & Pagliaro, A. M. (1992b). Phenomenon of drug and substance abuse among the elderly. Part 1: An overview. *Journal of Pharmacy Technology*, 8, 65–73.

Pagliaro, L. A., & Pagliaro, A. M. (1998). *The pharmacologic basis of psychotherapeutics: An introduction for psychologists*. Washington, DC: Brunner/Mazel.

Pagliaro, L. A., & Pagliaro, A. M. (1999). *PPDR: Psychologists' psychotropic drug reference*. Philadelphia, PA: Brunner/Mazel.

Pagliaro, L. A., & Pagliaro, A. M. (2004). *Pagliaros' comprehensive guide to drugs and substances of abuse* (1st ed.). Washington, DC: American Pharmacists Association.

Pagliaro, L. A., & Pagliaro, A. M. (2009). *Pagliaros' comprehensive guide to drugs and substances of abuse* (2nd ed.). Washington, DC: American Pharmacists Association.

Pagliaro, L. A., & Pagliaro, A. M. (2012). *Handbook of child and adolescent drug and substance abuse*. Hoboken, NJ: Wiley & Sons.

Pan, W., & Bai, H. (2009). A multivariate approach to a meta-analytic review of the effectiveness of the D.A.R.E. program. *International Journal of Environmental Research and Public Health*, 6(1), 267–277. doi:10.3390/ijerph6010267

Panebianco, D., Gallupe, O., & Carrington, P. J. (2016, January). Personal support networks, social capital, and risk of relapse among individuals treated for substance use issues. *The International Journal on Drug Policy*, 27, 146–153. doi:10.1016/j.drugpo.20125.09.009

Pang, R. D., Bello, M. S., & Stone, M. D. (2016). Premenstrual symptoms and smoking-related expectancies. *Addictive Behaviors*, 57, 38–41. doi:10.1016/j.addbeh.2016.01.015

Paris, R., Herriott, A., & Holt, M. (2015, December). Differential responsiveness to a parenting intervention for mothers in substance abuse treatment. *Child Abuse & Neglect*, 50, 206–217. doi:10.1016/j.chiabu.2015.09.007

Passik, S. D. (2014). Tamper-resistant opioid formulations in the treatment of acute pain. *Advances in Therapy*, 31(3), 264–275. doi:10,1007/s12325-014-0099-7

Passik, S. D., Hays, L., & Eisner, N. (2006). Psychiatric and pain characteristics of prescription drug abusers entering drug rehabilitation. *Journal of Pain and Palliative Care Pharmacotherapy*, 20(2), 5–13.

Patnode, C. D., Henderson, J. T., & Thompson, J. T. (2015). Behavioral counseling and pharmacotherapy interventions for tobacco cessation in adults, including pregnant women: A review of reviews for the U.S. Preventive Services Task Force. *Annals of Internal Medicine*, 163, 608–621. doi:10.7326/M15-0171

Pearson, M. R. (2013). Use of alcohol protective behavioral strategies among college students: A critical review. *Clinical Psychology Review*, 33(8), NP. doi:10.1016/j.cpr.2013.08.006

Pearson, M. R., D'Lima, G. M., & Kelley, M. L. (2013). Daily use of protective behavioral strategies and alcohol-related outcomes among college students. *Psychology of Addictive Behaviors*, 27(3), NP. doi:10.1037/a0032516

Pechmann, C., & Reibling, E. T. (2000). Anti-smoking advertising campaigns targeting youth: Case studies from USA and Canada. *Tobacco Control*, 9(Supplement 2), 1118–1131. doi:10.1136/tc.9.suppl_2.ii18

Peralta, R. L., & Jauk, D. (2011). A brief feminist review and critique of the sociology of alcohol-use and substance-abuse treatment approaches. *Sociology Compass*, 5(10), 882–897. doi:10.1111/j.1751-9020.2011.00414.x

Perry, A. E., Neilson, M., & Martyn-St James, M. (2014). Interventions for female drug-using offenders. *Cochrane Database of Systematic Reviews*, 1, CD010910. doi:10.1002/14651858.CD010910

Philip Morris. (1986, January 21). *Discussion draft sociopolitical strategy.* Retrieved from http:/legacy.library.ucsf.edu/tid/aba84e00

Pinkerton, J. V., Guico-Pabia, C. J., & Taylor, H. S. (2010). Menstrual cycle-related exacerbation of disease. *American Journal of Obstetrics & Gynecology*, 202(3), 221–231. doi:10.1016/j.ajog.2009.07.061

Postolache, P., Nemes, R. M., & Serban, R. I. (2015). Electronic cigarette—A way of smoking cessation? *Revista medico-chirurgicala a Societatii de Medici si Naturalisti din lasi*, 119(2), 510–516.

Powell, C., Stevens, S., & Lo Dolce, B. (2012). Outcomes of a trauma-informed Arizona family drug court. *Journal of Social Work Practice in the Addictions*, 12(3), 219–241. doi:10.1080/1533256X.2012.702624

Powers, M. B., Vedel, E., & Emmelkamp, P. M. (2008). Behavioral couples therapy (BCT) for alcohol and drug use disorders: A meta-analysis. *Clinical Psychology Review*, 28(6), 952–962.

Pritham, U. A. (2013). Breastfeeding promotion for management of neonatal abstinence. *Journal of Obstetric, Gynecologic, & Neonatal Nursing*, 42(5), 517–526. doi:10.1111/1552–6909.12242

Prochaska, J. J., & Hilton, J. F. (2012). Risk of cardiovascular serious adverse events associated with varenicline use for tobacco cessation: Systematic review and meta-analysis. *BMJ*, 344, e2856. doi:10.1136/bmj.e2856

Project Match (Matching Alcoholism Treatment to Client Hetergeneity): Rationale and methods for a multisite clinical trial matching patients to alcoholism treatment. (1993). *Alcoholism, Clinical & Experimental Research*, 17, 1130–1145.

Quanbeck, A., Chih, M. Y., & Isham, A. (2016). Mobile delivery of treatment for alcohol use disorders: A review of the literature. *Alcohol Research: Current Reviews*, 36(1), 111–122.

Raisch, D. W., Fye, C. L., & Boardman, K. D. (2002). Opioid dependence treatment, including buprenorphine/naloxone. *Annals of Pharmacotherapy*, 36(2), 312–321.

Ranney, L., Melvin, C., & Lux, L. (2006, June). Tobacco use: Prevention, cessation, and control. *Evidence Report—Technology Assessment*(140), 1–120.

Rasmussen, H. F., Borelli, J. L., & Decoste, C. (2016). A longitudinal examination of toddlers' behavioral cues as a function of substance-abusing mothers' disengagement. *Infant Mental Health Journal*, 37(2), 140–150. doi:10.1002/imhj.21552

Reback, C. J., & Fletcher, J. B. (2014). HIV prevalence, substance use, and sexual risk behaviors among transgender women recruited through outreach. *AIDS and Behavior*, 18(7), 1359–1367. doi:10.1007/s10461-013-0657-z

Reid, M. S., & Thakkar, V. (2009). Valproate treatment and cocaine cue reactivity in cocaine dependent individuals. *Drug and Alcohol Dependence*, 102(1–3), 144–150.

Richter, K. P., Shireman, T. I., & Ellerbeck, E. F. (2015). Comparative and cost effectiveness of telemedicine versus telephone counseling for smoking cessation. *Journal of Medical Internet Research*, 17(5), e113. doi:10.2196/jmir.3975

Ritter, A., & Cameron, J. (2006, November). A review of the efficacy and effectiveness of harm reduction strategies for alcohol, tobacco and illicit drugs. *Drug and Alcohol Review*, 25(6), 611–624. doi:10.1080/09595230600944529

Roberts, A., Jackson, M. S., & Carlton-LaNey, I. (2000). Revising the need for feminism and afrocentric theory when treating African-American female substance abusers. *Journal of Drug Issues*, 30(4), 901–918.

Roberts, N. P., Roberts, P. A., & Jones, N. (2016, April 4). Psychological therapies for post-traumatic stress disorder and comorbid substance use disorder. *Cochrane Database Systematic Reviews*, 4, CD010204. doi:10.1002/14651858.CD010204.pub2

Robinson, S. E. (2006). Buprenorphine-containing treatments: Place in the management of opioid addiction. *CNS Drugs*, 20(9), 697–712.

Robles, G. I., Singh-Franco, D., & Ghin, H. L. (2008). A review of the efficacy of smoking-cessation pharmacotherapies in nonwhite populations. *Clinical Therapeutics*, 30(5), 800–812. doi:10.1016/j.clinthera.2008.05.010

Room, R., & Greenfield, T. (1993). Alcoholics Anonymous, other 12-step movements and psychotherapy in the US population, 1990. *Addiction*, 88, 555–562.

Rosner, S., Hackl-Herrwerth, A., & Leucht, S. (2010). Acamprosate for alcohol dependence. *Cochrane Database of Systematic Reviews*, 9, CD004332.

Roth, M. E., Cosgrove, K. P., & Carroll, M. E. (2004). Sex differences in the vulnerability to drug abuse: A review of preclinical studies. *Neuroscience & Biobehavior Reviews*, 28(6), 533–546.

Ruff, S., McComb, J. L., & Coker, C. J. (2010). Behavioral couples therapy for the treatment of substance abuse: A substantive and methodological review of O'Farrell, Fals-Stewart, and colleagues' program of research. *Family Process*, 49(4), 439–456. doi:10.1111/j.1545-5300.2010.01333.x

Ruglass, L. M., Hien, D. A., & Hu, M. C. (2014). Associations between posttraumatic stress symptoms, stimulant use, and treatment outcomes: A secondary analysis of NIDA's Women and Trauma Study. *The American Journal on Addictions*, 23(1), 1–10. doi:10.1111/j.1521-0391.2013.12068.x

Saladin, M. E., McClure, E. A., & Baker, N. L. (2015). Increasing progesterone levels are associated with smoking abstinence among free-cycling women smokers who receive brief pharmacotherapy. *Nicotine & Tobacco Research*, 17(4), 398–406. doi:10.1093/ntr/ntu262

Saladin, M. E., Wray, J. M., & Carpenter, M. J. (2015). Menstrual cycle phase effects in the gender dimorphic stress cue reactivity of smokers. *Nicotine & Tobacco Research*, 17(5), 607–611. doi:10.1093/ntr/ntu203

SAMHSA, Substance Abuse and Mental Health Services Administration. (2015). *Clinical use of extended-release injectable naltrexone in the treatment of opioid use disorder: A brief guide.* Health and Human Services. Rockville, MD: Substance Abuse and Mental Health Services Administration.

Santos, G. M., Rapues, J., & Wilson, E. C. (2014). Alcohol and substance use among transgender women in San Francisco: Prevalence and association with human immunodeficiency virus infection. *Drug and Alcohol Review*, 33(3), 287–295. doi:10.1111/dar.12116

Schaeffer, C. M., Swenson, C. C., & Tuerk, E. H. (2013). Comprehensive treatment for co-occurring child maltreatment and parental substance abuse: Outcomes from a 24-month pilot study of the MST-Building Stronger Families Program. *Child Abuse & Neglect*, 37(8), 596–607. doi:10.1016/j.chiabu.2013.04.004

Schaeffer, T. (2012). Abuse-deterrent formulations, an evolving technology against the abuse and misuse of opioid analgesics. *Journal of Medical Toxicology*, 8, 400–407. doi:10.1007/s13181-012-0270-y

Seger, D. L. (2004). Flumazenil—Treatment or toxin. *Journal of Toxicology—Clinical Toxicology*, 42(2), 209–216.

Sellers, E. M., Perrino, P. J., & Colucci, S. V. (2013). Attractiveness of reformulated OxyContin(R) tablets: Assessing comparative preferences and tampering potential. *Journal of Psychopharmacology*, 27(9), 808–816. doi:10.1177/0269881113493364

Shaw, M. R., Grant, T., & Barbosa-Leiker, C. (2015). Intervention with substance-abusing mothers: Are there rural-urban differences? *The American Journal on Addictions*, 24(2), 144–152. doi:10.1111/ajad.12155

Shinn, A. K., & Greenfield, S. F. (2010). Topiramate in the treatment of substance-related disorders: A critical review of the literature. *The Journal of Clinical Psychiatry*, 71(5), 634–648.

Singh, S., Loke, Y. K., & Spangler, J. G. (2011). Risk of serious adverse cardiovascular events associated with varenicline: A systematic review and meta-analysis. *CMAJ, Canadian Medical Association Journal*, 183(12), 1359–1366. doi:10.1503/cmaj.110218

Siu, A. L. (2015). Behavioral and pharmacotherapy interventions for tobacco smoking cessation in adults, including pregnant women: U.S. Preventive Services Task Force recommendation statement. *Annals of Internal Medicine*, 163(8), 622–634. doi:10.7326/M15-2023

Slesnick, N., & Erdem, G. (2012). Intervention for homeless, substance abusing mothers: Findings from a non-randomized pilot. *Behavioral Medicine*, 38(2), 36–48. doi:10.1080/08964289.2012.657724

Slesnick, N., & Erdem, G. (2013). Efficacy of ecologically-based treatment with substance-abusing homeless mothers: Substance use and housing outcomes. *Journal of Substance Abuse Treatment*, 45(5), 416–425. doi:10.1016/j.jsat.2013.05.008

Slesnick, N., Glassman, M., & Katafiasz, H. (2012). Experiences associated with intervening with homeless, substance-abusing mothers: The importance of success. *Social Work*, 57(4), 343–352.

Slesnick, N., & Prestopnik, J. L. (2005). Ecologically based family therapy outcome with substance abusing runaway adolescents. *Journal of Adolescence*, 28, 277–298.

Slesnick, N., & Zhang, J. (2016). Family systems therapy for substance-using mothers and their 8- to 16-year-old children. *Psychology of Addictive Behaviors*, 30(6), 619–629.

Sloboda, Z., Stephens, R. C., & Stephens, P. C. (2009, June 1). The Adolescent Substance Abuse Prevention Study: A randomized field trial of a universal substance abuse prevention program. *Drug and Alcohol Dependence*, 102(1–3), 1–10. doi:10.1016/j.drugalcdep.2009.01.015

Smith, H. S. (2011). Morphine sulfate and naltrexone hydrochloride extended release capsules for the management of chronic, moderate-to-severe pain, while reducing morphine-induced subjective effects upon tampering by crushing. *Expert Opinion on Pharmacotherapy*, 12(7), 1111–1125. doi:10.1517/14656566.2011.571205

Smith, J. P., & Randall, C. L. (2012). Anxiety and alcohol disorders – Comorbidity and treatment considerations. *ARCR, Alcohol Research Current Reviews*, 34(4), 414–431.

Smith, L. A., Gates, S., & Foxcroft, D. (2006, January 25). Therapeutic communities for substance related disorder. *Cochrane Database of Systematic Reviews*, 1, CD005338.

Smith, T. T., Sved, A. F., & Hatsukami, D. K. (2014). Nicotine reduction as an increase in the unit price of cigarettes: A behavioral economics approach. *Preventive Medicine*, 68, 23–28. doi:10.1016/j.ypmed.2014.07.005

Soares, B. G., Lima, M. S., & Reisser, A. A. (2003). Dopamine agonists for cocaine dependence. *Cochrane Database of Systematic Reviews*, 2, CD003352.

Soares, B., Lima Reisser, A. A., & Farrell, M. (2010, February 17). WITHDRAWN: Dopamine agonists for cocaine dependence. *The Cochrane Database of Systematic Reviews*, 2, CD003352. doi:10.1002/14651858.CD003352.pub2

Somers, J. M., Currie, L., & Moniruzzaman, A. (2012). Drug treatment court of Vancouver: An empirical evaluation of recidivism. *International Journal of Drug Policy*, 23(5), 393–400. doi:10.1016/j.drugpo.2012.01.011

Soyka, M., & Rosner, S. (2010). Nalmefene for treatment of alcohol dependence. *Expert Opinion on Investigational Drugs*, 19(11), 1451–1459.

Stanley, K. M., Worrall, C. L., & Lunsford, S. L. (2005). Experience with an adult alcohol withdrawal syndrome practice guideline in internal medicine patients. *Pharmacotherapy*, 25(8), 1073–1083. doi:10.1592/phco.2005.25.8.1073

Stead, L. F., Koilpillai, P., & Fanshawe, T. R. (2016, March 24). Combined pharmacotherapy and behavioural interventions for smoking. *Cochrane Database Systematic Reviews*, 24, CD008286. doi:10.1002/14651858,CD008286.pub3

Stead, L. F., & Lancaster, T. (2005, April 18). Group behavior therapy programmes for smoking cessation. *Cochrane Database of Systematic Reviews*, 2, CD001007.

Steiner, M. (2000). Premenstrual syndrome and premenstrual dysphoric disorder: Guidelines for management. *Journal of Psychiatry & Neuroscience*, 25(5), 459–468.

Stevens, S. (2012). Meeting the substance abuse treatment needs of lesbian, bisexual and transgender women: Implications from research to practice. *Substance Abuse and Rehabilitation*, 3(Supplement 1), 27–36.

Stevens-Watkins, D., Knighton, J.-S., & Allen, K. (2016, April). John Henryism active coping as a cultural correlate of substance abuse treatment participation among African American women. *Journal of Substance Abuse Treatment*, 63, 54–60. doi:10.1016/j.jsat.2016.01.004

Stoops, W. W., & Rush, C. R. (2013). Agonist replacement for stimulant dependence: A review of clinical research. *Current Pharmaceutical Design*, 19(40), 7026–7035.

Stover, M. W., & Davis, J. M. (2015). Opioids in pregnancy and neonatal abstinence syndrome. *Seminars in Perinatology*, 39, 5612–565.

Suchman, N. E., Decoste, C., & Rosenberger, P. (2012). Attachment-based intervention for substance-using mothers: A preliminary test of the proposed mechanisms of change. *Infant Mental Health Journal*, 33(4), 360–371. doi:10.1002/imhj.21311

Sullivan, M., Bisaga, A., & Pavlicova, M. (2017, January 10). Long-acting injectable naltrexone induction: A randomized trial of outpatient opioid detoxification with naltrexone versus buprenorphine. *The American Journal of Psychiatry*. Retrieved from http://dx,doi.org/10.1176/appi.ajp.2016.16050548

Sun, A. P. (2012). Helping homeless individuals with co-occurring disorders: The four components. *Social Work*, 57(1), 23–37.

Sutter, M. B., Leeman, L., & Hsi, A. (2014). Neonatal opioid withdrawal syndrome. *Obstetrics and Gynecology Clinics of North America*, 41(2), 317–334. doi:10.1016/j.ogc.2014.02.010

Swift, R. (2007). Emerging approaches to managing alcohol dependence. *American Journal of Health-System Pharmacy*, 64(5, Supplement 3), S12–S22.

Syed, Y. Y., & Keating, G. M. (2013). Extended-release intramuscular naltrexone (VIVITROL): A review of its use in the prevention of relapse to opioid dependence in detoxified patients. *CNS Drugs*, 27(10), 851–861. doi:10.1007/s40263-013-0110-x

Szapocznik, J., & Williams, R. A. (2000). Brief Strategic Family Therapy: Twenty-five years of interplay among theory, research and practice in adolescent behavior problems and drug abuse. *Clinical Child and Family Psychological Review*, 3(2), 117–134.

Ta, V. M., & Chen, T. (2008, November). Substance abuse among native Hawaiian women in the United States: A review of current literature and recommendations for future research. *Journal of Psychoactive Drugs*(Supplement 5), 411–422.

Testa, M. F., & Smith, B. (2009). Prevention and drug treatment. *The Future of Children*, 19(2), 147–168.

Thomas, R., & Perera, R. (2006, July 19). School-based programmes for preventing smoking. *The Cochrane Database of Systematic Reviews*, 3, CD001293.

Tonstad, S., Tonnesen, P., & Hajek, P. (2006). Effect of maintenance therapy with varenicline on smoking cessation: A randomized controlled trial. *JAMA, The Journal of the American Medical Association*, 296(1), 64–71.

Tracy, E. M., Min, M. O., & Park, H. (2016, March). Personal network structure and substance use in women by 12 months post treatment intake. *Journal of Substance Abuse Treatment*, 62, 55–61. doi:10.1016/j.jstat.2015.11.002

Tuchman, E. (2010). Women and addiction: The importance of gender issues in substance abuse research. *Journal of Addictive Diseases*, 29(2), 127–138. doi:10.1080/10550881003684582

Tusa, A. L., & Burgholzer, J. A. (2013, October–December). Came to believe: Spirituality as a mechanism of change in Alcoholics Anonymous: A review of the literature from 1992 to 2012. *Journal of Addictions Nursing*, 24(4), 237–246. doi:10.1097/JAN.0000000000000003

U.S. Department of Health and Human Services. (2015, April). *Abuse-deterrent opioids–evaluation and labeling guidance for industry*, pp. 1–26. Retrieved August 3, 2016, from www.fda.gov/Drugs/GuidanceComplianceRegulatoryInformation/Guidances/default.htm

U.S. Department of Justice. (2016, May 13). Drug courts. *Office of Justice Programs*. National Institute of Justice. www.nij.gov/topics/courts/drug-courts/Pages/welcome.aspx

U.S. Preventive Services Task Force. (2015, September). Tobacco smoking cessation in adults, including pregnant women: Behavioral and pharmacotherapy interventions. *Final Update Summary*. U.S. Preventive Services Task Force. Retrieved from www.uspreventiveservicestaskforce.org/Page/Document/UpdateSummaryFinal/tobacco-use-in-adults-and-pregnant-women-counseling-and-interventions1

Vaillant, G. E. (2005). Alcoholics Anonymous: Cult or cure? *Australian and New Zealand Journal of Psychiatry*, 39(6), 431–436.

van der Meer, R. M., Willemsen, M. C., & Smit, F. (2013, August 21). Smoking cessation interventions for smokers with current or past depression. *Cochrane Database Systematic Reviews*, 8, CD006102. doi:10.1002/14651858.CD006102.pub2

Varenicline. (2009, October 1). *MedlinePlus*, 1–4. Retrieved from www.nlm.nih.gov/medlineplus/druginfo/meds/a606024.html

Vocci, F. J., & Chiang, C. N. (2001). Vaccines against nicotine: How effective are they likely to be in preventing smoking? *CNS Drugs*, 15(7), 505–514. doi:10.2165/00023210-200115070-00001

Volpicelli, J. R., Clay, K. L., & Watson, N. T. (1995). Naltrexone in the treatment of alcoholism: Predicting response to naltrexone. *The Journal of Clinical Psychiatry*, 56(Supplement 7), 39–44.

Vosburg, S. K., Jones, J. D., & Manubay, J. M. (2012). Assessment of a formulation designed to be crush-resistant in prescription opioid abusers. *Drug and Alcohol Dependence*, 126(0), 206–215. doi:10.1016/j.drugalcdep.2012.05.013

Wagenaar, A. C., Salois, M. J., & Komro, K. A. (2009). Effects of beverage alcohol price tax levels on drinking: A meta-analysis of 1003 estimates from 112 studies. *Addiction*, 104(2), 179–190. doi:10.1111/j.1360-0443.2008.02438.x

Wakefield, M., Flay, B., & Nichter, M. (2003, May–June). Effects of anti-smoking advertising on youth smoking: A review. *Journal of Health Communications*, 8(3), 229–247. doi:10.1080/10810730305686

Waldron, H. B., & Kaminer, Y. (2004). On the learning curve: The emerging evidence supporting cognitive-behavioral therapies for adolescent substance abuse. *Addiction*, 99(Supplement 2), 93–105.

Warren, C. S., Lindsay, A. R., & White, E. K. (2013). Weight-related concerns related to drug use for women in substance abuse treatment: Prevalence and relationships with eating pathology. *Journal of Substance Abuse Treatment*, 44(5), 494–501. doi:10.1016/j.jsat.2012.08.222

Washton, A. M., & Resnick, R. B. (1981). Clonidine in opiate withdrawal: Review and appraisal of clinical findings. *Pharmacotherapy*, 1(2), 140–146.

Webster, J. M., Rosen, P. J., & Krietemeyer, J. (2006). Gender, mental health, and treatment motivation in a drug court setting. *Journal of Psychoactive Drugs*, 38(4), 441–448.

Webster, L. R., Cochella, S., & Dasgupta, N. (2011). An analysis of the root causes for opioid-related overdose deaths in the United States. *Pain Medicine*, 12(Supplement 2), S26–S35.

Weinberger, A. H., Smith, P. H., & Allen, S. S. (2015). Systematic and meta-analytic review of research examining the impact of menstrual cycle phase and ovarian hormones on smoking and cessation. *Nicotine & Tobacco Research*, 17(4), 407–421. doi:10.1093/ntr/ntu249

Weisner, C., Greenfield, T., & Room, R. (1995). Trends in the treatment of alcohol problems in the US general population: 1979 through 1990. *American Journal of Public Health*, 85, 55–60.

Welch-Lazoritz, M. L., Whitbeck, L. B., & Armenta, B. E. (2015). Characteristics of mothers caring for children during episodes of homelessness. *Community Mental Health Journal*, 51(8), 913–920. doi:10.1007/s10597-014-9794-8

White, A., Kavanagh, D., & Stallman, H. (2010). Online alcohol interventions: A systematic review. *Journal of Medical Internet Research*, 12(5), e62. doi:10.2196/jmir.1479

White Hughto, J. M., Reisner, S. L., & Pachankis, J. E. (2015, December). Transgender stigma and health: A critical review of stigma determinants, mechanisms, and interventions. *Social Science & Medicine*, 147, 222–231. doi:10.1016/j.socscimed.2015.11.010

Williams, A. R., & Bisaga, A. (2016). From AIDS to opioids—How to combat an epidemic. *The New England Journal of Medicine*, 375(9), 813–815. doi:10.1056/NEJMp1604223

Wilson, E. C., Chen, Y. H., & Arayasirikul, S. (2014). Connecting the dots: Examining transgender women's utilization of transition-related medical care and associations with mental health, substance use, and HIV. *Journal of Urban Health: Bulletin of the New York Academy of Medicine*, 92(1), 182–192. doi:10.1007/s11524-014-9921-4

Winter, M. (2014, February 21). Utah, Colorado move to hike smoking age to 21. *USA Today*, p. 1.

Witbrodt, J., & Delucchi, K. (2011). Do woman differ from men on Alcoholics Anonymous participation and abstinence? A multi-wave analysis of treatment seekers. *Alcoholism: Clinical and Experimental Research*, 35(12), 2231–2241. doi:10.1111/j.1530-0277.2011.01

Wittouck, C., Dekkers, A., & De Ruyver, B. D. (2013). The impact of drug treatment courts on recovery: A systematic review. *The Scientific World Journal*, 2013, 1–12. doi:10.1155/2013/493679

Worcel, S., Furrer, C., & Green, B. (2008). Effects of family treatment drug courts on substance abuse and child welfare outcomes. *Child Abuse Review*, 17, 427–443.

Wu, L.-T., & Blazer, D. G. (2011). Illicit and nonmedical drug use among older adults: A review. *Journal of Aging Health*, 23(3), 481–504. doi:10.1177/0898264310386224

Wu, L. T., & Blazer, D. G. (2014, April). Substance use disorders and psychiatric comorbidity in mid and later life: A review. *International Journal of Epidemiology*, 43(2), 304–317. doi:10.1093/ije/dyt173

York, J., Lamis, D. A., & Garfinkel, P. W. (2012). Family drug treatment courts and social determinants of health. *Family Court Review*, 50(1), 137–149. doi:10.1111/j.1744-1617.2011.01435.x

Young-Wolff, K. C., Kasza, K. A., & Hyland, A. J. (2014). Increased cigarette tax is associated with reductions in alcohol consumption in a longitudinal U.S. sample. *Alcoholism: Clinical and Experimental Research*, 38(1), 241–248. doi:10.1111/acer.12226

Zedler, B. K., Mann, A. L., & Kim, M. M. (2016). Buprenorphine compared with methadone to treat pregnant women with opioid use disorder: A systematic review and meta-analysis of safety in the mother, fetus and child. *Addiction*, 111, 2115–2128. doi:10.1111/add.13462

Zemore, S. E., Kaskutas, L. A., & Mericle, A. (2017, February). Comparison of 12-step groups to mutual help alternatives for AUD in a large, national study: Differences in membership characteristics and group participation, cohesion, and satisfaction. *Journal of Substance Abuse Treatment*, 73, 16–26. doi:10.1016/j.jsat.2016.10.004

INDEX

Note: f, followed by the figure number, indicates that the index entry is to be found within the identified figure; fn, followed by the footnote number, indicates that the index entry is to be found within the identified footnote at the bottom of the identified page; t, followed by the table number, indicates that the index entry is to be found within the identified table; tn, followed by the table note number, indicates that the index entry is to be found within the identified table note at the bottom of the identified table.

For Product Safety Concerns and Information please contact our EU
representative GPSR@taylorandfrancis.com
Taylor & Francis Verlag GmbH, Kaufingerstraße 24, 80331 München, Germany

www.ingramcontent.com/pod-product-compliance
Ingram Content Group UK Ltd.
Pitfield, Milton Keynes, MK11 3LW, UK
UKHW022113190926
475702UK00013B/1417
9781138908383